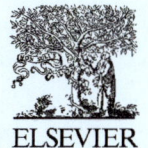

多囊卵巢综合征
从基础医学到全生命周期健康管理新进展

Polycystic Ovary Syndrome
Basic Science to Clinical Advances Across the Lifespan

主 编　[巴基] 瑞哈娜·拉赫曼（Rehana Rehman）
　　　　[巴基] 艾莎·谢赫（Aisha Sheikh）
主 译　郁　琦　陈　蓉　甄璟然　郭艺红

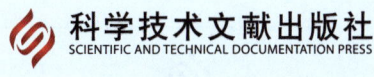

·北京·

图书在版编目（CIP）数据

多囊卵巢综合征：从基础医学到全生命周期健康管理新进展 /（巴基）瑞哈娜·拉赫曼（Rehana Rehman），（巴基）艾莎·谢赫（Aisha Sheikh）主编；郁琦等主译. -- 北京：科学技术文献出版社，2025. 7. -- ISBN 978-7-5235-2481-7

Ⅰ．R711.75

中国国家版本馆 CIP 数据核字第 2025VX5026 号

著作权合同登记号 图字：01-2024-2200

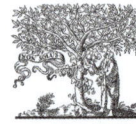

Elsevier (Singapore) Pte Ltd.
3 Killiney Road,
#08-01 Winsland House I,
Singapore 239519
Tel: (65) 6349-0200; Fax: (65) 6733-1817

Polycystic Ovary Syndrome: Basic Science to Clinical Advances Across the Lifespan

Copyright © 2024 by Elsevier, Inc. All rights are reserved, including those for text and data mining, AI training, and similar technologies.

Publisher's note: Elsevier takes a neutral position with respect to territorial disputes or jurisdictional claims in its published content, including in maps and institutional affiliations.

ISBN: 978-0-323-87932-3

This Translation of Polycystic Ovary Syndrome: Basic Science to Clinical Advances Across the Lifespan by Rehana Rehman and Aisha Sheikh was undertaken by Scientific and Technical Documentation Press Co., Ltd and is published by arrangement with Elsevier (Singapore) Pte Ltd.

Polycystic Ovary Syndrome: Basic Science to Clinical Advances Across the Lifespan by Rehana Rehman and Aisha Sheikh 由科学技术文献出版社进行翻译，并根据科学技术文献出版社与爱思唯尔（新加坡）私人有限公司的协议约定出版。

多囊卵巢综合征：从基础医学到全生命周期健康管理新进展（郁琦 陈蓉 甄璟然 郭艺红 主译）

ISBN：978-7-5235-2481-7

Copyright © 2025 by Elsevier (Singapore) Pte Ltd. and Scientific and Technical Documentation Press Co., Ltd.

All rights reserved.No part of this publication may be reproduced or transmitted in any form or by any means, electronic or mechanical, including photocopying, recording,or any information storage and retrieval system, without permission in writing from Elsevier (Singapore) Pte Ltd. and Scientific and Technical Documentation Press Co., Ltd.

声明

本译本由科学技术文献出版社独立完成。相关从业及研究人员必须凭借其自身经验和知识对文中描述的信息数据、方法策略、搭配组合、实验操作进行评估和使用。由于医学科学发展迅速，临床诊断和给药剂量尤其需要经过独立验证。在法律允许的最大范围内，爱思唯尔、译文的原文作者、原文编辑及原文提供者均不对译文或因产品责任、疏忽或其他操作造成的人身及(或)财产伤害及(或)损失承担责任，亦不对由于使用文中提到的方法、产品、说明或思想而导致的人身及（或）财产伤害及（或）损失承担责任。

Printed in China by Scientific and Technical Documentation Press Co., Ltd. under special arrangement with Elsevier (Singapore) Pte Ltd. This edition is authorized for sale in the People's Republic of China only, excluding Hong Kong SAR, Macau SAR and Taiwan.

多囊卵巢综合征：从基础医学到全生命周期健康管理新进展

策划编辑：袁婴婴	责任编辑：袁婴婴	责任校对：张永霞	责任出版：张志平

出 版 者	科学技术文献出版社
地　　址	北京市复兴路15号　邮编 100038
编 务 部	（010）58882938，58882087（传真）
发 行 部	（010）58882868，58882870（传真）
邮 购 部	（010）58882873
官方网址	www.stdp.com.cn
发 行 者	科学技术文献出版社发行　全国各地新华书店经销
印 刷 者	北京地大彩印有限公司
版　　次	2025 年 7 月第 1 版　2025 年 7 月第 1 次印刷
开　　本	787×1092　1/16
字　　数	420千
印　　张	21.75
书　　号	ISBN 978-7-5235-2481-7
定　　价	168.00元

版权所有　违法必究

购买本社图书，凡字迹不清、缺页、倒页、脱页者，本社发行部负责调换

译者委员会

主　　译　郁　琦　陈　蓉　甄璟然　郭艺红

译　　者　（按姓氏笔画排序）

马晓楠　王　阳　王　芳　王　雪　王亚平

史　昊　冯鹏辉　李　婧　杨可扬　杨灵津

何西彦　张多多　陈　蓉　范宇博　郁　琦

罗　敏　桂　婷　高　辉　郭艺红　郭载欣

唐瑞怡　陶　陶　黄　凯　谢卓霖　甄璟然

熊　巍

主译简介

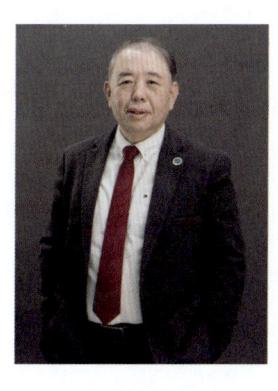

郁琦

医学博士，主任医师，教授，博士研究生导师，北京协和医院妇科内分泌与生殖中心教研室主任、学科带头人。

曾任亚太绝经联盟主席，兼任中华医学会妇产科学分会绝经学组组长，中国医药教育协会副会长、生殖内分泌专业委员会主任委员，中国老年保健协会更年期与妇科内分泌分会主任委员，中国妇幼健康研究会生殖内分泌学专业委员会副主任委员，北京医学会生殖医学分会常务委员，国际绝经学会 *Climacteric* 杂志副主编，《中华妇产科杂志》《中华骨质疏松和骨矿盐疾病杂志》《实用妇产科杂志》《中国实用妇科与产科杂志》《生殖医学杂志》编委会委员。

从事妇科内分泌相关工作30余年，专注于不育、月经相关疾病、绝经和性发育异常等疾病的临床诊治与科学研究，以及辅助生殖技术等相关技术的研发。承担国家自然科学基金、"十五"至"十四五"国家重点研发计划／科技支撑计划项目等课题，累计发表学术论文200余篇。

主译简介

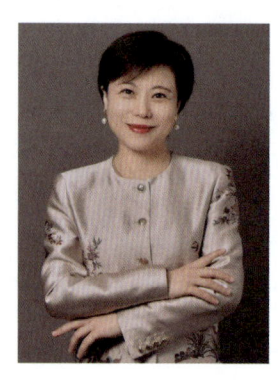

陈蓉

医学博士，主任医师，博士研究生导师，北京协和医院妇产科学系副主任、妇科内分泌与生殖中心副主任。

兼任中华医学会妇产科学分会绝经学组副组长，中国医药教育协会更年期医学教育专业委员会主任委员、生殖内分泌专业委员会副主任委员，中国老年保健协会更年期与妇科内分泌分会副主任委员，中国妇幼健康研究会第二届更年期保健专业委员会副主任委员，北京医学会乳腺疾病分会第二届委员会副主任委员。

主要研究方向为妇科内分泌及绝经相关疾病。主持和参与国家自然科学基金项目、国家重点研发计划等10余项国家级及省部级科研项目。发表文章100余篇，其中被SCI收录30余篇。

主译简介

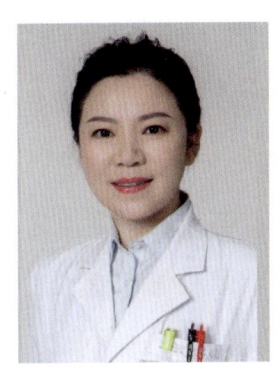

甄璟然

医学博士，主任医师，副教授，硕士研究生导师。

兼任中国医药教育协会生殖内分泌专业委员会秘书长、常务委员、科普中心副主任委员，中国医师协会生殖医学分会北京青年委员会副主任委员，中国老年保健协会健康医学培训专业委员会常务委员，中国女医师协会第一届生殖医学专业委员会委员，北京妇幼保健与优生优育协会生殖与遗传学组委员，全国卫生产业企业管理协会健康医学分会理事。

从事妇科内分泌相关工作 20 余年，在女性不孕不育、月经失调、高泌乳素血症，以及更年期激素替代治疗方面具有丰富的临床经验。亚临床专业为生殖医学，擅长试管婴儿技术中的临床促排卵及相关实验室工作。参编图书 8 部。承担包括北京协和医院在内的多项科研课题，曾作为主要参与者获得高等学校科学研究优秀成果奖（科学技术）二等奖。长期致力于大众健康科普工作，多次受邀参与中央电视台《职场健康课》、北京卫视《我是大医生》、贵州卫视《最强大夫》等节目。

主译简介

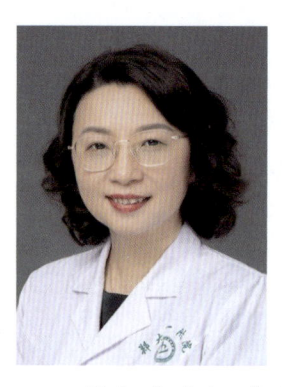

郭艺红

医学博士，主任医师，博士研究生导师，郑州大学第一附属医院生殖与遗传专科医院常务副院长，郑州大学第一附属医院生殖医学部副主任（主持工作），河南省罕见病医疗质量控制中心主任。国家卫生健康突出贡献中青年专家，2022年度"中原英才计划（育才系列）"中原医疗卫生领军人才。

兼任中华医学会生殖医学分会委员，中国医师协会生殖医学专业委员会委员，中国医药教育协会生殖内分泌专业委员会副主任委员，河南省医学会生殖医学分会副主任委员，河南省医师协会生殖医学分会副会长，《中华生殖与避孕杂志》《生殖医学杂志》等杂志编委会委员。

主持国家自然科学基金面上项目2项及省部级课题多项，以第一作者和通信作者在SCI收录期刊发表论文40余篇，获河南省科学技术进步奖二等奖2项。

原著编者名单

Tauseef Ahmad, MSc, PhD
  Researcher
  Department of Epidemiology and Health Statistics
  School of Public Health
  Southeast University
  Nanjing, China

Intisar Ahmed, MBBS
  Fellow
  Aga Khan University
  Medicine
  Aga Khan University, Karachi
  Sindh
  Pakistan

Faiza Alam, MBBS, MPHIL, PHD
  Assistant Professor Clinical Academia
  Medicine
  PAPRSB Institute of Health Sciences
  Muara, Bandar Seri Begawan
  Brunei Darussalam

Sobia Sabir Ali, MBBS, FCPS, MRCP(UK), FRCP(Edin), MHPE
  Professor
  Diabetes & Endocrinology
  Peshawar Medical College, Peshawar
  KPK
  Pakistan

Azra Amerjee, MBBS, FCPS, MCPS(HPE)
  Doctor, Assistant Professor
  Obstetrics & Gynecology
  The Aga Khan University Hospital, Karachi
  Sindh
  Pakistan

Muzna Arif, MBBS, FCPS Pediatrics
  Fellow
  Pediatrics and Child Health
  Aga Khan University, Karachi
  Sindh
  Pakistan

Nargis Asad
  Chair, Associate Professor
  Department of Psychiatry
  Aga Khan University Hospital, Karachi
  Sindh
  Pakistan

Mukhtiar Baig, MBBS, MPhil, PhD
  Professor
  Clinical Biochemistry
  King Abdulaziz University
  Jeddah
  Saudi Arabia

Sumera Batool, MBBS, FCPS (Medicine), FCPS (Endocrinology & Diabetes)
  Consultant Endocrinologist & Diabetologist
  Department of Medicine
  Dr. Ziauddin University Hospital, Karachi
  Sindh
  Pakistan

Amna Subhan Butt, MBBS, FCPS (Medicine), FCPS (Gastroenterology), MSc Clinical Researcher, WGO Fellow in ERCP
  Associate Professor
  Medicine
  The Aga Khan University Hospital, Karachi
  Sindh
  Pakistan

Bhagwan Das, MBBS, FCPS (Medicine), FCPS (Endocrinology), SCE-Endocrine and Diabetes, Diabetes, Endocrine, and Metabolism Fellow
  Consultant Physician and Endocrinologist
  Medicine and Endocrine
  Aster Sanad Hospital
  Riyadh
  KSA

Jalpa Devi, MBBS
  Postgraduate Trainee
  Gastroenterology
  Liaquat University of Medical and Health Sciences
  Hyderabad
  Pakistan

Raj HT Dodia, MBChB, MMEd, MRCOG
  Obstetrics & Gynecology
  MPShah Hospital
  Nairobi
  Kenya

Rubia Farid, MBBS, FCPS
  PCOS Phenotypes
  Family Medicine
  Aga Khan University Hospital, Karachi
  Sindh
  Pakistan

Mahwish Fatima, Pharm-D, MPhil (Pharmacology), PhD Scholar (Pharmacology)
  Program Coordinator (Diabetes and Hypertension)
  The Indus Hospital and Health Network
  Karachi
  Pakistan

Tehseen Fatima, MBBS, FCPS (Medicine)
  Assistant Professor and consultant
  Endocrinologist, Hamdard University, Karachi
  Sindh
  Pakistan

Shayana Rukhsar Hashmani, MBBS
  Resident
  Dermatology
  Aga Khan Hospital, Karachi
  Sindh
  Pakistan

Muhammad Faisal Hashmi, MBBS
  Clinical Fellow
  Internal Medicine
  The Royal Wolverhampton NHS Trust
  Wolverhampton
  United Kingdom

Khadija Nuzhat Humayun, MBBS, FCPS, Adv. DHPE
  Paediatrics Endocrinologist
  Associate Professor
  Paediatrics and Child Health
  Aga Khan University, Karachi
  Sindh
  Pakistan

Zaheena Islam, MBBS, FCPS
  Assistant Professor
  Obstetrics & Gynecology
  Aga Khan University Hospital, Karachi
  Sindh
  Pakistan

Sumerah Jabeen, FCPS(Medicine), FCPS (Endocrinology)
  Consultant Endocrinologist
  Medicine Department
  Patel Hospital, Karachi
  Sindh
  Pakistan

Muhammad Abdullah Javed
  Medical Student
  Medical College
  Aga Khan University, Karachi
  Sindh
  Pakistan

Hafi z S. Kamran, MBBS, FCPS, MRCP
  Registrar
  Acute Medicine
  Royal Preston Hospital
  Dudley
  United Kingdom

Rakhshaan Khan, MBBS, MPH, MBA
  MEd Hearing Impairment
  Doctor
  Public Health
  ICAT, Karachi
  Sindh
  Pakistan

Unab I. Khan, MBBS, MS
  Associate Professor
  Family Medicine
  Aga Khan University, Karachi
  Sindh
  Pakistan

Kimmee Khan, MBBS, BSc, MRCOG
  Doctor
  Obstetrics & Gynaecology
  St Georges Hospital NHS Trust
  London
  United Kingdom

Zareen Kiran, MBBS, FCPS (Med), MRCP (UK), FCPS (Endo)
  Assistant Professor Endocrinology
  Endocrinology, Medicine
  National Institute of Diabetes and Endocrinology
  Dow University of Health Sciences, Karachi
  Sindh
  Pakistan
  Consultant Endocrinologist
  Endocrinology, Medicine
  Aga Khan University Hospital, Karachi
  Sindh
  Pakistan

Sadia Masood, MBBS, FCPS, MHPE
  Assistant Professor
  Medicine
  Aga Khan University, Karachi
  Sindh
  Pakistan

原著编者名单

Malik Hassan H. Mehmood, BPharm, MPhil, PhD
Associate Professor and Chairperson
Department of Pharmacology
Government College University,
Faisalabad, Faisalabad
Punjab
Pakistan

Fozia Memon, MBBS, FCPS
Instructor Pediatric Endocrinology
Pediatrics and Child Health
Aga Khan University, Karachi
Sindh
Pakistan

Asma Altaf Hussain Merchant, MBBS
Research Fellow, Dean's Office
Aga Khan Medical College
Karachi
Pakistan

Ahmed Sayed Mohammed Sayed Mettawi, MSc, DIP, MB ChB
Clinical Nutrition Specialist
Clinical Nutrition & Endocrine Service
CareZone Clinics, Giza
Egypt
Interim Clinical Director & Chief Physician Nutrition
Specialist
Clinical Nutrition Department
Al Haram Hospital, Giza
Egypt

Sarah Nadeem, MD, FACE
Director, CCBP, Assistant Professor
Section of Endocrinology
Department of Medicine
Aga Khan University, Karachi
Sindh
Pakistan
Tania Nadeem, MBBS
Clinical Associate Professor
Psychiatry
Aga Khan University, Karachi
Sindh
Pakistan

Nida Najmi, MRCOG, FCPS, MHPE, MSc. Clinical Research
Assistant Professor
Obstetrics & Gynaecology
Aga Khan University, Karachi
Sindh
Pakistan

Sumaira Naz, MBBS, FCPS
Senior Instructor
Obstetrics & Gynecology
Aga Khan University Hospital, Karachi
Sindh
Pakistan

Aisha Noorullah, MBBS, FCPS
Senior Instructor
Department Of Psychiatry
Aga Khan University Hospital, Karachi
Sindh
Pakistan

Kamal Ojha, MD FRCOG
Obstetrics & Gynaecology
St Georges Hospital
London
United Kingdom

Ouma Pillay
Doctor
St George's University Hospitals NHS Foundation Trust
Blackshaw Road
Tooting
London
SW17 0QT

Rahat Najam Qureshi, MBBS, FRCOG
Consultant
Obstetrics & Gynecology
Aga Khan University, Karachi
Sindh
Pakistan

Muhammad Hassan Raza Raja
Medical Student
Medical College
Aga Khan University, Karachi
Sindh
Pakistan

Muhammad Owais Rashid, MBBS, FCPS(Medicine), FCPS(Endocrinology)
Assistant Professor
Diabetes & Endocrinology
Liaquat National Hospital, Karachi
Sindh
Pakistan
Consultant Endocrinologist
Department of Medicine (Section of Endocrinology)
Aga Khan University Hospital, Karachi
Sindh
Pakistan

Rehana Rehman, MBBS, MPhil, PhD, FHEA, MHPE
   Associate Professor and Director Graduate Studies
   Department of Biological & Biomedical Sciences
   Aga Khan University, Karachi
   Sindh
   Pakistan

Tamar Saeed, MBBS, MRCP(UK), MRCP (Endocrine & Diabetes)
   CCT Endocrine & Diabetes (UK), FRCP(Glasg) RCP(London)
   Consultant in Endocrinology and Diabetes Mellitus
   Foundation Training Programme Director
   MTI Lead in Department of Medicine
   Diabetes and Endocrine Centre, North Wing
   Th e Dudley Group NHS Foundation Trust
   Russells Hall Hospital
   Dudley
   United Kingdom

Zainab Samad, MBBS, MHS
   Professor & Chair
   Department of Medicine
   Aga Khan University, Karachi
   Sindh
   Pakistan

Maheen Shahid, MBBS
   Research Scholar & Teaching Assistant
   Department of Biological & Biomedical Sciences
   Aga Khan University, Karachi
   Sindh
   Pakistan

Pirbhat Shams, MBBS
   Resident Cardiology
   Department of Medicine
   Aga Khan University, Karachi
   Sindh
   Pakistan

Aisha Sheikh, MBBS, FCPS, FACE, PGDipDiab, PGDipEndocrine
   Lecturer & Consultant Endocrinologist
   Department of Medicine
   Th e Aga Khan University Hospital, Karachi
   Sindh
   Pakistan
   Tutor, University of South Wales, Cardiff , United Kingdom

Lumaan Sheikh
   Associate Professor & Chair
   Department of Obstetrics & Gynecology
   Aga Khan University Hospital, Karachi
   Sindh
   Pakistan

Rida Siddique Pharm D, MPhil and PhD (Pharmacology)
   Department of Pharmacology
   Faculty of Pharmaceutical Sciences
   Government College University
   Faisalabad
   Punjab
   Pakistan

Sairabanu Mohamed Rashid Sokwala, MBBS, MMed(Internal Medicine)
   PGDip(Diabetes), PGDip(Endocrinology)
   Consultant
   Diabetes and Endocrinology
   Aga Khan University Hospital
   Nairobi
   Kenya

Saba Tariq, MBBS, MPhil, PhD
   Professor/ Head of Department
   Pharmacology & Th erapeutics
   University Medical and Dental College
   Th e University of Faisalabad, Faisalabad
   Punjab
   Pakistan

Syeda Muneela Wajid, MBBS, MAIUM, MCPS
   Gynecologist, Obstetrician
   Marium General Hospital, Karachi
   Sindh
   Pakistan

Farheen Yousuf, FRCOG, FCPS, MCPS(HPE), MCPS(OBGYN)
   Assistant Professor
   Obstetrics & Gynecology
   Aga Khan University, Karachi
   Sindh
   Pakistan

Nadeem Zuberi, MBBS, FCPS
   Associate Professor
   Department of Obstetrics & Gynecology
   The Aga Khan University, Karachi
   Sindh
   Pakistan

序

《多囊卵巢综合征：从基础医学到全生命周期健康管理新进展》一书对多囊卵巢综合征（polycystic ovary syndrome, PCOS）这一常见而又复杂的疾病所阐述的深度和广度令人印象深刻。本书全面覆盖了PCOS的流行病学、临床表现（涉及躯体和心理）、病理生理相关的交叉学科（如遗传学、胰岛素抵抗、炎症、内分泌疾病、表观遗传学），并在疾病负担方面提出了针对性策略。同时，本书对PCOS的患病率和临床特点在全球（不同国家和地区）的细微差别进行了独树一帜的阐述。书中重新审视了男性类PCOS的可能性，阐述了相关补充和替代治疗方案，对当前和未来未解决的需求进行了反思，内容发人深省。

本书的编者们在整本书的撰写过程中精益求精，呈现出全面翔实的内容，无疑是值得赞扬的。对广大读者而言，无论是医学生、临床医师、研究人员还是政策制定者，都会从中获益。我希望本书能够号召大家共同努力，收集基于人群的数据，以明确南亚女性PCOS的患病率、临床表现和诊疗难题。本书编者所倾注的努力令人钦佩，我很荣幸能为本书作序，以表达我的支持，并祝愿该团队取得圆满成功。

Lubna Pal MBBS, FRCOG, MS
Professor of Obstetrics Gynecology &
Reproductive Sciences
Director, Program for PCOS, Yale Reproductive
Endocrinology & Infertility
Yale School of Medicine
New Haven, CT, USA

前言

多囊卵巢综合征（PCOS）是育龄期女性最常见的内分泌代谢疾病，从初潮到闭经都有可能发病。PCOS 在世界不同地区的患病率、病因、诊断、临床实践、治疗方案，以及对社会心理健康的影响都十分复杂，需要干预。与之相关的合并症，比如肥胖、糖耐量减低、痤疮、多毛症、无排卵及遗传疾病等，常与 PCOS 共存，可能导致临床关注点偏移至这些相关合并症，而非疾病本身。由于目前使用的诊断标准不一致，PCOS 的确切患病率仍不清楚；然而，在过去十年中，患者的比例是有所增加的。《国际 PCOS 循证指南》（International Evidence-Based PCOS Guidelines）指出，PCOS 的高患病率、不明确的病因和发病机制，以及在种族和地域上的差异限制了 PCOS 的终身管理方式。

为了更好地了解 PCOS，我们付出了巨大的努力来回顾和汇编所有有关 PCOS 的信息，特别是关于其病因、患病率、诊断、发展趋势和世界不同地区的管理方法，并将研究结果分为 4 个篇章进行阐述。第一篇对 PCOS 进行了概述，重点介绍了其在青春期和成年后的患病率、分类和表型。第二篇详细讨论了该病的发病机制、临床表现、各种相关合并症的相互作用，以及生育问题。第三篇详细介绍了 PCOS 的管理，包括一般健康问题、生育问题，以及相关合并症的管理。由于 PCOS 的患病率和特征在不同地域各不相同，并且不同遗传和环境因素似乎对治疗方案的效果有影响，因此第四篇介绍了 PCOS 在世界不同地区流行的全面情况，以及影响该疾病发展趋势的因素。这些因素可能包括特定地区的医疗体系、民众的健康与文化信仰、求医行为与生活方式、传统治疗方法、疾病流行趋势、当地女性健康状况、公共卫生政策侧重点、相关问题的遗传易感性，以及影响该地区民众社会心理健康的各种因素之间的相互作用。此外，诊断筛查、生育检测与生育管理的可及性是贯穿上述各领域的共性特征。

我们希望本书能为读者提供关于该疾病在全球范围内的全面了解。书中重点阐述了该疾病对卫生保健预算造成的负担，并强调为应对其日益增长的患病率，应尽早发现和预防 PCOS。

我们非常感谢 Lubna Pal 博士为本书撰写序言，真诚地感谢所有贡献者付出的努力，他们对分配给各自的主题内容进行了明确而翔实的撰述。

Dr. Rehana Rehman
Associate Professor & Director-Graduate Studies
Department of Biological & Biomedical Sciences
Aga Khan University

Dr. Aisha Sheikh
Lecturer & Consultant Endocrinologist
Department of Medicine
Aga Khan University Hospital
Tutor, University of South Wales, Cardiff,
United Kingdom

献 词

本书献给所有患有多囊卵巢综合征的优秀女性（她们一生都在与这种疾病做斗争），希望她们的生活充满微笑。

致 谢

感谢我们的父母、丈夫和孩子,没有他们的支持,本书很难出版。

我们还要特别感谢:

- 阿迦汗大学生物与医学系(内分泌学)各部门主任,以及 Kulsoom Ghias 博士和 Zainab Samad 博士的激励与全力支持。
- Rakhshaan Khan 博士,感谢她校对文稿、绘制图表,并始终鼓励我们完成这项研究。
- Saira Sokawala 博士,感谢她对部分手稿的审阅。
- 感谢所有让我们工作轻松愉快的同事和朋友。

我们还要向所有为本研究工作给予直接或间接帮助的作者及各界人士致以诚挚的谢意。

Dr. Rehana Rehman
Dr. Aisha Sheikh

目 录

第一篇 多囊卵巢综合征概述

第一章 多囊卵巢综合征简介 1
　　一、引言 1
　　二、多囊卵巢综合征的健康问题 3
　　三、多囊卵巢综合征的历史 3
　　四、多囊卵巢综合征的定义 4
　　五、多囊卵巢综合征的流行病学 5

第二章 多囊卵巢综合征表型 7
　　一、引言 7
　　二、不同种族人群的多囊卵巢综合征患病率和临床表现存在差异 7
　　三、诊断标准的演变 7
　　四、多囊卵巢综合征表型中的胰岛素抵抗 9
　　五、多囊卵巢综合征表型间代谢并发症和心血管疾病风险的差异 10
　　六、多囊卵巢综合征表型对生育力的影响差异 10
　　七、基于表型的治疗方法 10

第三章 青春期多囊卵巢综合征 15
　　一、引言 15
　　二、青春期多囊卵巢综合征的病因与风险因素 16
　　三、青春期多囊卵巢综合征的诊断挑战 16
　　四、青春期多囊卵巢综合征的鉴别诊断 17
　　五、青春期多囊卵巢综合征的诊断 18
　　六、青春期多囊卵巢综合征的临床表现 18
　　七、青春期多囊卵巢综合征患者的生活质量 21
　　八、青春期多囊卵巢综合征的诊断方法 22
　　九、青春期多囊卵巢综合征的治疗方案 24
　　十、总结 27

第二篇 多囊卵巢综合征的发病机制和临床表现

第四章 多囊卵巢综合征的病理生理学 30
　　一、引言 30
　　二、激素异常 30
　　三、血管内皮生长因子 34

	四、维生素 D	34
	五、表观遗传学	35
	六、遗传学	37

第五章 脂肪细胞因子与多囊卵巢综合征的相互作用 ... 45
	一、引言	45
	二、脂连蛋白	47
	三、瘦素	48
	四、抵抗素	49
	五、内脂素	49
	六、趋化素	52
	七、白脂素	53
	八、结论	53

第六章 多囊卵巢综合征发病机制中氧化应激和慢性炎症的相互作用 ... 59
	一、引言	59
	二、氧化和抗氧化系统	59
	三、氧化应激和慢性炎症	59
	四、氧化应激与多囊卵巢综合征	60
	五、活性氧对多囊卵巢综合征患者细胞功能的影响	62
	六、多囊卵巢综合征中检测到的氧化应激生物标志物	63
	七、识别和预防氧化应激的增强因素	65
	八、结论	66

第七章 多囊卵巢综合征和低生育力：排卵调节障碍和生育力问题（临床特征和病理生理学） ... 69
	一、引言	69
	二、正常排卵生理学	69
	三、多囊卵巢综合征的病理学	71
	四、结论	73

第八章 多囊卵巢综合征的临床特征及表现 ... 75
| | 一、引言 | 75 |
| | 二、临床特征 | 76 |

第九章 多囊卵巢综合征的诊断标准 ... 82
	一、引言	82
	二、成人多囊卵巢综合征的诊断	82
	三、绝经后女性多囊卵巢综合征的诊断	89
	四、青少年多囊卵巢综合征的诊断	90
	五、多囊卵巢综合征的鉴别诊断	91
	六、青少年多囊卵巢综合征的鉴别诊断	92
	七、转诊至专科医师	93
	八、随访	94
	九、结论	95

第十章 多囊卵巢综合征和代谢综合征：后期生活中的风险 ... 102
一、引言 ... 102
二、多囊卵巢综合征和肥胖 ... 102
三、多囊卵巢综合征和胰岛素抵抗 ... 103
四、多囊卵巢综合征和代谢综合征 ... 105
五、多囊卵巢综合征中的糖耐量异常和糖尿病 ... 110
六、晚年风险 ... 111
七、代谢综合征的筛查 ... 112
八、临床意义 ... 113
九、未来研究需求 ... 113

第十一章 多囊卵巢综合征和心理健康 ... 118
一、引言 ... 118
二、抑郁症和焦虑症 ... 118
三、身体形象 ... 118
四、文化、病耻感 ... 118
五、性与婚姻生活 ... 119
六、生活质量 ... 119
七、应对策略 ... 119
八、进食障碍 ... 120
九、双相情感障碍 ... 120
十、肥胖、多囊卵巢综合征和心理问题之间的复杂关系 ... 120
十一、多囊卵巢综合征患者的心理健康管理 ... 120
十二、抑郁症和焦虑症的特殊管理 ... 121
十三、多囊卵巢综合征心境障碍的药物治疗 ... 122
十四、转诊至精神专科 ... 122
十五、结论 ... 122

第十二章 多囊卵巢综合征和非酒精性脂肪性肝病 ... 125
一、多囊卵巢综合征与非酒精性脂肪性肝病之间是否存在关联 ... 125
二、多囊卵巢综合征与非酒精性脂肪性肝病之间可能存在的关联是什么 ... 125
三、结论 ... 130

第十三章 男性类多囊卵巢综合征 ... 138
一、引言 ... 138
二、有关多囊卵巢综合征女性患者的男性亲属的研究发现 ... 139
三、早发性雄激素性脱发：可能是男性类多囊卵巢综合征的标志吗 ... 141
四、结论和结语 ... 146

第三篇 多囊卵巢综合征及其相关并发症的管理

第十四章 多囊卵巢综合征的药物治疗：月经不规律 ... 153
一、定义 ... 153
二、病理生理学 ... 153

三、多囊卵巢综合征患者月经不规律的含义 ... 155
　　四、多囊卵巢综合征患者月经不规律的管理 ... 155
　　五、总结 ... 158

第十五章　多囊卵巢综合征的药物治疗：多毛症和痤疮 ... 161
　　一、引言 ... 161
　　二、多毛症的治疗 ... 161
　　三、寻常痤疮的治疗 ... 163
　　四、活动性痤疮的治疗设备和物理疗法 ... 165
　　五、结论 ... 166

第十六章　多囊卵巢综合征的药物治疗：减重 ... 168
　　一、体重的重要性 ... 168
　　二、体重管理 ... 169
　　三、药物干预 ... 171
　　四、减重术 ... 174

第十七章　胰岛素增敏剂在多囊卵巢综合征管理中的作用 ... 179
　　一、引言 ... 179
　　二、胰岛素增敏剂在多囊卵巢综合征中的作用机制 ... 179
　　三、治疗多囊卵巢综合征的胰岛素增敏剂 ... 179
　　四、不同胰岛素增敏剂的比较研究 ... 185
　　五、结论 ... 185

第十八章　降低多囊卵巢综合征患者的心血管疾病风险 ... 187
　　一、引言 ... 187
　　二、多囊卵巢综合征中的心血管疾病风险因素 ... 187
　　三、多囊卵巢综合征和心血管疾病 ... 189
　　四、多囊卵巢综合征患者的心血管疾病风险管理 ... 190
　　五、降低多囊卵巢综合征患者心血管疾病风险的主要策略 ... 191
　　六、结论 ... 191

第十九章　多囊卵巢综合征患者低生育力的管理 ... 195
　　一、引言 ... 195
　　二、促性腺激素刺激卵巢的生理学原则 ... 196
　　三、病理生理学：多囊卵巢综合征对生育力的影响 ... 198
　　四、多囊卵巢综合征患者不孕症的检查 ... 199
　　五、多囊卵巢综合征患者无排卵性不孕的治疗原则 ... 200
　　六、治疗管理 ... 200
　　七、结论 ... 215

第二十章　多囊卵巢综合征患者妊娠相关风险的管理 ... 221
　　一、多囊卵巢综合征女性妊娠期病理生理变化的可能潜在机制 ... 221
　　二、多囊卵巢综合征相关的妊娠风险 ... 222
　　三、多囊卵巢综合征患者妊娠并发症的管理 ... 224
　　四、结论 ... 225

| 第二十一章 | 生活方式干预的重要性 | 228 |

- 一、引言 228
- 二、病理生理学/机制 228
- 三、饮食调整 229
- 四、运动 229
- 五、行为策略 230
- 六、维生素 D 231
- 七、环境内分泌干扰物 231
- 八、总结 231

第二十二章 补充和替代治疗在多囊卵巢综合征中的作用 235

- 一、引言 235
- 二、病因学 235
- 三、治疗方法 236
- 四、补充和替代治疗 237

第二十三章 基于循证的临床实践推荐（未来的研究与实践方向） 248

- 一、引言 248
- 二、关于多囊卵巢综合征诊断标准的探讨与建立的问题 248
- 三、关于改善多囊卵巢综合征治疗和干预措施的问题 249
- 四、关于识别多囊卵巢综合征患者身心共病的问题 249
- 五、关于影响多囊卵巢综合征预后的环境因素和社会因素问题 249
- 六、关于加强卫生系统能力建设、满足多囊卵巢综合征患者或易感人群服务需求和组织准备的问题 250
- 七、结束语 250

第四篇　多囊卵巢综合征的全球治疗方式

第二十四章 南亚多囊卵巢综合征的现状分析 253

- 一、多囊卵巢综合征的遗传学研究 254
- 二、多囊卵巢综合征女性的代谢疾病及其他疾病 255
- 三、多囊卵巢综合征患者的生育力和妊娠 256
- 四、多囊卵巢综合征患者的身体特征及其对生活的影响 257

第二十五章 中亚和东亚多囊卵巢综合征的现状分析 261

- 一、引言 261
- 二、发病率、诊断和治疗的影响因素 261
- 三、中亚地区 262
- 四、东亚地区 263
- 五、结论 269

第二十六章 东南亚多囊卵巢综合征的现状分析 273

- 一、文莱 273
- 二、柬埔寨 274

三、东帝汶 275
　　四、印度尼西亚 275
　　五、老挝 276
　　六、马来西亚 276
　　七、缅甸 277
　　八、菲律宾 278
　　九、新加坡 278
　　十、泰国 279
　　十一、越南 280
　　十二、结论 280

第二十七章　西亚多囊卵巢综合征的现状分析 283
　　一、位于西亚北部的国家 284
　　二、位于西亚新月沃地的国家 285
　　三、位于阿拉伯半岛的国家 290

第二十八章　欧洲多囊卵巢综合征的现状分析 297
　　一、引言 297
　　二、多囊卵巢综合征的现状 297
　　三、多囊卵巢综合征患者的文化信仰和生活方式 299
　　四、心理影响 300

第二十九章　非洲多囊卵巢综合征的全球应对方式 302
　　一、引言 302
　　二、患病率 302
　　三、临床表现 303
　　四、治疗方式 306
　　五、建议和结论 308

第三十章　北美洲多囊卵巢综合征的现状分析 313
　　一、引言 313
　　二、美国女性的多囊卵巢综合征相关疾病 313
　　三、诊断 317
　　四、治疗（根据美国生殖医学协会的建议） 317
　　五、并发症及族群构成 318
　　六、美国青少年多囊卵巢综合征 318
　　七、北美洲多囊卵巢综合征与肥胖 319

第一篇 多囊卵巢综合征概述

第一章 多囊卵巢综合征简介

一、引言

多囊卵巢综合征（polycystic ovary syndrome，PCOS）是一种内分泌疾病，全世界育龄期女性的发病率为 5%～15%，是不孕症和妊娠相关并发症的主要原因。70%～80% 患有 PCOS 的女性不能生育，并伴有各种形式的月经不规律和无排卵问题。PCOS 因其高患病率及与生殖、心血管和代谢问题的相关性而备受关注。

有趣的是，PCOS 遗传特征复杂。Stein 和 Leventhal 首次报道了该疾病。他们描述了 7 名具有不同表型特征（即多毛症、痤疮、肥胖和闭经）的双侧多囊卵巢患者，这些患者的表型多样性很明显。

认知上的差异和共识的缺乏会影响诊断的正确性。无法正确诊断或延迟诊断不仅会加剧患者的痛苦、削弱其对医疗体系的信任，还会使医疗保健系统错失开展患者教育、早期预防和早期干预的机会。深受延迟诊断或诊断不足困扰的患者强调，医师可以通过深入理解患者的抱怨和担忧来避免这种不幸情况的发生。研究还表明，最让患者感到困扰的并不是确切的诊断结果，而是缺乏对相关合并症的理解和认知。

此外，过度诊断不仅会给未患病女性带来不必要的困扰，还可能使其对糖尿病、不孕症、心血管损伤及肥胖等潜在健康风险产生过度担忧与焦虑。误诊还会引发其他问题：其一，被误诊女性服用治疗 PCOS 的药物（如口服避孕药、二甲双胍或螺内酯）后，可能出现不良反应，需进一步处理；其二，误诊导致健康保险分类错误，进而影响保险覆盖范围。

PCOS 在疾病初期表现为月经不规律、痤疮和多囊卵巢形态，这些症状可能在青春期出现，且与青春期发育特征相似，容易被误诊。因此，医务人员应该进行全面检查以发现这些易被忽视的问题。

鉴于青春期 PCOS 的认知及管理存在一些深层问题，国际儿科内分泌组织加强了对 PCOS 的关注。人们意识到建立 PCOS 全生命周期指导方针的必要性。随后，在 71 个国家的多个协会共同努力下，适用于不同生命阶段 PCOS 评估和管理的国际循证指南得以制定。制定指南的多学科小组分析了现有数据，提出了可行的建议，并进行了严格审查，制定了基于证据的指导方针。该方针涵盖以下 PCOS 相关主题。

- 育龄期女性潜在风险的调查、鉴别和评估。
- 患者疾病相关情绪问题的有效处理方法。
- 生活方式干预。
- 除生育力之外问题的治疗措施。
- 生育力相关问题的诊断及治疗方案。

这些建议对 PCOS 相关疾病进行了精准识别，并强调了预防、筛查、诊断与规范管理的重要性（图 1.1）。

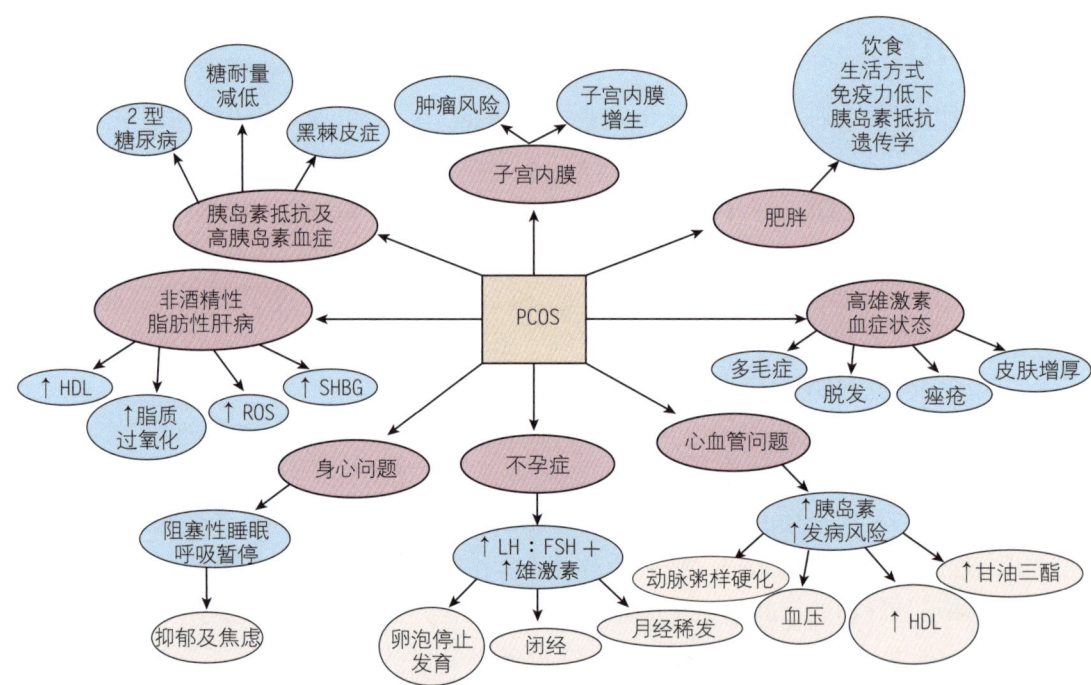

FSH（follicle-stimulating hormone）：卵泡刺激素；HDL（high density lipoprotein）：高密度脂蛋白；LH（luteinizing hormone）：黄体生成素；ROS（reactive oxygen species）：活性氧；SHBG（sex hormone–binding globulin）：性激素结合球蛋白。

图 1.1 多囊卵巢综合征的影响概述

二、多囊卵巢综合征的健康问题

PCOS 对健康的影响主要体现在生殖、代谢和心理 3 个方面，且应对 PCOS 相关问题的医疗成本及情感负担也较大（图 1.2）。目前国际上有很多推荐的临床实践标准，这些标准为医疗工作者及普通女性提供了详细的相关信息。鉴于 PCOS 对患者健康的长远影响，在临床工作中，强调疾病诊断、临床表现、患者教育，并预防患者全生命周期内并发症，具有非常重要的意义。

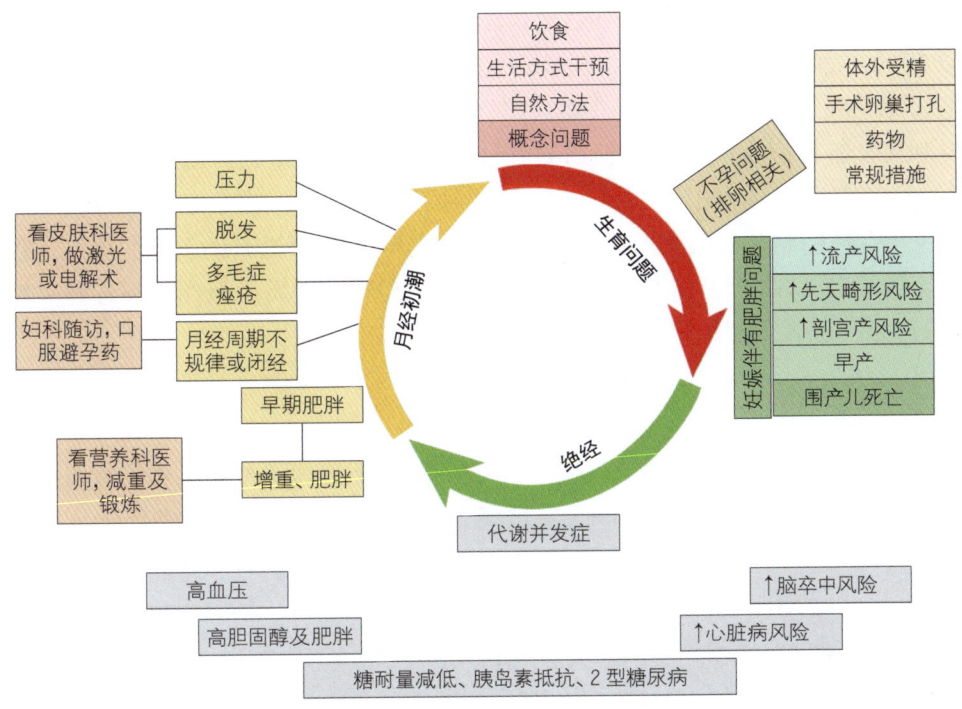

图 1.2　多囊卵巢综合征的影响：女性健康模式中的"健康和预算"问题（从月经初潮到绝经）

三、多囊卵巢综合征的历史

自 1935 年 Stein 和 Leventhal 首次描述 PCOS 以来，其定义和诊断标准不断发生变化。尽管在 20 世纪 50 年代末至 20 世纪 80 年代末，在对该综合征的特征描述方面取得了相当大的进展，但由于"诊断标准"缺乏共识，如何以整体方式来定义该综合征仍存在很大争议。1990 年 4 月，美国国立卫生研究院（National Institutes of Health，NIH）召开了一次会议，旨在通过对参会者的调查来消除这一歧义。在这次会议中，PCOS 的"经典"定义产生了。

2003 年 5 月，欧洲妇产科医师及专家在鹿特丹举行了第二次会议，重新审查和定义了 PCOS。他们进一步扩大了诊断标准的范围，使定义更加全面。

最后，在 2006 年 11 月，雄激素过多和多囊卵巢综合征协会（Androgen Excess and PCOS Society，AE-PCOS）发布了关于 PCOS 的诊断建议，这项建议主要基于 PCOS 标准与相关健康风险（如代谢问题）之间的关系而制定。

对 PCOS 的认识迈出的重要一步，是根据以下 3 个主要临床和（或）生化特征将 PCOS 分为 4 种表型：

- 高雄激素血症。
- 慢性无排卵。
- 超声显示多囊卵巢形态。

2003 年的"鹿特丹标准"和 2006 年的 AE-PCOS 建议只是"NIH 1990"标准的延伸，这也加深了我们对该综合征的理解。建立全面的 PCOS 定义有助于我们加深对全球范围内 PCOS 流行病学的认识。但需要强调的是，在克服障碍并制定全球可接受的 PCOS 标准及其定义的过程中，"共识科学"起到了关键作用。由于 PCOS 的临床表现及潜在的病理生理机制存在极大变异性，因此，进行科学的讨论有助于我们更好地理解该综合征。尽管过去 50 年 PCOS 的相关研究已取得实质性进展，但在诊断各种类型的 PCOS 并管理相关患者方面，仍需做大量的工作。

四、多囊卵巢综合征的定义

PCOS 的定义一直存在着巨大的争议。目前，它被理解为一种卵巢功能障碍和内分泌疾病的综合征，其主要特征包括雄激素过多、高胰岛素血症和代谢综合征。2003 年在鹿特丹召开的欧洲人类生殖与胚胎学协会（European Society of Human Reproduction and Embryology，ESHRE）/美国生殖医学协会（American Society for Reproductive Health，ASRM）联合会议提出，在排除了雄激素过多和月经不规律的其他可能原因后，在推荐的以下 3 项标准中至少有 2 项存在时才能确诊 PCOS。

- 稀发排卵和（或）无排卵，表现为月经稀发和（或）闭经。
- 临床或生化高雄激素血症。
- 超声检查提示多囊卵巢。

稀发排卵或无排卵是指月经周期少于 21 天或多于 35 天，有诊断意义的多囊卵巢形态是至少有 12 个直径为 2～9 mm 的卵泡或卵巢容积大于 10 mL。然而，这些诊断标准在青少年中容易被忽略，因为青春期相关的生理变化与 PCOS 的病理变化之间存在重叠。

目前，除了慢性无排卵和高雄激素血症，卵巢形态被作为新的诊断依据，使 PCOS 的表型更加多样化。NIH 专家组保留了更具包容性的鹿特丹诊断标准，但强调要持续记录 PCOS 患者表型。这些标准的组合构成了以下 PCOS 的表型：

- H-CA：临床或生化高雄激素血症，慢性无排卵。
- H-PCOM：高雄激素血症，超声显示多囊卵巢，但无排卵问题。

- CA-PCOM：慢性无排卵，超声显示多囊卵巢，但无高雄激素血症。
- H-CA-PCOM：高雄激素血症，慢性无排卵，超声显示多囊卵巢。

五、多囊卵巢综合征的流行病学

PCOS 影响着绝经前女性，其通常发病于青春期前后。尽管如此，PCOS 常常出现诊断延迟，PCOS 相关的月经不规律、多毛症等症状也常常被忽略，因为这些症状与月经初潮后 2 年的性成熟表现相似。此外，具有 PCOS 遗传倾向的体形偏瘦女性在体重增加时也可能表现出该综合征。

不同国家之间的 PCOS 患病率存在差异。美国育龄女性中 PCOS 的患病率为 4%～12%；而欧洲地区的调查显示 PCOS 患病率为 6.5%～8.0%；伊朗和中国分别观察到 3% 和 2.2% 的患病率。此外，在巴西、斯里兰卡、巴勒斯坦、英国、希腊和西班牙等国家也发现了 5%～10% 的患病率。而丹麦、土耳其和澳大利亚的患病率更高，为 15%～20%。2017 年，印度博帕尔的一项研究发现 17～24 岁女大学生 PCOS 患病率为 8.2%；而根据 NIH 标准，克什米尔地区女性的 PCOS 患病率为 28.9%，以 AE-PCOS 作为诊断标准甚至可高达 34.3%，这可能是全球报道的最高水平。

全球不同地区的 PCOS 患病率差异巨大主要是由多种因素造成：首先数据收集地点不同会对选定人群民族、种族及年龄分布产生显著影响，这些因素会影响雄激素症状的表达程度及超声检查下卵泡外观、数量等特征。此外，在许多国家/地区中，PCOS 女性并不能获得诊断或需要花费数年时间才能被诊断，这可能是因为医护人员缺乏相关培训或认识所致。

参考文献

1. Azziz R, Carmina E, Dewailly D, et al. The Androgen Excess and PCOS Society criteria for the polycystic ovary syndrome: the complete task force report. Fertil Steril. 2009;91(2):456-488. Available at: https://doi.org/10.1016/j.fertnstert.2008.06.035.
2. Franks S. Diagnosis of polycystic ovarian syndrome: in defense of the Rotterdam criteria. J Clin Endocrinol Metab. 2006;91(3):786-789. Available at: https://doi.org/10.1210/jc.2005-2501.
3. Wild S, Pierpoint T, McKeigue P, Jacobs H. Cardiovascular disease in women with polycystic ovary syndrome at long-term follow-up: a retrospective cohort study. Clin Endocrinol. 2000;52(5):595-600.
4. Legro RS. The genetics of obesity Lessons for polycystic ovary syndrome. Ann N Y Acad Sci. 2000;l900(1):193-202.
5. Azziz R. How polycystic ovary syndrome came into its own. F S Sci. 2021;2(1):2-10. Available at: https://doi.org/10.1016/j.xfss.2020.12.007.
6. Stein IF, Leventhal ML. Amenorrhea associated with bilateral polycystic ovaries. Am J Obstet Gynecol. 1935;29(2):181-191. Available at: https://doi.org/10.1016/S0002-9378(15)30642-6.
7. Gibson-Helm M, Teede H, Dunaif A, Dokras A. Delayed diagnosis and a lack of information associated with dissatisfaction in women with polycystic ovary syndrome. J Clin Endocrinol Metab. 2017;102(2):604-612. Available at: https://doi.org/10.1210/jc.2016-2963.
8. Rowlands IJ, Teede H, Lucke J, Dobson AJ, Mishra GD. Young women's psychological distress after a diagnosis

of polycystic ovary syndrome or endometriosis. Hum Reprod. 2016;31(9):2072-2081. Available at: https://doi.org/10.1093/humrep/dew174.
9. Dokras A, Witchel SF. Are young adult women with polycystic ovary syndrome slipping through the healthcare cracks? J Clin Endocrinol Metab. 2014;99(5):1583-1585. Available at: https://doi.org/10.1210/jc.2013-4190.
10. Ibáñez L, Oberfield SE, Witchel S, et al. An international consortium update: pathophysiology, diagnosis, and treatment of polycystic ovarian syndrome in adolescence. Horm Res Paediatr. 2017;88(6):371-395. Available at: https://doi.org/10.1159/000479371.
11. Teede HJ, Misso ML, Costello MF, et al. Recommendations from the international evidence-based guideline for the assessment and management of polycystic ovary syndrome. Hum Reprod. 2018;33(9):1602-1618. Available at: https://doi.org/10.1093/humrep/dey256.
12. Cooney LG, Lee I, Sammel MD, Dokras A. High prevalence of moderate and severe depressive and anxiety symptoms in polycystic ovary syndrome: a systematic review and meta-analysis. Hum Reprod. 2017;32(5):1075-1091. Available at: https://doi.org/10.1093/humrep/dex044.
13. Ding T, Hardiman PJ, Petersen I, Baio G. Incidence and prevalence of diabetes and cost of illness analysis of polycystic ovary syndrome: a Bayesian modelling study. Hum Reprod. 2018;33(7):1299-1306. Available at: https://doi.org/10.1093/humrep/dey093.
14. Gilbert EW, Tay CT, Hiam DS, Teede HJ, Moran LJ. Comorbidities and complications of polycystic ovary syndrome: an overview of systematic reviews. Clin Endocrinol (Oxf). 2018;89(6):683-699. Available at: https://doi.org/10.1111/cen.13828.
15. Rotterdam ESHRE/ASRM-Sponsored PCOS Consensus Workshop Group. Revised 2003 consensus on diagnostic criteria and long-term health risks related to polycystic ovary syndrome (PCOS). Hum Reprod. 2004;19(1):41-47. Available at: https://doi.org/10.1093/humrep/deh098.
16. Varanasi LC, Subasinghe A, Jayasinghe YL, et al. Polycystic ovarian syndrome: prevalence and impact on the wellbeing of Australian women aged 16-29 years. Aust N Z J Obstet Gynaecol. 2018;58(2):222-233. Available at: https://doi.org/10.1111/ajo.12730.
17. Fauser BC, Tarlatzis BC, Rebar RW, et al. Consensus on women's health aspects of polycystic ovary syndrome (PCOS): the Amsterdam ESHRE/ASRM-Sponsored 3rd PCOS Consensus Workshop Group. Fertil Steril. 2012;97(1):28-38.e25. Available at: https://doi.org/10.1016/j.fertnstert.2011.09.024.
18. Barber TM, Hanson P, Weickert MO, Franks S. Obesity and polycystic ovary syndrome: implications for pathogenesis and novel management strategies. Clin Med Insights Reprod Health. 2019;13:1179558119874042. Available at: https://doi.org/10.1177/1179558119874042.
19. Azziz R, Woods KS, Reyna R, Key TJ, Knochenhauer ES, Yildiz BO. The prevalence and features of the polycystic ovary syndrome in an unselected population. J Clin Endocrinol Metab. 2004;89(6):2745-2749. Available at: https://doi.org/10.1210/jc.2003-032046.
20. Asunción M, Calvo RM, San Millán JL, Sancho J, Avila S, Escobar-Morreale HCF. A prospective study of the prevalence of the polycystic ovary syndrome in unselected Caucasian women from Spain. J Clin Endocrinol Metab. 2000;85(7):2434-2438. Available at: https://doi.org/10.1210/jcem.85.7.6682.
21. Ding T, Hardiman PJ, Petersen I, Wang FF, Qu F, Baio G. The prevalence of polycystic ovary syndrome in reproductive-aged women of different ethnicity: a systematic review and meta-analysis. Oncotarget. 2017;8(56):96351-96358. Available at: https://doi.org/10.18632/oncotarget.19180.
22. Gupta M, Singh D, Toppo M, Priya A, Sethia S, Gupta P. A cross sectional study of polycystic ovarian syndrome among young women in Bhopal, Central India. Int J Community Med Public Health. 2018;5(1):95-100.
23. Ganie MA, Rashid A, Sahu D, Nisar S, Wani IA, Khan J. Prevalence of polycystic ovary syndrome (PCOS) among reproductive age women from Kashmir valley: a cross-sectional study. Int J Gynecol Obstet. 2020;149(2):231-236. Available at: https://doi.org/10.1002/ijgo.13125.

第二章 多囊卵巢综合征表型

一、引言

多囊卵巢综合征（PCOS）是最常见的内分泌疾病之一，影响着 5%～8% 的育龄期女性。PCOS 的病理生理变化受到多重因素和基因的影响。此外，受生活方式影响的表观遗传变化可导致卵泡发育异常和排卵功能障碍（ovulatory dysfunction，OD），同时脂肪组织异常引起的胰岛素抵抗也在该疾病的发生发展中发挥着重要作用。

PCOS 的临床表现在代谢和生殖方面具有多样性特征。虽然卵巢功能障碍、高雄激素血症（hyperandrogenism，HA）和多囊卵巢形态仍然是主要特征，但 PCOS 患者表现出的超重和腹部脂肪增加也可能是由胰岛素抵抗和高胰岛素血症导致，二者与长期不良的心血管代谢事件（如 2 型糖尿病、高血压、血脂异常和心血管疾病的发展）相关联。这种临床表现的多样性使得 PCOS 的诊断标准难以明确定义，这不仅会导致该疾病在评估和管理上存在不一致的情况，而且在流行病学和临床研究中也会存在差异。

在本章中，我们将讨论随着表型定义的演变，不同的临床表现如何被纳入诊断标准。然后，我们将讨论 PCOS 表型之间的重要差异，这种认识不仅可以实现更有效的临床护理、改善健康结局，还可以为全球研究提供一个标准化的平台。

二、不同种族人群的多囊卵巢综合征患病率和临床表现存在差异

无论使用何种定义，PCOS 的患病率在种族之间存在广泛差异。欧洲和美国的前瞻性研究报道，育龄期女性中的 PCOS 患病率为 4%～8%，但巴基斯坦的一项横断面研究估计，在接受不孕症治疗的女性中，PCOS 的患病率可达 20%。此外，从发展中国家移民至发达国家的女性 PCOS 患病率更高。墨西哥裔美国女性的患病率估计为 13%，而英国的一项研究报道称，南亚裔女性的患病率为 52%，而白种女性为 20%。

PCOS 的临床表现也因种族和族群而异，不同种族间多毛症、痤疮、卵巢多囊样改变、肥胖和胰岛素抵抗的发生频率不同。南亚裔患者代谢综合征的患病率较高，有很高的 2 型糖尿病风险，而韩国 PCOS 患者出现月经不规律伴多囊卵巢而无 HA 的情况更为普遍。

理解 PCOS 不同的临床表现不仅可以更准确地评估该疾病对健康的影响，还可以揭示可能影响 PCOS 患病率、严重程度和并发症的潜在环境或种族因素。

三、诊断标准的演变

自 1935 年首次被描述为"Stein-Leventhal 综合征"以来，PCOS 的诊断标准已经

发生了演变。Irving Stein 和 Michael Leventhal 将该综合征描述为"二三十岁年轻女性出现继发性闭经、不育、双侧多囊卵巢和多毛症"。定义标准一经引入，临床医师和科学家几乎立即报告了患者特征的差异。自那时起，诊断标准已根据科学进展进行了修订，如可以使用量化激素水平的方式和超声检查对卵巢形态进行评估。但不管使用哪种定义，PCOS 的关键特征包括：①排卵功能障碍；②生化/临床 HA；③多囊卵巢。

1990 年，美国国立卫生研究院（NIH）的诊断标准将 PCOS 定义为：在没有已知的内分泌障碍的情况下表现为 HA 的一种疾病，存在稀发排卵或无排卵和生化/临床 HA。

2003 年，欧洲人类生殖与胚胎学协会（ESHRE）和美国生殖医学协会（ASRM）在鹿特丹召开了一次专家会议，建议将多囊卵巢（polycystic ovaries，PCO）的存在作为第三个标准。因此，根据 2003 年鹿特丹标准，在没有其他可以解释 HA 的内分泌异常的情况时，需要符合 3 条标准（稀发排卵或无排卵、HA 和 PCO）中的 2 条才可诊断 PCOS。这种诊断标准的扩大导致了更多的表型被加到该综合征中，从而使得全球 PCOS 的患病率增加。

2006 年，雄激素过多和多囊卵巢综合征协会（AE-PCOS）的任务小组进行了一项系统回顾，汇总了有关 PCOS 流行病学和表型表现的现有证据。该任务小组得出的结论是，HA（及其各种临床表现）仍然是 PCOS 患者中的核心异常表现，不应在没有其临床或生化证据的情况下确定诊断；并且 HA 伴有多囊卵巢形态和（或）排卵功能障碍（及其各种表现，包括月经不规律）应被视为具有诊断意义。根据这些特征的各种组合，该任务小组确定了 9 种 PCOS 的表型，但同时也认识到，同一患者的表型表现可能会随体重变化和生命阶段不同而改变。

在 2012 年，NIH 举办了一次关于 PCOS 循证研讨会，专家们不仅讨论了不同诊断标准的利弊，还讨论了最佳的预防和治疗策略，并就未来研究重点提出了建议。该小组认识到，使用不同标准会影响临床护理和研究进展。该任务小组推荐继续使用鹿特丹标准，但建议再添加一种表型分类，以便临床医师了解该综合征对患者的临床表现严重程度、相关并发症和生殖健康问题的影响，以及对患者生活质量的整体影响。

PCOS 表型包括以下 4 种。
- A 型（经典表型/明显 PCOS），其特征是高雄激素水平/HA、月经不规律/排卵迟缓和多囊卵巢（HA + OD + PCO）。
- B 型（非 PCO 表型），其特征是高雄激素水平/HA、月经不规律/排卵迟缓和正常卵巢（HA + OD）。
- C 型（排卵表型），其特征是高雄激素水平/HA、月经规律（35 天或更短周期）/定期排卵和多囊卵巢（HA + PCO）。
- D 型（非 HA 表型），被认为是较轻的表型，其特征是雄激素水平正常、月经不规律/排卵迟缓和多囊卵巢（OD + PCO）。

下面我们将讨论这些表型的临床特征和相关异常。

（一）A 型和 B 型表型

在 PCOS 患者中，A 型和 B 型表型更为常见，据报道二者患病率分别为 50%～68% 和 8%～11%。大多数患者表现为月经不规律、低生育力和不孕症，并且有 HA 的临床表现，包括多毛症。尽管 A 型表型患者被认为是心脑血管不良事件发生风险最高的一类人群，但在没有排卵障碍的情况下出现 HA，如 B 型表型中所见，也可能导致代谢异常和胰岛素抵抗（insulin resistance，IR）。前脂肪细胞含有雄激素受体，而脂肪细胞功能受雄激素调节。因此，HA 会促进腹型肥胖，从而加重 IR。此外，已经有研究证明，在培养的脂肪细胞中加入雄激素会诱导出现选择性 IR。因此，A 型和 B 型表型患者具有更高的肥胖率，以及 IR、血脂异常、肝脂肪变性和代谢综合征发生率，这也使这类患者更容易发生潜在的代谢和心血管不良事件。

（二）C 型表型

排卵性 PCOS 的女性表现为 HA 和多囊卵巢，但没有排卵功能障碍。他们占 PCOS 患者的 20%～30%。与 A 型和 B 型表型患者相比，那些排卵性 PCOS 患者不仅有中等程度的雄激素水平异常，其体重指数（body mass index，BMI）更低并且伴有高胰岛素血症和 IR。然而，研究表明，排卵性 PCOS 中的 IR 减轻很大程度上与腹部脂肪减少有关。与 BMI 匹配的 A 型或 B 型表型 PCOS 女性相比，C 型表型 PCOS 女性的腹部脂肪和 IR 水平更高，而脂连蛋白水平更低。此外，当 BMI 和腹部肥胖相匹配时，C 型表型患者与 A 型和 B 型表型患者有着相同的心脑血管不良事件发生风险。

（三）D 型表型

非 HA PCOS 的女性占 PCOS 女性的 3%～5%。她们表现出月经周期不规律和与多囊卵巢相关的排卵功能障碍。她们的特征是黄体生成素（LH）和 LH∶FSH 升高，但睾酮和其他雄激素的增加很少。然而，与没有患 PCOS 的女性相比，D 型表型的 PCOS 女性被报道具有更高的雄激素水平，这可能影响她们的 BMI，造成脂代谢异常，并促进 IR 发生。此外，与 A 型和 B 型表型的女性相比，她们的代谢风险相对降低，脂肪总量和腹部脂肪较低，代谢综合征的患病率也较低。

造成这种情况的可能原因是 PCOS 女性的 HA 严重程度不同，尽管在大多数表型（A、B、C 型表型）中雄激素过多会驱动 PCOS 发生，但在雄激素轻微异常（D 型或非 HA PCOS）的女性中，需要更多遗传或环境因素诱导腹部肥胖相关的 IR，进而引发生殖和卵巢功能障碍。

四、多囊卵巢综合征表型中的胰岛素抵抗

Burghen 等首次提出了胰岛素在卵巢功能中的作用，他们观察到高胰岛素血症与 HA 相关联。无论肥胖程度如何，IR 是 PCOS 发生的内在因素。50%～80% 的 PCOS 患者可表现出 IR。高水平的胰岛素与 LH 协同作用促进了卵泡膜细胞产生雄激素，导致

血脂异常。此外，升高的胰岛素水平抑制了性激素结合球蛋白在肝脏中的合成，导致游离睾酮量增加，从而在 PCOS 的发病机制中起到直接和间接作用。

经典表型（A 型和 B 型表型）的女性比排卵表型（C 型表型）或正常雄激素表型（D 型表型）的女性表现出更严重的 IR 特征。此外，超重 / 肥胖的 A 型表型患者比 B 型表型患者有着更高的循环雄激素水平。有意思的是，尽管没有 HA，超重 / 肥胖的 D 型表型患者也可表现出 IR。

五、多囊卵巢综合征表型间代谢并发症和心血管疾病风险的差异

PCOS 女性的雄激素过多与代谢综合征和冠状动脉疾病发生率增加直接相关。PCOS 女性患代谢综合征的风险是其同龄女性的 11 倍。通过不同表型的定义，我们能够区分哪些表型具有较高的心血管代谢风险，并且更有可能发展成糖尿病、血脂异常和心血管疾病。研究表明，A、B、C 型表型的女性患代谢综合征的风险是非 PCOS 女性的 6～8 倍。因此，这些表型的女性不仅应该治疗生殖方面的问题，还必须定期进行心血管代谢异常的筛查和治疗。

BMI 高和月经不规律程度是 PCOS 女性代谢功能不良的独立预测因子。多囊卵巢本身并不与代谢异常相关。

六、多囊卵巢综合征表型对生育力的影响差异

PCOS 可以通过多种方式影响生育力。睾酮水平增加和卵泡不成熟是排卵功能障碍的常见原因。在排卵周期中，激素失衡可能阻止子宫内膜正常发育，从而影响着床。不可预测的月经周期也可能导致计划怀孕变得困难。虽然现有的循证指南可供评估和管理患有 PCOS 的不孕症患者，但这些指南并没有考虑表型分类。目前仍然很少有研究探讨不同 PCOS 表型中不孕症的患病率和不同表型对治疗方式的影响。据报道，A 型表型的女性对氯米芬的反应较其他表型更差。

七、基于表型的治疗方法

PCOS 及其相关临床症状的治疗需在正确识别表型后开始。治疗目标的建立应基于多重获益的方法，以确保满足患者的意愿（如治疗不孕症、调节月经以保护子宫内膜、控制多毛症和痤疮等 HA 特征）。与此同时，临床医师的目标是筛查、监测和降低已知心血管代谢风险。

治疗方法可以总结如下：

• 生活方式干预对所有患有 PCOS 的女性都有帮助，尤其是对于超重或肥胖的患者。具有较高心血管代谢风险的 A 型和 B 型表型患者需要进行血压、血脂和血糖水平的筛查和定期监测。此外，D 型表型的患者通过减重可以改善月经不规律而不受雄激素水平

变化的影响。

- 对于在 A 型、B 型和 D 型表型中出现的月经不规律，可使用口服避孕药和胰岛素增敏剂（如二甲双胍）。
- 对于生育问题，包括低生育力和不孕症，可以使用胰岛素增敏剂、枸橼酸氯米芬、来曲唑、促性腺激素和腹腔镜卵巢打孔术等方法。
- 在 A 型、B 型和 C 型表型中出现的 HA 表现，如多毛症和痤疮，可使用口服避孕药、抗雄激素类药、美容手术、盐酸依氟鸟氨酸和促性腺激素释放激素激动剂（GnRH-agonist）进行治疗。

从青春期到绝经后期，PCOS 临床表型可能会在整个生命周期中重叠或改变，这很大程度上受肥胖、代谢改变和种族背景的影响。不过，使用表型方法对 PCOS 患者有一些实际意义。在临床实践中，可以及早识别最有可能发生长期心血管代谢不良事件的女性（A 型和 B 型表型），并且制定筛查和治疗方案。同样，D 型表型的患者应通过减重改善月经不规律的情况。

随着我们对 PCOS 理解的不断深入，表型分类将使研究重点放在每个亚组的发病机制、治疗和不良事件上，并实现更加个性化的管理。

参考文献

1. Azziz R, Woods KS, Reyna R, Key TJ, Knochenhauer ES, Yildiz BO. The prevalence and features of the polycystic ovary syndrome in an unselected population. J Clin Endocrinol Metab. 2004;89(6):2745-2749.
2. Shen HR, Qiu LH, Zhang ZQ, Qin YY, Cao C, Di W. Genome-wide methylated DNA immunoprecipitation analysis of patients with polycystic ovary syndrome. PLoS One. 2013;8(5):e64801.
3. Diamanti-Kandarakis E. Polycystic ovarian syndrome: pathophysiology, molecular aspects and clinical implications. Expert Rev Mol Med. 2008;10:e3.
4. Ilie IR, Georgescu CE. Polycystic ovary syndrome-epigenetic mechanisms and aberrant microRNA. Adv Clin Chem. 2015;71:25-45.
5. Kokosar M, Benrick A, Perfilyev A, et al. Erratum: epigenetic and transcriptional alterations in human adipose tissue of polycystic ovary syndrome. Sci Rep. 2016;6:25321.
6. Haffner SM, D'Agostino R, Festa A, et al. Low insulin sensitivity (Si=0) in diabetic and nondiabetic subjects in the insulin resistance atherosclerosis study: is it associated with components of the metabolic syndrome and nontraditional risk factors? Diabetes Care. 2003;26(10):2796-2803.
7. Li L, Yang D, Chen X, Chen Y, Feng S, Wang L. Clinical and metabolic features of polycystic ovary syndrome. Int J Gynecol Obstet. 2007;97(2):129-134.
8. Allahbadia GN, Merchant R. Polycystic ovary syndrome in the Indian Subcontinent. Semin Reprod Med. 2008;26(1):22-34.
9. Moran C, Tena G, Moran S, Ruiz P, Reyna R, Duque X. Prevalence of polycystic ovary syndrome and related disorders in Mexican women. Gynecol Obstet Invest. 2010;69(4):274-280.
10. Diamanti-Kandarakis E, Kouli CR, Bergiele AT, et al. A survey of the polycystic ovary syndrome in the Greek island of Lesbos: hormonal and metabolic profile. J Clin Endocrinol Metab. 1999;84(11):4006-4011.
11. Azziz R, Woods KS, Reyna R, Key TJ, Knochenhauer ES, Yildiz BO. The prevalence and features of the polycystic ovary syndrome in an unselected population. J Clin Endocrinol Metab. 2004;89(6):2745-2749.

12. Baqai Z, Khanam M, Parveen S. Prevalence of PCOS in infertile patients. Med Channel. 2010;16(3):437-440.
13. Goodarzi MO, Quiñones MJ, Azziz R, Rotter JI, Hsueh WA, Yang H. Polycystic ovary syndrome in Mexican-Americans: prevalence and association with the severity of insulin resistance. Fertil Steril. 2005;84(3):766-769.
14. Mirza SS, Shafique K, Shaikh AR, Khan NA, Qureshi MA. Association between circulating adiponectin levels and polycystic ovarian syndrome. J Ovarian Res. 2014;7(1):1-7.
15. Zhao Y, Qiao J. Ethnic differences in the phenotypic expression of polycystic ovary syndrome. Steroids. 2013;78(8):755-760.
16. Wang S, Alvero R, eds. Racial and Ethnic Differences in Physiology and Clinical Symptoms of Polycystic Ovary Syndrome. Seminars in Reproductive Medicine. New York, NY. USA: Thieme Medical Publishers; 2013.
17. Amato MC, Verghi M, Galluzzo A, Giordano C. The oligomenorrhoic phenotypes of polycystic ovary syndrome are characterized by a high visceral adiposity index: a likely condition of cardiometabolic risk. Hum Reprod. 2011;26(6):1486-1494.
18. Stein E, Leventhal ML. Polycystic ovary syndrome. Am J Obstet Gynecol. 1935;29:181.
19. Leventhal ML. Amenorrhea and sterility caused by bilateral polycystic ovaries. Am J Obstet Gynecol. 1941;41(3):516-517.
20. Hofmeister FJ, Byce KR. Clinical aspects of the Stein-Leventhal syndrome. Obstet Gynecol. 1966;28(2):264-267.
21. Ibrahim MS, Zaki S, Girgis S. The diagnostic problem of the Stein-Leventhal syndrome. A review of the literature and report on 9 cases. J Egypt Med Assoc. 1966;49(9):629-638.
22. Raj SG, Thompson I, Berger M, Talert L, Taymor M. Diagnostic value of androgen measurements in polycystic ovary syndrome. Obstet Gynecol. 1978;52(2):169-171.
23. Adams J, Polson D, Franks S. Prevalence of polycystic ovaries in women with anovulation and idiopathic hirsutism. Br Med J (Clin Res Ed). 1986;293(6543):355-359.
24. Azziz R, Carmina E, Dewailly D, et al. The Androgen Excess and PCOS Society criteria for the polycystic ovary syndrome: the complete task force report. Fertil Steril. 2009;91(2):456-488.
25. ESHRE TR, Group A-SPCW. Revised 2003 consensus on diagnostic criteria and long-term health risks related to polycystic ovary syndrome. Fertil Steril. 2004;81(1):19-25.
26. Azziz R, Carmina E, Dewailly D, et al. Criteria for defining polycystic ovary syndrome as a predominantly hyperandrogenic syndrome: an androgen excess society guideline. J Clin Endocrinol Metab. 2006;91(11):4237-4245.
27. Johnson T, Kaplan L, Ouyang P, Rizza R. Final Report: Evidence-based Methodology Workshop on Polycystic Ovary Syndrome. https://prevention.nih.gov/workshops/2012/pcos/docs/PCOS_Final_Statement.pdf. National Institute of Health. December 3-5, 2012.
28. Guastella E, Longo RA, Carmina E. Clinical and endocrine characteristics of the main polycystic ovary syndrome phenotypes. Fertil Steril. 2010;94(6):2197-2201.
29. Sachdeva G, Gainder S, Suri V, Sachdeva N, Chopra S. Comparison of the different PCOS phenotypes based on clinical metabolic, and hormonal profile, and their response to clomiphene. Indian J Endocrinol Metab. 2019;23(3):326.
30. Jamil AS, Alalaf SK, Al-Tawil NG, Al-Shawaf T. Comparison of clinical and hormonal characteristics among four phenotypes of polycystic ovary syndrome based on the Rotterdam criteria. Arch Gynecol Obstet. 2016;293(2):447-456.
31. Romualdi D, Di Florio C, Tagliaferri V, et al. The role of anti-Müllerian hormone in the characterization of the different polycystic ovary syndrome phenotypes. Reprod Sci. 2016;23(5):655-661.
32. Sahmay S, Atakul N, Oncul M, Tuten A, Aydogan B, Seyisoglu H. Serum anti-Mullerian hormone levels in the main phenotypes of polycystic ovary syndrome. Eur J Obstet Gynecol Reprod Biol. 2013;170(1):157-161.
33. Hsu MI, Liou TH, Chou SY, Chang CY, Hsu CS. Diagnostic criteria for polycystic ovary syndrome in Taiwanese Chinese women: comparison between Rotterdam 2003 and NIH 1990. Fertil Steril. 2007;88(3):727-729.

34. Kim JJ, Hwang KR, Choi YM, et al. Complete phenotypic and metabolic profiles of a large consecutive cohort of untreated Korean women with polycystic ovary syndrome. Fertil Steril. 2014;101(5):1424-1430.e3.
35. Welt C, Gudmundsson J, Arason G, et al. Characterizing discrete subsets of polycystic ovary syndrome as defined by the Rotterdam criteria: the impact of weight on phenotype and metabolic features. J Clin Endocrinol Metab. 2006;91(12):4842-4848.
36. Escobar-Morreale HF, San Millán JL. Abdominal adiposity and the polycystic ovary syndrome. Trends Endocrinol Metab. 2007;18(7):266-272.
37. Corbould A, Dunaif A. The adipose cell lineage is not intrinsically insulin resistant in polycystic ovary syndrome. Metabolism. 2007;56(5):716-722.
38. Moran L, Teede H, Moran L, Teede H. Metabolic features of the reproductive phenotypes of polycystic ovary syndrome. Hum Reprod Update. 2009;15(4):477-488.
39. Diamanti-Kandarakis E, Panidis D. Unravelling the phenotypic map of polycystic ovary syndrome (PCOS): a prospective study of 634 women with PCOS. Clin Endocrinol. 2007;67(5):735-742.
40. Carmina E, Orio F, Palomba S, et al. Endothelial dysfunction in PCOS: role of obesity and adipose hormones. Am J Med. 2006;119(4):356.e1-356.e6.
41. Jones H, Sprung VS, Pugh CJ, et al. Polycystic ovary syndrome with hyperandrogenism is characterized by an increased risk of hepatic steatosis compared to nonhyperandrogenic PCOS phenotypes and healthy controls, independent of obesity and insulin resistance. J Clin Endocrinol Metab. 2012;97(10):3709-3716.
42. Goverde A, Van Koert A, Eijkemans M, et al. Indicators for metabolic disturbances in anovulatory women with polycystic ovary syndrome diagnosed according to the Rotterdam consensus criteria. Hum Reprod. 2009;24(3):710-717.
43. Mehrabian F, Khani B, Kelishadi R, Kermani N. The prevalence of metabolic syndrome and insulin resistance according to the phenotypic subgroups of polycystic ovary syndrome in a representative sample of Iranian females. J Res Med Sci. 2011;16(6):763.
44. Pehlivanov B, Orbetzova M. Characteristics of different phenotypes of polycystic ovary syndrome in a Bulgarian population. Gynecol Endocrinol. 2007;23(10):604-609.
45. Moran L, Teede H. Metabolic features of the reproductive phenotypes of polycystic ovary syndrome. Hum Reprod Update. 2009;15(4):477-488.
46. Carmina E, Bucchieri S, Mansueto P, Rini G, Ferin M, Lobo RA. Circulating levels of adipose products and differences in fat distribution in the ovulatory and anovulatory phenotypes of polycystic ovary syndrome. Fertil Steril. 2009;91(4):1332-1335.
47. Dewailly D, Catteau-Jonard S, Reyss AC, Leroy M, Pigny P. Oligoanovulation with polycystic ovaries but not overt hyperandrogenism. J Clin Endocrinol Metab. 2006;91(10):3922-3927.
48. Norman RJ, Masters SC, Hague W, Beng C, Pannall P, Wang JX. Metabolic approaches to the subclassification of polycystic ovary syndrome. Fertil Steril. 1995;63(2):329-335.
49. Dilbaz B, Özkaya E, Cinar M, Cakir E, Dilbaz S. Cardiovascular disease risk characteristics of the main polycystic ovary syndrome phenotypes. Endocrine. 2011;39(3):272-277.
50. Burghen GA, Givens JR, Kitabchi AE. Correlation of hyperandrogenism with hyperinsulinism in polycystic ovarian disease. J Clin Endocrinol Metab. 1980;50(1):113-116.
51. Stepto NK, Cassar S, Joham AE, et al. Women with polycystic ovary syndrome have intrinsic insulin resistance on euglycaemic–hyperinsulaemic clamp. Hum Reprod. 2013;28(3):777-784.
52. Diamanti-Kandarakis E, Dunaif A. Insulin resistance and the polycystic ovary syndrome revisited: an update on mechanisms and implications. Endocr Rev. 2012;33(6):981-1030.
53. Dunaif A. Drug insight: insulin-sensitizing drugs in the treatment of polycystic ovary syndrome-a reappraisal. Nat Clin Pract Endocrinol Metab. 2008;4(5):272-283.
54. Nestler JE, Jakubowicz DJ, Falcon de Vargas A, Brik C, Quintero N, Medina F. Insulin stimulates testosterone biosynthesis by human thecal cells from women with polycystic ovary syndrome by activating its own

receptor and using inositolglycan mediators as the signal transduction system. J Clin Endocrinol Metab. 1998;83(6):2001-2005.
55. Poretsky L, Smith D, Seibel M, Pazianos A, Moses A, Flier J. Specific insulin binding sites in human ovary. J Clin Endocrinol Metab. 1984;59(4):809-811.
56. Yilmaz M, Isaoglu U, Delibas IB, Kadanali S. Anthropometric, clinical and laboratory comparison of four phenotypes of polycystic ovary syndrome based on Rotterdam criteria. J Obstet Gynaecol Res. 2011;37(8):1020-1026.
57. Shroff R, Syrop CH, Davis W, Van Voorhis BJ, Dokras A. Risk of metabolic complications in the new PCOS phenotypes based on the Rotterdam criteria. Fertil Steril. 2007;88(5):1389-1395.
58. March WA, Moore VM, Willson KJ, Phillips DI, Norman RJ, Davies MJ. The prevalence of polycystic ovary syndrome in a community sample assessed under contrasting diagnostic criteria. Hum Reprod. 2010;25(2):544-551.
59. Rizzo M, Longo R, Guastella E, Rini G, Carmina E. Assessing cardiovascular risk in Mediterranean women with polycystic ovary syndrome. J Endocrinol Invest. 2011;34(6):422-426.
60. Orio Jr F, Palomba S, Spinelli L, et al. The cardiovascular risk of young women with polycystic ovary syndrome: an observational, analytical, prospective case-control study. J Clin Endocrinol Metab. 2004;89(8):3696-3701.
61. Wild RA, Painter P, Coulson PB, Carruth KB, Ranney G. Lipoprotein lipid concentrations and cardiovascular risk in women with polycystic ovary syndrome. J Clin Endocrinol Metab. 1985;61(5):946-951.
62. Shroff R, Syrop CH, Davis W, Van Voorhis BJ, Dokras A. Risk of metabolic complications in the new PCOS phenotypes based on the Rotterdam criteria. Fertil Steril. 2007;88(5):1389-1395.
63. Ehrmann DA, Liljenquist DR, Kasza K, et al. Prevalence and predictors of the metabolic syndrome in women with polycystic ovary syndrome. J Clin Endocrinol Metab. 2006;91(1):48-53.
64. Brower M, Brennan K, Pall M, Azziz R. The severity of menstrual dysfunction as a predictor of insulin resistance in PCOS. J Clin Endocrinol Metab. 2013;98(12):E1967-E1971.
65. Legro RS, Chiu P, Kunselman AR, Bentley CM, Dodson WC, Dunaif A. Polycystic ovaries are common in women with hyperandrogenic chronic anovulation but do not predict metabolic or reproductive phenotype. J Clin Endocrinol Metab. 2005;90(5):2571-2579.
66. Costello M, Misso M, Balen A, et al. Evidence summaries and recommendations from the international evidence-based guideline for the assessment and management of polycystic ovary syndrome: assessment and treatment of infertility. Human Reprod Open. 2019;2019(1):hoy021.
67. Moran C, Arriaga M, Rodriguez G, Moran S. Obesity differentially affects phenotypes of polycystic ovary syndrome. Int J Endocrinol. 2012;2012:317241.
68. Papadakis G, Kandaraki EA, Garidou A, et al. Tailoring treatment for PCOS phenotypes. Expert Rev Endocrinol Metab. 2021;16(1):9-18.

第三章 青春期多囊卵巢综合征

一、引言

多囊卵巢综合征（PCOS）是女性中极为常见的一种疾病。它是一种异质性疾病，通常表现为月经不规律、高雄激素血症（HA）和多囊卵巢形态。在青少年中诊断PCOS是很困难的，虽然早期诊断PCOS可以更早地治疗，从而预防长期并发症，但草率的诊断会增加不必要的治疗风险和心理困扰。

在成年人中，PCOS的诊断有5种不同的标准（表3.1）：1990年美国国立卫生研究院（NIH）标准、2003年鹿特丹标准、2006年雄激素过多和多囊卵巢综合征协会（AE-PCOS）标准、2012年阿姆斯特丹标准和2013年美国内分泌学会标准。NIH标准将PCOS定义为：

- 存在临床或生化HA。
- 月经稀发/无排卵。

表3.1 多囊卵巢综合征的不同诊断标准

标准	高雄激素血症	慢性无排卵	多囊卵巢
1990年NIH标准	+	+	−
2003年鹿特丹标准[a]	+/−	+/−	+/−
2006年AE-PCOS标准[b]	+	+/−	+/−
2012年阿姆斯特丹标准	+	+	+
2013年美国内分泌学会标准	+	+	+
儿科内分泌学会标准[c]	+	+[d]	−

来源：Akgül S, Düzçeker Y, Kanbur N, Derman O. Do different diagnostic criteria impact polycystic ovary syndrome diagnosis for adolescents? J Pediatr Adolesc Gynecol. 2018; 31(3): 258–262.

注：[a] 3条中必须达到2条。
[b] 高雄激素血症及其他2项中至少有1项达标。
[c] 生化高雄激素血症：血清睾酮水平持续超过成年人正常标准。临床高雄激素血症：中到重度的多毛症或中到重度的炎症性寻常痤疮。
[d] 育龄期异常子宫出血持续1～2年。
+：需包括的定义标准。
+/−：可有可无的定义标准。

Akgül等将表3.1中列出的所有不同PCOS标准应用于可能患有PCOS的青少年，并发现当评估方法为阿姆斯特丹标准和儿科内分泌学会（Pediatric Endocrine Society, PES）标准时，根据鹿特丹标准诊断的青少年数量减少了30%以上，因此引发了对漏诊或过度诊断的担忧。此外，令人担忧的是，目前没有为青少年使用的特定诊断标准。2013年，美国内分泌学会的临床实践指南建议，如果排除其他病理性原因后，青少年女性持续存在月经稀发，临床和（或）生化证据表明存在 HA，则可以诊断 PCOS。

由于无排卵症状和多囊卵巢（PCO）形态可能出现在生殖系统成熟的早期阶段，美国内分泌学会的指南建议在给青少年贴上 PCOS 标签之前要谨慎，尤其是在月经初潮后的 2 年内。2015 年，PES 共识认可了美国内分泌学会的标准，并进行了一些修改，如针对持续的高雄激素源性稀发排卵 / 无排卵的月经异常阶段，建议采用适当的年龄标准，具体将在下文中详细讨论。

二、青春期多囊卵巢综合征的病因与风险因素

PCOS 是一种多因素疾病。文献支持 PCOS 的发生甚至可以追溯到宫内阶段。临床表现的多样性最好通过遗传与环境的相互作用来解释，其中最重要的是遗传与生活方式和饮食的相互作用。

尽管 PCOS 的病因尚不清楚，但有足够的证据表明，它是遗传、代谢和环境因素的综合结果，包括胰岛素抵抗（IR）、肾上腺和卵巢的类固醇激素生成和代谢异常、胰岛素产生的变化、神经内分泌影响及复杂的表观遗传机制。目前已经确认，HA 青春期女性的促性腺激素分泌模式与成年 PCOS 女性是相似的。

在患有 PCOS 的青春期女性中，由于对黄体生成素（LH）过度反应，下丘脑 – 垂体 -GnRH 轴（该轴促进卵泡发育）出现了失衡。研究表明，与正常女性血清相比，PCOS 患者被促性腺激素释放激素（gonadotropin releasing hormone，GnRH）刺激后的 LH 释放明显更高。

三、青春期多囊卵巢综合征的诊断挑战

由于多种因素存在，青春期 PCOS 的诊断比成年人群更具挑战性。

（一）下丘脑 – 垂体 – 卵巢轴未成熟与月经不规律

在下丘脑 – 垂体 – 卵巢轴正常发育的早期阶段，月经不规律和无排卵周期很常见。在正常的青春期发育过程中，月经稀发在初潮后非常常见，因此对 PCOS 青少年患者来说并不具有特异性。在月经初潮后的第 1 年、第 3 年和第 6 年，无排卵周期的发生率分别为 85%、59% 和 25%，并且人们发现这种现象与血清雄激素和 LH 水平高相关。大约 75% 的 PCOS 患者在青春期出现月经问题。因此，很难区分月经稀发是由 PCOS 引起的还是青春期生理性月经稀发。但 16 岁时仍没有月经来潮或在乳房发育后 2～3 年仍未出现月经，以及月经初潮后 2 年以上持续的月经稀发可能需要进行额外的评估。

（二）高雄激素血症

HA 是青少年中最常见的特征，因为正常的青春期变化与 PCOS 非常相似。单独出现多毛症和（或）痤疮不应被视为 PCOS HA 的临床证据，但严重的痤疮和多毛症可能是 PCOS 的迹象。几乎一半的青少年会出现 HA 相应的皮肤征象。如果临床或生化指标

异常，青少年应该评估是否有其他原因引发了 HA（方框 3.1）。此外，对青少年来说，没有标准化的分级系统，其生化 HA 的定义也会很模糊，因为缺乏青春期生理性发育过程中雄激素水平的临界值。

方框 3.1 青春期高雄激素血症的鉴别诊断	
• 肾上腺功能初现过强	• 肢端肥大症
• 迟发型先天性肾上腺皮质增生症	• 雄激素作用或代谢异常
• 雄性化瘤	• Hair-An 综合征（高雄激素血症、胰岛素抵抗、黑棘皮症）
• 库欣综合征	• 卵巢类固醇合成受阻
• 高催乳素血症	• 雄激素药物性高雄激素血症
• 性发育异常	• 癫痫（使用丙戊酸治疗）
• 糖皮质激素抵抗	• 特发性高雄激素血症

改编自：Oliveira A, Sampaio B, Teixeira A, Castro-Correia C, Fontoura M, Luís Medina J. Síndrome del ovario poliquístico: retos en la adolescencia. Endocrinol y Nutr. 2010; 57(7): 328–336.

（三）青春期多囊卵巢综合征患者中的生理性胰岛素抵抗和肥胖的叠加效应

与健康的成年人相比，健康青少年的 IR 和高胰岛素血症更为常见。这种青春期的 IR 状态通常是由生长激素增加引起的。

此外，与正常体重的女性相比，肥胖的女性在青春期具有较高的雄激素水平，这表明肥胖会加重 HA。

四、青春期多囊卵巢综合征的鉴别诊断

根据美国内分泌学会的观点，首先应该排除与 PCOS 相关的疾病，包括甲状腺功能减退症、高催乳素血症和非经典型先天性肾上腺皮质增生症。此外，根据青少年 PCOS 的表现，还应该排除其他诊断，如库欣综合征、妊娠、原发性卵巢功能不全、下丘脑性闭经、肾上腺肿瘤和肢端肥大症等。需明确 PCOS 是一种排除性诊断。在评估怀疑患有 PCOS 的青少年时，医师应注意其他可能存在的疾病，如高催乳素血症、甲状腺功能异常、高皮质醇血症和其他引起雄激素过多的疾病，如起源于附件或肾上腺的分泌雄激素的肿瘤，或先天性肾上腺皮质增生症（nonclassic congenital adrenal hyperplasia, NCCAH）。临床上，垂体和肾上腺疾病常常在初潮期出现，并且需要通过临床评估排除。在呈现 PCOS 症状的青少年女性中，筛查非经典型 NCCAH 非常重要。NCCAH 可能占高雄激素性无排卵育龄期女性的 1% ～ 4%。表 3.2 总结了青春期 PCOS 鉴别诊断中需考虑的因素。

表 3.2 青春期多囊卵巢综合征的鉴别诊断

异常表现	提示多囊卵巢综合征的症状和体征	参考文献
青春期生理性无排卵	生理性无排卵月经周期	2, 12
非经典型先天性肾上腺皮质增生症	高雄激素性无排卵、多毛症、阴蒂增大	15

续表

异常表现	提示多囊卵巢综合征的症状和体征	参考文献
甲状腺功能异常	月经不规律；甲状腺功能减退症也能导致卵巢多囊样改变，SHBG下降、毛发变粗会被认为是多毛症表现	12
催乳素过多	月经周期紊乱与乳溢	18
库欣综合征	紫纹、肥胖、水牛背，少数病例有多毛症表现，并且与高雄激素性无排卵相关	19
肢端肥大症	月经稀发、多毛症和IR状态	20
分泌雄激素的肿瘤/雄激素过多	男性化、雄激素性脱发、变声、阴蒂增大	21
妊娠	继发性闭经	22
卵巢功能不全或卵巢早衰	原发或继发的月经稀发/闭经	23

注：IR，胰岛素抵抗；PCOS，多囊卵巢综合征；SHBG，性激素结合球蛋白。

五、青春期多囊卵巢综合征的诊断

根据国际共识和PES指南，青少年PCOS的诊断仅取决于两个标准：
- 临床或生化的HA迹象。
- 稀发排卵/无排卵的功能障碍。

更多有关信息请参阅表3.3。如果青春期女性被诊断为PCOS是基于不明原因的持续性高雄激素性稀发排卵/无排卵症状，那这可能是不正确的。多达80%被诊断为PCOS的女性表现出高雄激素的生化特征。对于任何表现出月经不规律、多毛症、耐药性痤疮、脱发、黑棘皮症和雄激素升高的青少年女性，都应该考虑PCOS。对于被评估为肥胖的女性，应特别注意这些症状和体征。

表3.3　依据国际共识、指南制定的青春期多囊卵巢综合征诊断标准

症状名称	症状描述
1.异常子宫出血	a.对于特定年龄或者育龄女性来说异常的出血模式 b.症状持续1~2年
2.高雄激素血症表现	a.血清睾酮水平超过了正常成年人上限 b.中到重度的多毛症 c.中到重度的寻常痤疮

来源：Witchel S, F, Oberfield S, Rosenfield R, L, et al., The Diagnosis of Polycystic Ovary Syndrome during Adolescence. Horm Res Paediatr 2015; 83: 376-389. doi: 10.1159/000375530.

六、青春期多囊卵巢综合征的临床表现

（一）稀发排卵或无排卵的功能障碍

大约2/3的PCOS青少年存在月经症状，但稀发排卵/无排卵和月经周期不规律见于下丘脑-垂体-卵巢（hypothalamic-pituitary-ovarian，HPO）轴生理成熟的早期阶段。在月经初潮后的第一年，约85%的月经周期是稀发排卵/无排卵的，6年后降至25%。在初潮后的一年（妇科意义上的一年）内，约75%的青少年月经周期持续21~45天，预计95%的青少年在初潮后3~5年达到成人月经周期的持续时间（21~40天）。月

经周期不规律是稀发排卵/无排卵的特征，如果这种症状一直持续，表明为 PCOS。区分由 PCOS 引起的月经稀发和正常的 HPO 轴生理性不成熟引起的月经稀发是困难的，因此，月经周期持续超过或少于 19～90 天，15 岁前无月经或在乳房发育后 2～3 年无月经，以及月经初潮后持续月经稀发超过 2 年，都需要进一步评估。

至少有 5% 的青少年会发生异常排卵，表现为异常子宫出血模式（表 3.4）。

表 3.4 青春期多囊卵巢综合征患者异常子宫出血的类型

异常子宫出血的类型	月经不规律的定义
原发性闭经	青春期发育正常者到 15 岁无月经，或乳房发育后 3 年内无月经
继发性闭经	月经初潮后超过 3 个月未行经
月经稀发（较少出现异常子宫出血）	月经初潮后 1 年：平均月经周期超过 90 天（每年少于 4 个月经周期）。月经初潮后 2 年：平均月经周期超过 60 天（每年少于 6 个月经周期）。月经初潮后 3～5 年：平均月经周期超过 45 天（每年少于 8 个月经周期）。月经初潮后 6 年以上：平均月经周期超过 38 天（每年少于 9 个月经周期）
无排卵性异常子宫出血过多	月经周期短于 21 天（行经超过 7 天或每 1～2 小时就需要更换超过 1 片卫生巾或卫生棉条）

青少年女性通常因月经不规律、皮肤表现（如痤疮或多毛症）求医，因为这个时期在与同龄人面前保持外貌正常对她们来说至关重要。

表现为闭经、月经稀发或子宫出血异常等的月经失调往往是 PCOS 的首发临床症状。大量月经稀发青少年的生化标志与 PCOS 相符，并随着年龄增长最终发展成综合征的临床特征。

（二）高雄激素血症的临床表现

体格检查结果包括多毛症、痤疮、脱发、肥胖、IR 和黑棘皮症。

1. 多毛症

多毛症是在与雄激素相关的身体部位出现过度毛发生长（类似男性的终毛增生）的一种疾病，50%～76% 患有 PCOS 的青少年女性有多毛症。多毛症的确切病因尚不清楚，但据推测是多因素的。已知性毛和皮脂腺的发育依赖于雄激素。PCOS 是多毛症最常见的原因，并且通常在青春期前后出现。中度至重度多毛症是雄激素过多最可靠的临床证据。毛发生长通常见于面部（上唇和下巴）、乳晕周围、脐周和下腹部；可以使用改良 Ferriman-Gallwey（modified Ferriman-Gallwey，mFG）评分系统（图 3.1）对其进行评估，有助于指导对其进行合理的管理。评分为 6～8 分表示轻度多毛症，8～15 分表示中度多毛症，大于 15 分表示重度多毛症。患有多毛症的青少年女性通常具有更严重的代谢紊乱。

2. 痤疮

痤疮在青春期的女性中很常见，但当它与不断加重的月经失调同时出现时，提示存在 HA。HA 引起皮脂分泌增加，导致囊肿性痤疮和粉刺形成。在肾上腺功能初现时皮脂分泌增加，而PCOS女孩的痤疮则代表了一种严重的肾上腺功能异常。痤疮严重程度可以根据病变类型和数量分为轻度、中度或重度。20%～50%的PCOS青少年患有寻常痤疮，通常对传统的局部治疗不易产生反应。局部治疗对中到重度炎症性寻常痤疮（表3.5）不起作用是测试HA的指征。粉刺性痤疮在青少年女性中很常见，但在月经初潮期间，中度或重度的炎症性痤疮并不常见。

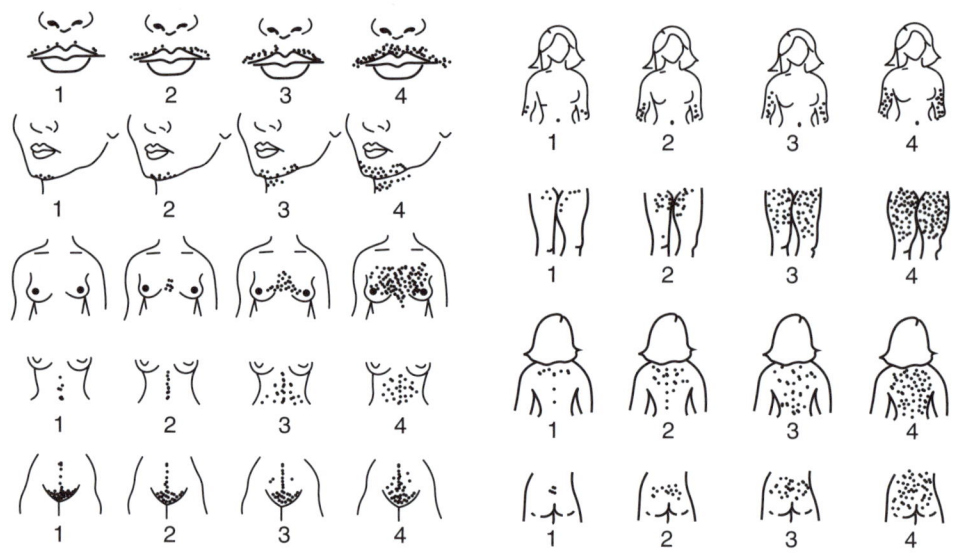

图3.1 面部和身体终毛的改良Ferriman-Gallwey（mFG）评分系统

来源：Ferriman, D., and Gallwey, J. D.: Clinical assessment of body hair growth in women, J. Clin. Endocrinol. Metab. 21: 1440. 1961 and Lorenzo, E. M.: Familial study of hirsutism, J. Clin. Endocrinol. Metab. 31: 556, 1970.

表3.5 青春期痤疮的评分

严重程度	粉刺性痤疮（分）	炎症性痤疮（分）
轻度	1～10	1～10
中度	11～25	11～25
重度	>25	>25

来源：Rosenfield RL. The diagnosis of polycystic ovary syndrome in adolescents. Pediatrics. 2015; 136(6): 1154–65.

3. 脱发

由HA引起的脱发类似于男性型脱发，常见于头顶、冠部、额部和颞部区域。脱发相对少见，在青少年中研究得不够充分。局部性痤疮和脱发不应作为青少年PCOS的诊断标准。

4. 黑棘皮症

黑棘皮症是高胰岛素血症和雄激素过多的皮肤表现，皮肤上会出现较粗糙的深色斑块，具有天鹅绒般的外观和质地，通常位于腋窝、颈部、背部、阴唇和腹股沟。由于继发于高胰岛素血症的表皮和真皮角化过度，色素沉着更常发生在深色皮肤人群中。

（三）肥胖与胰岛素抵抗

胰岛素抵抗、高胰岛素血症和肥胖虽然在患有 PCOS 的青少年女性中相对常见，但不能作为青少年 PCOS 的诊断标准。肥胖是 PCOS 的一个普遍特征，约 40%～60% 的 PCOS 患者存在肥胖。目前尚不清楚肥胖是 PCOS 的病因，还是肥胖增加了 PCOS 的患病风险；然而，肥胖或短期内体重迅速增加，是约 50% 的青春期 PCOS 患者的首发表现。肥胖还可能进一步加重 PCOS 相关的月经不规律。PCOS 中的高胰岛素血症似乎与向心性肥胖有关，与体重指数（BMI）无关，这种过度的脂肪含量进一步增加了脂肪沉积和胰岛素抵抗。过量的胰岛素促进了 LH 的分泌，并可能加重 LH 的失调。过量的胰岛素和 LH 反过来又导致雄激素产生增加、月经不规律的稀发排卵/无排卵、肥胖，并增加未来心血管代谢异常的风险。

代谢综合征是由于胰岛素抵抗与肥胖和年龄相互作用而导致的血糖异常、向心性（男性型）肥胖、高血压和血脂异常的组合。它在肥胖者中发生率最高，大约有 25% 的患有 PCOS 的青春期少女存在代谢综合征。代谢综合征的存在作为合并症，使得 PCOS 成为 2 型糖尿病早期发生、睡眠呼吸障碍的风险因素，并最终成为心血管疾病的威胁。

PCOS 中出现的胰岛素抵抗主要是胰岛素对糖代谢的影响。在 PCOS 中，其他胰岛素作用相对不受影响，结果导致了代偿性的胰岛素抵抗和高胰岛素血症。高胰岛素血症是雄激素过多的根本原因，因为胰岛素直接促进了 LH 的作用，间接提高了 GnRH 的水平，此外还降低了性激素结合球蛋白（SHBG）水平，而 SHBG 是控制睾酮水平的主要结合蛋白。由于 SHBG 减少，游离雄激素水平升高，进而导致痤疮、多毛症和脱发等雄激素过多的临床表现。胰岛素抵抗还可能导致血脂异常、黑棘皮症，并增加心血管疾病和糖尿病风险。代谢综合征和 PCOS 的临床特征通常相似，如胰岛素抵抗、肥胖、2 型糖尿病、高脂血症和高血压。这些症状不是 PCOS 诊断标准的一部分，在做出 PCOS 的最终诊断时不应考虑进去。但有大量证据表明 PCOS 是代谢综合征的危险因素。

国际上 PCOS 诊断和管理的循证指南强调识别和筛查 PCOS 导致的代谢异常。肥胖和（或）胰岛素抵抗的迹象，以及黑棘皮症的存在，应促使医师考虑 PCOS 及代谢综合征相关合并症的可能性。

七、青春期多囊卵巢综合征患者的生活质量

PCOS 患者所面临的心理健康问题与健康相关生活质量（health-related quality of life, HRQoL）下降有关。越来越多的证据表明，在患有 PCOS 的青少年女性中，多毛症、痤疮、脱发等皮肤表现，以及 HRQoL 下降常致使患者出现多种心理合并症，如焦虑症、进食障碍、抑郁症，同时还会导致患者产生不良的身体形象认知。高胰岛素血症、HA 和肥胖也加剧了这种关联。因此心理压力筛查应包含在被诊断为 PCOS 的青少年中。

八、青春期多囊卵巢综合征的诊断方法

诊断青春期 PCOS 非常具有挑战性,因为基于证据支持的国际指南中的诊断标准与生理性的青春期发育相似。出现月经问题(包括月经稀发/闭经)的青春期女性需要适当的筛查和意识教育,以及适当的医疗干预,以改善其生殖健康和 HRQoL。一种有效的诊断方法是识别具有临床特征的女性,对其进行筛查、生化和影像检查以利于诊断。对于有中重度痤疮和多毛症,特别是进展迅速的病例,以及伴有黑棘皮症、月经不规律和向心性肥胖的青春期女性,需要进一步评估。

针对青春期女性,建议采用分步诊断方法。在做出 PCOS 诊断之前,详细的病史询问和体格检查对识别雄激素过多的潜在原因必不可少。病史应包括 HA 的发生时间和持续时间、详细的月经史(初潮、闭经和月经稀发)、类固醇/雄激素类药物暴露史(宫内或外源)及药物(抗癫痫或精神疾病)使用史,因为一些药物可能会导致类似 PCOS 的临床特征。应检查家族史是否有 PCOS、糖尿病、甲状腺疾病或早发的心血管疾病。许多青少年女性可能使用药物治疗痤疮,而导致 PCOS 的一些特征消失或被掩盖。

体格检查应包括对体毛分布、脱发或头发稀疏、痤疮、阴蒂及卵巢是否增大进行评估。应寻找胰岛素抵抗的征象,如黑棘皮症、向心性肥胖和高血压。

(一)生化高雄激素血症的实验室检测

生化检测有助于诊断 PCOS 并排除 HA 和月经不规律的其他原因。具有高雄激素迹象和症状的青春期女性是评估 HA 的适宜人群。HA 的初始内分泌评估包括总睾酮、游离睾酮、SHBG、硫酸脱氢表雄酮(dehydroepiandrosterone sulfate,DHEAS)和清晨 17- 羟孕酮(17-hydroxyprogesterone,17-OHP)水平。肾上腺或卵巢分泌肿瘤患者血液中的 DHEAS 水平会显著升高,但在患有 PCOS 的个体中,DHEAS 仅轻度升高(20%~30%)。血清总睾酮水平在有分泌性肿瘤的患者中也会显著升高。用于测量睾酮的商用试剂盒对于 PCOS 患者的低睾酮水平并不敏感。液相色谱-串联质谱法是所有类固醇测量的金标准,但价格昂贵且普及率较低。循环中的睾酮与 SHBG 结合;因此,SHBG 浓度是调节游离睾酮水平的主要因素。游离睾酮的测定缺乏标准,尤其是在儿童人群中的测定经常不可靠。游离睾酮或游离雄激素指数可以通过总睾酮和 SHBG 浓度计算得出。睾酮水平在青春期开始上升,并在几年后达到峰值水平。没有绝对的睾酮切割值可以诊断 HA。促性腺激素测定不用于 PCOS 的诊断。LH∶FSH 升高常见于 PCOS,但不具有诊断性。

抗米勒管激素(anti-Müllerian hormone,AMH)与睾酮水平相关。与正常排卵的青春期女性相比,PCOS 患者的 AMH 水平升高,但对于使用 AMH 水平诊断 PCOS 尚无统一标准,主要是因为分析前和分析过程中存在一些问题。

通常情况下,下列生化检测(表 3.6)应作为疑似青春期 PCOS 检查的一部分,并且应排除其他已存在的病理因素和其他可能与 PCOS 重叠的 HA 原因。

表 3.6 青春期多囊卵巢综合征患者的生化评估

评估项目	诊断依据
雌二醇	卵巢功能
17-OHP	怀疑 NCCAH
FSH	PCOS 患者中正常至升高 原发性性腺功能减退症（这是原发性闭经的一种病因）中处于偏高水平
LH	PCOS 患者中升高 低促性腺激素性性腺功能减退症中较低
催乳素	如怀疑存在垂体肿瘤或垂体肿物
睾酮	雄激素过多
DHEAS	分泌雄激素的肿瘤
促甲状腺激素	甲状腺功能异常
空腹血脂	血脂异常
2 小时 OGTT	胰岛素抵抗与 2 型糖尿病
血清与尿皮质醇	库欣综合征

注：17-OHP，17-羟孕酮；DHEAS，硫酸脱氢表雄酮；FSH，卵泡刺激素；LH，黄体生成素；NCCAH，非经典型先天性肾上腺皮质增生症；OGTT，口服葡萄糖耐量试验；PCOS，多囊卵巢综合征。

尽管 NCCAH 仅占高雄激素性无排卵的 5%，但所有指南都支持对其进行筛查，因为该疾病与 PCOS 非常相似。推荐筛查甲状腺功能，因为甲状腺功能异常可能导致月经不规律和头发粗糙（与多毛症不同）。据报道，高催乳素血症在患有 PCOS 的年轻女性中的发生率高达 14%～16%。PCOS 患者出现的多毛症和向心性肥胖/躯干肥胖可能会让人怀疑库欣综合征的诊断，但其他特征还是有很多不同。

由于昼夜变化，17-羟孕酮随机值不能完全排除 NCCAH，应测量并分析清晨的 17-羟孕酮水平。应该在 PCOS 患者中进行 2 型糖尿病和代谢综合征的评估，尤其是那些肥胖并具有家族风险因素的青春期患者。

（二）超声检查

在成人中，经典的多囊卵巢形态（polycystic ovary morphology，PCOM）超声定义为卵巢具有增厚的囊壁、较大的体积（体积 > 10 cm³），以及多个小卵泡或至少一个卵巢中有 12 个或更多的直径为 2～9 mm 的窦状卵泡。然而在青春期女性，尤其是月经初潮后不满 8 年的女性中，很少需要进行盆腔超声检查以诊断 PCOM。这些标准在年轻女性中不确定且存在问题，因为在月经初潮前后通常会看到具有多个卵泡的卵巢，如果将 PCOM 用作 PCOS 诊断的标准，约有 50% 的青春期女性会符合这些标准，从而导致这些年轻女性被错误地诊断为 PCOS。如果临床结果表明存在雄性化瘤，患者出现如多毛症快速发展、盆腔包块、阴蒂增大、总睾酮水平大于 200 ng/dL 或性发育障碍等特征，则应进行超声检查。美国内分泌学会指南也反对在青春期女性中将 PCOM 作为 PCOS 诊断标准。

在月经初潮后不满 8 年的青春期女性中使用盆腔超声作为诊断方法会过度诊断 PCOS。建议将月经初潮后满 8 年作为截止年龄,因为卵巢体积在 20 岁时达到最大值。

九、青春期多囊卵巢综合征的治疗方案

到目前为止,尚无能够完全治愈 PCOS 的特定药物,但有药物可用于治疗与 PCOS 相关的临床症状。每位 PCOS 年轻女性患者的治疗策略因其临床表现和潜在病因不同而存在差异。治疗的两个主题包括控制 HA 症状(多毛症、痤疮、月经不规律和不孕症),以及改善和预防 PCOS 患者长期存在的合并症(代谢综合征、心血管异常、2 型糖尿病、血脂异常,以及情绪和自尊心问题)。治疗应考虑青少年女性的感受,这对患者长期配合治疗至关重要。可选的治疗方法包括生活方式干预、复方口服避孕药(combined oral contraceptive,COC)、抗雄激素类药、胰岛素增敏剂、减重术和局部美容治疗(表 3.7)。

表 3.7 青春期多囊卵巢综合征的治疗方案

症状	治疗方案
高雄激素血症	一线治疗药物是 COC
	美容治疗(激光、脱毛、电解);依氟鸟氨酸外用乳膏
	联合治疗:螺内酯与 COC 可改善中到重度的多毛症
痤疮	COC
	局部抗生素、维 A 酸和水杨酸
	全身多发的痤疮应系统性使用抗生素和异维 A 酸
月经稀发/闭经	生活方式干预:减重 5%~10%,健康饮食。可以降低雄激素水平、减轻 IR 和降低心血管疾病风险
	COC 使 LH 下降、减少雄激素合成,从而使睾酮水平下降并提高多毛症评分;也可周期性使用孕酮
	二甲双胍:改善排卵,规律月经周期
代谢综合征	减重是改善胰岛素抵抗和高雄激素血症的关键,同时也可以降低心血管疾病风险和抑制卵巢分泌雄激素,从而降低代谢综合征和 2 型糖尿病风险
	用二甲双胍治疗胰岛素抵抗相关症状

来源:Ibáñez L, Oberfield SE, Witchel S, et al. An international consortium update: pathophysiology, diagnosis, and treatment of polycystic ovarian syndrome in adolescence. *Horm Res Paediatr*. 2017; 88(6): 371–395; Fitzgerald S, Divasta A, Gooding H. An update on PCOS in adolescents. *Curr Opin Pediatr*. 2018; 30(4): 459–465; and Teede HJ, Misso ML, Costello MF, et al. Recommendations from the international evidence-based guideline for the assessment and management of polycystic ovary syndrome. Hum Reprod. 2018; 33(9): 1602–1618.

注:COC,复方口服避孕药;IR,胰岛素抵抗;LH,黄体生成素;PCOS,多囊卵巢综合征。

(一)生活方式干预

生活方式干预是治疗 PCOS 首要的而又简单的方法,因为 PCOS 是一种长期慢性疾病,且伴随 2 型糖尿病等其他并发症。研究发现,肥胖的 PCOS 患者中多毛症和排卵功能障碍的发生率更高、症状更严重。在青少年中进行的随机对照试验表明,包括均衡饮食和锻炼在内的生活方式干预对降低体重、减轻胰岛素抵抗、降低睾酮水平、规律月

经周期、减少睾酮量（伴随着 SHBG 数量的增加），以及降低多毛症评分（mFGS）均有积极影响。肥胖的青少年女性在 6 个月内仅减轻 5%～10% 的体重就可以显示出良好效果。然而，长期进行生活方式干预对青少年来说具有挑战性，并且存在可能回到之前的生活状态和停止改变生活习惯的较高风险。家庭支持对于确保这些干预措施的可持续性是至关重要的。

（二）复方口服避孕药

COC 含有雌激素和孕酮，是青春期 PCOS 患者的一线治疗方案。这种药物不仅可以控制高雄激素症状，还可以使月经周期规律。COC 中的雌激素成分提高了 SHBG 水平，降低了游离雄激素水平。COC 中的孕激素抑制了 LH 的分泌，从而通过抑制垂体和卵巢的反馈来减少雄激素的分泌。COC 的这种降雄激素作用对治疗高雄激素的临床表现（如多毛症和痤疮）非常有效。像屈螺酮这样的新型孕激素具有更强的孕激素作用和较弱的抗雄激素作用，可用于治疗 PCOS。COC 的最佳组合和治疗时间仍存在争议。与这类药物相关的主要不良反应包括心脏代谢指标的恶化、甘油三酯水平升高、胰岛素敏感性降低，以及血栓栓塞事件风险增加。屈螺酮导致静脉血栓形成的风险较高，可能不适用于病态性肥胖的女性。建议使用最低有效日剂量的雌激素（20～30 μg 炔雌醇或其等效物）或天然雌激素类似物——共轭马雌激素。应根据患者的风险等级选择性使用 COC，并且如果有任何禁忌证，应立即停止使用。

（三）抗雄激素类药

雄激素受体拮抗剂，如螺内酯、氟他胺或第三代孕激素（醋酸环丙孕酮），以及 5α- 还原酶抑制剂，如非那雄胺，是用于治疗多毛症的抗雄激素类药。螺内酯是一种醛固酮拮抗剂，常用剂量为 25 mg/d，最大剂量可增加至 200 mg/d。螺内酯的一些副作用包括乳房胀痛、经间期出血和脱发。氟他胺由于在大剂量（大于 250 mg/d）使用时具有肝毒性而没有被广泛使用，但 1 mg/（kg·d）的低剂量长期使用并不具有肝毒性，而且与螺内酯疗效相似。它与二甲双胍联合使用可减轻其肝毒性，并相较于二甲双胍单药疗法能够显著减轻多毛症。抗雄激素类药与复方口服避孕药或二甲双胍联合使用时疗效显著。对于青春期性活跃的女性，应避免使用抗雄激素药物治疗，以防止妊娠后对男性胎儿产生女性化影响。醋酸环丙孕酮具有强效的抗雄激素和孕激素活性，常与炔雌醇联合使用治疗痤疮和多毛症。非那雄胺是一种 5α- 还原酶抑制剂，可降低多毛症评分，但由于其具有致畸作用，使用受到限制。

（四）胰岛素增敏剂

这类药物用于治疗与 PCO 相关的代谢并发症，因为它们可以通过降低胰岛素抵抗和使胰岛素水平恢复正常来发挥作用。当胰岛素抵抗减少时，雄激素水平降低，从而使月经周期规律。

1. 二甲双胍

二甲双胍是最常用的胰岛素增敏剂，用于改善 IR 和高胰岛素血症，从而降低 PCOS 患者的雄激素水平。二甲双胍联合生活方式干预时，可改善代谢指标，尤其是可以通过增加外周组织对葡萄糖的摄取与利用、减少肝脏葡萄糖生成、降低 BMI 和皮下与内脏脂肪堆积，进而提高胰岛素敏感性和糖耐量，并缓解无排卵性月经失调。研究表明，二甲双胍可改善肥胖或非肥胖 PCOS 青少年的糖耐量异常及其他代谢综合征相关表现。18%～24% 的 PCOS 青少年患者存在糖代谢异常。二甲双胍治疗亦能改善月经不规律。对于存在 COC 禁忌证的女性，二甲双胍是理想的替代选择。但是，它没有直接抗雄激素作用，对多毛症或痤疮的改善效果有限。

目前，除剂量依赖性的胃肠道不适外，尚无二甲双胍导致严重副作用的报道。国际共识指南建议，对明确诊断为 PCOS 或已出现 PCOS 症状的青少年，可在生活方式干预的基础上联合使用二甲双胍。

此外，二甲双胍对预防长期 PCOS 相关合并症（如子宫内膜癌、2 型糖尿病、心血管疾病和高血压）具有积极作用。

2. 噻唑烷二酮类药物

噻唑烷二酮类药物（thiazolidinediones，TZD）通常被称为"格列酮"，包括罗格列酮和吡格列酮。TZD 降低了 11β-HSD 酶的活性，该酶负责将无活性的皮质酮转化为有活性的皮质醇。它们被认为是 PCOS 患者的二线治疗药物，在二甲双胍之后用于改善胰岛素抵抗。TZD 可以提高 SHBG 水平并减少过量的雄激素。二甲双胍和 TZD 在增加排卵、减少胰岛素抵抗和规律月经周期方面的疗效相当，但在青春期患者中使用的相关研究较少。

3. 联合治疗

生活方式干预是所有 PCOS 患者的一线治疗，特别是那些超重或肥胖的患者。在 BMI > 25 kg/m^2 的 PCOS 患者中，当服用 COC 和生活方式干预不能达到预期目标时，可以考虑使用 COC 和二甲双胍的联合治疗。在经过 6 个月的 COC 和美容治疗无效后，也可以考虑将抗雄激素类药与 COC 联合使用，以治疗 PCOS 患者严重的多毛症。与 COC 相比，低剂量的二甲双胍、氟他胺和吡格列酮的三联药物组合对青春期 PCOS 患者的雄激素水平没有改善作用，但改善了血脂水平、颈动脉内膜中层厚度和身体成分参数。

（五）减肥治疗（减重术）

减肥药物未被批准用于儿童和青少年。为改善 PCOS 和不孕症而行减重术也暂不予考虑。

（六）避孕

每 10 名月经稀发的女性中就有 1 名可以自发排卵，因此，建议性活跃的青少年女性遵循一般的避孕原则。对于 PCOS 的青少年患者，没有特定的避孕方法/药物推荐。

（七）皮肤症状的管理

美容方面的问题可以通过短期和长期疗法来解决。多毛症可以通过短期的物理方法（如化学脱毛、拔毛和蜡脱毛）和长期的方法（如电解和激光治疗）来处理。此外，可以使用 13.9% 的依氟鸟氨酸溶液来减少面部毛发生长，但只有短期效果，且需要每天使用。

十、总结

由于 PCOS 会降低青春期女性的 HRQoL，它已逐渐成为青少年生殖健康中的重要问题。由于在青少年中诊断 PCOS 具有挑战性，专家建议为青少年设计不同的诊断标准。由于将早期青春期女性诊断为 PCOS 会对代谢、心血管、心理健康和生殖健康产生长期影响，因此，建议至少在月经来潮 2 年后再进行 PCOS 诊断。不管他们是否被诊断为 PCOS，针对这些患者的治疗均包含生活方式干预。对于超重和肥胖的青少年，建议采用限制热量摄入和运动等减重策略。青少年 PCOS 的药物治疗仍然存在争议，但应该在具有合并症风险、确诊 PCOS 或对其他治疗抵抗的病例中使用。

参考文献

1. Çelebier M, Kaplan O, Özel Ş, Engin-Üstün Y. Polycystic ovary syndrome in adolescents: Q-TOF LC/MS analysis of human plasma metabolome. J Pharm Biomed Anal. 2020;191:113543.
2. Legro RS, Arslanian SA, Ehrmann DA, et al. Diagnosis and treatment of polycystic ovary syndrome: an Endocrine Society clinical practice guideline. J Clin Endocrinol Metab. 2013;98(12):4565-4592.
3. Nicandri KF, Hoeger K. Diagnosis and treatment of polycystic ovarian syndrome in adolescents. Curr Opin Endocrinol Diabetes Obes. 2012;19(6):497-504.
4. Akgül S, Bonny AE. Metabolic syndrome in adolescents with polycystic ovary syndrome: prevalence on the basis of different diagnostic criteria. J Pediatr Adolesc Gynecol. 2019;32(4):383-387.
5. Akgül S, Düzçeker Y, Kanbur N, Derman O. Do different diagnostic criteria impact polycystic ovary syndrome diagnosis for adolescents? J Pediatr Adolesc Gynecol. 2018;31(3):258-262.
6. Oliveira A, Sampaio B, Teixeira A, Castro-Correia C, Fontoura M, Luís Medina J. Síndrome del ovario poliquístico: retos en la adolescencia. Endocrinol y Nutr. 2010;57(7):328-336.
7. Dabadghao P. Polycystic ovary syndrome in adolescents. Best Pract Res Clin Endocrinol Metab. 2019;33(3):101272. Available at: https://doi.org/10.1016/j.beem.2019.04.006.
8. Shayya R, Chang RJ. Reproductive endocrinology of adolescent polycystic ovary syndrome. BJOG. 2010;117(2):150-155.
9. Patel K, Coffler MS, Dahan MH, Malcom PJ, Deutsch R, Chang RJ. Relationship of GnRH-stimulated LH release to episodic LH secretion and baseline endocrine-metabolic measures in women with polycystic ovary syndrome. Clin Endocrinol (Oxf). 2004;60:67-74.
10. Rothenberg SS, Beverley R, Barnard E, Baradaran-Shoraka M, Sanfilippo JS. Polycystic ovary syndrome in adolescents. Best Pract Res Clin Obstet Gynaecol. 2018;48:103-114.

11. Roe AH, Prochaska E, Smith M, Sammel M, Dokras A. Using the androgen excess-PCOS society criteria to diagnose polycystic ovary syndrome and the risk of metabolic syndrome in adolescents. J Pediatr. 2013;162(5):937-941. Available at: http://dx.doi.org/10.1016/j.jpeds.2012.11.019.
12. Rosenfield RL. The diagnosis of polycystic ovary syndrome in adolescents. Pediatrics. 2015;136(6):1154-1165.
13. Rosner W, Auchus RJ, Azziz R, Sluss PM, Raff H. Position statement: utility, limitations, and pitfalls in measuring testosterone: an Endocrine Society position statement. J Clin Endocrinol Metab. 2007;92(2):405-413.
14. Dewailly D, Lujan ME, Carmina E, et al. Definition and significance of polycystic ovarian morphology: a task force report from the Androgen Excess and Polycystic Ovary Syndrome Society. Hum Reprod Update. 2014;20(3):334-352.
15. Rosenfield RL. The diagnosis of polycystic ovary syndrome in adolescents. Pediatrics. 2015;136(6):1154-1165.
16. Kamboj MK, Bonny AE. Polycystic ovary syndrome in adolescence: diagnostic and therapeutic strategies. Transl Pediatr. 2017;6(4):248-255.
17. Hachey LM, Kroger-Jarvis M, Pavlik-Maus T, Leach R. Clinical implications of polycystic ovary syndrome in adolescents. Nurs Womens Health. 2020;24(2):115-126. Available at: https://doi.org/10.1016/j.nwh.2020.01.011.
18. Melmed S, Casanueva FF, Hoffman AR, et al. Diagnosis and treatment of hyperprolactinemia: an Endocrine Society clinical practice guideline method of development of evidence-based clinical practice guidelines. J Clin Endocrinol Metab. 2011;96:273-288.
19. Kaltsas GA, Korbonits M, Isidori AM, et al. How common are polycystic ovaries and the polycystic ovarian syndrome in women with Cushing's syndrome? Clin Endocrinol. 2000;53(4):493-500.
20. Melmed S, Colao A, Barkan A, et al. Guidelines for acromegaly management: an update. J Clin Endocrinol Metab. 2009;94(5):1509-1517.
21. Carmina E, Rosato F, Jannı, A, Rizzo JM, Longo RA. Extensive clinical experience relative prevalence of different androgen excess disorders in 950 women referred because of clinical hyperandrogenism. J Clin Endocrinol Metab. 2006;91(1):2-6.
22. Klein DA, Poth MA. Amenorrhea: an approach to diagnosis and management. Am Fam Physician. 2013;87(11):781-788.
23. Peña AS, Witchel SF, Hoeger KM, et al. Adolescent polycystic ovary syndrome according to the international evidence-based guideline. BMC Med. 2020;18(1):1-16.
24. Trent M, Gordon CM. Diagnosis and management of polycystic ovary syndrome in adolescents. Pediatrics. 2020;145(suppl 2):S210-S218.
25. Nicolaides NC, Matheou A, Vlachou F, Neocleous V, Skordis N. Polycystic ovarian syndrome in adolescents: from diagnostic criteria to therapeutic management. Acta Biomed. 2020;91(3):1-13.
26. Legro RS. Ovulation induction in polycystic ovary syndrome: current options. Best Pract Res Clin Obstet Gynaecol. 2016;37:152-159. Available at: http://dx.doi.org/10.1016/j.bpobgyn.2016.08.001.
27. Ibáñez L, Oberfield SE, Witchel S, et al. An international consortium update: pathophysiology, diagnosis, and treatment of polycystic ovarian syndrome in adolescence. Horm Res Paediatr. 2017;88(6):371-395.
28. Rosenfield RL, Ehrmann DA. The Pathogenesis of Polycystic Ovary Syndrome (PCOS): the hypothesis of PCOS as functional ovarian hyperandrogenism revisited. Endocr Rev. 2016;37(5):467-520.
29. Lizneva D, Gavrilova-Jordan L, Walker W, Azziz R. Androgen excess: investigations and management. Best Pract Res Clin Obstet Gynaecol. 2016;37:98-118. Available at: http://dx.doi.org/10.1016/j.bpobgyn.2016.05.003.
30. Mihailidis J, Dermesropian R, Taxel P, Luthra P, Grant-Kels JM. Endocrine evaluation of hirsutism. Int J Women's Dermatology. 2017;3(1):S6-S10. Available at: http://dx.doi.org/10.1016/j.ijwd.2017.02.007.
31. Escobar-Morreale HF, Carmina E, Dewailly D, et al. Epidemiology, diagnosis and management of hirsutism: a consensus statement by the androgen excess and polycystic ovary syndrome society. Hum Reprod Update. 2012;18(2):146-170.
32. Fitzgerald S, Divasta A, Gooding H. An update on PCOS in adolescents. Curr Opin Pediatr. 2018;30(4):459-465.

33. Muscogiuri G, Colao A, Orio F. Insulin-mediated diseases: adrenal mass and polycystic ovary syndrome. Trends Endocrinol Metab. 2015;26(10):512-514. Available at: http://dx.doi.org/10.1016/j.tem.2015.07.010.
34. Witchel SF, Burghard AC, Tao RH, Oberfield SE. The diagnosis and treatment of PCOS in adolescents: an update. Curr Opin Pediatr. 2019;31(4):562-569.
35. Bulsara J, Patel P, Soni A, Acharya S. A review: brief insight into Polycystic Ovarian syndrome. Endocr Metab Sci. 2021;3:100085.
36. Diamanti-Kandarakis E, Dunaif A. Insulin resistance and the polycystic ovary syndrome revisited: an update on mechanisms and implications. Endocr Rev. 2012;33(6):981-1030.
37. Eek D, Paty J, Black P, Celeste Elash C, Reaney M. A comprehensive disease model of Polycystic Ovary Syndrome (PCOS). Value Heal. 2015;18(7):A722.
38. Jain P, Jain S, Singh A, Goel S. Pattern of dermatologic manifestations in polycystic ovarian disease cases from a tertiary care hospital. Int J Adv Med. 2018;5(1):197.
39. Dokras A, Sarwer DB, Allison KC, et al. Weight loss and lowering androgens predict improvements in health-related quality of life in women with PCOS. J Clin Endocrinol Metab. 2016;101(8):2966-2974.
40. Teede H, Misso M, Costello M, et al. International Evidence-Based Guideline for the Assessment and Management of Polycystic Ovary Syndrome 2018. Monash University, Melbourne Australia: National Health and Medical Research Council (NHMRC); 2018:1-198.
41. Conway G, Dewailly D, Diamanti-Kandarakis E, et al. The polycystic ovary syndrome: a position statement from the European Society of Endocrinology. Eur J Endocrinol. 2014;171(4):P1-P29.
42. Rocha AL, Oliveira FR, Azevedo RC, et al. Recent advances in the understanding and management of polycystic ovary syndrome[version 1; peer review: 3 approved]. F1000Res. 2019;8(565):1-11.
43. Guleken Z, Bulut H, Bulut B, Depciuch J. Assessment of the effect of endocrine abnormalities on biomacromolecules and lipids by FT-IR and biochemical assays as biomarker of metabolites in early polycystic ovary syndrome women. J Pharm Biomed Anal. 2021;204:114250. Available at: https://doi.org/10.1016/j.jpba.2021.114250.
44. Legro RS, Arslanian SA, Ehrmann DA, et al. Diagnosis and treatment of polycystic ovary syndrome: an Endocrine Society clinical practice guideline. J Clin Endocrinol Metab. 2013;98(12):4565-4592.
45. Teede HJ, Misso ML, Costello MF, et al. Recommendations from the international evidence-based guideline for the assessment and management of polycystic ovary syndrome. Hum Reprod. 2018;33(9):1602-1618.
46. Peña AS, Witchel SF, Hoeger KM, et al. Adolescent polycystic ovary syndrome according to the international evidence-based guideline. BMC Med. 2020;18(1):1-16.
47. Hoeger K, Davidson K, Kochman L, Cherry T, Kopin L, Guzick DS. The impact of Metformin, oral contraceptives, and lifestyle modification on polycystic ovary syndrome in obese adolescent women in two randomized, placebo-controlled clinical trials. J Clin Endocrinol Metab. 2008;93(11):4299-4306.
48. Kavitha VJ, Devi MG, Puvaneswari N Clinical presentation, risk assessment and management of Polycystic Ovary Syndrome [PCOS]. International Journal of Biomedical and Advance Research. 2017;8(3):66-71.
49. Sebastian MR, Wiemann CM, Bacha F, Alston Taylor SJ. Diagnostic evaluation, comorbidity screening, and treatment of polycystic ovary syndrome in adolescents in 3 specialty clinics. J Pediatr Adolesc Gynecol. 2018;31(4):367-371. Available at: https://doi.org/10.1016/j.jpag.2018.01.007.
50. Dokras A, Feldman Witchel S. Are young adult women with polycystic ovary syndrome slipping through the healthcare cracks? J Clin Endocrinol Metab. 2014;99(5):1583-1585.

第二篇 多囊卵巢综合征的发病机制和临床表现

第四章 多囊卵巢综合征的病理生理学

一、引言

多囊卵巢综合征（PCOS）是由多种病因导致育龄期女性内分泌紊乱的一种疾病，广义的定义为满足以下3种条件中的2种即可诊断：稀发排卵或无排卵、多囊卵巢和高雄激素血症（HA）。目前普遍认为这是一种排除性诊断，PCOS仍然是导致育龄期女性无排卵相关不孕症的主要原因，估计高达20%的育龄女性受到了PCOS的影响。由于PCOS具有复杂的病理生理学，不仅涉及激素异常之间的相互作用，还涉及遗传因素、后天因素和环境因素，PCOS往往表现为从轻症到重症的一系列疾病。

二、激素异常

（一）雄激素过多

HA是PCOS的典型特征，可以导致多种临床表现。在生理状态下，育龄女性的卵巢和肾上腺各自分泌相同量的雄激素（主要是雄烯二酮和睾酮）；而在PCOS的患者中，由于功能失调，卵巢（在某些情况下为肾上腺）在类固醇合成过程中会产生更多的雄激素（图4.1）。

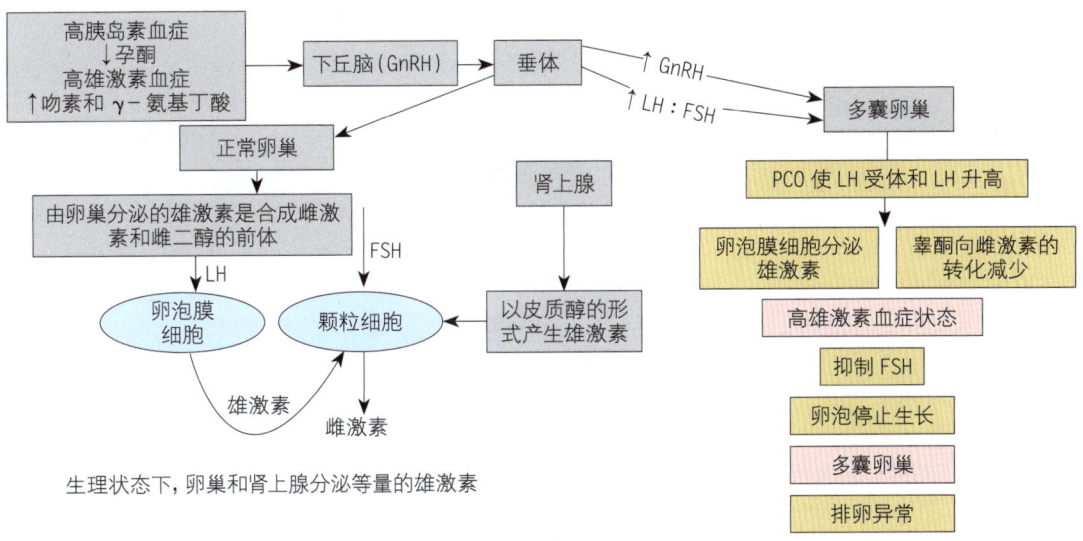

FSH，卵泡刺激素；GnRH，促性腺激素释放激素；LH，黄体生成素；PCO，多囊卵巢。

图4.1　多囊卵巢综合征的激素异常（雄激素过多）

1. 功能性卵巢高雄激素血症

卵泡膜细胞是卵巢分泌雄激素的主要来源，它主要分泌雄烯二酮（图4.1）。雄烯二酮在卵泡膜细胞中可以被直接转化为睾酮，也有可能分泌至血液中并在周围组织中被转化。PCOS患者的HA是由内因和外因双向驱动的。在PCOS患者中，卵泡膜细胞中CYP17A1和CYP11A酶高表达而颗粒细胞中的CYP19低表达。

CYP17A1是卵泡膜细胞中生物合成的限速酶。这个酶是以17α-羟化酶和17,20-裂解酶发挥作用，其中孕烯醇酮在这两个酶的作用下生成了脱氢雄酮，孕酮生成了雄烯二酮。Rosenfield等发现在PCOS患者的卵泡膜细胞中CYP17A1过表达，因此导致了雄激素产生过多。卵泡膜细胞经过长期的体外培养也会出现CYP17A1表达增加，因此也表明卵巢内存在失调的机制。CYP11A/P450scc表达上调可以使胆固醇生成更多的孕烯醇酮，然而，颗粒细胞中CYP19表达下调导致睾酮转化为雌激素的量下降，从而产生了HA（图4.2）。

不断有证据表明，类固醇生物合成过程失调可能引起功能性卵巢HA，可能影响到胎儿。已证实恒河猴和母羊在宫内时高雄激素暴露会发生一系列不可逆事件，如在青春期和成年时期出现无排卵和卵巢HA。妊娠期间，一定水平的性激素结合球蛋白（SHBG）和胎盘内源性芳香化酶活性可保护胎儿免受母体雄激素的伤害。导致胎儿雄激素暴露增加的可能机制有：母亲患有先天性肾上腺皮质增生症，基因表达差异导致SHBG和（或）芳香化酶水平降低，或者是母体高胰岛素血症抑制了芳香化酶活性和（或）SHBG的分泌。

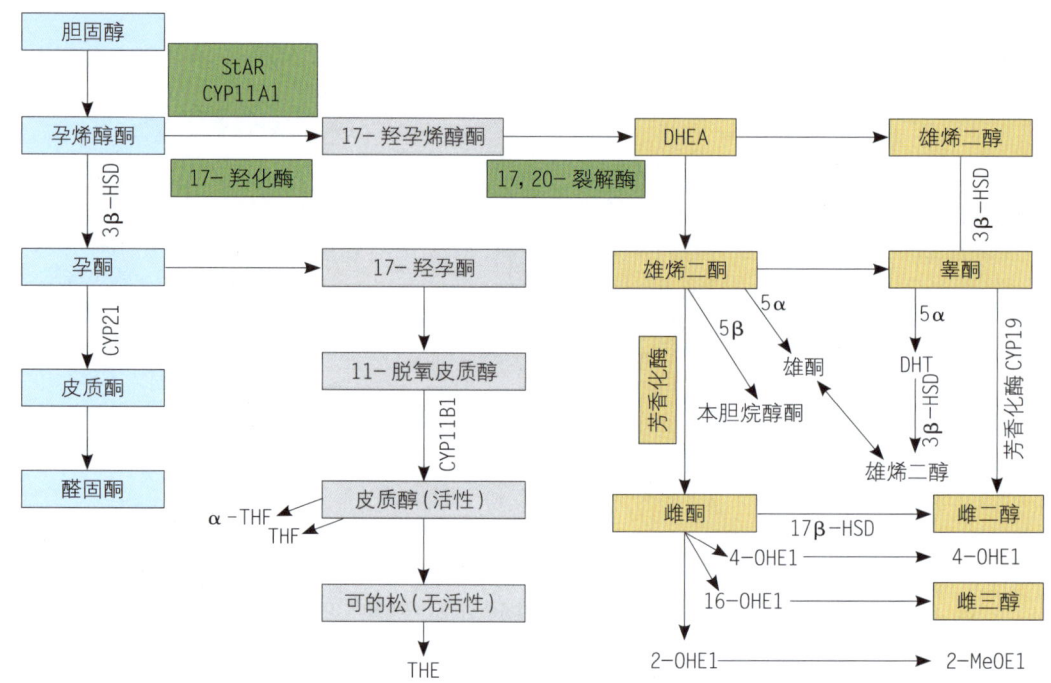

3β-HSD，3β-羟基类固醇脱氢酶；CYP11B1，11β-羟化酶；α-THF，α-四氢呋喃；THF，四氢呋喃；THE，四氢可的松；DHEA，脱氢表雄酮；DHT，双氢睾酮；17β-HSD，17β-羟基类固醇脱氢酶；4-OHE1，4-羟基雌酮；4-MeOE1，4-甲氧基雌酮；16-OHE1，16-羟基雌酮；2-OHE1，2-羟基雌酮；2-MeOE1，2-甲氧基雌酮。

图 4.2　类固醇生物合成途径

2. 下丘脑－垂体－卵巢轴失调

正如上述内容所强调的，尽管卵巢自身的因素可以导致 HA，一些外在的因素，如下丘脑－垂体－卵巢（HPO）轴调节失调，同样也可以导致 HA。下丘脑的促性腺激素释放激素（GnRH）呈脉冲样释放进入正中隆起的门脉系统，促使垂体促性腺激素（包括 FSH 和 LH）的释放。FSH 和 LH 都对调节卵巢功能至关重要。FSH 主要刺激卵泡发育，同时也可以促进颗粒细胞中的雄激素转化为雌激素。此外，LH 是产生雄激素和排卵的关键刺激因素，而且在黄体期促进孕酮的产生。在月经周期的每个阶段，FSH 和 LH 的水平仍然受到 GnRH 脉冲振幅和频率变化的严格控制。

在 PCOS 患者中，LH 和 FSH 水平有明显的异常，LH 水平显著升高，FSH 水平显著降低，导致大多数女性的 LH：FSH 增加。LH 上游的 GnRH 脉冲频率增加使得 LH 脉冲的频率和振幅增加，似乎是造成这一现象的原因。虽然这种频率变化背后的潜在机制尚不清楚，但也有人提出了以下几种机制：

- 高胰岛素血症增强了垂体对 GnRH 和内在 GnRH 神经元活动的反应。
- PCOS 患者由于无排卵，孕酮水平降低，破坏了 GnRH 的负反馈回路，导致 GnRH 分泌增加。

- HA 直接破坏了孕酮和雌激素对 GnRH/LH 产生的负反馈回路。

HPO 轴的功能障碍可以通过下丘脑水平的神经内分泌生理学改变来解释。一种称为吻素的下丘脑调节肽是由 *KISS1* 基因编码的。之前大多数文献表明，患有 PCOS 的女性吻素水平较高，并且通过升高 GnRH 脉冲频率和振幅来影响 HPO 轴。此外，越来越多的证据表明，γ-氨基丁酸（γ-aminobutyric acid，GABA）也在 PCOS 的病理生理学中起着一定的作用。虽然 GABA 是一种中枢神经系统抑制性神经递质，但 GABA 在下丘脑似乎可以通过 GABA 受体增加 GnRH 神经元的活性。因此，GABA 的增加会导致 GnRH 分泌增加及 LH：FSH 升高。

3. 功能性肾上腺高雄激素血症

虽然功能性卵巢 HA 仍然是导致 PCOS 患者 HA 的主要机制，但肾上腺引起的类固醇生成功能障碍也能起到一定的作用。先前的文献表明，在 PCOS 患者中功能性肾上腺 HA 的患病率为 20%～65%，只有不到 3% 的 PCOS 病例仅归因于功能性肾上腺 HA。功能性肾上腺 HA 的显著特征是肾上腺皮质分泌的血清硫酸脱氢表雄酮（DHEAS）水平升高。肾上腺雄激素产生增加的潜在机制尚不清楚，但是也有假设认为，导致功能性卵巢 HA 发生的类似机制也会导致功能性肾上腺 HA，从而导致类固醇生物合成途径功能障碍。此外，也有研究表明，肾上腺对促肾上腺皮质激素的敏感性升高，PCOS 患者的高胰岛素状态也会增强 17α-羟化酶和 17，20-裂解酶的活性。肾上腺网状带和卵巢由于酶的表达差异而产生的雄激素不同。肾上腺中 3β-羟基类固醇脱氢酶（3β-hydroxysteroid dehydrogenase，3β-HSD）2 活性降低和 SULT2A1 磺基转移酶表达增加导致脱氢表雄酮（DHEA）转化为硫酸脱氢表雄酮（而不是卵巢中的雄烯二酮）。

（二）胰岛素抵抗和高胰岛素血症

除了 HA，IR 和高胰岛素血症是近 2/3 胰岛素敏感性降低患者的关键特征；PCOS 患者的高胰岛素状态可归因于 IR，其引发机制是胰岛素受体和胰岛素受体底物-1 的丝氨酸磷酸化异常导致受体后信号转导缺陷。这种过度磷酸化的原因是细胞内丝氨酸激酶活性增加。此外，高胰岛素血症与 PCOS 中的高雄激素状态密切相关，而且通常这 2 个因素具有协同作用。由于高胰岛素血症，肝脏的 SHBG 产生减少，从而游离的雄激素水平升高。此外，胰岛素可以直接作为一种生殖激素，促进 GnRH 介导的促性腺激素从垂体中释放，随后在与 LH 的协同作用下，诱导卵泡膜细胞产生雄激素。PCOS 患者的卵巢中存在胰岛素受体，可以刺激颗粒细胞和卵泡膜细胞生成类固醇。令人惊讶的是，IR 似乎具有选择性，它只影响 PCOS 患者的糖代谢并导致随后一系列的代谢紊乱，而对卵巢没有任何影响。然而，目前仍不清楚的是，IR 和高胰岛素血症是否有助于促成 PCOS，是否只是 PCOS 的代谢效应，在这方面还需要进一步研究。

三、血管内皮生长因子

血管内皮生长因子（vascular endothelial growth factor，VEGF）是一种结合内皮细胞上的特定受体、诱导血管生成的蛋白质。在卵巢组织中，血管发生是周期性的，VEGF 在介导血管生成和血管通透性中起着重要作用，而且对排卵和黄体的发育至关重要。

VEGF 及其受体在多种卵巢细胞上表达，包括卵泡膜细胞和颗粒细胞。卵泡液中 VEGF 的水平明显高于血清中的水平。有研究报道，接受体外受精（in vitro fertilization，IVF）的 PCOS 受试者有很高的 VEGF 水平。另有研究发现，在卵泡膜细胞、颗粒细胞和黄体细胞中，VEGF 的表达增加。多普勒研究显示，卵巢中血流速度增加与 VEGF 水平呈正相关，而 VEGF 水平升高继发的血管生成增加可能是导致卵巢增大的一个因素，也是该疾病的一个标志。高表达的 VEGF 可导致卵泡膜细胞的异常生长。大量的研究发现 *VEGF* 基因多态性在 PCOS 病理过程中发挥着一定作用。Bao 等发现 rs1570360 单核苷酸多态性与 PCOS 风险增加有显著相关性，而 rs3025020 和 rs833061 与 PCOS 风险增加相关性甚微。上述发现表明，高水平的 VEGF 确实有助于在 PCOS 患者中观察到许多表型特征。

四、维生素 D

维生素 D 是一种重要的类固醇激素，以维生素 D_2（麦角钙化醇）和维生素 D_3（胆钙化醇）的形式存在，通过维生素 D 受体发挥作用。维生素 D 的主要功能是调节体内的钙和磷的代谢，从而影响骨代谢。

维生素 D 除了在骨代谢中发挥作用外，还在卵巢功能和 PCOS 发病机制中发挥着重要作用（图 4.3）。维生素 D 缺乏在 PCOS 患者中非常普遍，患病率为 67%～85%。PCOS 与抗米勒管激素（AMH）水平密切相关。据推测，AMH 具有以下主要功能并起到抑制作用：

- 卵泡的激活和生长。
- FSH 促进生长。
- 颗粒细胞生长。
- 抑制芳香化酶活性。

在 PCOS 患者中，高水平的 AMH 可能会导致卵泡对 FSH 的敏感性降低，从而损害卵巢功能。而且，PCOS 患者体内雌激素水平降低可能是因为 AMH 对芳香化酶抑制作用增强导致的。AMH 可以直接刺激卵泡膜细胞合成更多的雄激素。一项研究显示，维生素 D 水平与 AMH 和 AMH 受体的 mRNA 水平呈负相关，因此，给予 PCOS 患者补充维生素 D，可以使 AMH 水平降低，从而改善卵泡发育。

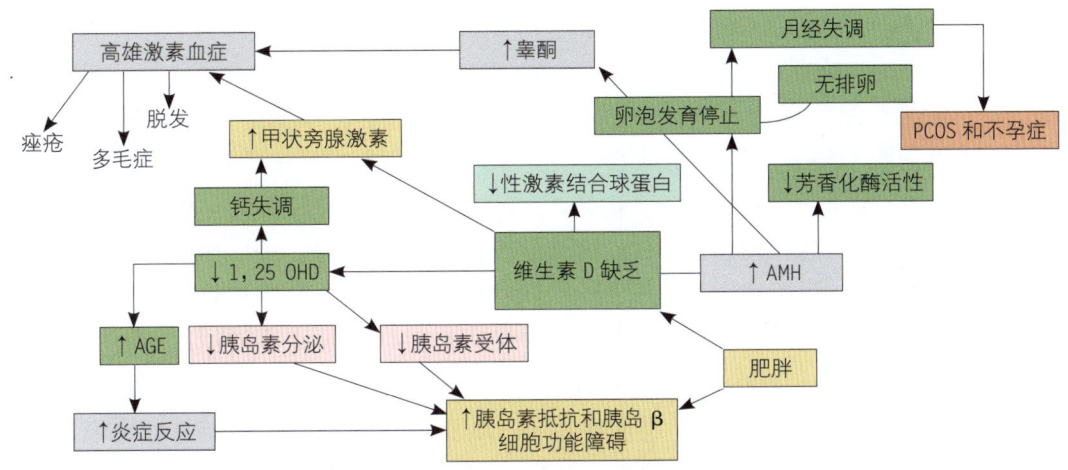

1, 25 OHD, 1,25 双羟维生素 D；AGE, 晚期糖基化终末产物；AMH, 抗米勒管激素。

图 4.3　维生素 D 缺乏和多囊卵巢综合征

晚期糖基化终末产物（advanced glycation end products，AGE）是 PCOS 中发现的可能导致卵泡功能障碍的促炎分子。AGE 的可溶性受体（soluble receptors for AGEs，sRAGE）可以与 AGE 结合，从而中和其有害影响。研究发现，补充维生素 D 与血液循环中 sRAGE 的水平升高存在着一定关联，从而也能减少 AGE 带来的有害效应。

伴有胰岛素抵抗的 PCOS 患者与维生素 D 水平下降显著相关。维生素 D 可以调节许多基因的表达，包括参与脂代谢和糖代谢的基因。因此，维生素 D 缺乏与胰岛素抵抗、游离睾酮指数增加有关。如前所述，血管内皮生长因子高表达是 PCOS 的一个危险因素，而补充维生素 D 可以降低血清中血管内皮生长因子的水平。

五、表观遗传学

表观遗传学变化是基因表达的可遗传变化，受环境和行为改变的影响，而潜在的基因组序列仍被保留下来。修饰基因表达的表观遗传学变化包括 DNA 甲基化、组蛋白修饰和微 RNA（microRNA，miRNA）水平的变化，这些修饰已被证明可以改变 PCOS 的发展和临床严重程度。

（一）微 RNA

miRNA 是由 21～22 个核苷酸组成的非编码小 RNA 分子。它们通过 mRNA 的衰减、分裂和最终抑制翻译来调节基因表达的转录和翻译阶段。miRNA 与 mRNA 上的位点（最常见的是 3′ 非翻译区）相互作用，通过诱导 mRNA 降解来减少翻译。miRNA 还可以与 mRNA 的其他位点结合，包括 5′ 非翻译区、基因启动子和编码序列。除细胞质外，miRNA 还存在于多种体液中，包括唾液、血浆、尿液、母乳、精液和泪液。

人们在 PCOS 患者的颗粒细胞、卵泡膜细胞、脂肪和血清中发现了 miRNA 的畸变，这表明它们有可能在 PCOS 的发病机制中发挥着作用。多种 miRNA 与 PCOS 的发病机制有关，包括 miRNA21、miRNA27b、miRNA-320 和 miR-376a。虽然对受 miRNA 影响的所有生化通路的阐述不属于本章讨论的范畴，但是已证明 PCOS 患者的 miRNA 异常可诱导细胞增殖、抑制细胞凋亡、促进 IR、下调雌激素分泌及改变类固醇生成。表 4.1 为我们列出了一些已知的在 PCOS 患者中常见的失调 miRNA。例如，miR-93 在颗粒细胞中过表达，通过抑制 *cdk1a* 基因导致颗粒细胞增殖。而 miRs-126-5p、miRs-29a-5p 和 miRs-92b 低表达会导致颗粒细胞凋亡。前两项陈述可能显得相互矛盾，但这可能有一个简单的解释。在 PCOS 患者中，一方面，细胞快速增殖，导致原始卵泡向初级卵泡转化加速，最终卵泡比例增加；另一方面，颗粒细胞凋亡也可能随之增加，导致闭锁卵泡、卵巢功能不全，进而导致 PCOS 患者无排卵。在卵泡膜细胞中，miR-92a 和 miR-92b 表达不足，分别导致 *GATA6* 基因和 *IRS-2* 基因产物的活性增加，导致 CYP17 和 17α-羟化酶的活性增加，从而导致雄激素产生增加。研究发现，miR-376a 通过调节增殖细胞核抗原的表达来增加原始卵泡的数量、抑制卵母细胞的凋亡。此外，miR-155 是一种通过调节 PCNA 起作用的 miRNA，通过抑制 PCNA 来抑制睾酮的释放，而且在 PCOS 患者中高表达，所以可作为一种潜在的生物标志物来监测 PCOS 患者的治疗效果。针对 PCOS 的特定 miRNA 的靶向疗法已被广泛研究，并且十分有研究前景。还有 miR-145，它通过抑制 IRS1 的表达，进而抑制 MAPK/EPK 信号通路来抑制颗粒细胞的增殖。这些研究表明，miR-145 可能是改善颗粒细胞不规则性的潜在治疗靶点。另外，miR-30d-5p 可以通过靶向 Smad 2 诱导颗粒细胞凋亡来实现 PCOS 治疗的目的。

表 4.1 卵巢内显著失调的 miRNA

miRNA	位置	在多囊卵巢综合征中的改变
miR-93 miR-483-5p miR-320 miR-145 miR-126-5p miR-29a-5p miR-92b	颗粒细胞	上调 下调
miR-92b miR-92a	卵泡膜细胞	下调
miR-233 miR-93	脂肪组织	上调 下调
miR-30a miR-320 miR-132 miR-140 let-7b	卵泡液	上调 下调

正如前文所说，在体液中同样发现了 miRNA，并且可以作为 PCOS 的潜在无创生化标志物。目前还没有发现哪一种 miRNA 可以具体影响 PCOS 的发病机制，但 miRNA

可以作为未来筛选和检测的生物标志物。一项病例对照研究结果表明，与对照组相比，PCOS 患者的血清中 miR-222、miR-146a 和 miR-30c 的水平显著升高，这也证实了它们可以作为潜在生物标志物使用。在另一项研究中，与对照组相比，PCOS 患者血清中的 miR-320 水平显著降低，由于 miR-320 对血清中内皮素产生负调控作用，因此内皮素水平显著升高，两者呈负相关。此外，对卵泡液中 miRNA 的水平也进行了研究。一项研究分析了 176 种 miRNA，发现 PCOS 患者与对照组之间有 29 种 miRNA 存在显著差异。在 29 种 miRNA 中，12 种与生殖相关，12 种与疾病过程中的炎症相关，6 种与良性盆腔疾病有关。另一项研究发现，PCOS 患者中 miR-132 的水平显著降低。因为 miRNA 能够调节体内雌二醇浓度，miRNA 较低的水平也解释了 PCOS 患者雌二醇水平较低的原因。

（二）DNA 甲基化

DNA 甲基化是通过 DNA 甲基转移酶将 S-腺苷甲硫氨酸基团添加到 DNA 分子中的过程。这个过程可能涉及不同的 DNA 序列，但主要发生在 CpG 二核苷酸序列上。DNA 甲基化降低了相关基因的转录，因为这些基因不能再被 RNA 聚合酶识别。

DNA 甲基化变化对 PCOS 发病机制影响的相关研究揭示了一些有趣的结果。国内的一项研究得出结论，基因的低甲基化可能导致基因表达的增加，从而导致包括雄激素在内的类固醇激素的合成增加，从而解释了在 PCOS 中的 HA。编码芳香化酶的 *CYP19A1* 启动子区域的高甲基化使得 PCOS 患者芳香化酶的活性降低，从而导致雌激素产生减少。还有一项研究发现，PCOS 患者的高瘦素水平可归因于相关基因的甲基化减少。全基因组关联研究表明，在 PCOS 患者中，胸腺细胞选择相关高迁移率群盒（thymocyte selection–associated high mobility group box，*TOX3*）被低甲基化或去甲基化，另一项研究也证明了这一点，PCOS 患者中 *TOX3* 甲基化水平、TOX3 mRNA 和蛋白水平较低。而且 PCOS 患者的 LH、促甲状腺激素（thyroid stimulating hormone，TSH）、睾酮和雌二醇水平较高，而 FSH 和催乳素水平较低。有一项研究中发现了一个有趣的现象，PCOS 患者的子宫环境可以改变与代谢、生殖相关的某些基因的甲基化水平，这些紊乱都会遗传给子代。

六、遗传学

几十年来，基因在 PCOS 发展中的作用一直是人们关注的话题，因此有很多学者在做关于这两者关系的研究。1968 年，Cooper 等首次证实了 PCOS 是常染色体显性遗传疾病；然而，对 11 对单卵双胎和双卵双胎进行的研究表明，PCOS 与 X 连锁的多基因遗传相关。这种基因遗传的发生被认为是多种基因与宫内、宫外环境因素相互作用的结果。

这种遗传关联性反映在家族中 PCOS 患病率较高上。研究报道，PCOS 患者的女性亲属（母亲、姐妹）患病率为 24% ～ 32%。同样，男性亲属也会有该综合征中的 IR 和内皮细胞功能障碍的特征。研究还表明，男性亲属更容易患上代谢综合征、血脂异常和高血压。PCOS 患者的兄弟姐妹中 DHEAS 水平显著升高，表明他们可能具有类固醇生成缺陷。

PCOS 的复杂性是显而易见的，其发病机制与许多基因相关（图 4.4）。

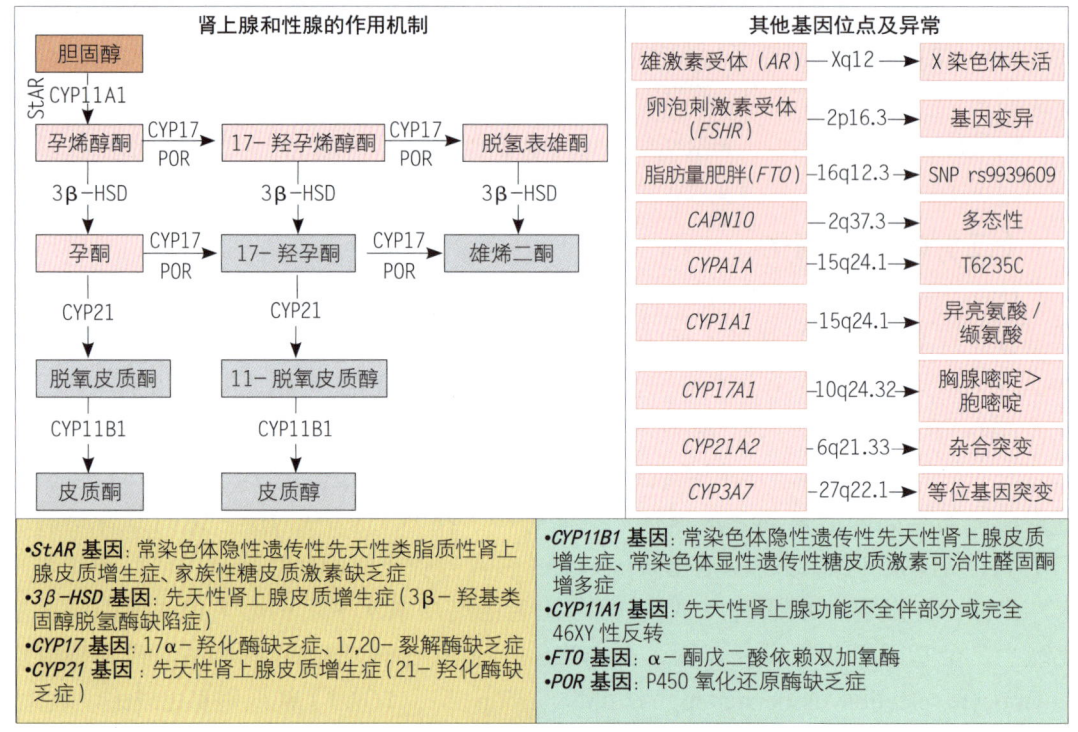

图 4.4　基因在多囊卵巢综合征发生发展中的作用

• *CYP11a*（胆固醇侧链裂解酶的基因——译者注）通过编码细胞色素 p450，将胆固醇转化为孕烯醇酮，此为类固醇生成的限速步骤。Gharani 等表明，*CYP11a* 的变化与 HA 有关，而 HA 是 PCOS 的典型特征。在国内进行的另一项病例对照研究得出结论：*CYP11A1* 的多态性与 PCOS 密切相关。

• *CYP21* 通过编码细胞色素 p450，将 17- 羟孕酮转化为 11- 脱氧皮质醇。一项研究显示：在 HA 女性中，*CYP21* 的杂合度增加。

• *CYP17* 编码 17α- 羟化酶，该酶将孕烯醇酮和孕酮分别转化为 17- 羟孕烯醇酮和17- 羟孕酮。这些产物通过 17，20- 裂解酶转化为 DHEA 和雄烯二酮。Rahimi 等得出结论，*CYP17 TC* 基因型患者对 PCOS 的易感性是对照组的 2.31 倍。*CYP17* 的 A2 等位基因变异是改变多囊卵巢表达的重要因素。

• *CYP19* 编码芳香化酶，将雄激素转化为女性性激素，特别是雌激素。多项研究发现，*CYP19* 基因中的单核苷酸多态性（single nucleotide polymorphisms，SNP）2414096 与 PCOS 发生风险增加相关。

- StAR 是类固醇生成急性调节蛋白（steroidogenic acute regulatory protein，StAR）的缩写。类固醇生物合成的第一步始于胆固醇，StAR 是一种负责通过线粒体膜转运胆固醇的转运蛋白。Melissa 等证实，PCOS 患者出现 HA 可能与类固醇生成限速步骤中 StAR 活性增强有关。

- 雄激素受体（androgen receptor，*AR*）基因编码雄激素受体，位于 X 染色体上的 Xq11-12。多聚谷氨酰胺链的延伸由 CAG 三核苷酸重复序列编码，且 AR 的活性与 CAG 重复序列数量呈负相关。因此，雄激素水平正常的患者出现 HA 的原因可能是 CAG 重复序列较少，导致 AR 活性增加。

- *SHBG* 基因编码一种血清蛋白，可结合雄激素并控制体内循环激素水平。它位于 17 号染色体上的 p12～p13 条带上。一项对 62 篇文章进行的荟萃分析发现，与对照组相比，PCOS 患者的 SHBG 水平显著降低，突出了 SHBG 在 PCOS 发病机制中的作用。

- *DENDD1A* 是一种在卵泡膜细胞中发现的蛋白质编码基因。该基因以前被认为与 PCOS 患者的代谢和生殖有关。*DENDD1A* 编码有两种变体，即 V1 和 V2，它们通过提高雄激素生物合成途径中某些酶的表达来增加雄激素的分泌。一项研究对 62 个家庭进行了全基因组测序，每个家庭中至少有一例 PCOS 患者，发现一半的家庭中至少有一种 *DEND1A* 变异。

参与 PCOS 发病机制的基因还有编码 LH 和 FSH 受体的基因。LH 是卵巢产生雄激素的重要调节因子，它在卵泡发育、诱导排卵和雌激素产生过程中发挥作用。LH 通过作用于多个卵巢细胞上的 LH 受体发挥作用，包括卵泡膜细胞、黄体细胞和颗粒细胞。LH 升高是 PCOS 的典型特征，而 LH 升高会导致雄激素分泌增加。LHβ 和 LH 受体的多态性与 PCOS 有关，而且大多数受影响的女性 LH 水平升高。此外，研究还发现 PCOS 患者的卵泡膜细胞和颗粒细胞中 LH 受体高表达。同样，FSH 编码基因的多态性与 PCOS 表型改变有关。研究还发现，负责胰岛素产生和作用的基因，如胰岛素 *VNTR*（可变数量串联重复序列）基因、*IGF-2* 基因和钙蛋白酶-10 等都与 PCOS 的发病机制有关。

参考文献

1. Kirschner MA, Bardin CW. Androgen production and metabolism in normal and virilized women. Metabolism. 1972;21(7):667-688. doi:10.1016/0026-0495(72)90090-x.
2. Dadachanji R, Shaikh N, Mukherjee S. Genetic variants associated with hyperandrogenemia in PCOS pathophysiology. Genet Res Int. 2018;2018:7624932. doi:10.1155/2018/7624932.
3. Rosenfield RL, Ehrmann DA. The Pathogenesis of Polycystic Ovary Syndrome (PCOS): the hypothesis of PCOS as functional ovarian hyperandrogenism revisited. Endocr Rev. 2016;37(5):467-520. doi:10.1210/er.2015-1104.
4. Abbott DH, Dumesic DA, Eisner JR, Colman RJ, Kemnitz JW. Insights into the development of polycystic ovary syndrome (PCOS) from studies of prenatally androgenized female rhesus monkeys. Trends Endocrinol Metab. 1998;9(2):62-67. doi:10.1016/s1043-2760(98)00019-8.

5. Padmanabhan V, Veiga-Lopez A. Reproduction symposium: developmental programming of reproductive and metabolic health. J Anim Sci. 2014;92(8):3199-3210. doi:10.2527/jas.2014-7637.
6. Morel Y, Roucher F, Plotton I, Goursaud C, Tardy V, Mallet D. Evolution of steroids during pregnancy: maternal, placental and fetal synthesis. Ann Endocrinol (Paris). 2016;77(2):82-89. doi:10.1016/j.ando.2016.04.023.
7. Puttabyatappa M, Cardoso RC, Padmanabhan V. Effect of maternal PCOS and PCOS-like phenotype on the offspring's health. Mol Cell Endocrinol. 2016;435:29-39. doi:10.1016/j.mce.2015.11.030.
8. Clarke IJ, Cummins JT. GnRH pulse frequency determines LH pulse amplitude by altering the amount of releasable LH in the pituitary glands of ewes. J Reprod Fertil. 1985;73(2):425-431. doi:10.1530/jrf.0.0730425.
9. Liao B, Qiao J, Pang Y. Central regulation of PCOS: abnormal neuronal-reproductive-metabolic circuits in PCOS pathophysiology. Front Endocrinol (Lausanne). 2021;12:667422. doi:10.3389/fendo.2021.667422.
10. Ohtaki T, Shintani Y, Honda S, et al. Metastasis suppressor gene KiSS-1 encodes peptide ligand of a G-protein-coupled receptor. Nature. 2001;411(6837):613-617. doi:10.1038/35079135.
11. Tang R, Ding X, Zhu J. Kisspeptin and polycystic ovary syndrome. Front Endocrinol (Lausanne). 2019;10:298. doi:10.3389/fendo.2019.00298.
12. Ruddenklau A, Campbell RE. Neuroendocrine impairments of polycystic ovary syndrome. Endocrinology. 2019;160(10):2230-2242. doi:10.1210/en.2019-00428.
13. Carmina E, Koyama T, Chang L, Stanczyk FZ, Lobo RA. Does ethnicity influence the prevalence of adrenal hyperandrogenism and insulin resistance in polycystic ovary syndrome? Am J Obstet Gynecol. 1992;167(6):1807-1812. doi:10.1016/0002-9378(92)91779-a.
14. Kumar A, Woods KS, Bartolucci AA, Azziz R. Prevalence of adrenal androgen excess in patients with the polycystic ovary syndrome (PCOS). Clin Endocrinol (Oxf). 2005;62(6):644-649. doi:10.1111/j.1365-2265.2005.02256.x.
15. Rosenfield RL. Evidence that idiopathic functional adrenal hyperandrogenism is caused by dysregulation of adrenal steroidogenesis and that hyperinsulinemia may be involved. J Clin Endocrinol Metab. 1996;81(3):878-880. doi:10.1210/jcem.81.3.8772543.
16. Rainey WE, Carr BR, Sasano H, Suzuki T, Mason JI. Dissecting human adrenal androgen production. Trends. Endocrinol Metab. 2002;13(6):234-239. doi:10.1016/s1043-2760(02)00609-4.
17. Tosi F, Bonora E, Moghetti P. Insulin resistance in a large cohort of women with polycystic ovary syndrome: a comparison between euglycaemic-hyperinsulinaemic clamp and surrogate indexes. Hum Reprod. 2017;32(12):2515-2521. doi:10.1093/humrep/dex308.
18. Corbould A, Kim YB, Youngren JF, et al. Insulin resistance in the skeletal muscle of women with PCOS involves intrinsic and acquired defects in insulin signaling. Am J Physiol Endocrinol Metab. 2005;288(5):E1047-E1054. doi:10.1152/ajpendo.00361.2004.
19. Dunaif A, Xia J, Book CB, Schenker E, Tang Z. Excessive insulin receptor serine phosphorylation in cultured fibroblasts and in skeletal muscle. A potential mechanism for insulin resistance in the polycystic ovary syndrome. J Clin Invest. 1995;96(2):801-810. doi:10.1172/jci118126.
20. Poretsky L, Cataldo NA, Rosenwaks Z, Giudice LC. The insulinrelated ovarian regulatory system in health and disease. Endocr Rev. 1999;20(4):535-582. doi:10.1210/edrv.20.4.0374.
21. Pugeat M, Crave JC, Elmidani M, et al. Pathophysiology of sex hormone binding globulin (SHBG): relation to insulin. J Steroid Biochem Mol Biol. 1991;40(4-6):841-849. doi:10.1016/0960-0760(91)90310-2.
22. Munir I, Yen HW, Geller DH, et al. Insulin augmentation of 17alpha-hydroxylase activity is mediated by phosphatidyl inositol 3-kinase but not extracellular signal-regulated kinase-1/2 in human ovarian theca cells. Endocrinology. 2004;145(1):175-183. doi:10.1210/en.2003-0329.
23. Nestler JE, Strauss JF III. Insulin as an effector of human ovarian and adrenal steroid metabolism. Endocrinol Metab Clin North Am. 1991;20(4):807-823.
24. Baptiste CG, Battista MC, Trottier A, Baillargeon JP. Insulin and hyperandrogenism in women with polycystic ovary syndrome. J Steroid Biochem Mol Biol. 2010;122(1-3):42-52. doi:10.1016/j.jsbmb.2009.12.010.

25. Rice S, Christoforidis N, Gadd C, et al. Impaired insulin-dependent glucose metabolism in granulosa-lutein cells from anovulatory women with polycystic ovaries. Hum Reprod. 2005;20(2):373-381. doi:10.1093/humrep/deh609.
26. Geva E, Jaffe RB. Role of vascular endothelial growth factor in ovarian physiology and pathology. Fertil Steril. 2000;74(3):429-438. doi:10.1016/s0015-0282(00)00670-1.
27. Li Y, Fang L, Yu Y, et al. Association between vascular endothelial growth factor gene polymorphisms and PCOS risk: a metaanalysis. Reprod Biomed Online. 2020;40(2):287-295. doi:10.1016/j.rbmo.2019.10.018.
28. Agrawal R, Conway G, Sladkevicius P, et al. Serum vascular endothelial growth factor and Doppler blood flow velocities in in vitro fertilization: relevance to ovarian hyperstimulation syndrome and polycystic ovaries. Fertil Steril. 1998;70(4):651-658. doi:10.1016/s0015-0282(98)00249-0.
29. Bao L, Syed R, Aloahd MS. Analysis of VEGF gene polymorphisms and serum VEGF protein levels contribution in polycystic ovary syndrome of patients. Mol Biol Rep. 2019;46(6):5821-5829. doi:10.1007/s11033-019-05015-y.
30. Mu Y, Cheng D, Yin TL, Yang J. Vitamin D and polycystic ovary syndrome: a narrative review. Reprod Sci. 2021;28(8):2110-2117. doi:10.1007/s43032-020-00369-2.
31. Lin MW, Wu MH. The role of vitamin D in polycystic ovary syndrome. Indian J Med Res. 2015;142(3):238-240. doi:10.4103/0971-5916.166527.
32. Zec I, Tislaric-Medenjak D, Megla ZB, Kucak I. Anti-Müllerian hormone: a unique biochemical marker of gonadal development and fertility in humans. Biochem Med (Zagreb). 2011;21(3):219-230. doi:10.11613/bm.2011.031.
33. Pigny P, Jonard S, Robert Y, Dewailly D. Serum anti-Mullerian hormone as a surrogate for antral follicle count for definition of the polycystic ovary syndrome. J Clin Endocrinol Metab. 2006;91(3):941-945. doi:10.1210/jc.2005-2076.
34. Diamanti-Kandarakis E. Polycystic ovarian syndrome: pathophysiology, molecular aspects and clinical implications. Expert Rev Mol Med. 2008;10:e3. doi:10.1017/s1462399408000598.
35. Kuyucu Y, Çelik LS, Kendirlinan Ö, Tap Ö, Mete U. Investigation of the uterine structural changes in the experimental model with polycystic ovary syndrome and effects of vitamin D treatment: an ultrastructural and immunohistochemical study. Reprod Biol. 2018;18(1):53-59. doi:10.1016/j.repbio.2018.01.002.
36. Merhi Z. Advanced glycation end products and their relevance in female reproduction. Hum Reprod. 2014;29(1):135-145. doi:10.1093/humrep/det383.
37. Irani M, Minkoff H, Seifer DB, Merhi Z. Vitamin D increases serum levels of the soluble receptor for advanced glycation end products in women with PCOS. J Clin Endocrinol Metab. 2014;99(5):E886-E890. doi:10.1210/jc.2013-4374.
38. Irani M, Merhi Z. Role of vitamin D in ovarian physiology and its implication in reproduction: a systematic review. Fertil Steril. 2014;102(2):460-468.e3. doi:10.1016/j.fertnstert.2014.04.046.
39. Irani M, Seifer DB, Grazi RV, Irani S, Rosenwaks Z, Tal R. Vitamin D decreases serum VEGF correlating with clinical improvement in vitamin D-deficient women with PCOS: a randomized placebo-controlled trial. Nutrients. 2017;9(4):334. doi:10.3390/nu9040334.
40. Xu N, Azziz R, Goodarzi MO. Epigenetics in polycystic ovary syndrome: a pilot study of global DNA methylation. Fertil Steril. 2010;94(2):781-783.e1. doi:10.1016/j.fertnstert.2009.10.020.
41. Jin Z, Liu Y. DNA methylation in human diseases. Genes Dis.2018;5(1):1-8. doi:10.1016/j.gendis.2018.01.002.
42. Chen B, Xu P, Wang J, Zhang C. The role of MiRNA in polycystic ovary syndrome (PCOS). Gene. 2019;706:91-96. Available at: https://doi.org/10.1016/j.gene.2019.04.082.
43. O'Brien J, Hayder H, Zayed Y, Peng C. Overview of microRNA biogenesis, mechanisms of actions, and circulation. Front Endocrinol (Lausanne). 2018;9:402. doi:10.3389/fendo.2018.00402.
44. Butler AE, Ramachandran V, Sathyapalan T, et al. MicroRNA expression in women with and without polycystic ovarian syndrome matched for body mass index. Front Endocrinol (Lausanne). 2020;11:206. doi:10.3389/

fendo.2020.00206.
45. Zhang H, Jiang X, Zhang Y, et al. MicroRNA 376a regulates follicle assembly by targeting PCNA in fetal and neonatal mouse ovaries. Reproduction (Cambridge, England). 2014;148(1):43-54. doi:10.1530/rep-13-0508.
46. Jiang L, Huang J, Li L, et al. MicroRNA-93 promotes ovarian granulosa cells proliferation through targeting CDKN1A in polycystic ovarian syndrome. J Clin Endocrinol Metab. 2015;100(5):E729-E738. doi:10.1210/jc.2014-3827.
47. Mao Z, Fan L, Yu Q, et al. Abnormality of klotho signaling is involved in polycystic ovary syndrome. Reprod Sci. 2018;25(3):372-383. doi:10.1177/1933719117715129.
48. Xu B, Zhang YW, Tong XH, Liu YS. Characterization of microRNA profile in human cumulus granulosa cells: identification of microRNAs that regulate Notch signaling and are associated with PCOS. Mol Cell Endocrinol. 2015;404:26-36. doi:10.1016/j.mce.2015.01.030.
49. Das M, Djahanbakhch O, Hacihanefioglu B, et al. Granulosa cell survival and proliferation are altered in polycystic ovary syndrome. J Clin Endocrinol Metab. 2008;93(3):881-887. doi:10.1210/jc.2007-1650.
50. Worku T, Rehman ZU, Talpur HS, et al. MicroRNAs: new insight in modulating follicular atresia: a review. Int J Mol Sci. 2017;18(2):333. doi:10.3390/ijms18020333.
51. Ho CKM, Wood JR, Stewart DR, et al. Increased transcription and increased messenger ribonucleic acid (mRNA) stability contribute to increased GATA6 mRNA abundance in polycystic ovary syndrome theca cells. J Clin Endocrinol Metab. 2005;90(12):6596-6602. doi:10.1210/jc.2005-0890.
52. Arancio W, Calogero Amato M, et al. Serum miRNAs in women affected by hyperandrogenic polycystic ovary syndrome: the potential role of miR-155 as a biomarker for monitoring the estroprogestinic treatment. Gynecol Endocrinol. 2018;34(8):704-708. doi:10.1080/09513590.2018.1428299.
53. Cai G, Ma X, Chen B, et al. MicroRNA-145 negatively regulates cell proliferation through targeting IRS1 in isolated ovarian granulosa cells from patients with polycystic ovary syndrome. Reprod Sci. 2017;24(6):902-910. doi:10.1177/1933719116673197.
54. Yu M, Liu J. MicroRNA-30d-5p promotes ovarian granulosa cell apoptosis by targeting Smad2. Exp Ther Med. 2020;19(1):53-60. doi:10.3892/etm.2019.8184.
55. Yin M, Wang X, Yao G, et al. Transactivation of micrornA-320 by microRNA-383 regulates granulosa cell functions by targeting E2F1 and SF-1 proteins. J Biol Chem. 2014;289(26):18239-18257. doi:10.1074/jbc.M113.546044.
56. Zhang CL, Wang H, Yan CY, Gao XF, Ling XJ. Deregulation of RUNX2 by miR-320a deficiency impairs steroidogenesis in cumulus granulosa cells from polycystic ovary syndrome (PCOS) patients. Biochem Biophys Res Commun. 2017;482(4):1469-1476. doi:10.1016/j.bbrc.2016.12.059.
57. Lin L, Du T, Huang J, Huang LL, Yang DZ. Identification of differentially expressed microRNAs in the ovary of polycystic ovary syndrome with hyperandrogenism and insulin resistance. Chin Med J (Engl). 2015;128(2):169-174. doi:10.4103/0366-6999.149189.
58. Chuang TY, Wu HL, Chen CC, et al. MicroRNA-223 expression is upregulated in insulin resistant human adipose tissue. J Diabetes Res. 2015;2015;943659. doi:10.1155/2015/943659.
59. Scalici E, Traver S, Mullet T, et al. Circulating microRNAs in follicular fluid, powerful tools to explore in vitro fertilization process. Sci Rep. 2016;6(1):24976. doi:10.1038/srep24976.
60. Sang Q, Yao Z, Wang H, et al. Identification of microRNAs in human follicular fluid: characterization of microRNAs that govern steroidogenesis in vitro and are associated with polycystic ovary syndrome in vivo. J Clin Endocrinol Metab. 2013;98(7):3068-3079. doi:10.1210/jc.2013-1715.
61. Abdalla M, Deshmukh H, Atkin SL, Sathyapalan T. MiRNAs as a novel clinical biomarker and therapeutic targets in polycystic ovary syndrome (PCOS): a review. Life Sci. 2020;259:118174. doi:10.1016/j.lfs.2020.118174.
62. Long W, Zhao C, Ji C, et al. Characterization of serum microRNAs profile of PCOS and identification of novel non-invasive biomarkers. Cell Physiol Biochem. 2014;33(5):1304-1315. doi:10.1159/000358698.

63. Rashad NM, Ateya MA, Saraya YS, et al. Association of miRNA - 320 expression level and its target gene endothelin-1 with the susceptibility and clinical features of polycystic ovary syndrome. J Ovarian Res. 2019;12(1):39. doi:10.1186/s13048-019-0513-5.
64. Butler AE, Ramachandran V, Hayat S, et al. Expression of microRNA in follicular fluid in women with and without PCOS. Sci Rep. 2019;9(1):16306. doi:10.1038/s41598-019-52856-5.
65. Pan JX, Tan YJ, Wang FF, et al. Aberrant expression and DNA methylation of lipid metabolism genes in PCOS: a new insight into its pathogenesis. Clin Epigenetics. 2018;10(1):6. doi:10.1186/s13148-018-0442-y.
66. Yu YY, Sun CX, Liu YK, Li Y, Wang L, Zhang W. Promoter methylation of CYP19A1 gene in Chinese polycystic ovary syndrome patients. Gynecol Obstet Invest. 2013;76(4):209-213. doi:10.1159/000355314.
67. Liu L, He D, Wang Y, Sheng M. Integrated analysis of DNA methylation and transcriptome profiling of polycystic ovary syndrome. Mol Med Rep. 2020;21(5):2138-2150. doi:10.3892/mmr.2020.11005.
68. Ning Z, Jiayi L, Jian R, Wanli X. Relationship between abnormal TOX3 gene methylation and polycystic ovarian syndrome. Eur Rev Med Pharmacol Sci. 2017;21(9):2034-2038.
69. Echiburú B, Milagro F, Crisosto N, et al. DNA methylation in promoter regions of genes involved in the reproductive and metabolic function of children born to women with PCOS. Epigenetics. 2020;15(11):1178-1194. doi:10.1080/15592294.2020.1754674.
70. Cooper HE, Spellacy W, Prem K, Cohen WD. Hereditary factors in the Stein-Leventhal syndrome. Am J Obstet Gynecol. 1968;100(3):371-387.
71. Jahanfar S, Eden JA, Warren P, Seppälä M, Nguyen TV. A twin study of polycystic ovary syndrome. Fertil Steril. 1995;63(3):478-486.
72. Kahsar-Miller MD, Nixon C, Boots LR, Go RC, Azziz R. Prevalence of polycystic ovary syndrome (PCOS) in first-degree relatives of patients with PCOS. Fertil Steril. 2001;75(1):53-58. doi:10.1016/s0015-0282(00)01662-9.
73. Kaushal R, Parchure N, Bano G, Kaski JC, Nussey SS. Insulin resistance and endothelial dysfunction in the brothers of Indian subcontinent Asian women with polycystic ovaries. Clin Endocrinol (Oxf). 2004;60(3):322-328. doi:10.1111/j.1365-2265.2004.01981.x.
74. Coviello AD, Sam S, Legro RS, Dunaif A. High prevalence of metabolic syndrome in first-degree male relatives of women with polycystic ovary syndrome is related to high rates of obesity. J Clin Endocrinol Metab. 2009;94(11):4361-4366. doi:10.1210/jc.2009-1333.
75. Legro RS, Kunselman AR, Demers L, Wang SC, Bentley-Lewis R, Dunaif A. Elevated dehydroepiandrosterone sulfate levels as the reproductive phenotype in the brothers of women with polycystic ovary syndrome. J Clin Endocrinol Metab. 2002;87(5):2134-2138. doi:10.1210/jcem.87.5.8387.
76. Payne AH, Hales DB. Overview of steroidogenic enzymes in the pathway from cholesterol to active steroid hormones. Endocr Rev. 2004;25(6):947-970. doi:10.1210/er.2003-0030.
77. Gharani N, Waterworth DM, Batty S, et al. Association of the steroid synthesis gene CYP11a with polycystic ovary syndrome and hyperandrogenism. Hum Mol Genet. 1997;6(3):397-402. doi:10.1093/hmg/6.3.397.
78. Zhang CW, Zhang XL, Xia YJ, et al. Association between polymorphisms of the CYP11A1 gene and polycystic ovary syndrome in Chinese women. Mol Biol Rep. 2012;39(8):8379-8385. doi:10.1007/s11033-012-1688-7.
79. Witchel SF, Aston CE. The role of heterozygosity for CYP21 in the polycystic ovary syndrome. J Pediatr Endocrinol Metab. 2000;13(suppl 5):1315-1317.
80. Rahimi Z, Mohammadi MSE. The CYP17 MSP AI (T-34C) and CYP19A1 (Trp39Arg) variants in polycystic ovary syndrome: a case-control study. Int J Reprod Biomed. 2019;17(3):201-208. doi:10.18502/ijrm.v17i3.4519.
81. Carey AH, Waterworth D, Patel K, et al. Polycystic ovaries and premature male pattern baldness are associated with one allele of the steroid metabolism gene CYP17. Hum Mol Genet.1994;3(10):1873-1876. doi:10.1093/hmg/3.10.1873.
82. Ashraf S, Rasool SUA, Nabi M, Ganie MA, Masoodi SR, Amin S. Impact of rs2414096 polymorphism of CYP19 gene on susceptibility of polycystic ovary syndrome and hyperandrogenism in Kashmiri women. Sci

Rep. 2021;11(1):12942. doi:10.1038/s41598-021-92265-1.
83. Mehdizadeh A, Kalantar SM, Sheikhha MH, Aali BS, Ghanei A. Association of SNP rs.2414096 CYP19 gene with polycystic ovarian syndrome in Iranian women. Int J Reprod Biomed. 2017;15(8):491-496.
84. Miller WL. Steroidogenic acute regulatory protein (StAR), a novel mitochondrial cholesterol transporter. Biochim Biophys Acta. 2007;1771(6):663-676. doi:10.1016/j.bbalip.2007.02.012.
85. Kahsar-Miller MD, Conway-Myers BA, Boots LR, Azziz R. Steroidogenic acute regulatory protein (StAR) in the ovaries of healthy women and those with polycystic ovary syndrome. Am J Obstet Gynecol. 2001;185(6):1381-1387. doi:10.1067/mob.2001.118656.
86. Trapman J, Klaassen P, Kuiper GG, et al. Cloning, structure and expression of a cDNA encoding the human androgen receptor. Biochem Biophys Res Commun. 1988;153(1):241-248. doi:10.1016/s0006-291x(88)81214-2.
87. Chamberlain NL, Driver ED, Miesfeld RL. The length and location of CAG trinucleotide repeats in the androgen receptor N-terminal domain affect transactivation function. Nucleic Acids Res. 1994;22(15):3181-3186. doi:10.1093/nar/22.15.3181.
88. Mifsud A, Ramirez S, Yong EL. Androgen receptor gene CAG trinucleotide repeats in anovulatory infertility and polycystic ovaries. J Clin Endocrinol Metab. 2000;85(9):3484-3488. doi:10.1210/jcem.85.9.6832.
89. Deswal R, Yadav A, Dang AS. Sex hormone binding globulin - an important biomarker for predicting PCOS risk: a systematic review and meta-analysis. Syst Biol Reprod Med. 2018;64(1):12-24. doi:10.1080/19396368.2017.1410591.
90. Bérubé D, Séralini GE, Gagné R, Hammond GL. Localization of the human sex hormone-binding globulin gene (SHBG) to the short arm of chromosome 17 (17p12-p13). Cytogenet Cell Genet. 1990;54(1-2):65-67. doi:10.1159/000132958.
91. Dapas M, Sisk R, Legro RS, Urbanek M, Dunaif A, Hayes MG. Family-based quantitative trait meta-analysis implicates rare noncoding variants in DENND1A in polycystic ovary syndrome. J Clin Endocrinol Metab. 2019;104(9):3835-3850. doi:10.1210/jc.2018-02496.
92. Deswal R, Nanda S, Dang AS. Association of Luteinizing hormone and LH receptor gene polymorphism with susceptibility of polycystic ovary syndrome. Syst Biol Reprod Med. 2019;65(5):400-408. doi:10.1080/19396368.2019.1595217.
93. Laven JSE. Follicle stimulating hormone receptor (FSHR) polymorphisms and polycystic ovary syndrome (PCOS). Front Endocrinol (Lausanne). 2019;10:23. doi:10.3389/fendo.2019.00023.
94. Howles CM. Role of LH and FSH in ovarian function. Mol Cell Endocrinol. 2000;161(1-2):25-30. doi:10.1016/s0303-7207(99)00219-1.
95. Choi J, Smitz J. Luteinizing hormone and human chorionic gonadotropin: origins of difference. Mol Cell Endocrinol. 2014;383(1-2):203-213. doi:10.1016/j.mce.2013.12.009.
96. Jakimiuk AJ, Weitsman SR, Navab A, Magoffin DA. Luteinizing hormone receptor, steroidogenesis acute regulatory protein, and steroidogenic enzyme messenger ribonucleic acids are overexpressed in thecal and granulosa cells from polycystic ovaries. J Clin Endocrinol Metab. 2001;86(3):1318-1323. doi:10.1210/jcem.86.3.7318.
97. Ajmal N, Khan SZ, Shaikh R. Polycystic ovary syndrome (PCOS) and genetic predisposition: a review article. Eur J Obstet Gynecol Reprod Biol X. 2019;3:100060. doi:10.1016/j.eurox.2019.100060.
98. Ferk P, Perme MP, Gersak K. Insulin gene polymorphism in women with polycystic ovary syndrome. J Int Med Res. 2008;36(6):1180-1187. doi:10.1177/147323000803600603.

第五章 脂肪细胞因子与多囊卵巢综合征的相互作用

一、引言

脂肪组织从根本上维持着人体的平衡。脂肪组织释放的生物活性物质可调节葡萄糖和脂质代谢,以及能量和免疫系统活动。脂肪组织炎症会激活一些信号通路,这些信号通路已被证明会破坏代谢平衡。此外,生物活性物质的失调也会导致代谢异常和慢性疾病,尤其是在肥胖人群中。

脂肪因子是仅由脂肪组织产生的生物活性物质,而脂肪细胞因子则由包括脂肪细胞在内的多种细胞产生。产生脂肪细胞因子的其他组织器官包括卵巢、胎盘、肝脏、肾脏、肌肉、心脏、骨髓,此外,外周单核细胞也可以产生脂肪细胞因子。不过,为了避免混淆,在本综述中,"脂肪因子"这一名称指的是这些生物活性分子。

脂肪因子既可以促炎也可以抗炎。研究发现,肥胖会增加促炎性脂肪因子,减少抗炎性脂肪因子,从而长期维持低水平的炎症反应。全球大量研究表明,脂肪因子在多种全身性疾病的发病机制中发挥核心作用。此外,研究还证实,脂肪因子在肥胖和肥胖相关疾病的病因中起着关键作用。脂肪因子的各种特征见表5.1和图5.1。

表5.1 脂肪因子的产生部位及其与炎症、生殖功能和代谢功能的关系

脂肪因子	产生部位	与炎症的关系	与生殖功能的关系	与代谢功能的关系
脂连蛋白	胎盘脂肪细胞、成骨细胞、心肌细胞	抗炎	青春期启动与调节	脂肪酸氧化、胰岛素敏感性、糖代谢
瘦素	胎盘脂肪组织	调节免疫反应	促性腺激素分泌的调节	调节食物摄入量、脂代谢和糖代谢
抵抗素	外周血单核细胞、胎盘	调节炎症反应	卵巢功能与PCOS	胰岛素抵抗
内脂素	脂肪组织、肝脏、肌肉、肾脏、心脏、骨髓、胎盘	调节炎症反应	卵巢功能与PCOS	胰岛素抵抗、糖代谢
爱帕琳肽	大脑、子宫、卵巢、肺、内皮小动脉	调节炎症反应	卵巢功能与PCOS	促进雌二醇和孕酮的分泌
网膜素	内脏脂肪组织库	在促炎条件下上调	卵巢功能与PCOS	胰岛素抵抗、糖代谢
趋化素	脂肪组织G蛋白偶联受体	卵巢类固醇生成的负控因子	卵巢功能与PCOS	抑制FSH诱导的p450酶的表达

注:FSH,卵泡刺激素;PCOS,多囊卵巢综合征。

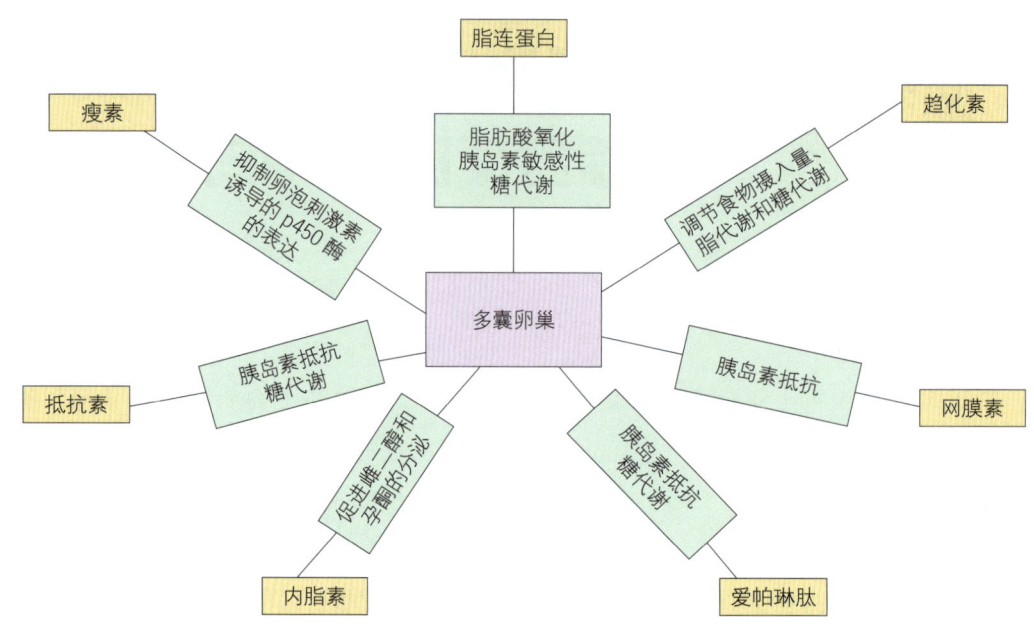

图 5.1　各种脂肪细胞因子对多囊卵巢综合征的影响示意

多囊卵巢综合征（PCOS）是育龄女性最常见的内分泌代谢疾病。PCOS 患者更容易出现代谢问题，如 2 型糖尿病（type 2 diabetes mellitus，T2DM）、胰岛素抵抗（IR）和脂肪组织功能障碍。PCOS 患者合并 T2DM 的患病率是普通人群的 10 倍，肥胖的 PCOS 患者的葡萄糖耐受不良率比普通人群高 30%～50%。10%～25% 的普通人群有 IR，而 PCOS 患者出现 IR 的风险要比前者高出 2～3 倍。此外，PCOS 患者的肥胖率也高于非 PCOS 患者。若 PCOS 合并肥胖，症状会明显加重，但其发病机制尚不清楚。许多研究证实，肥胖的 PCOS 患者经常会出现脂肪组织功能失调，从而导致脂肪因子水平改变，这表明脂肪因子对 PCOS 患者有一定的作用。

一种理论认为，PCOS 患者体内脂肪因子水平的变化是由肥胖而非 PCOS 引起的。这体现在脂肪因子水平与体重指数（BMI）成正比，而 PCOS 患者的 BMI 更高。此外，一项荟萃分析（meta-analysis，MA）发现，患有 PCOS 的女性超重肥胖和向心性肥胖的发病率更高。一项 MA 纳入了非肥胖 PCOS 患者的数据，以证实肥胖对脂肪因子水平的影响，并评估 PCOS 与脂肪因子水平之间的联系。研究结果表明，非肥胖型 PCOS 患者的脂肪因子水平发生了变化；因此，研究结果否定了肥胖而非 PCOS 导致 PCOS 患者脂肪因子水平变化的理论。这意味着，无论体重如何，脂肪因子都可能在 PCOS 患者中发挥作用；然而，脂肪因子导致 PCOS 发生的确切机制尚不清楚。

越来越多的研究热衷于测定 PCOS 患者体内循环脂肪因子水平的变化。人们还推测，这些脂肪因子可能是 PCOS 的病因之一。在已有的系统性回顾性研究和荟萃分析中，内脏脂肪特异性丝氨酸蛋白酶抑制剂（vaspin）、抵抗素（resistin）、瘦素（leptin）、趋化素（chemerin）、网膜素（omentin）、脂连蛋白（adiponectin）和内脂素（visfatin）与 PCOS 有关（表 5.2）。

表 5.2　脂肪因子在多囊卵巢综合征中作用的荟萃分析结果

研究项目	研究数量	受试者人数（病例组/对照组）	在多囊卵巢综合征中的研究发现	结论
Lin 等，2021 年	71	5015（2495/2520）	血清脂连蛋白＝较低 血清趋化素和抵抗素＝较高 爱帕琳肽和网膜素＝无变化	无论肥胖程度如何，脂肪因子水平失调都可能在 PCOS 的发生和发展过程中起到关键作用
Mehrabani 等，2021 年	77	8239	血清 vaspin、趋化素和抵抗素＝较高 血清爱帕琳肽水平＝无变化	血清 vaspin、趋化素和抵抗素的水平可用来预测 PCOS 的发生
Mansoori 等，2022 年	22	2256（1191/1065）	血清和卵泡液中趋化素及 mRNA 表达＝较高	趋化素可能与 PCOS 和 BMI 都有关联
Wang 等，2022 年	8	897（524/373）	血清趋化素＝较高	趋化素可能是 PCOS 的病因之一
Raeisi 等，2021 年	38	4328（2424/1904）	血清抵抗素＝较高	血清抵抗素可能在 PCOS 发病机制中发挥作用
Seth 等，2021 年	35	3782（2015/1767）	血清瘦素＝无变化（在方法学质量较高的研究中） 血清瘦素＝较高（在方法学质量较低的研究中）	在方法学质量较高的研究中，血清瘦素与患 PCOS 的风险无关。需要进行更多的研究
Zheng 等，2017 年	19	1889（991/898）	血清瘦素＝较高	瘦素水平较高与 PCOS 患者的 IR、代谢紊乱、不孕症甚至心血管疾病风险有关，这表明瘦素可能在 PCOS 的发生和发展中发挥作用
Tang 等，2017 年	10	1264（733/531）	血清网膜素 -1＝较低	血清网膜素 -1 可能与 PCOS 的发病机制有关
Li 等，2014 年	38	3598（1944/1654）	血清脂连蛋白＝较低	血液中的脂连蛋白水平可能在 PCOS 的发病过程中起到一定的作用
Sun 等，2015 年		1341（695/646）	血清内脂素＝较高	血清内脂素可作为 PCOS 的生物标志物

注：BMI，体重指数；IR，胰岛素抵抗；PCOS，多囊卵巢综合征；vaspin，内脏脂肪特异性丝氨酸蛋白酶抑制剂。

尽管如此，相关文献仍然很少，而且不完整，结果也不一致。研究人员仍在努力弄清每种脂肪因子在 PCOS 中的作用。因此，脂肪因子在 PCOS 中的作用是目前的研究热点。脂肪因子与 PCOS 之间相互作用的研究结果可能有助于临床医师更好地诊断和管理 PCOS 及其相关问题。本章将对脂肪因子与 PCOS 之间相互作用有关的现有证据进行综述。

二、脂连蛋白

脂连蛋白是一种 30 kDa 的蛋白质，主要由脂肪细胞分泌，但也有一部分由成骨细胞、胎盘和心肌细胞产生。它具有抗炎、抗动脉粥样硬化和胰岛素增敏的特性。肥胖是 PCOS 的一个特征，它会通过改变脂连蛋白受体的表达来影响脂连蛋白的敏感性。肥胖会引起 IR，从而加剧 PCOS 女性的高胰岛素血症。此外，脂连蛋白基因多态性在 PCOS 中更为普遍。

在患有 PCOS 的肥胖女性中，低水平的脂连蛋白大多与 PCOS 和肥胖的存在或相互作用有关。胰岛素抵抗与脂连蛋白水平相关，有荟萃分析进一步证实了这一点。与此相反，还有几项研究报告称血清脂连蛋白水平与 IR 之间没有联系。这些相互矛盾的研究结果很可能是因为不同人群在肥胖和 IR 方面存在遗传差异。

超重/肥胖的 PCOS 患者血清中的脂连蛋白水平明显较低。同样，克罗地亚的 PCOS 患者血清中的脂连蛋白水平也明显低于健康女性。一项荟萃分析表明，非肥胖的 PCOS 女性的脂连蛋白水平也较低。

有关脂连蛋白的遗传学和功能学研究表明，脂连蛋白水平降低是导致代谢综合征（metabolic syndrome，MetS）、T2DM、IR、PCOS，甚至动脉粥样硬化发生的原因之一。由于发现脂连蛋白具有抗炎作用，因此在肥胖和 PCOS 等低度慢性炎症的情况下，脂连蛋白可能会减少。据报道，脂连蛋白能刺激白细胞介素-10（interleukin-10，IL-10）和 IL-1 受体拮抗剂的分泌，这两种物质都具有抗炎作用，同时还能抑制细胞因子（促炎）的产生。此外，脂连蛋白还能通过抑制肝糖异生来促进胰岛素分泌。因此，在肥胖和 PCOS 等炎症情况下，低水平的脂连蛋白可能可以解释炎症的发生。不过，PCOS 女性患者体内脂连蛋白的作用机制还需要进一步探索。

三、瘦素

瘦素是一种由 167 个氨基酸组成的产物，主要由白色脂肪组织分泌，但其他器官也会分泌。已证实瘦素具有多种功能，包括调节食物摄入量、促进肝细胞葡萄糖和促性腺激素分泌、调节免疫反应，以及抑制脂肪组织内的脂肪生成。血液循环中的瘦素水平取决于脂肪组织的含量。瘦素水平与黄体生成素（LH）和促性腺激素释放激素（GnRH）的分泌相关。

根据一项荟萃分析，非肥胖型 PCOS 患者血液循环中的瘦素水平要明显高于正常人。数项研究发现，PCOS 患者的瘦素浓度高于对照组。还有一项研究报道，PCOS 患者与对照组患者的血清瘦素水平没有差异。

一项研究发现，与对照组相比，PCOS 患者血液中的瘦素水平明显高于正常人，而与 BMI 分层无关，这意味着 PCOS 患者血清瘦素水平升高的原因并非体重增加。作为一种抗肥胖激素，瘦素在减少食物摄入、促进脂肪氧化、提高胰岛素敏感性方面发挥着中枢和外周调节作用。患有 PCOS 的肥胖女性体内瘦素水平升高可能与肥胖及 PCOS 相关的高胰岛素血症状态有关。瘦素通过促进类固醇生成和阻断 GnRH 的神经肽 Y 分泌，导致 GnRH 和 LH 水平升高，进而诱发高雄激素血症（HA）。

多项研究表明，肥胖者体内瘦素的作用模式被打乱；尽管血液中这种激素的水平升高，但食欲却得不到控制，因此产生了瘦素抵抗。IR 或高胰岛素血症可能是影响血清瘦素水平的诱发因素。据观察，胰岛素可直接诱导体外脂肪组织中瘦素 mRNA 的生成，这表明胰岛素可能是 PCOS 患者体内瘦素分泌的刺激因素。高胰岛素血症和胰岛素抵抗常与瘦素抵抗有关，从而导致能量平衡问题和各种代谢紊乱的发生。

不过，目前还没有确切的证据表明瘦素在 PCOS 的发病过程中扮演了什么角色。Escobar-Morreale 等（1997）发现 HA 可提高瘦素水平，而瘦素可影响 PCOS 患者的性腺轴。此外，瘦素浓度升高会降低胰岛素基因启动子的转录活性和外周器官中胰岛素受体的磷酸化水平，从而抑制胰岛素原 mRNA 的表达。

四、抵抗素

抵抗素是一种脂肪细胞因子，主要产生于人类的巨噬细胞和脂肪细胞。最初的报道称，抵抗素可以促进 IR，从而导致糖尿病；然而，人们对其在肥胖、胰岛素敏感性和 T2DM 中的作用还不完全了解。研究发现，在肥胖和代谢性疾病（如 PCOS）患者中，循环中的抵抗素水平会升高。许多已发表的研究数据表明抵抗素与胰岛素抵抗之间有联系。还有一些研究表明，抵抗素会直接导致内皮功能障碍。后者可刺激 IL-6 和 TNX-α 等促炎细胞因子的分泌。

在最近的一项荟萃分析中，Lin 等（2021）报道，非肥胖型 PCOS 患者的抵抗素水平明显升高。一项研究报告称，经二甲双胍治疗后，PCOS 患者的血清抵抗素水平明显降低。同样，另一项荟萃分析表明，PCOS 组的血清抵抗素水平明显高于对照组。

克罗地亚的一项研究报告显示，患有 PCOS 的女性体内抵抗素水平明显高于健康女性。同一项研究发现，PCOS 患者体内的抵抗素水平与稳态模型评估-胰岛素抵抗指数（homeostasis model assessment-IR，HOMA-IR）或雄激素水平之间没有相关性。

抵抗素基因与 PCOS 相关的 D19S884 多态性标记很接近，两者可能都是 PCOS 的易感位点。印度的一项研究表明，抵抗素基因中的 420 C G（启动子区域）和 299 G A 多态性与 PCOS 的发生有关。这两种多态性与 T2DM 患者的脑血管疾病和 IR 的发生有明显关系，这也解释了 PCOS 患者出现 IR 的原因。目前，有关脂肪因子基因多态性及其在 PCOS 中功能的研究很少，而且结果不一致，需要进行更多的研究来确定其意义。

考虑到 PCOS 患者的肥胖问题，研究发现脂肪细胞表达的抵抗素 mRNA 大幅增加。此外，研究还观察到，在培养的人类卵泡膜细胞中，抵抗素可以增强 17α-羟化酶活性，而 17α-羟化酶活性增强是 PCOS 患者卵巢 HA 的标志；因此，抵抗素可能在 PCOS 的发病机制中发挥部分作用。尽管如此，要确定它在 PCOS 中的作用，还需要进行更多的研究。

五、内脂素

内脂素被认为是与 IL-6 和肿瘤坏死因子（tumor necrosis factor，TNF）相关的一种促炎性脂肪因子，而 IL-6 和 TNF 可能会导致与肥胖相关的胰岛素抵抗的发生。在生理环境下，一方面，内脂素的作用与胰岛素类似，可降低血糖水平；另一方面，过量的内脂素表达对预防肥胖、T2DM 和 PCOS 患者的高血糖和 IR 没有明显的效果。内脂素还能通过增加 TNF-α 和 IL-6 的释放来促进炎症活性，从而进一步提高 IR。土耳其的一项研究报告称，PCOS 患者的血清内脂素水平大大高于对照组。与基线值相比，二甲双胍治疗可以显著降低内脂素水平。血清内脂素水平与 BMI、腰围、甘油三酯、HOMA-IR 和胰岛素水平呈正相关。波兰的一项研究报告称，PCOS 患者血清内脂素水平与对照组相比无明显差异。一项荟萃分析发现，非肥胖型 PCOS 患者的血清内脂素水平明显升高。与此类似，另一项荟萃分析显示，PCOS 患者的血清内脂素水平显著高于对照组。分层分析和单因素分析表明，内脂素水平升高与 BMI、IR 或总睾酮率无关。

Behboudi-Gandevani 等（2017）证明超重/肥胖的 PCOS 女性体内的内脂素水平明显高于正常体重女性。这意味着 PCOS 女性的内脂素水平与肥胖有关。这种升高可以弥补内脂素信号的减少，从而增强靶组织对胰岛素的敏感性。此外，还有人提出，PCOS 女性体内的内脂素与炎症有关。Ozkaya 等（2010）发现，二甲双胍治疗 3 个月可降低 PCOS 患者的循环内脂素水平。其关键机制是二甲双胍提高了 PCOS 患者的胰岛素敏感性。因此，PCOS 患者的内脂素分泌增加可能是避免 IR 的一种补偿机制。此外，胰岛素敏感性越高，循环中的内脂素水平越低。一项研究发现，PCOS 患者无论消瘦还是肥胖，内脂素分泌量都有所增加，这表明内脂素升高是 PCOS 的固有特征。因此，内脂素可作为治疗 PCOS 的一种可能的生物标志物，并有助于识别高风险的 PCOS 患者。

胰岛素和糖代谢通过磷脂酰肌醇 3-激酶和蛋白激酶 B 途径影响内脂素的分泌。此外，内脂素和雄激素的增加共同形成了一个恶性循环，从而增加了患 PCOS 和其他内分泌相关疾病的风险。如要更好地了解内脂素的调控及其在肥胖和 PCOS 病理生理学中可能产生的影响，还需要进行更多的研究。

（一）爱帕琳肽

爱帕琳肽（Apelin）是一种由 36 个氨基酸构成的多肽（Apelin 最常见的异构体），最初源于（牛）胃提取物，是 G 蛋白偶联受体（即 APJ）的内源性配体。然而，除了胃，Apelin 的表达还见于脑、子宫、卵巢、肺等多种器官，甚至小动脉内皮。这表明，APJ/Apelin 系统可能在各种生理过程中发挥着重要作用。Apelin 与代谢疾病的进展、食欲中枢活动的调节、脂肪组织的生长及肥胖的发病机制有关。Apelin 通过增强肌肉和脂肪组织对葡萄糖的摄取和吸收来降低血糖水平。它还能提高细胞对胰岛素的敏感性。

脂肪组织中 Apelin 的表达和血液循环中的 Apelin 水平在 IR 和肥胖患者中更高。先前的研究已经证实，胰岛素会刺激 Apelin 的分泌，而 Apelin 却会抑制胰岛素的分泌。此外，炎症可在 Apelin 合成和受体调节中发挥积极作用。一项荟萃分析发现，PCOS 组和对照组的 Apelin 水平在统计学上没有显著差异。

PCOS 患者血清中的 Apelin 水平与 IR 之间是否存在关联仍有争议，但已发表的少量数据显示，Apelin 是 PCOS 卵巢功能障碍的一种特征，而不是胰岛素敏感性的标志。在人类卵泡、卵泡膜细胞、颗粒细胞和卵母细胞中已观察到 APJ 和 Apelin 的表达，体外研究也证明了 Apelin 在控制卵巢各种功能中的潜在作用。Apelin 还被证明能调节黄体溶解过程和卵母细胞的成熟。据观察，颗粒细胞中 Apelin 的 mRNA 水平与血浆卵泡刺激素水平呈负相关。虽然 Apelin 与月经周期的长短呈正相关，但它也可能扰乱激素水平，成为 PCOS 发病的根本原因。

人们在卵巢卵泡和颗粒细胞中发现了 Apelin 及其受体的表达。它们在血管生成和卵巢激素代谢中发挥着重要作用。这表明 Apelin 及其受体可能在卵泡发育过程中起着至关重要的作用。在 PCOS 中，Apelin 及其受体表达升高，从而引起月经周期紊乱，进而导致月经失调甚至无排卵。此外，据报道，在代谢紊乱（如 T2DM 和肥胖）的情况下，Apelin 也会增加，而这两种疾病都是 PCOS 的危险因素。

Kolan 等（2021）报告称 PCOS 组的 Apelin 水平明显低于健康组。PCOS 组的 Apelin 水平不受 BMI 或碳水化合物代谢因素的影响。然而，有关 Apelin 的研究结果并不全都一致，有的甚至是相互矛盾的。部分研究结果表明，在与 PCOS 相关的代谢异常疾病（如糖代谢异常）中，Apelin 具有预测作用。

PCOS 患者体内的脂肪因子含量明显较低，这可能有助于预测 PCOS 导致的代谢异常。为了证实这一观点，我们需要对 Apelin 进行更多研究。

（二）网膜素

网膜素又称内凝集素 -1，是一种新型脂肪因子，主要由内脏脂肪分泌。有报道称，与对照组相比，PCOS 女性的颗粒细胞和卵泡液中网膜素的表达量要高得多。大多数研究报告称，PCOS 女性血浆中网膜素水平和网膜素 mRNA 水平均较低。已发表的数据观察到血清网膜素与 HOMA-IR/ 空腹胰岛素呈反比关系。体外研究证实，高胰岛素血症可降低脂肪组织中网膜素的表达。激素水平的紊乱，主要是 HA，被认为是导致 PCOS 女性网膜素合成减少的一个关键因素。

网膜素的调控也可能是由炎症引起的，因为在炎症中网膜素的表达水平往往会发生变化，而 PCOS 被认为是一种促炎性疾病。颗粒细胞和卵泡液中网膜素表达增加，这表明卵巢水平的网膜素生成与胰岛素的作用无关，而是由其他机制调节的。据报道，与月经周期正常的女性相比，月经周期不规律的 PCOS 女性血清中网膜素的水平更高。这表明，脂肪因子的表达与排卵功能障碍之间呈正相关，这在 PCOS 中表现得尤为明显。

在人体脂肪细胞中，网膜素是一种胰岛素增敏激素。它还能减少 TNF 诱导的超氧化物的释放，从而起到抗炎作用。在患有 PCOS 的女性中，HA 和高胰岛素血症也可能导致网膜素浓度降低。

与体重正常的 PCOS 女性相比，超重 / 肥胖 PCOS 女性的网膜素水平要低得多。然而，在健康女性的不同 BMI 组别中，网膜素水平基本一致。尽管如此，有研究表明，肥胖和 PCOS 之间并没有统计学意义上的显著关联性，因此研究人员假设，除了 PCOS 和肥胖外，还有多种因素可能参与调节循环中网膜素-1 的水平。因此，还需要更多的研究来明确这种模糊的联系。

由于肥胖 PCOS 患者的网膜素水平发生了变化，网膜素水平的降低可能与 PCOS 患者的代谢异常有关。在某些研究中，网膜素与 PCOS 有关联，但要充分了解两者之间的联系，还需要做更多的工作。

六、趋化素

趋化素是一种多面性的脂肪细胞因子，存在于 G 蛋白偶联受体 CMKLR1 的配体中，是一种主要参与固有免疫和适应性免疫的促炎细胞因子。研究报告显示，在 PCOS 女性患者中，趋化素和 CMKLR1 在卵泡液和颗粒细胞中的 mRNA 水平都较高。趋化素在炎症和代谢综合征中的作用可能是 IR 和体内脂肪储存的病理生理机制。此外，作为一种脂肪因子，趋化素能调节胰岛素的敏感性和分泌，而胰岛素反过来又能增加脂肪组织中趋化素的释放。研究表明，肥胖的 PCOS 患者体内的趋化素水平较高，而且 PCOS 患者皮下和网膜脂肪组织储库中的趋化素 mRNA 表达量也大幅增加。其他几项研究也发现，肥胖的 PCOS 患者体内的趋化素水平较高，而这些患者同时还存在 IR。根据最近的一项荟萃分析，PCOS 组的血清趋化素水平大大高于对照组。

此外，趋化素水平还与胰岛素调节功能有关。脂肪量是趋化素水平高低的最重要的决定因素。Tan 等（2009）的研究表明，二甲双胍治疗 6 个月后，PCOS 患者的血清趋化素水平显著下降，同时 IR 也有所缓解。

一项研究发现，超重和体重正常的 PCOS 患者与对照组之间的血清趋化素水平没有明显的统计学差异。相比之下，另一项研究报告称，超重 PCOS 患者的趋化素水平大大高于体重正常的 PCOS 患者。研究发现，在 PCOS 患者中，趋化素与 BMI、甘油三酯、胰岛素和 HOMA-IR 呈正相关。这些研究结果表明，BMI 本身并不是循环趋化素水平的可靠预测指标。

这些研究结果的差异可能是由于在不同的 PCOS 患者人群中脂肪含量和脂肪组织的化学炎症反应不同，以及检测设置和卵巢体积较大的 PCOS 患者表型不同。此外，还有人提出，趋化素血清水平不一定代表不同类型和不同数量的脂肪组织所引起的变化。由于不同研究的结果差异很大，建议进一步详细研究趋化素、肥胖和 PCOS 之间的关系。

尽管在 PCOS 模型中得出的结果并不一致，但大多数研究都报告称，PCOS 女性脂肪组织和血浆中的趋化素水平都有所增加。已发表的文献表明，趋化素可能参与抑制窦状卵泡的生长，后者与高雄激素促炎状态相关，而高雄激素促炎状态正是 PCOS 的特征。

已提出的涉及 PCOS 的趋化素分子机制包括趋化素及其受体 chemR23 的转录和翻译，后者在 PCOS 患者的卵巢中明显升高。趋化素与 PCOS 参数，以及与其他过程之间的复杂联系值得进一步研究。

七、白脂素

白脂素是一种新发现的由白色脂肪组织产生的多肽。它能激活 G 蛋白 -cAMP-PKA 通路，促进肝脏产生葡萄糖，其水平在 IR 或肥胖时会异常升高。在患有 T2DM 的受试者中，白脂素水平明显高于对照组，而 IR 也与 T2DM 患者的白脂素水平有关。

土耳其的一项研究发现，PCOS 患者体内的白脂素含量大大高于对照组。相比之下，另一项研究发现，PCOS 患者和对照组之间的血清白脂素水平没有明显的统计学差异。不过，与同等的非 HA 和非 IR PCOS 组相比，HA 和 IR PCOS 组患者的血清白脂素水平明显较低。还有 2 项调查发现，PCOS 女性体内的白脂素水平大大高于对照组。根据 Chang 等（2019）的研究，PCOS 女性的白脂素水平与对照组相当。Alan 等（2019）假设白脂素通过干扰 IR 和炎症等病理生理途径，对 PCOS 的发展有重要作用。

白脂素的发现是针对 IR 相关的多种代谢疾病治疗的未来研究中最重要课题之一。尽管如此，目前的研究仍处于起步阶段，无法断定白脂素是否与 PCOS、胰岛素抵抗和代谢参数有关。因此，建议进行更多的调查。

八、结论

人们对脂肪因子在 PCOS 中的作用还没有明确的认识。关于它们在该疾病的病理生理学中的作用，还有很多东西需要学习。有趣的是，少部分研究发现，在 PCOS 中的脂肪因子（如白脂素和瘦素）水平会升高、降低或没有变化。关于它们在 PCOS 中的功能，已经得出了一些结论：

- 有些脂肪因子在卵巢上有受体，因此能直接发挥作用。
- 有几种脂肪因子是通过与雄激素和胰岛素相互作用而间接产生作用的。
- 由于大多数 PCOS 患者都是肥胖的，许多脂肪因子水平都不相同。
- 卵泡膜细胞和颗粒细胞参与了某些脂肪因子的合成。
- 促炎和抗炎脂肪因子的失衡可能会加重 PCOS 的症状。
- 脂肪因子的多态性可能会影响 PCOS 患者的脂肪因子水平。
- 脂肪因子也可能不是 PCOS 的病因，但 IR 和 HA 等代谢改变可能会导致脂肪组织失调，从而导致脂肪因子水平的变化。
- 从 PCOS 中恢复可能需要达到最佳的脂肪因子水平；因此需要进一步了解异常脂肪因子水平及其与 PCOS 的关系。
- 据报道，二甲双胍可通过平衡异常的脂肪因子水平（如趋化素、抵抗素、鸢尾素和内脂素）来治疗 PCOS 及其症状。二甲双胍可改善睾酮水平和提高胰岛素敏感性，而由于这些生化指标恢复正常，脂肪因子水平也会恢复正常。不过，二甲双胍对这些脂肪因子没有直接影响。为了确定二甲双胍是否能通过调节失调的脂肪因子水平来帮助治疗 PCOS，还需要开展更多的研究。

• 由于PCOS的确切机制尚不清楚，脂肪因子很可能在该疾病的发生和发展过程中起到了一定的作用。

脂肪因子似乎在健康和疾病中发挥着至关重要的作用，尤其是在PCOS中。脂肪因子与IR、肥胖、类固醇激素、血脂状况、肿瘤发病机制、内皮功能障碍、骨骼病理和不孕症之间的联系，说明这些生物活性物质在多种疾病的病理生理学中发挥着重要的作用。因此，需要进行更多的研究，以确定脂肪因子与PCOS之间的相互作用，并就脂肪因子参与PCOS得出结论。

参考文献

1. Xu X, Grijalva A, Skowronski A, van Eijk M, Serlie MJ, Ferrante Jr AW. Obesity activates a program of lysosomal-dependent lipid metabolism in adipose tissue macrophages independently of classic activation. Cell Metab. 2013;18(6):816-830.
2. Ezeh U, Chen IY, Chen YH, Azziz R. Adipocyte insulin resistance in PCOS: relationship with GLUT-4 expression and whole-body glucose disposal and β-cell function. J Clin Endocrinol Metab. 2020;105(7):e2408-e2420.
3. Reilly SM, Saltiel AR. Adapting to obesity with adipose tissue inflammation. Nat Rev Endocrinol. 2017;13(11):633-643.
4. Azamar-Llamas D, Hernandez-Molina G, Ramos-Avalos B, Furuzawa-Carballeda J. Adipokine contribution to the pathogenesis of osteoarthritis. Mediators Inflamm. 2017;2017:5468023.
5. Achari AE, Jain SK. Adiponectin, a therapeutic target for obesity, diabetes, and endothelial dysfunction. Int J Mol Sci. 2017;18(6):1321.
6. Shibata R, Ouchi N, Ohashi K, Murohara T. The role of adipokines in cardiovascular disease. J Cardiol. 2017;70(4):329-334.
7. Ouchi N, Parker JL, Lugus JJ, Walsh K. Adipokines in inflammation and metabolic disease. Nat Rev Immunol. 2011;11(2):85-97.
8. Maximus PS, Al Achkar Z, Hamid PF, Hasnain SS, Peralta CA. Adipocytokines: are they the theory of everything? Cytokine. 2020;133:155144.
9. Chen T, Wang F, Chu Z, et al. Serum CTRP3 levels in obese children: a potential protective adipokine of obesity, insulin sensitivity and pancreatic cell function. Diabetes Metab Syndr Obes. 2019;12:1923.
10. Baldani DP, Skrgatic L, Kasum M, Zlopasa G, Kralik Oguic S, Herman M. Altered leptin, adiponectin, resistin and ghrelin secretion may represent an intrinsic polycystic ovary syndrome abnormality. Gynecol Endocrinol. 2019;35(5):401-405.
11. Arikan Ş, Bahceci M, Tuzcu A, Kale E, Gökalp D. Serum resistin and adiponectin levels in young non-obese women with polycystic ovary syndrome. Gynecol Endocrinol. 2010;26(3):161-166.
12. Jahromi BN, Dabaghmanesh MH, Parsanezhad ME, Fatehpoor F. Association of leptin and insulin resistance in PCOS: a casecontrolled study. Int J Reprod Biomed. 2017;15(7):423.
13. Borsuk A, Biernat W, Zieba D. Multidirectional action of resistin in the organism. Postepy Hig Med Dosw. 2018;72:327-338.
14. Góralska M, Majewska-Szczepanik M, Szczepanik M. Immunological mechanisms involved in obesity and their role in metabolic syndrome. Postepy Hig Med Dosw. 2015;69:1384-1404.
15. Lin K, Sun X, Wang X, Wang H, Chen X. Circulating adipokine levels in nonobese women with polycystic ovary syndrome and in nonobese control women: a systematic review and meta-analysis. Front Endocrinol. 2021;11:537809.
16. Sarray S, Madan S, Saleh LR, Mahmoud N, Almawi WY. Validity of adiponectin-to-leptin and adiponectin-to-

resistin ratios as predictors of polycystic ovary syndrome. Fertil Steril. 2015;104(2):460-466.
17. Kralisch S, Klein J, Lossner U, et al. Interleukin-6 is a negative regulator of visfatin gene expression in 3T3-L1 adipocytes. Am J Physiol Heart Circ Physiol. 2005;289(4):E586-E590.
18. Sun Y, Wu Z, Wei L, Liu C, Zhu S, Tang S. High-visfatin levels in women with polycystic ovary syndrome: evidence from a meta-analysis. Gynecol Endocrinol. 2015;31(10):808-814.
19. Rak A, Drwal E, Rame C, et al. Expression of apelin and apelin receptor (APJ) in porcine ovarian follicles and in vitro effect of apelin on steroidogenesis and proliferation through APJ activation and different signaling pathways. Theriogenology. 2017;96:126-135.
20. Roche J, Ramé C, Reverchon M, et al. Apelin (APLN) regulates progesterone secretion and oocyte maturation in bovine ovarian cells. Reproduction. 2017;153(5):589-603.
21. Altinkaya SÖ, Nergiz S, Küçük M, Yüksel H. Apelin levels in relation with hormonal and metabolic profile in patients with polycystic ovary syndrome. Eur J Obstet Gynecol Reprod Biol. 2014;176:168-172.
22. Yang HY, Ma Y, Lu XH, et al. The correlation of plasma omentin-1 with insulin resistance in non-obese polycystic ovary syndrome. Ann Endocrinol (Paris). 2015;76(5):620-627.
23. Tang YL, Yu J, Zeng ZG, Liu Y, Liu JY, Xu JX. Circulating omentin-1 levels in women with polycystic ovary syndrome: a meta-analysis. Gynecol Endocrinol. 2017;33(3):244-249.
24. Özgen İT, Oruçlu Ş, Selek S, Kutlu E, Guzel G, Cesur Y. Omentin-1 level in adolescents with polycystic ovarian syndrome. Pediatr Int. 2019;61(2):147-151.
25. Fatima SS, Rehman R, Baig M, Khan TA. New roles of the multidimensional adipokine: chemerin. Peptides. 2014;62:15-20.
26. Wang Q, Leader A, Tsang BK. Inhibitory roles of prohibitin and chemerin in FSH-induced rat granulosa cell steroidogenesis. Endocrinology. 2013;154(2):956-967.
27. Bongrani A, Mellouk N, Rame C, et al. Ovarian expression of adipokines in polycystic ovary syndrome: a role for chemerin, omentin, and apelin in follicular growth arrest and ovulatory dysfunction? Int J Mol Sci. 2019;20(15):3778.
28. Spritzer PM, Lecke SB, Satler F, Morsch DM. Adipose tissue dysfunction, adipokines, and low-grade chronic inflammation in polycystic ovary syndrome. Reproduction. 2015;149(5):R219-R227.
29. Legro RS, Kunselman AR, Dodson WC, Dunaif A. Prevalence and predictors of risk for type 2 diabetes mellitus and impaired glucose tolerance in polycystic ovary syndrome: a prospective, controlled study in 254 affected women. J Clin Endocrinol Metab. 1999;84(1):165-169.
30. Jakubowicz D, Wainstein J, Homburg R. The link between polycystic ovarian syndrome and type 2 diabetes: preventive and therapeutic approach in Israel. Isr Med Assoc J. 2012;14(7):442-447.
31. Sirmans SM, Pate KA. Epidemiology, diagnosis, and management of polycystic ovary syndrome. Clin Epidemiol. 2014;6:1-13.
32. Lim SS, Davies MJ, Norman RJ, Moran LJ. Overweight, obesity and central obesity in women with polycystic ovary syndrome: a systematic review and meta-analysis. Hum Reprod Update. 2012;18(6):618-637.
33. Itoh H, Kawano Y, Furukawa Y, Matsumoto H, Yuge A, Narahara H. The role of serum adiponectin levels in women with polycystic ovarian syndrome. Clin Exp Obstet Gynecol. 2021;40(4):531-535.
34. Kumawat M, Ram M, Agarwal S, Singh V. Role of serum Leptin, insulin and other hormones in women with Polycystic ovarian syndrome. Indian J Clin Biochem. 2018;33:S88-S89.
35. Barrea L, Arnone A, Annunziata G, et al. Adherence to the Mediterranean diet, dietary patterns and body composition in women with polycystic ovary syndrome (PCOS). Nutrients. 2019;11(10):2278.
36. Mehrabani S, Arab A, Karimi E, Nouri M, Mansourian M. Blood circulating levels of adipokines in polycystic ovary syndrome patients: a systematic review and meta-analysis. Reprod Sci. 2021;28:3032-3050.
37. Raeisi T, Rezaie H, Darand M, et al. Circulating resistin and follistatin levels in obese and non-obese women with polycystic ovary syndrome: a systematic review and meta-analysis. PLoS One. 2021;16(3):e0246200.
38. Seth MK, Gulati S, Gulati S, et al. Association of leptin with polycystic ovary syndrome: a systematic review

and meta-analysis. J Obstet Gynaecol India. 2021;71:567-576.

39. Zheng SH, Du DF, Li XL. Leptin levels in women with polycystic ovary syndrome: a systematic review and a meta-analysis. Reprod Sci. 2017;24(5):656-670.
40. Wang X, Zhang Q, Zhang L, et al. Circulating chemerin levels in women with polycystic ovary syndrome: a meta-analysis. Gynecol Endocrinol. 2022;38:22-27.
41. Mansoori A, Amoochi-Foroushani G, Zilaee M, Hosseini SA, Azhdari M. Serum and follicular fluid chemerin and chemerin mRNA expression in women with polycystic ovary syndrome: systematic review and meta-analysis. Endocrinol Diabetes Metab. 2022;5:e00307.
42. Li S, Huang X, Zhong H, et al. Low circulating adiponectin levels in women with polycystic ovary syndrome: an updated meta-analysis. Tumour Biol. 2014;35(5):3961-3973.
43. Sun X, Wu X, Zhou Y, Yu X, Zhang W. Evaluation of apelin and insulin resistance in patients with PCOS and therapeutic effect of drospirenone-ethinylestradiol plus metformin. Med Sci Monit. 2015;21:2547.
44. Drolet R, Bélanger C, Fortier M, et al. Fat depot-specific impact of visceral obesity on adipocyte adiponectin release in women. Obesity. 2009;17(3):424-430.
45. Xita N, Georgiou I, Chatzikyriakidou A, et al. Effect of adiponectin gene polymorphisms on circulating adiponectin and insulin resistance indexes in women with polycystic ovary syndrome. Clin Chem. 2005;51(2):416-423.
46. Behboudi-Gandevani S, Tehrani FR, Yarandi RB, Noroozzadeh M, Hedayati M, Azizi F. The association between polycystic ovary syndrome, obesity, and the serum concentration of adipokines. J Endocrinol Invest. 2017;40(8):859-866.
47. Toulis KA, Goulis DG, Farmakiotis D, et al. Adiponectin levels in women with polycystic ovary syndrome: a systematic review and a meta-analysis. Hum Reprod Update. 2009;15:297-307.
48. Oliveira BS, Costa JA, Gomes ET, et al. Expression of adiponectin and its receptors (AdipoR1 and AdipoR2) in goat ovary and its effect on oocyte nuclear maturation in vitro. Theriogenology. 2017;104:127-133.
49. Febriza A, Ridwan R, As'ad Suryani, Kasim VN, Idrus HH. Adiponectin and its role in inflammatory process of obesity. Mol Cell Biomed Sci. 2019;3(2):60-66.
50. Kolan E, Boinska J, Socha MW. Adipokine levels and carbohydrate metabolism in patients diagnosed de novo with polycystic ovary syndrome. Qatar Med J. 2021;2021(2):34.
51. Baig M, Rehman R, Tariq S, Fatima SS. Serum leptin levels in polycystic ovary syndrome and its relationship with metabolic and hormonal profile in Pakistani females. Int J Endocrinol. 2014;2014:132908.
52. Veldhuis JD, Pincus SM, Garcia-Rudaz MC, Ropelato MG, Escobar ME, Barontini M. Disruption of the synchronous secretion of leptin, LH, and ovarian androgens in nonobese adolescents with the polycystic ovarian syndrome. J Clin Endocrinol Metab. 2001;86(8):3772-3778.
53. Escobar-Morreale HF, Serrano-Gotarredona J, Varela C, Garcia-Robles R, Sancho J. Circulating leptin concentrations in women with hirsutism. Fertil Steril. 1997;68(5):898-906.
54. Tan BK, Adya R, Farhatullah S, et al. Omentin-1, a novel adipokine, is decreased in overweight insulin-resistant women with polycystic ovary syndrome: ex vivo and in vivo regulation of omentin-1 by insulin and glucose. Diabetes. 2008;57(4):801-808.
55. Tarkun İ, Dikmen E, Çetinarslan B, Cantürk Z. Impact of treatment with metformin on adipokines in patients with polycystic ovary syndrome. Eur Cytokine Netw. 2010;21(4):272-277.
56. Urbanek M, Du Y, Silander K, et al. Variation in resistin gene promoter not associated with polycystic ovary syndrome. Diabetes. 2003;52(1):214-217.
57. Nambiar V, Vijesh VV, Lakshmanan P, Sukumaran S, Suganthi R. Association of adiponectin and resistin gene polymorphisms in South Indian women with polycystic ovary syndrome. Eur J Obstet Gynecol Reprod Biol. 2016;200:82-88.
58. Kunnari A, Ukkola O, Kesäniemi YA. Resistin polymorphisms are associated with cerebrovascular disease in Finnish Type 2 diabetic patients. Diabet Med. 2005;22(5):583-589.

59. Pine GM, Batugedara HM, Nair MG. Here, there and everywhere: resistin-like molecules in infection, inflammation, and metabolic disorders. Cytokine. 2018;110:442-451.
60. Kralisch S, Klein J, Lossner U, et al. Hormonal regulation of the novel adipocytokine visfatin in 3T3-L1 adipocytes. J Endocrinol. 2005;185(3):R1-R8.
61. Kern PA, Ranganathan S, Li C, Wood L, Ranganathan G. Adipose tissue tumor necrosis factor and interleukin-6 expression in human obesity and insulin resistance. Am J Physiol Endocrinol Metab. 2001;280(5):E745-E751.
62. Farshchian F, Tehrani FR, Amirrasouli H, et al. Visfatin and resistin serum levels in normal-weight and obese women with polycystic ovary syndrome. Int J Endocrinol Metab. 2014;12(3):e15503.
63. Tan BK, Chen J, Digby JE, Keay SD, Kennedy CR, Randeva HS. Increased visfatin mRNA and protein levels in adipose tissue and adipocytes in women with polycystic ovary syndrome (PCOS): parallel increase in plasma visfatin. J Clin Endocrinol Metab. 2006;91:5022-5028.
64. Lajunen TK, Purhonen AK, Haapea M, et al. Full-length visfatin levels are associated with inflammation in women with polycystic ovary syndrome. Eur J Clin Invest. 2012;42(3):321-328.
65. Ozkaya M, Cakal E, Ustun Y, Engin-Ustun Y. Effect of metformin on serum visfatin levels in patients with polycystic ovary syndrome. Fertil Steril. 2010;93(3):880-884.
66. Nawrocka J, Starczewski A. Effects of metformin treatment in women with polycystic ovary syndrome depends on insulin resistance. Gynecol Endocrinol. 2007;23(4):231-237.
67. Jiang T, Pan J, Ying SU, Zhou H, Qiu M, Xiaoyi LI. The relationship between polycystic ovary syndrome and vaspin, apelin and leptin. J Kunming Med Univ. 2016;37(10):41-46.
68. Zhu S, Sun F, Li W, et al. Apelin stimulates glucose uptake through the PI3K/Akt pathway and improves insulin resistance in 3T3-L1 adipocytes. Mol Cell Biochem. 2011;353(1):305-313.
69. Ma WY, Yu TY, Wei JN, et al. Plasma apelin: a novel biomarker for predicting diabetes. Clin Chim Acta. 2014;435:18-23.
70. Xu S, Tsao PS, Yue P. Apelin and insulin resistance: another arrow for the quiver? J Diabetes. 2011;3(3):225-231.
71. Karimi E, Moini A, Yaseri M, et al. Effects of synbiotic supplementation on metabolic parameters and apelin in women with polycystic ovary syndrome: a randomised double-blind placebo-controlled trial. Br J Nutr. 2018;119(4):398-406.
72. Kanwal S, Allahwasaya A, Anjum N, Fatima SS. Serum apelin levels in polycystic ovary syndrome and its relationship with adiposity profile in females. Prof Med J. 2021;28(6):902-906.
73. Chang CL, Huang SY, Hsu YC, Chin TH, Soong YK. The serum level of irisin, but not asprosin, is abnormal in polycystic ovary syndrome patients. Sci Rep. 2019;9(1):1-11.
74. Kurowska P, Barbe A, Różycka M, Chmielińska J, Dupont J, Rak A. Apelin in reproductive physiology and pathology of different species: a critical review. Int J Endocrinol. 2018;2018:9170480.
75. Zabetian-Targhi F, Mirzaei K, Keshavarz SA, Hossein-Nezhad A. Modulatory role of omentin-1 in inflammation: cytokines and dietary intake. J Am Coll Nutr. 2016;35(8):670-678.
76. Guvenc Y, Var A, Goker A, Kuscu NK. Assessment of serum chemerin, vaspin and omentin-1 levels in patients with polycystic ovary syndrome. J Int Med Res. 2016;44(4):796-805.
77. Kazama K, Usui T, Okada M, Hara Y, Yamawaki H. Omentin plays an anti-inflammatory role through inhibition of TNF- induced superoxide production in vascular smooth muscle cells. Eur J Pharmacol. 2012;686(1-3):116-123.
78. Yang X, Yao J, Wei Q, et al. Role of chemerin/CMKLR1 in the maintenance of early pregnancy. Front Med. 2018;12(5):525-532.
79. Fatima SS, Bozaoglu K, Rehman R, Alam F, Memon AS. Elevated chemerin levels in Pakistani men: an interrelation with metabolic syndrome phenotypes. PLoS One. 2013;8(2):e57113.
80. Bauer S, Bala M, Kopp A, et al. Adipocyte chemerin release is induced by insulin without being translated to higher levels in vivo. Eur J Clin Invest. 2012;42(11):1213-1220.

81. Tan BK, Chen J, Farhatullah S, et al. Insulin and metformin regulate circulating and adipose tissue chemerin. Diabetes. 2009;58(9):1971-1977.
82. Guzel EC, Celik C, Abali R, et al. Omentin and chemerin and their association with obesity in women with polycystic ovary syndrome. Gynecol Endocrinol. 2014;30(6):419-422.
83. Martínez-García MÁ, Montes-Nieto R, Fernández-Durán E, Insenser M, Luque-Ramírez M, Escobar-Morreale HF. Evidence for masculinization of adipokine gene expression in visceral and subcutaneous adipose tissue of obese women with polycystic ovary syndrome (PCOS). J Clin Endocrinol Metab. 2013;98(2):E388-E396.
84. Kort DH, Kostolias A, Sullivan C, Lobo RA. Chemerin as a marker of body fat and insulin resistance in women with polycystic ovary syndrome. Gynecol Endocrinol. 2015;31(2):152-155.
85. Romere C, Duerrschmid C, Bournat J, et al. Asprosin, a fasting-induced glucogenic protein hormone. Cell. 2016;165(3):566-579.
86. Zhang L, Chen C, Zhou N, Fu Y, Cheng X. Circulating asprosin concentrations are increased in type 2 diabetes mellitus and independently associated with fasting glucose and triglyceride. Clin Chim Acta. 2019;489:183-188.
87. Wang Y, Qu H, Xiong X, et al. Plasma asprosin concentrations are increased in individuals with glucose dysregulation and correlated with insulin resistance and first-phase insulin secretion. Mediators Inflamm. 2018;2018:9471583.
88. Deniz R, Yavuzkir S, Ugur K, et al. Subfatin and asprosin, two new metabolic players of polycystic ovary syndrome. J Obstet Gynaecol. 2021;41(2):279-284.
89. Jiang Y, Liu Y, Yu Z, Yang P, Zhao S. Serum asprosin level in different subtypes of polycystic ovary syndrome: a cross-sectional study. Rev Assoc Med Bras. 2021;67:590-596.
90. Alan M, Gurlek B, Yilmaz A, et al. Asprosin: a novel peptide hormone related to insulin resistance in women with polycystic ovary syndrome. Gynecol Endocrinol. 2019;35(3):220-223.
91. Li X, Liao M, Shen R, et al. Plasma asprosin levels are associated with glucose metabolism, lipid, and sex hormone profiles in females with metabolic-related diseases. Mediators Inflamm. 2018;2018:7375294.

第六章 多囊卵巢综合征发病机制中氧化应激和慢性炎症的相互作用

一、引言

生殖过程需要卵泡的不断发育。为了实现这种发育，每个动情周期都会发生包括卵巢、子宫和子宫内膜的一系列结构变化。除了这些变化外，基础体温也有波动，与子宫内膜厚度的改变相对应。此外，精子进入女性生殖系统后，如果在 24 小时内有卵子存在，就会发生三步过程，这一过程被称为卵子的"受精"或妊娠。着床是一个非常重要的过程，它是受精后成功怀孕的关键。从颗粒细胞成熟到受精卵着床的整个过程都需要特定的环境来获得生殖能力。在卵泡发育、卵母细胞成熟和胚胎发育过程中，适度的活性氧（reactive oxidant species，ROS）对信号转导途径至关重要。

二、氧化和抗氧化系统

适度生成的 ROS 是卵母细胞成熟所必需的；然而，不适当的氧化剂水平会使卵母细胞质量下降，对生殖结果产生负面影响。

线粒体在产生能量的过程中会产生自由基，这些自由基如果被抗氧化剂对抗，就不会产生有害影响。因此，氧化环境的平衡和恢复对卵母细胞的自然渐进生长、细胞完整性和生殖活动所需的激素平衡至关重要。

卵母细胞随女性年龄增长而老化和持续的心理压力是影响卵母细胞受精能力的两个主要风险因素。临近绝经期时，卵巢储备功能会下降，导致激素的稳定性和卵母细胞的功能下降，而这两者对生育力来说是至关重要的。普遍认为，随着卵母细胞年龄的增加，氧化应激（oxidative stress，OS）也会增加，并导致卵母细胞质量下降。大量研究表明，多囊卵巢综合征（PCOS）患者存在 OS，血清中氨基酰脯氨酸二肽酶的表达和活性升高，总氧化剂水平升高。PCOS 通常与炎症、OS、胰岛素抵抗（IR）（无论患者是否肥胖）和卵泡成熟度差有关。

三、氧化应激和慢性炎症

慢性炎症的定义是，组织损伤造成持续且不受控制的细胞因子的产生和分泌，导致炎症未得到解决。慢性炎症会产生过量的 ROS，使细胞的抗氧化能力下降，从而诱发 OS。在持续的炎症过程中，NF-κB-p65 磷酸化的增加会促进还原型烟酰胺腺嘌呤二核苷酸磷酸（reduced nicotinamide adenine dinucleotide phosphate，NADPH）氧化酶的表达，进而产生大量的氧自由基。这些自由基通过超氧化物歧化酶（superoxide dismutase，SOD）的酶促作用转化为 H_2O_2，然后 H_2O_2 自由地进入细胞的细胞质，激活 NF-κB-p65 磷酸化，导致促炎细胞因子［肿瘤坏死因子-α（TNF-α）和白细胞介素-6（IL-6）］过度产生。

某些细胞因子已被证实会导致卵母细胞成熟缺陷。代谢综合征（包括肥胖、高胰岛素血症和 IR）伴随着慢性炎症状态和细胞因子水平的升高。体重指数（BMI）的增加已被证明会对 PCOS 患者的生殖结果产生负面影响。肥胖是一种低度慢性炎症，会导致 OS 并引发代谢疾病和神经系统慢性疾病。众所周知，OS 可诱导局部炎症，导致细胞因子的产生增加。从肥胖的角度来看，沉积在脂肪细胞中的循环甘油三酯增加导致脂肪细胞肥大。这导致脂肪细胞因缺氧而坏死。因此，单核细胞趋化因子 1（MCP-1/CCL2）和烟酰胺磷酸核糖转移酶（nicotinamide phosphoribosyltransferase，NAMPT）的分泌促使巨噬细胞和辅助性 T 细胞等免疫细胞从血液循环中渗入脂肪组织。巨噬细胞相继产生促炎细胞因子和促炎白细胞介素（分别为 TNF-α 和 IL-6）。这些细胞因子激活了 NF-κB 信号转导通路，细胞因子的产生开始了恶性循环。瘦素和脂质运载蛋白等其他脂肪因子也会分泌，以促进 TNF-α 和 IL-6 的释放。血液循环中存在的细胞因子和脂肪因子会引发包括卵巢在内的身体其他组织产生炎症的级联反应。

胰岛素信号通过招募蛋白酪氨酸激酶受体发挥作用，从而维持胰岛素敏感性。在 PCOS 患者中，过度的丝氨酸磷酸化活动会抑制酪氨酸激酶受体的功能，导致 PCOS 患者出现 IR。此外，它还会影响 P450c17 酶的活性，从而导致 PCOS 女性体内产生高雄激素血症（HA）。高胰岛素血症还会增强黄体生成素（LH）对卵巢间质细胞的作用，导致雄激素分泌增加。在 PCOS 患者中，IR 的发生率相当高，为 50%～70%。由于高血糖和游离脂肪酸升高会产生 ROS，因此 IR 也会促进 OS 的产生。

四、氧化应激与多囊卵巢综合征

ROS 经常被认为是一把"双刃剑"。它们作为第二信使的功能对于细胞内信号级联的发生至关重要，但过量的 ROS 又会对细胞过程产生影响。常见的 ROS 有超氧阴离子（O_2^-）、过氧化氢（H_2O_2）和羟基（–OH）。线粒体是产生 ROS 的主要细胞器，因为它参与了电子传递链反应的能量产生途径。H_2O_2 本身并无害处，但它很容易穿过生物细胞膜，分解成高活性的 -OH 自由基。

人体确实可以通过抗氧化剂［如 SOD、过氧化氢酶（catalase，CAT）、谷胱甘肽过氧化物酶（glutathione peroxidase，GPx）和谷胱甘肽还原酶（glutathione reductase，GSR）］来抵御体内产生的 ROS。除 GPx 外，它们都是主要的防御蛋白。GPx 具有过氧化物酶活性，与氧化还原酶、核酶和维生素 E（vitamin E，VE）一起作为二级防御蛋白保护机体。

ROS 是细胞功能顺利运行的一个重要因素，但它也能通过与细胞中的各种蛋白

第六章　多囊卵巢综合征发病机制中氧化应激和慢性炎症的相互作用

质相互作用诱发细胞氧化损伤。细胞膜、细胞器，特别是 DNA 中的大分子很容易成为 ROS 的攻击目标。大量产生的 OS 常常通过各种途径影响卵母细胞的成熟。

在 PCOS 患者中，OS 可能会导致 IR 的发生。高氧化环境会激活蛋白激酶，诱导胰岛素受体底物（insulin receptor substrate，IRS）的丝氨酸/苏氨酸成分磷酸化，并抑制其典型的酪氨酸磷酸化，从而诱导 IRS 的降解。

DNA 氧化可能是 PCOS 的另一个特征。与胞嘧啶、胸腺嘧啶和腺嘌呤相比，鸟嘌呤残基具有更高的氧化潜能。产生能量的电子传递链产生的 O_2^- 引起的 ROS 暴发，组蛋白防御功能的缺失，以及现有不存在或微不足道的修复机制，都对线粒体 DNA 构成了极大的威胁。过氧化氢的大量增加会导致 DNA 链断裂，使 PCOS 女性的卵母细胞成熟失败。

另一种观点认为，OS 与 PCOS 之间呈负相关。PCOS 所表现出的因素会导致 OS，而 OS 又会导致 IR 和高胰岛素血症。这一理论尚未得到很好的证实；然而，PCOS 的病因被认为是多因素的，而 PCOS 的发病机制是基因变异导致细胞的生理功能无法保持。在这些临床病例中，氧化剂和 ROS 之间的失衡会产生明显的影响，如糖耐量减低、2 型糖尿病，以及高血压、血脂异常和内皮功能障碍的风险增加（图 6.1）。

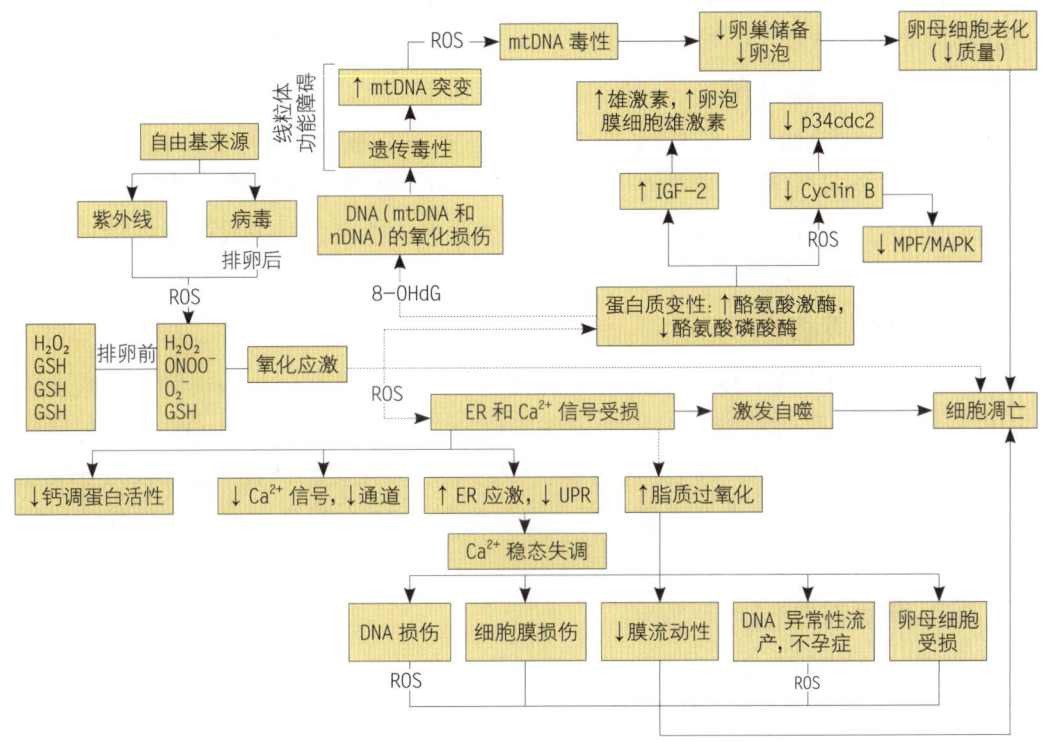

H_2O_2，过氧化氢；GSH，谷胱甘肽；$ONOO^-$，过氧亚硝基阴离子；O_2^-，超氧阴离子；mtDNA，线粒体 DNA；nDNA，核 DNA；8-OHdG，8-羟基脱氧鸟苷；ER，内质网；IGF-2，胰岛素样生长因子 -2；Cyclin B，细胞周期蛋白 B；MPF，M 期促进因子；MAPK，丝裂原活化蛋白激酶；ROS，活性氧；UPR，未折叠蛋白反应。

图 6.1　氧化应激对卵母细胞发育的影响

五、活性氧对多囊卵巢综合征患者细胞功能的影响

（一）转录因子激活

促炎细胞因子和脂肪因子的表达、细胞分化和凋亡都受转录因子（AP-1、p53 和 NF-κB）的调控。如前所述，PCOS 是一种同时存在低度炎症和炎性细胞因子升高的状态，通常以 C 反应蛋白（C-reactive protein，CRP）、TNF-α、IL-6 和 IL-18 来衡量。

（二）蛋白激酶激活

细胞通过激活蛋白激酶对各种细胞外信号和压力做出反应，促使细胞损伤或死亡（坏死或凋亡）。

增加的 ROS 会触发丝裂原活化蛋白激酶信号通路，通过增强酪氨酸激酶受体、蛋白酪氨酸激酶、细胞因子受体和生长因子受体的活性，成为基因转录的主要调节因子。ROS 还能激活其他通路，如 c-Jun N-末端激酶（c-Jun N-terminal kinases，JNK）和 p38 通路，它们通过影响各种细胞因子、生长因子、炎症酶、基质金属蛋白酶和免疫球蛋白的基因转录来调节其表达。

在 PCOS 患者中，OS 会激活蛋白激酶，进而通过诱导丝氨酸/苏氨酸磷酸化和抑制 IRS 的酪氨酸磷酸化来降解 IRS（图 6.2）。

（三）离子通道开放

随着 ROS 的增加，Ca^{2+} 从内质网释放出来，导致细胞内 Ca^{2+} 稳态失调。细胞质 Ca^{2+} 过高会对线粒体膜的稳定性产生不利影响，导致腺苷三磷酸（adenosine triphosphate，ATP）合成减少，使细胞陷入坏死状态。这可能是 PCOS 患者卵母细胞不能有效成熟的原因之一。

（四）蛋白质氧化

OS 可直接氧化氨基酸侧链，将其转化为羰基产物，从而轻易地破坏氨基酸。羰基产物无法发挥蛋白质的功能，因此会出现蛋白质功能障碍，这也是 OS 和疾病导致蛋白质功能障碍的一个原因。PCOS 患者血清中的晚期氧化蛋白产物（advanced oxidation protein products，AOPP）水平明显升高，被认为是 ROS 介导蛋白质损伤的新型生物标志物。

（五）脂质过氧化

ROS 会引发细胞膜和含脂细胞器（线粒体）中多不饱和脂肪酸侧链的脂质过氧化反应。这种损伤会导致细胞死亡。

在血清过氧化脂质浓度较高的 PCOS 患者中，氧化的低密度脂蛋白和丙二醛等生物标志物的水平会升高。

第六章　多囊卵巢综合征发病机制中氧化应激和慢性炎症的相互作用

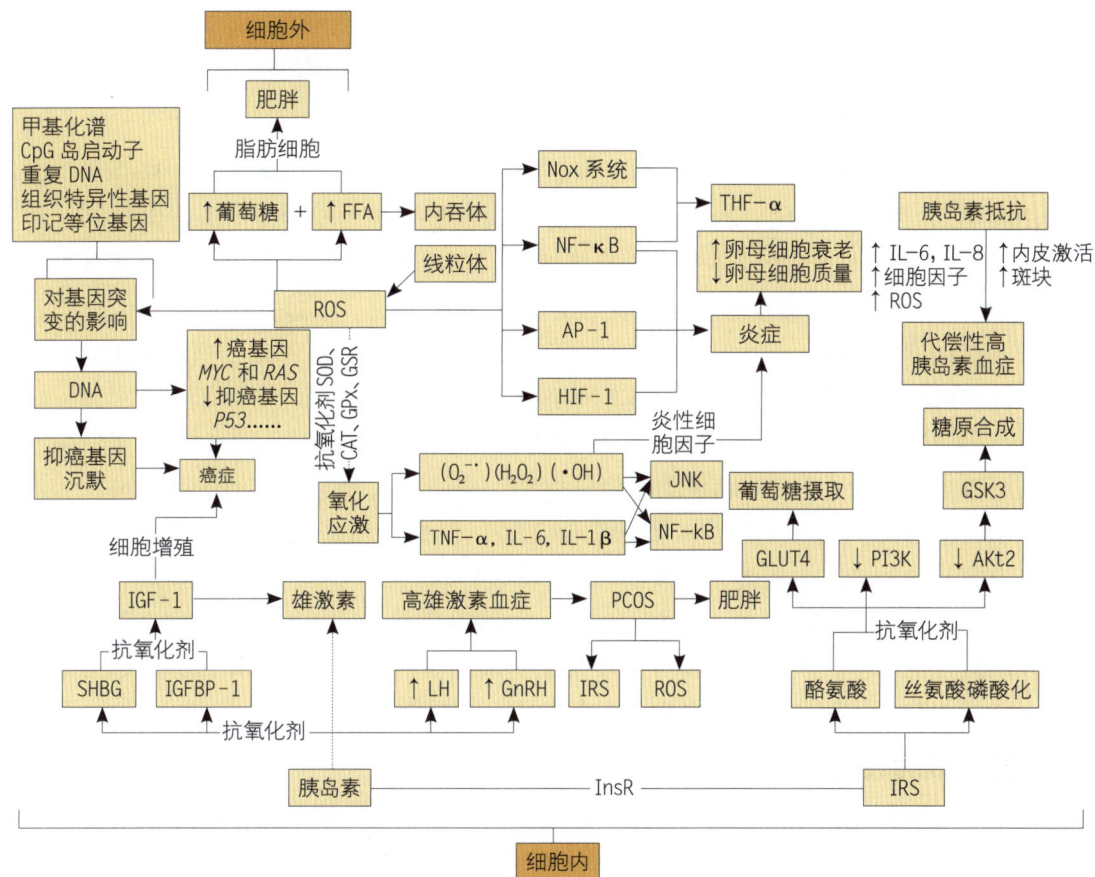

Akt，蛋白激酶 B；AP-1，激活蛋白-1；FFA，游离脂肪酸；GLUT4，葡萄糖转运体-4；GnRH，促性腺激素释放激素；HIF-1，缺氧诱导因子-1；IGFBP-1，胰岛素样生长因子结合蛋白-1；IGF-1，胰岛素样生长因子-1；IL，白细胞介素；InsR，胰岛素受体；IRS，胰岛素受体底物；JNK，c-Jun N-末端激酶；LH，黄体生成素；NF-κB，细胞核因子-κB；Nox，烟酰胺腺嘌呤二核苷酸磷酸氧化酶系统；PI3K，磷脂酰肌醇 3-激酶；ROS，活性氧；SHBG，性激素结合球蛋白；TNF-α，肿瘤坏死因子-α。

图 6.2　多囊卵巢综合征中氧化应激、炎症、胰岛素抵抗和高雄激素血症的相互作用

六、多囊卵巢综合征中检测到的氧化应激生物标志物

公认的与 PCOS 发病机制有关的生物标志物是丙二醛和一氧化氮（氧化剂）。不过，科学家们对总抗氧化能力（total antioxidant capacity，TAC）、SOD、GPx、VE、VC 和 GSR 等指标和抗氧化剂也进行了研究。

（一）丙二醛

多不饱和脂肪酸的脂质过氧化是 OS 和 PCOS 的常见机制，丙二醛（malondialdehyde，MDA）是这种脂质过氧化反应的产物。因此，MDA 不仅在血清中，而且在 PCOS 患者的卵泡液中都可作为 OS 的生物标志物。肥胖和非肥胖 PCOS 患者的血清 MDA 浓度都

会升高。MDA 与肥胖、BMI 和年龄无关，是一种首选的生物标志物。PCOS 患者的卵泡 MDA 较高可能是由于孕酮分泌较低，而 LH : FSH 较高所致。

（二）一氧化氮

一氧化氮（nitric oxide，NO）是一种重要的自由基，也是一种细胞信号分子，所有生理和病理过程都需要适量的 NO。NO 合酶利用氧气和 NADPH 作为辅助因子，将 L-精氨酸转化为 NO。在免疫过程中，单核细胞、巨噬细胞和中性粒细胞也会通过吞噬活动释放 NO。NO 的半衰期很短，因此很难在体内检测到。不过，它在血管中充当神经递质，在调节血管张力、血压、血管修复和炎症方面发挥重要作用。当 NO 达到毒性水平时，它可能会与其他炎症因子一起影响细胞结构。

在代谢良好的年轻 PCOS 患者中，高浓度 NO（低浓度亚硝酸盐）和纤维蛋白原水平升高可能成为 IR 相关血管病变的生物标志物。亚硝酸盐与硝酸盐的浓度比可作为内皮源性 NO 的指标。这些机制与年龄和肥胖无关，但是，当高 BMI 和 IR 同时存在时，就会成为容易导致 PCOS 的混杂因素。

此外，人们还发现 NO 与 OS 共存。饮食中硝酸盐摄入量的增加会影响血浆中亚硝酸盐和硝酸盐的水平，反映为内源性 NO 生成的增加。因此可以得出结论，亚硝酸盐水平低可能是 OS 的致病因素，导致 PCOS 患者的内皮损伤。

（三）晚期糖基化终末产物

晚期糖基化终末产物（AGE）又称"糖毒素"，是在美拉德反应（Maillard reaction）中产生的。在美拉德反应中，碳水化合物的羰基与脂质或蛋白质的氨基发生非酶促反应，诱发 OS，导致炎症和组织损伤。这进一步加强了美拉德反应，形成了一个恶性循环。在这些作用下，AGE 可能会改变酶的功能，诱发炎症改变，并通过 PCOS 患者多囊卵巢中的类固醇生物合成引起 IR。PCOS 女性体内发生的这种非典型类固醇生成导致雄激素合成旺盛和卵泡发育功能障碍。研究发现，PCOS 患者的血清 AGE 浓度和单核细胞中 AGE 受体的表达均有所升高，血清 AGE 的升高与睾酮呈正相关。

（四）黄嘌呤氧化酶

黄嘌呤氧化酶（xanthine oxidase，XO）通过酶促作用将次黄嘌呤氧化为黄嘌呤，并通过氧化过程将黄嘌呤催化为尿酸。这使得 XO 成为产生超氧阴离子自由基的潜在来源，导致了 OS。在心血管疾病、糖尿病、代谢综合征和 PCOS 患者中，都观察到了 XO 在人体中分解嘌呤和产生 ROS 的作用。研究发现，随着 OS 生物标志物的升高，抗氧化剂也随之下降。

（五）总抗氧化能力

总抗氧化能力（TAC）是指血液中存在的抗氧化剂抵御自由基的能力。TAC 与 PCOS 的关系尚未确定，一些研究发现 PCOS 患者的 TAC 充足，而另一些研究则表明

PCOS 患者的 TAC 水平较低。尽管如此，有一种理论认为，PCOS 患者体内 TAC 水平较高是对 OS 增加的一种补偿或反应性增加。

（六）超氧化物歧化酶

报道显示，SOD 与 PCOS 的关系是复杂的。与对照组相比，患有 PCOS 的女性体内 SOD 水平升高，这表明在 PCOS 女性患者体内氧化损伤的副产物会增加。SOD 是一种重要的抗氧化剂，它能识别并消除超氧阴离子（O_2^-），通过酶的作用将其转化为 H_2O_2，然后通过 GPx 将其转化为水。

科学家们对 PCOS 患者血清和卵泡液中的 SOD 进行了研究。PCOS 患者血清中的 SOD 水平可能会降低，但卵泡液中的 SOD 水平可能会升高。PCOS 患者血清中的 SOD 浓度随着 SOD 活性的增加而降低，这是因为 SOD 的消耗量增加了，而 ROS 的产生是由 IR 和肥胖等并存的混杂因素引起的。在卵泡液中，SOD 试图抵消 ROS 介导的细胞凋亡。此外，SOD 水平的降低还可能影响卵母细胞第二信使系统的功能。由于 PCOS 的特点是卵巢中有大量的大卵泡，因此也需要大量细胞凋亡。PCOS 患者的卵泡液 SOD 浓度下降及颗粒细胞 mRNA 表达下降，表明退化或死亡的颗粒细胞的更替频繁，这表明 SOD 在卵母细胞成熟的过程和维持中具有重要意义。

（七）谷胱甘肽过氧化物酶

GPx 属于酶家族，可防止氧化损伤。它通过将脂质氢过氧化物还原成各自的醇类，然后将 H_2O_2 转化为水。然而，研究人员一直未能报告 PCOS 患者体内 GPx 水平下降的情况。这可能是因为 GPx 对 ROS 的补偿性增加。需要进一步研究以找出因果关系。

（八）维生素 E

VE 是一种脂溶性分子，被称为生育酚。由于其抗氧化和抗炎特性，它对女性怀孕、分娩和整体生殖结果具有至关重要的作用。VE 具有抗氧化特性，因为它是一种过氧自由基清除剂。它能防止自由基在膜和血浆脂蛋白中增殖，从而起到"断链型抗氧化剂"的作用。此外，由于其脂溶性，它还能防止多不饱和脂肪酸过氧化。卵泡液中可耐受的 VE 水平可提高卵母细胞成熟率，从而改善卵胞质内单精子注射的效果。VE 可改善 PCOS 患者的 OS，有助于减少人绝经期促性腺激素（human menopausal gonadotrophin，HMG）用量（对卵泡发育无影响）、减小子宫内膜厚度和降低雌二醇水平。它还能提高血清中 TAC 水平，降低 MDA 水平。

七、识别和预防氧化应激的增强因素

PCOS 被认为是一种复合疾病，可由 OS 和慢性炎症的几种前兆因素引发。识别日常生活方式的各种因素，并了解它们对 PCOS 病情加重的影响，对预防该疾病的发展起着至关重要的作用。肥胖和 IR 是 OS 和慢性炎症的主要结果。潜在的 PCOS 患者需要改变不健康的饮食、运动和睡眠缺乏、情绪压力（累积）和吸烟等生活方式，有助于获得更好的生殖结果（图6.3）。

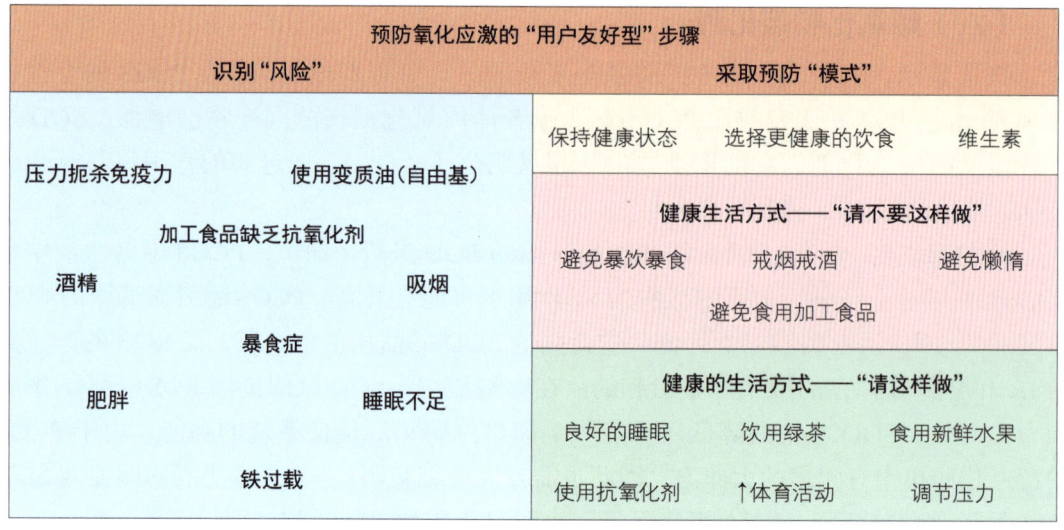

图6.3 "防患于未然"——氧化应激的风险与预防

八、结论

PCOS通常表现为激素分泌失调、卵母细胞成熟障碍、IR、糖尿病、内皮功能障碍，以及高血压和血脂异常风险增加。无论相关疾病是什么，其根本原因都在于OS和慢性炎症之间的相互影响。评估OS和细胞因子/脂肪因子对炎症等级的影响在PCOS患者的治疗中发挥重要作用。

参考文献

1. Agarwal A, Gupta S, Sharma RK. Role of oxidative stress in female reproduction. Reprod Biol Endocrinol. 2005;3:28.
2. Pandey AN, Tripathi A, Premkumar KV, Shrivastav TG, Chaube SK. Reactive oxygen and nitrogen species during meiotic resumption from diplotene arrest in mammalian oocytes. J Cell Biochem. 2010;111(3):521-528. doi:10.1002/jcb.22736.
3. Tatemoto H, Sakurai N, Muto N. Protection of porcine oocytes against apoptotic cell death caused by oxidative stress during In vitro maturation: role of cumulus cells. Biol Reprod. 2000;63(3):805-810.
4. Ishii T, Miyazawa M, Takanashi Y, et al. Genetically induced oxidative stress in mice causes thrombocytosis, splenomegaly and placental angiodysplasia that leads to recurrent abortion. Redox Biol. 2014;2:679-685.
5. Shkolnik K, Tadmor A, Ben-Dor S, Nevo N, Galiani D, Dekel N. Reactive oxygen species are indispensable in ovulation. Proc Natl Acad Sci U S A. 2011;108(4):1462-1467. doi:10.1073/pnas.1017213108.
6. Eichenlaub-Ritter U. Oocyte ageing and its cellular basis. Int J Dev Biol. 2012;56(10-12):841-852.
7. Landskron G, De la Fuente M, Thuwajit P, Thuwajit C, Hermoso MA. Chronic inflammation and cytokines in the tumor microenvironment. J Immunol Res. 2014;2014:149185.

8. Biswas SK. Does the interdependence between oxidative stress and inflammation explain the antioxidant paradox? Oxid Med Cell Longev. 2016;2016:5698931.
9. Hussain T, Tan B, Yin Y, Blachier F, Tossou MC, Rahu N. Oxidative stress and inflammation: what polyphenols can do for us? Oxid Med Cell Longev. 2016;2016:7432797.
10. Bedard K, Krause KH. The NOX family of ROS-generating NADPH oxidases: physiology and pathophysiology. Physiol Rev. 2007;87(1):245-313.
11. Lu X, Murphy TC, Nanes MS, Hart CM. PPARγ regulates hypoxia-induced Nox4 expression in human pulmonary artery smooth muscle cells through NF-kB. Am J Physiol Lung Cell Mol Physiol. 2010;299(4):L559-L566.
12. Oliveira-Marques V, Marinho HS, Cyrne L, Antunes F. Role of hydrogen peroxide in NF-kB activation: from inducer to modulator. Antioxid Redox Signal. 2009;11(9):2223-2243.
13. Yin J, Duan J, Cui Z, Ren W, Li T, Yin Y. Hydrogen peroxide-induced oxidative stress activates NF-kB and Nrf2/Keap1 signals and triggers autophagy in piglets. RSC Adv. 2015;5(20):15479-15486.
14. Rehman R, Mehmood M, Ali R, Shaharyar S, Alam F. Influence of body mass index and polycystic ovarian syndrome on ICSI/IVF treatment outcomes: a study conducted in Pakistani women. Int J Reprod Biomed. 2018;16(8):529.
15. Piya MK, McTernan PG, Kumar S. Adipokine inflammation and insulin resistance: the role of glucose, lipids and endotoxin. J Endocrinol. 2013;216(1):T1-T15.
16. Ouchi N, Parker JL, Lugus JJ, Walsh K. Adipokines in inflammation and metabolic disease. Nat Rev Immunol. 2011;11(2):85-97.
17. Wang Y, Huang F. N-3 polyunsaturated fatty acids and inflammation in obesity: local effect and systemic benefit. Biomed Res Int. 2015;2015:581469.
18. Xie F, Anderson CL, Timme KR, Kurz SG, Fernando SC, Wood JR. Obesity-dependent increases in oocyte mRNAs are associated with increases in proinflammatory signaling and gut microbial abundance of Lachnospiraceae in female mice. Endocrinology. 2016;157(4):1630-1643.
19. Yeon Lee J, Baw CK, Gupta S, Aziz N, Agarwal A. Role of oxidative stress in polycystic ovary syndrome. Curr Womens Health Rev. 2010;6(2):96-107.
20. Pollak M. The insulin and insulin-like growth factor receptor family in neoplasia: an update. Nat Rev Cancer. 2012;12(3):159-169.
21. Zhang D, Luo WY, Liao H, Wang CF, Sun Y. The effects of oxidative stress to PCOS. Sichuan Da Xue Xue Bao Yi Xue Ban. 2008;39(3):421-423.
22. Cooke MS, Evans MD, Dizdaroglu M, Lunec JJ. Oxidative DNA damage: mechanisms, mutation, and disease. FASEB J. 2003;17(10):1195-1214.
23. Dinger Y, Akcay T, Erdem T, Ilker Saygili E, Gundogdu S. DNA damage, DNA susceptibility to oxidation and glutathione level in women with polycystic ovary syndrome. Scand J Clin Lab Invest. 2005;65(8):721-728.
24. Amato G, Conte M, Mazziotti G, et al. Serum and follicular fluid cytokines in polycystic ovary syndrome during stimulated cycles. Obstet Gynecol. 2003;101(6):1177-1182.
25. Kelly CC, Lyall H, Petrie JR, Gould GW, Connell JM, Sattar N. Low grade chronic inflammation in women with polycystic ovarian syndrome. J Clin Endocrinol Metab. 2001;86(6):2453-2455.
26. Wang X, Martindale JL, Liu Y, Holbrook N. The cellular response to oxidative stress: influences of mitogen-activated protein kinase signalling pathways on cell survival. Biochem J. 1998;333(2):291-300.
27. Boutros T, Chevet E, Metrakos PJ. Mitogen-activated protein (MAP) kinase/MAP kinase phosphatase regulation: roles in cell growth, death, and cancer. Pharmacol Rev. 2008;60(3):261-310.
28. Brown MD, Sacks DB. Protein scaffolds in MAP kinase signalling. Cell Signal. 2009;21(4):462-469.
29. Diamanti-Kandarakis E, Dunaif A. Insulin resistance and the polycystic ovary syndrome revisited: an update on mechanisms and implications. Endocr Rev. 2012;33(6):981-1030.

30. Kaya C, Erkan AF, Cengiz SD, et al. Advanced oxidation protein products are increased in women with polycystic ovary syndrome: relationship with traditional and nontraditional cardiovascular risk factors in patients with polycystic ovary syndrome. Fertil Steril. 2009;92(4):1372-1377.
31. Nur Torun A, Vural M, Cece H, Camuzcuoglu H, Toy H, Aksoy N. Paraoxonase-1 is not affected in polycystic ovary syndrome without metabolic syndrome and insulin resistance, but oxidative stress is altered. Gynecol Endocrinol. 2011;27(12):988-992.
32. Yildirim B, Demir S, Temur I, Erdemir R, Kaleli B. Lipid peroxidation in follicular fluid of women with polycystic ovary syndrome during assisted reproduction cycles. J Reprod Med. 2007;52(8):722-726.
33. Stichtenoth D, Frölich JC. Nitric oxide and inflammatory joint diseases. Br J Rheumatol. 1998;37(3):246-257.
34. Meng C. Nitric oxide (NO) levels in patients with polycystic ovary syndrome (PCOS): a meta-analysis. J Int Med Res. 2019;47(9):4083-4094.
35. Sprung VS, Atkinson G, Cuthbertson DJ, et al. Endothelial function measured using flow-mediated dilation in polycystic ovary syndrome: a meta-analysis of the observational studies. Clin Endocrinol (Oxf). 2013;78(3):438-446.
36. Garg D, Merhi Z. Relationship between advanced glycation end products and steroidogenesis in PCOS. Reprod Biol Endocrinol. 2016;14(1):1-13.
37. Puddu P, Puddu GM, Cravero E, Vizioli L, Muscari A. The relationships among hyperuricemia, endothelial dysfunction, and cardiovascular diseases: molecular mechanisms and clinical implications. J Cardiol. 2012;59(3):235-242.
38. Galassetti P. Inflammation and oxidative stress in obesity, metabolic syndrome, and diabetes. Exp Diabetes Res. 2012;2012:943706.
39. Miric DJ, Kisic BB, Zoric LD, Mitic RV, Miric BM, Dragojevic IM. Xanthine oxidase and lens oxidative stress markers in diabetic and senile cataract patients. J Diabetes Complications. 2013;27(2):171-176.
40. Verit FF, Erel O. Oxidative stress in nonobese women with polycystic ovary syndrome: correlations with endocrine and screening parameters. Gynecol Obstet Invest. 2008;65(4):233-239.
41. Talat A, Satyanarayana P, Anand P. Association of superoxide dismutase level in women with polycystic ovary syndrome. J Obstet Gynaecol India. 2022;72:6-12.
42. Seleem AK, El Refaeey AA, Shaalan D, Sherbiny Y, Badawy A. Superoxide dismutase in polycystic ovary syndrome patients undergoing intracytoplasmic sperm injection. J Assist Reprod Genet. 2014;31(4):499-504.
43. Savic-Radojevic A, Antic IB, Coric V, et al. Effect of hyperglycemia and hyperinsulinemia on glutathione peroxidase activity in non-obese women with polycystic ovary syndrome. Hormones (Athens). 2015;14(1):101-108.
44. Shamim AA, Schulze K, Merrill RD, et al. First-trimester plasma tocopherols are associated with risk of miscarriage in rural Bangladesh. Am J Clin Nutr. 2015;101(2):294-301.
45. Lebold KM, Traber MG. Interactions between α-tocopherol, polyunsaturated fatty acids, and lipoxygenases during embryogenesis. Free Radic Biol Med. 2014;66:13-19.
46. Ashraf M, Mustansir F, Baqir SM, Alam F, Rehman R. Changes in vitamin E levels as a marker of female infertility. J Pak Med Assoc. 2020;70(10):1762-1766.

第七章 多囊卵巢综合征和低生育力：排卵调节障碍和生育力问题（临床特征和病理生理学）

一、引言

多囊卵巢综合征（PCOS）主要影响育龄期女性。根据种族不同，发病率可能在8%～13%，存在差异的原因是诊断标准不同。与PCOS相关的最常见问题是青春期女性的身体外观，但代谢异常、心血管危险因素和心理社会问题也是更广泛疾病谱的一部分。对中年女性来说，一个非常重要且令人苦恼的问题是低生育力/不孕症。尽管在不同的研究中尚未发现患有PCOS和未患有PCOS女性家庭规模的差异，但PCOS女性可能需要治疗或一些医疗帮助才能怀孕。为了解PCOS女性不孕症的病理生理过程，科研人员对多种因素进行了研究，其中慢性无排卵是其主要原因。而稀发排卵/无排卵也是PCOS的主要诊断标准之一。

低生育力是指试图怀孕的夫妇生育力降低，在持续12个月内无保护性交后未孕。有8%～12%的夫妇受此影响，而且在50%的病例中，不孕症的主要原因是男性不育。在排卵异常导致的不孕症女性中，最常见的诊断是PCOS，约占70%。美国生殖医学协会建议，如果患有PCOS的女性在无保护性交6个月后（前提是有规律的性交，每周2～3次）仍未受孕，则应进行不孕症的相关评估。

二、正常排卵生理学

排卵的特征是在每个月经周期中，从卵巢发育并排出一个优势卵泡。随后卵子进入输卵管，并在此受精。整个排卵过程需要功能完善的下丘脑-垂体轴。

在胚胎发育过程中原始卵泡形成，主要为停滞在减数分裂Ⅰ期的卵母细胞。每个卵巢中有100万～200万个原始卵泡。在青春期前的女性，卵泡发育到窦状卵泡期；此后，卵泡成熟主要依赖促性腺激素。在青春期，促性腺激素的分泌增加会刺激原始卵泡完成减数分裂Ⅰ期，形成次级卵泡。这些次级卵泡进入减数分裂Ⅱ期，并继续发育至排卵前期。其中一个卵泡被选为优势卵泡，继续发育并排卵。其余的卵泡则闭锁。在一个排卵周期中会损失大量卵泡，而损失的卵泡数量与年龄呈线性相关。两侧卵巢每个月交替排卵。随着绝经的到来，排卵功能会停止（图7.1）。

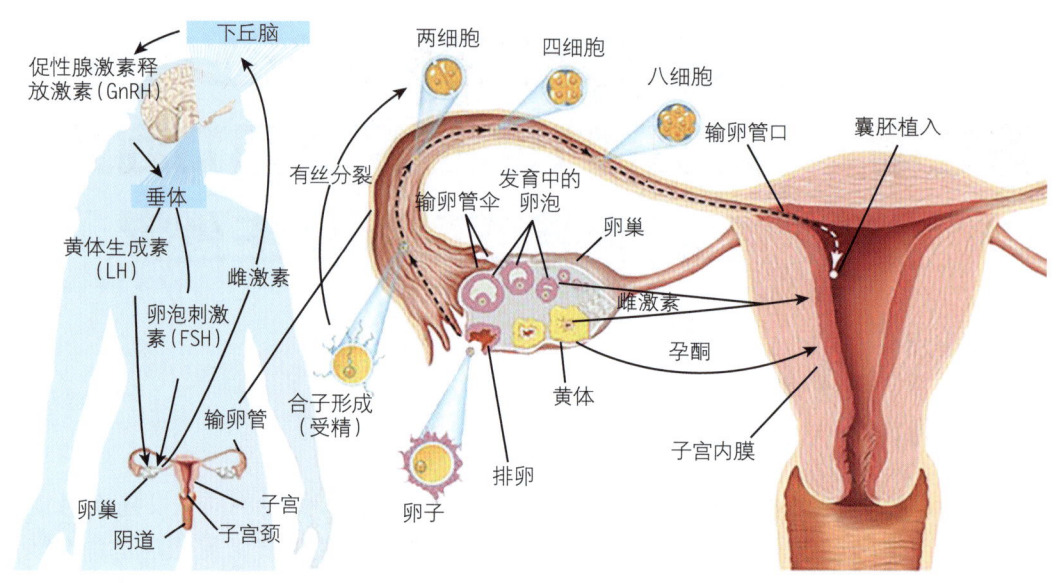

图 7.1 下丘脑-垂体-卵巢轴：从排卵到着床

促性腺激素释放激素（GnRH）由下丘脑弓状核分泌。它以脉冲形式分泌，调控垂体前叶分泌卵泡刺激素（FSH）和黄体生成素（LH）。GnRH 的低频脉冲刺激 FSH 分泌，而高频脉冲促进 LH 分泌。

促性腺激素是糖蛋白分子，有 2 个亚基（即 α 和 β）。所有糖蛋白，如促甲状腺激素和人绒毛膜促性腺激素，都有共同的 α 亚基，就像 FSH 和 LH 一样。β 亚基则是每种激素所特有的。

在女性中，FSH 与雌激素的分泌相关，调控优势卵泡的成熟。而 LH 会促进卵泡膜细胞产生雄激素。低水平的雌激素会对促性腺激素产生负反馈作用。

FSH 作用于颗粒细胞表面的 G 蛋白偶联受体，启动雌激素的分泌。雌激素是月经周期中卵泡发育和成熟所必需的激素，它还会促使颗粒细胞分泌更多的雌激素。当雌激素达到临界水平时，就会开始对 LH 产生正反馈，引发 LH 峰。

LH 峰引起优势卵泡破裂，诱发排卵和颗粒细胞黄体化，形成黄体。随后黄体分泌孕酮，标志着黄体期开始。如果没有受精，黄体就会自动退化，孕酮水平也会下降。这标志着子宫内膜开始脱落和月经开始。

GnRH、FSH 和 LH 之间复杂的相互作用对卵泡发育和成熟、排卵、子宫内膜的容受性改变或子宫内膜脱落至关重要（图 7.2）。

第七章　多囊卵巢综合征和低生育力：排卵调节障碍和生育力问题（临床特征和病理生理学）

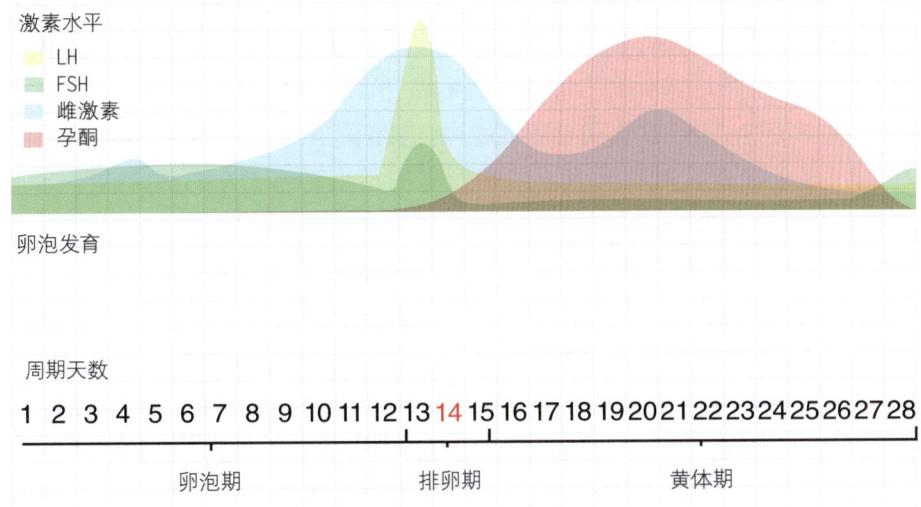

FSH，卵泡刺激素；LH，黄体生成素。

图 7.2　月经周期不同阶段的激素水平

（经内华达州生殖医学中心许可转载，https://nevadafertility.com/phasesofthemenstrualcycle/）

三、多囊卵巢综合征的病理学

PCOS 的病理复杂，涉及多种因素，包括高雄激素血症（HA）、排卵障碍、月经异常，以及超声检查多囊卵巢形态。卵巢或肾上腺雄激素分泌过多是由类固醇生成缺陷和胰岛素水平升高所致。大多数患有 PCOS 的女性（60%～80%）也有代谢异常，如超重/肥胖和胰岛素抵抗（IR）。

下面对下丘脑、垂体和卵巢不同程度的异常进行讨论。

（一）下丘脑 – 垂体轴

PCOS 患者下丘脑分泌过多的 GnRH，且 GnRH 的脉冲频率比正常增加 40%，一些证据表明垂体前叶对 GnRH 的作用更加敏感。较高的脉冲频率会促进 LH 的分泌，而较低的 GnRH 脉冲频率则会刺激 FSH 水平升高。因此，高脉冲频率的 GnRH 会导致相对较高的 LH 水平。因此，在 PCOS 患者中，LH : FSH 通常是正常值的 2～3 倍，但这并没有纳入 PCOS 的诊断标准。正常情况下，黄体分泌孕酮，对下丘脑的 GnRH 起负反馈作用，但是由于 PCOS 患者的 FSH 和雌二醇水平较低，且没有 LH 峰，所以不会排卵，也不会形成黄体，导致对下丘脑 GnRH 的负反馈缺失。此外，由于雄激素水平较高，下丘脑对雌二醇和孕酮的负反馈不敏感，从而形成恶性循环。

（二）卵巢层面的异常

LH 作用于卵巢卵泡膜细胞上的 LH 受体，引发卵泡膜细胞增生并产生大量雄激素。

正常情况下，卵泡膜细胞产生的雄激素通过芳香化酶转化为雌激素。芳香化酶由颗粒细胞产生，是雌激素产生的限速酶，可通过雌二醇：睾酮来评估。然而，在PCOS患者中，芳香化酶的活性降低或失调。具体原因有待进一步研究。

同样，IR和肥胖对芳香化酶活性的影响仍存在争议。高雄激素水平在临床上可表现为痤疮、多毛症或暂时性秃发。几乎所有的指南都将HA的临床或生化证据作为PCOS的主要诊断标准之一。

相对较低的雌二醇和FSH水平及较高的雄激素水平会影响卵泡成熟过程。多个卵泡同时开始生长，但生长过早停止，排卵受到抑制。这种无排卵是PCOS女性低生育力的主要原因，也是此类患者采用诱导排卵作为一线治疗方案的原因。

此外，一个重要的问题是月经不规律，这也是PCOS的主要诊断标准之一。这是PCOS女性的常见表现，不规律排卵使计划妊娠变得困难。75%～80%的PCOS女性存在一定程度的月经失调。此外，在PCOS患者中，即使月经周期规律，排卵也不规律，导致受孕机会减少。

PCOS患者体内的雄激素大部分由卵巢产生，但也有一些由肾上腺产生。

（三）肥胖与胰岛素抵抗

尽管对超重和肥胖患者的定义采用了不同的临界值，但大多数（35%～80%）PCOS女性都属于这两类。肥胖，尤其是向心性肥胖，会增强PCOS的临床和生化特征，并增加胰岛素抵抗。

高胰岛素血症会降低性激素结合球蛋白（SHBG）水平，导致游离睾酮水平升高，从而进一步引发HA。

PCOS的一个重要病理变化是IR，也是PCOS的一个标志，影响65%～70%的患者。IR的一个常见临床症状是黑棘皮症，常见于PCOS患者。另外，在PCOS患者中IR是瘦型PCOS的基础，甚至与肥胖程度无关或不成比例。IR与LH协同作用，促进卵巢雄激素的合成。IR能上调卵泡膜细胞表面的LH受体，并诱导酶参与类固醇生成。这被认为是一种功能性HA，因为它不涉及任何酶的缺乏。这些生化异常（HA和IR）也诱导了排列在卵巢外围的微囊形成，超声检查显示为特征性多囊形态。

（四）子宫内膜层面的异常

由于持续暴露于雌激素而缺乏足够的孕酮保护，与正常人群相比，PCOS女性的子宫内膜会发生增生，她们是子宫内膜癌的高危人群。然而，目前仍不建议对PCOS女性进行子宫内膜癌的常规筛查。此外，这些子宫内膜的变化会导致子宫不容易妊娠，着床失败或早期流产的发生率增加。约50%的PCOS女性经历过妊娠早期流产（图7.3）。

第七章 多囊卵巢综合征和低生育力：排卵调节障碍和生育力问题（临床特征和病理生理学）

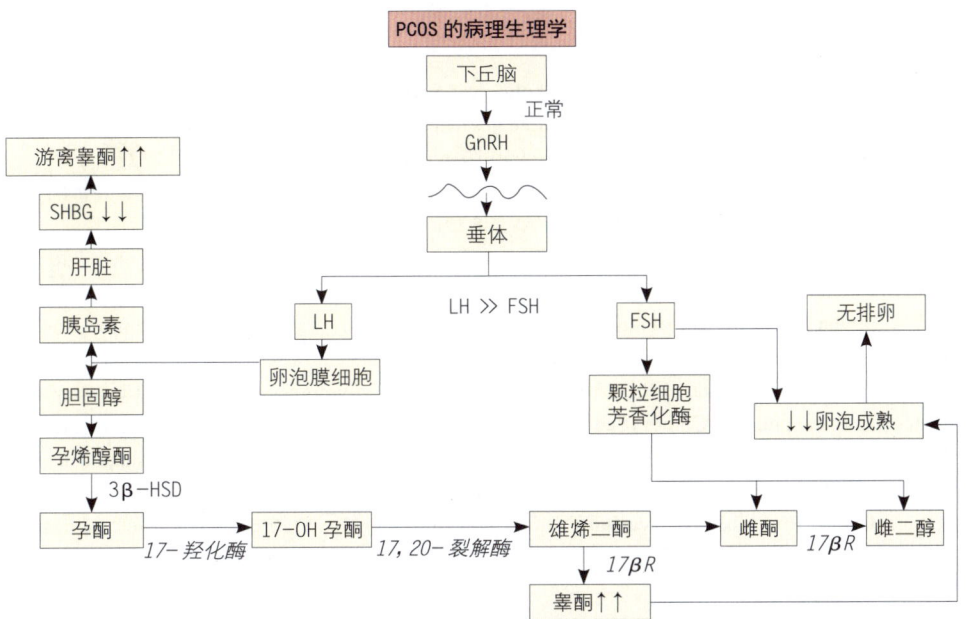

FSH，卵泡刺激素；GnRH，促性腺激素释放激素；LH，黄体生成素；SHBG，性激素结合球蛋白；3β-HSD，3β-羟基类固醇脱氢酶；17βR，17β受体。

图7.3 多囊卵巢综合征的多因素病理学

（五）宫内雄激素暴露

研究发现，如此广泛的疾病症状可能是多种环境和遗传因素长期相互作用造成的。遗传因素之所以被考虑在内，是因为该病有家族聚集现象。然而，研究发现只有少数基因与PCOS有关。一些重要的环境因素，如久坐不动的生活方式、超重/肥胖及产前暴露于雄激素等，可能在其中发挥了作用。

患有先天性肾上腺皮质增生症的母亲所生的女婴在宫内暴露于高水平的雄激素时，其卵巢会在青春期出现PCOS形态。在其他男性化疾病和肿瘤中也观察到同样的情况，这证明PCOS与产前雄激素暴露有关。

（六）其他因素

在PCOS女性中抑郁和心境障碍很常见（23%～64%的患者）。有报道称，在PCOS女性中性功能障碍的比例高达57.7%。这可能是由于焦虑、自卑，或者因肥胖、多毛症或痤疮等导致身体形象改变造成的心理问题。这些因素在有不孕症/低生育力相关问题的夫妇中很重要。另一个原因是雄激素水平过高会直接降低女性的性欲。

四、结论

总之，通过流行病学和观察性研究收集的数据表明，PCOS和低生育力的发病机制是多因素的。HA是主要的生化异常，但肥胖和IR常见于PCOS女性，并进一步加剧HA，对其生育潜力产生负面影响。

参考文献

1. Sanchez-Garrido MA, Tena-Sempere M. Metabolic dysfunction in polycystic ovary syndrome: pathogenic role of androgen excess and potential therapeutic strategies. Mol Metab. 2020;35:100937. Available at: https://www.ncbi.nlm.nih.gov/pmc/articles/PMC7115104/. doi:10.1016/j.molmet.2020.01.001.
2. Mohammad MB, Seghinsara AM. Polycystic ovary syndrome (PCOS), diagnostic criteria, and AMH. Asian Pac J Cancer Prev. 2017;18(1):17-21. doi:10.22034/APJCP.2017.18.1.17.
3. Vander Borght M, Wyns C. Fertility and infertility: definition and epidemiology. Clin Biochem. 2018;62:2-10. doi:10.1016/j.clinbiochem.2018.03.012.
4. Cunha A, Póvoa AM. Infertility management in women with polycystic ovary syndrome: a review. Porto Biomed J. 2021;6(1):e116. doi:10.1097/j.pbj.0000000000000116.
5. Melo AS, Ferriani RA, Navarro PA. Treatment of infertility in women with polycystic ovary syndrome: approach to clinical practice. Clinics (Sao Paulo). 2015;70(11):765-769. doi:10.6061/clinics/2015(11)09.
6. Holesh JE, Bass AN, Lord M. Physiology, ovulation. In: StatPearls [Internet]. Treasure Island (FL): StatPearls Publishing; 2021. Available at: http://www.ncbi.nlm.nih.gov/books/NBK441996/.
7. Cox E, Takov V. Embryology, Ovarian Follicle Development. In: StatPearls [Internet]. Treasure Island (FL): StatPearls Publishing; 2022 [cited 2022 Aug 24]. Available from: http://www.ncbi.nlm.nih.gov/books/NBK532300/
8. Richards JS, Russell DL, Robker RL, Dajee M, Alliston TN. Molecular mechanisms of ovulation and luteinization. Mol Cell Endocrinol. 1998;145(1-2):47-54. doi:10.1016/s0303-7207(98)00168-3.
9. Laven JSE. Follicle stimulating hormone receptor (FSHR) polymorphisms and polycystic ovary syndrome (PCOS). Front Endocrinol. 2019;10:23. doi:10.3389/fendo.2019.00023.
10. Gardner DG, Shoback D, eds. Greenspan's Basic & Clinical Endocrinology. 10th ed. McGraw Hill; 2017. Available at: https://accessmedicine.mhmedical.com/content.aspx?bookid=2178&sectionid=166246461.
11. Mikhael S, Punjala-Patel A, Gavrilova-Jordan L. Hypothalamic-pituitary-ovarian axis disorders impacting female fertility. Biomedicines. 2019;7(1):5. doi: 10.3390/biomedicines7010005.
12. Reed BG, Carr BR. The normal menstrual cycle and the control of ovulation. In: Feingold KR, Anawalt B, Boyce A, et al., eds. Endotext [Internet]. South Dartmouth (MA): MDText.com, Inc.; 2000. Available at: https://www.ncbi.nlm.nih.gov/books/NBK279054/.
13. Richards JS, Pangas SA. The ovary: basic biology and clinical implications. J Clin Invest. 2010;120(4)963-972. doi: 10.1172/JCI41350.
14. Abbara A, Dhillo WS. Targeting elevated GnRH pulsatility to treat polycystic ovary syndrome. J Clin Endocrinol Metab. 2021;106(10):e4275-e4277. doi:10.1210/clinem/dgab422.
15. Saadia Z. Follicle stimulating hormone (LH: FSH) ratio in polycystic ovary syndrome (PCOS) - obese vs. non-obese women. Med Arch. 2020;74(4):289-293. doi:10.5455/mearh.2020.74.289-293.
16. Chen J, Shen S, Tan Y, et al. The correlation of aromatase activity and obesity in women with or without polycystic ovary syndrome. J Ovarian Res. 2015;8:11. doi:10.1186/s13048-015-0139-1.
17. Harris HR, Titus LJ, Cramer DW, Terry KL. Long and irregular menstrual cycles, polycystic ovary syndrome, and ovarian cancer risk in a population-based case-control study. Int J Cancer. 2017;140(2):285-291. doi:10.1002/ijc.30441.
18. Li X, Feng Y, Lin JF, Billig H, Shao R. Endometrial progesterone resistance and PCOS. J Biomed Sci. 2014;21(1):2. doi:10.1186/1423-0127-21-2.
19. Ruddenklau A, Campbell RE. Neuroendocrine impairments of polycystic ovary syndrome. Endocrinology. 2019;160(10):2230-2242. doi:10.1210/en.2019-00428.
20. Eftekhar T, Sohrabvand F, Zabandan N, Shariat M, Haghollahi F, Ghahghaei-Nezamabadi A. Sexual dysfunction in patients with polycystic ovary syndrome and its affected domains. Iran J Reprod Med. 2014;12(8):539-546.

第八章 多囊卵巢综合征的临床特征及表现

一、引言

多囊卵巢综合征（PCOS）是一种具有系统性代谢表现的复杂疾病，影响全球 4%～20% 的育龄期女性。其症状或体征的特点是雄激素过多、月经周期无排卵和（或）一侧或两侧卵巢多囊样表现。PCOS 的表型是多样的，其潜在的病理生理机制尚未完全清楚。多种遗传和环境因素在这个异质性疾病的发生中起重要作用。PCOS 可以追溯到 1935 年，由两位著名的妇科医师首次提出了 7 名女性的病例系列，表现为月经不规律、不育和高雄激素血症（HA），当时被称为 "Stein-Leventhal 综合征"。1990 年，PCOS 的第一个国际定义问世，此后，该定义不断发展，并由各种专业机构进行分类。PCOS 虽然目前有 3 种不同的定义，但仍被认为是一种排除性诊断。

PCOS 有 3 种主要的诊断标准。HA 的临床或生化证据，以及伴有月经稀发或闭经的慢性无排卵，这两个经典特征是 3 个标准的共同组成部分，但鹿特丹标准将超声检查多囊卵巢形态作为附加特征。

2012 年，由美国国立卫生研究院主办的 PCOS 循证研讨会将 PCOS 分为以下 4 种主要表型：

- HA、排卵功能障碍和多囊卵巢形态。
- HA 伴排卵功能障碍。
- HA 和多囊卵巢形态。
- 排卵功能障碍伴多囊卵巢形态。

PCOS 的 HA 通常表现为多毛症、痤疮、雄激素性脱发和头发稀疏。男性化（如男性型秃发、声音低沉、肌肉量增加）不是 PCOS 的特征，但提示潜在的肾上腺或卵巢肿瘤，或严重的胰岛素抵抗（IR）。患有 PCOS 的女性容易出现体重增加，可能导致 IR，进而引起 HA，使 PCOS 的症状恶化。

月经周期不规律或无周期是 PCOS 最常见的症状之一。月经周期不规律定义为月经周期少于 21 天或超过 35 天，或每年少于 8 个周期。但青春期女性在 15 岁或 16 岁时表现为原发性闭经时，也应排除其他原因。同样，持续超过 90 天的继发性闭经也不常见，需要进一步评估。由于无排卵周期，PCOS 女性患不孕症的风险增加，肥胖 PCOS 的患者发生自然流产的概率比一般人群更高。

二、临床特征

PCOS 的详细临床特征可阐述为以下几点：
- 皮肤或外观表现。
    - i. 多毛症。
    - ii. 痤疮。
    - iii. 雄激素性脱发。
    - iv. 黑棘皮症。
    - v. 皮脂溢出。
- 排卵功能障碍。
    - i. 月经稀发。
    - ii. 不孕症。
- 代谢功能障碍。
    - i. 肥胖。
    - ii. IR。
    - iii. 血糖代谢障碍。
- 心理脆弱性。
- 与 PCOS 相关的其他疾病或症状。
    - i. 甲状腺功能异常。
    - ii. 子宫内膜癌。
    - iii. 脂代谢紊乱。
    - iv. 阻塞性睡眠呼吸暂停（obstructive sleep apnea，OSA）。
    - v. 非酒精性脂肪性肝病（nonalcoholic fatty liver disease，NAFLD）/非酒精性脂肪性肝炎（nonalcoholic steatohepatitis，NASH）。
    - vi. 不良妊娠结局。

（一）皮肤表现

高胰岛素血症和 IR 常见于女性 PCOS 患者。高胰岛素血症与黄体生成素（LH）协同作用，一方面可促进卵巢卵泡膜细胞分泌雄激素；另一方面降低肝脏分泌性激素结合球蛋白（SHBG），导致 HA，进而引起游离睾酮水平升高，临床表现为多毛症、痤疮、皮脂溢出和脱发。黑棘皮症和皮赘是 PCOS 的其他皮肤表现，提示这些患者有潜在的 IR。

雄激素在 PCOS 的皮肤表现中起着重要作用，但在没有 HA 生化指标的患者中也观察到雄激素的表现，这导致临床或生化 HA 被纳入 PCOS 标准，成为其中一个组成部分。

虽然肥胖容易引发高胰岛素血症，但 PCOS 女性患者显著的 IR 是独立于肥胖程度和雄激素浓度的。因此，PCOS 的皮肤表现是多种激素和代谢因素复杂相互作用的结果。

1. 多毛症

多毛症被定义为女性雄激素依赖区域的终毛呈雄性生长模式。多毛症仍然是HA最常见的临床特征。65%～75%的PCOS患者都有这种症状。多毛症应与毛发过多症（指全身毛发异常增多）鉴别。多毛症的发展受遗传和地域变化的影响，在亚洲人群中发病率较低。

HA临床表现的严重程度取决于循环和局部雄激素浓度及毛囊皮脂腺单位对雄激素的敏感性。在代谢性肥胖患者中，多毛症往往更严重。多毛症可能是PCOS代谢后遗症的标志，也可能预示着不孕症治疗期间受孕和妊娠相关的不良预后。

改良Ferriman-Gallwey评分系统是大多数临床医师评价多毛症时使用的工具，它包括全身9个对雄激素最敏感部位的评分，从0（没有毛发）到4（直白地说，男性化的），将每一项分数加起来就是激素性多毛症的分数。8分及以上的分数被认为是症状显著，8～15分是轻度多毛症，16～36分是中度到重度多毛症。然而，该评分系统有其自身的局限性，因为它取决于患者的主观性，并且不包括鬓角、颈背、指骨和肛周区域的毛发生长情况。上唇较厚的女性得分可能低于8分，因此不能反映患者的外观。

2. 痤疮

痤疮是PCOS的常见皮肤表现之一。据报道，其患病率为9.8%～34.0%，它形成的机制是粉刺和皮脂的积累，以及脱落的滤泡上皮细胞，为痤疮丙酸杆菌的定植提供了基质。PCOS女性的痤疮可出现在面部、颈部、上胸部、上背部和上臂。虽然雄激素（增加了毛囊皮脂腺单位内的皮脂分泌）在痤疮的病理生理中起着重要作用，但在青春期和青春期后的PCOS中，痤疮也可能是青春期正常生理表现，由肾上腺机能初现，肾上腺来源的雄激素激增导致的。因此雄激素依赖性和非雄激素依赖性痤疮都可能发生于女性PCOS患者。

3. 雄激素性脱发

据Ludwig描述，雄激素性脱发为保留前额发际线，头顶的头发逐渐变薄，这是PCOS的公认症状。雄激素性脱发在疾病进程中出现较晚，但它是女性心理困扰的重要原因。

它可以表现为几种类型，包括弥漫性发量减少和头发稀疏。据报道，PCOS中脱发的患病率在67.0%～77.8%，证实了PCOS与雄激素性脱发之间的联系。研究显示脱发与循环雄激素水平呈正相关。因此，与循环雄激素水平相比，局部雄激素可能是雄激素性脱发发展的重要媒介。Ludwig评分是一种众所周知的主观方法，用于雄激素性脱发的分级。

4. 黑棘皮症

黑棘皮症的定义是色素沉着、增厚、柔软的天鹅绒样斑块，主要出现在腋窝、颈部和肘关节的外侧面。这是女性PCOS的一个重要特征，且被认为是IR与2型糖尿病风险增加的临床指标。肥胖的女性更容易患黑棘皮症。印度的一项研究显示，PCOS女性患者的黑棘皮症患病率为56%，明显高于一般人群。这重申了生活方式干预的重要性，这些患者的查体指标明显且易识别，可以用来防止未来可能发生的代谢后遗症。

5. 皮脂溢出

皮脂溢出是一种常见的皮肤问题，可导致头皮和面部出现红色、瘙痒的皮疹和白色鳞屑，也被定义为 PCOS 的一种皮肤特征，一项研究显示其患病率为 34.7%。皮脂溢的临床表现与游离睾酮、空腹血糖和胰岛素水平较高有关。除了 HA，遗传易感性、气候和情绪因素也是影响皮脂溢发生的重要因素。因此，对于 PCOS 女性患者，临床、血清学和放射学检查对诊断与 PCOS 相关的皮脂溢非常重要。

（二）排卵功能障碍

排卵功能障碍是 PCOS 最常见的特征之一。由于 PCOS 被认为是一种 IR 状态，胰岛素水平升高会刺激卵巢类固醇激素的生成，导致女性卵巢功能障碍。

1. 月经稀发

排卵功能障碍包括月经稀发或月经频发，前者定义为一个月经周期持续时间超过 35 天或每年月经周期少于 8 个；后者定义为周期持续时间少于 21 天。也有一小部分患有 PCOS 的女性可能表现为月经正常，可通过测量黄体中期（第 21～23 天）孕酮水平进行更仔细的评估。

由于 PCOS 以非雌激素性慢性无排卵为特征，子宫内膜充分受到雌激素刺激，因此这类女性在使用孕酮后 5～10 天可诱发撤退性出血。继发性闭经的患者出现撤退性出血，可进一步支持继发于 PCOS 的无排卵，排除卵巢功能不全或低促性腺激素性性腺功能减退症等雌激素低下状态。

2. 不孕症

PCOS 仍然是无排卵性不孕的主要原因之一，在基于人群的不孕症研究中占 25%～40%。尽管稀发排卵 / 无排卵仍然是 PCOS 患者不孕的最常见原因，但还有其他潜在因素可能导致不孕，包括由于 PCOS 女性子宫内膜的雄激素受体增加而导致的卵母细胞能力降低和子宫内膜容受性降低。这类女性伴发的肥胖也导致延迟受孕和低生育力。排除上述因素后，在评估不孕症时还应考虑男性因素。

（三）代谢功能障碍

PCOS 是一种影响生殖和代谢功能的常见内分泌疾病。IR 与 PCOS 的其他代谢异常共同导致了肥胖、2 型糖尿病、血脂异常、高血压和心血管疾病的风险增加。

1. 肥胖

肥胖仍然是 PCOS 患者的一个共同特征。肥胖与 PCOS 之间的关系是复杂的。虽然有证据表明 PCOS 的女性肥胖患病率增加，但 PCOS 的发病率增加是否与肥胖患病率增加相一致是有争议的。

PCOS 女性上半身肥胖的比例更高，与体重指数（BMI）正常与否无关。与 BMI 匹配的对照女性相比，她们的腰围和腰臀比更高。

肥胖，特别是腹型肥胖，通过启动 SHBG 水平的降低和增加生物可利用的雄激素向靶组织的输送，导致相对 HA。非 SHBG 结合的脱氢表雄酮和雄烯二酮的产生速率也增加，这解释了为什么与正常体重的女性相比，超重和肥胖的成年女性月经异常和慢性无排卵更常见。

与正常体重的 PCOS 女性相比，肥胖的 PCOS 患者临床特征更严重，中心脂肪分布增加，代谢指标更高，HA、代谢异常更严重。因此，肥胖往往会加剧这些女性的生殖和代谢异常，包括无排卵性不孕的相对风险。肥胖也被证明会阻碍诱导排卵周期的刺激，需要更高的剂量和更长的刺激时间。

2. 胰岛素抵抗

IR 和高胰岛素血症在 PCOS 女性患者中很常见，特别是在多囊卵巢形态和慢性无排卵的女性中。与体重相当的非 PCOS 女性相比，患有 PCOS 的女性骨骼肌胰岛素介导的葡萄糖摄取减少了 35%～40%，这表明 IR 与肥胖无关。此外，肥胖通过抑制胰岛素介导的内源性肝糖异生而加剧 IR。因此，肥胖和 PCOS 共同对内源性葡萄糖生成产生了有害影响，这为葡萄糖耐受不良的发病机制奠定了基础。

3. 血糖代谢障碍

PCOS 患者出现糖代谢异常的风险比一般人群高 5～10 倍，发生时间稍早（大约在生命的第 3 个或第 4 个 10 年）。伴有高胰岛素血症的 IR 和部分 PCOS 的患者表现出 β 细胞功能改变，导致代谢异常，包括糖耐量减低、2 型糖尿病和血脂异常，这些是心血管疾病的重要危险因素。肥胖、2 型糖尿病阳性家族史和 HA 是导致 PCOS 代谢异常的其他因素。

（四）心理脆弱性

与 PCOS 相关的各种外貌、妇科和代谢方面的特征可能对个体的心理健康产生严重影响。PCOS 女性的外表可能会呈现非正常的女性特质，导致患者终身受到情绪困扰。这些患者容易出现焦虑、自卑、对身体形象不满、进食障碍和性障碍。因此，从治疗的一开始就解决心理问题与治疗他们的生理症状同样重要。

（五）其他相关特征

1. 甲状腺功能异常

PCOS 和自身免疫性甲状腺疾病是两种最常见的内分泌疾病。研究表明，与对照组相比，PCOS 患者甲状腺肿和亚临床甲状腺功能减退症的患病率明显更高。虽然这两种疾病之间的联系尚未明确定义，但 BMI 和 IR 增加是二者共同的特点。与对照组相比，PCOS 女性也显示出更高的甲状腺抗体水平、更大的甲状腺体积和甲状腺回声。PCOS 也增加了甲状腺以外器官的自身免疫疾病的风险。

2. 子宫内膜癌

有研究表明，PCOS 和子宫内膜癌之间存在关联。PCOS 被认为是发生子宫内膜癌的危险因素。一项研究表明，PCOS 的女性发生子宫内膜癌的风险增加了 3 倍。

3. 脂代谢紊乱

代谢异常是 PCOS 女性的共同特征。PCOS 患者具有特定的代谢特征，主要是胰岛素作用和 β 细胞功能缺陷，这大大增加了葡萄糖耐受不良和 2 型糖尿病的风险。研究表明，PCOS 女性的脂代谢发生改变，包括升高的甘油三酯和低密度脂蛋白（low-density lipoproteins，LDL）胆固醇，以及降低的高密度脂蛋白（high-density lipoproteins，HDL），并伴有 C 反应蛋白（CRP）水平升高，慢性轻度炎症使她们更容易患心血管疾病，如动脉粥样硬化。

4. 阻塞性睡眠呼吸暂停

OSA 是 PCOS 女性的一种并发症，主要是由 HA 和肥胖所致。但这两个因素不能完全解释发病机制，因为在控制 BMI 后，与对照组相比，PCOS 女性睡眠呼吸障碍和白天嗜睡的发生率增加了数倍。

5. 非酒精性脂肪性肝病 / 非酒精性脂肪性肝炎

由于 PCOS 潜在的代谢功能障碍，非酒精性脂肪性肝病 / 非酒精性脂肪性肝炎（NAFLD/NASH）也被证实是 PCOS 的潜在并发症，年龄增长、种族、肥胖、IR、血脂异常和葡萄糖耐受不良是潜在的复合致病因素。

6. 不良妊娠结局

PCOS 也被认为是无排卵性不孕的最常见原因之一。这些女性诱导排卵困难，需要更高剂量的药物和更长的时间来刺激排卵。有证据表明，PCOS 女性易合并早产、妊娠期糖尿病和先兆子痫等不良妊娠结局。一项荟萃分析表明，PCOS、妊娠期糖尿病和高血压之间存在独立的关联。

参考文献

1. Deswal R, Narwal V, Dang A, Pundir CS. The prevalence of polycystic ovary syndrome: a brief systematic review. J Hum Reprod Sci. 2020;13(4):261.
2. Legro RS, Arslanian SA, Ehrmann DA, et al. Diagnosis and treatment of polycystic ovary syndrome: an Endocrine Society clinical practice guideline. J Clin Endocrinol Metab. 2013;98:4565-4592.
3. Stein IF. Amenorrhea associated with bilateral polycystic ovaries. Am J Obstet Gynecol. 1935;29:181-191.
4. Johnson T, Kaplan L, Ouyang P, Rizza P. National Institutes of Health Evidence-Based Methodology Workshop on Polycystic Ovary Syndrome. NIH EbMW Reports. Bethesda, MD: National Institutes of Health. 2012;1:1-14. Available at: https://prevention.nih.gov/sites/default/files/2018-06/FinalReport.pdf.
5. Witchel SF, Oberfield SE, Peña AS. Polycystic ovary syndrome: pathophysiology, presentation, and treatment with emphasis on adolescent girls. J Endocr Soc. 2019;3(8):1545-1573.
6. Li L, Yang D, Chen X, Chen Y, Feng S, Wang L. Clinical and metabolic features of polycystic ovary syndrome. Int J Gynecol Obstet. 2007;97(2):129-134.
7. Dunaif A, Segal KR, Futterweit W, Dobrjansky A. Profound peripheral insulin resistance, independent of obesity, in polycystic ovary syndrome. Diabetes. 1989;38(9):1165-1174.
8. Bozdag G, Mumusoglu S, Zengin D, Karabulut E, Yildiz BO. The prevalence and phenotypic features of polycystic ovary syndrome: a systematic review and meta-analysis. Hum Reprod. 2016;31(12):2841-2855.
9. Özdemir S, Özdemir M, Görkemli H, Kiyici A, Bodur S. Specific dermatologic features of the polycystic ovary

syndrome and its association with biochemical markers of the metabolic syndrome and hyperandrogenism. Acta Obstet Gynecol Scand. 2010;89(2):199-204.
10. Rausch ME, Legro RS, Barnhart HX, et al. Predictors of pregnancy in women with polycystic ovary syndrome. J Clin Endocrinol Metab. 2009;94(9):3458-3466.
11. Azziz R, Sanchez LA, Knochenhauer ES, et al. Androgen excess in women: experience with over 1000 consecutive patients. J Clin Endocrinol Metab. 2004;89(2):453-462.
12. Cela E, Robertson C, Rush K, et al. Clinical study prevalence of polycystic ovaries in women with androgenic alopecia. Eur J Endocrinol. 2003;149(5):439-442.
13. Rathnakar U, Gopalakrishna H, Jagadish RP. Acanthosis nigricans in PCOS patients and its relation with type 2 diabetes mellitus and body mass at a tertiary care hospital in southern India. J Clin Diagn Res. 2013;7(2):317-319.
14. Trounson A, Wood C, Kausche A. In vitro maturation and the fertilization and developmental competence of oocytes recovered from untreated polycystic ovarian patients. Fertil Steril. 1994;62(2):353-362.
15. Apparao KB, Lovely LP, Gui Y, Lininger RA, Lessey BA. Elevated endometrial androgen receptor expression in women with polycystic ovarian syndrome. Biol Reprod. 2002;66(2):297-304.
16. Sam S. Obesity and polycystic ovary syndrome. Obes Manag. 2007;3(2):69-73.
17. Pasquali R. Obesity and androgens: facts and perspectives. Fertil Steril. 2006;85(5):1319-1340.
18. Pasquali R, Gambineri A, Pagotto U. The impact of obesity on reproduction in women with polycystic ovary syndrome. BJOG. 2006;113(10):1148-1159.
19. Dunaif A. Insulin action in the polycystic ovary syndrome. Endocrinol Metab Clin North Am. 1999;28(2):341-359.
20. Pelusi B, Gambineri A, Pasquali R. Type 2 diabetes and the polycystic ovary syndrome. Minerva Ginecol. 2004;56(1):41-51.
21. Farkas J, Rigó A, Demetrovics Z. Psychological aspects of the polycystic ovary syndrome. Gynecol Endocrinol. 2014;30(2):95-99.
22. Singla R, Gupta Y, Khemani M, Aggarwal S. Thyroid disorders and polycystic ovary syndrome: an emerging relationship. Indian J Endocrinol Metab. 2015;19(1):25.
23. Fénichel P, Gobert B, Carré Y, Barbarino-Monnier P, Hiéronimus S. Polycystic ovary syndrome in autoimmune disease. Lancet. 1999;353(9171):2210.
24. Chittenden BG, Fullerton G, Maheshwari A, Bhattacharya S. Polycystic ovary syndrome and the risk of gynaecological cancer: a systematic review. Reprod Biomed Online. 2009;19(3):398-405.
25. Haoula Z, Salman M, Atiomo W. Evaluating the association between endometrial cancer and polycystic ovary syndrome. Hum Reprod. 2012;27(5):1327-1331.
26. Alves AC, Valcarcel B, Mäkinen VP, et al. Metabolic profiling of polycystic ovary syndrome reveals interactions with abdominal obesity. Int J Obes. 2017;41(9):1331-1340.
27. Vgontzas AN. Legro RS, Bixler EO, Grayev A, Kales A, Chrousos GP. Polycystic ovary syndrome is associated with obstructive sleep apnea and daytime sleepiness: role of insulin resistance. J Clin Endocrinol Metab. 2001;86:517-520.
28. Setji TL, Holland ND, Sanders LL, Pereira KC, Diehl AM, Brown AJ. Nonalcoholic steatohepatitis and nonalcoholic fatty liver disease in young women with polycystic ovary syndrome. J Clin Endocrinol Metab. 2006;91(5):1741-1747.
29. Boomsma CM, Eijkemans MJ, Hughes EG, Visser GH, Fauser BC, Macklon NS. A meta-analysis of pregnancy outcomes in women with polycystic ovary syndrome. Hum Reprod Update. 2006;12(6):673-683.

第九章 多囊卵巢综合征的诊断标准

一、引言

多囊卵巢综合征（PCOS）是全球女性最常见的内分泌疾病之一。在育龄期女性中，它以高雄激素性无排卵为特征。Stein 和 Leventhal 于 1935 年发现了闭经、高雄激素血症（HA）和不孕症之间的联系，并首次描述了 PCOS。它涵盖了一系列的症状，包括多毛症、男性化、月经稀发、闭经、月经过少，甚至月经频发，以及低生育力甚至不孕症。由于这种综合征中激素相互作用，几乎所有病例都伴随或潜伏着代谢综合征的一些特征，存在患糖尿病和心血管疾病（cardiovascular disease，CVD）的风险。

PCOS 的异质性和复杂的临床表现使得该疾病的定义和术语一直难以界定。尽管现在使用 PCOS 这个术语来指代这一系列"多系统生殖-代谢紊乱"，但关于该病不同表型的演变提示了对更确切的诊断标准或更准确术语的需求。

二、成人多囊卵巢综合征的诊断

对于任何有月经不规律和 HA 症状（痤疮、多毛症、男性型脱发）的育龄女性，都可以怀疑其患有 PCOS。曾经出现突然或逐渐体重增加并符合明显超重或肥胖标准的女性应接受 PCOS 相关检查。在超声检查中发现多囊卵巢，但没有其他 PCOS 的临床特征（HA 或月经失调）的患者不应被认为患有 PCOS，并应避免对其进行过度检查。同时，对于 PCOS 保持高度警惕是很重要的，因为这些患者可能存在与 CVD 相关的危险因素，如葡萄糖耐受不良、血脂异常、脂肪肝和阻塞性睡眠呼吸暂停，而这些都需要进行相应的评估和治疗。

（一）临床特征

PCOS 被认为是一种具有多种潜在病因和不同临床表现的综合征。它以排卵功能障碍、雄激素过多和多囊卵巢形态为特征。不孕症或低生育力是患者的常见主诉。可以基于患者的病史和体格检查及鹿特丹标准（稍后详述）对其进行诊断。因此，为了更好地理解诊断方法，后文将更详细地描述这些区别特征。

1. 月经失调

（1）月经不规律

PCOS 患者可能会出现间隔短于 21 天的频繁月经，或间隔长于 35 天的不规律月经。有时，尽管间隔正常，出血可能是无排卵性的（25～35 天）。因此，PCOS 的月经失调可以表现为月经频发、月经稀发甚至闭经，后两者与排卵不规律或无排卵密切相关。在这种情况下，可以通过黄体中期孕酮来检测有无排卵。女性患者通常有轻微延迟或正常的月经初潮，随后出现月经周期不规律。因此，月经不规律可能是从围青春期开始的。也有患者可能在二十多岁或三十多岁时才出现症状，她们起初月经正常，之后出现月经不规律并伴随体重增加。

（2）促性腺激素的影响

PCOS 患者的平均黄体生成素（LH）水平较高，脉冲频率和振幅也较高。然而，在解释血清 LH 水平真正升高之前，必须考虑许多因素（方框 9.1）。因此，血清 LH 水平未升高并不能排除 PCOS 的可能性。此外，PCOS 患者的血清卵泡刺激素（FSH）水平可能正常或偏低；然而，诊断 PCOS 并不需要检测到血清 LH 浓度升高或 LH：FSH 升高。

方框 9.1 影响多囊卵巢综合征女性患者黄体生成素水平的因素
1. 相对于末次月经的标本采集时间 2. 卵巢活动 3. 口服避孕药的使用 4. 体重指数 5. 黄体生成素采样频率

（3）子宫内膜异型增生和子宫内膜癌

除了 PCOS 患者常见的月经稀发或闭经症状，无排卵导致的雌激素对子宫内膜的慢性无拮抗刺激，可能会增加子宫内膜增生和子宫内膜癌的风险。早在 1949 年，人们就首次提出了 PCOS 与子宫内膜癌之间的关联，但在文献中相关的科学证据一直存在争议。原因在于，尽管有多个内分泌和代谢因素被认为与子宫内膜癌的风险增加有关，但仍缺乏无排卵与癌症风险之间的独立关联。虽然在不同诊断标准的背景下缺乏共识，但最近对 5 项研究进行的一项荟萃分析发现，患有 PCOS 的女性患子宫内膜癌的风险增加［优势比（odds ratio, OR）：2.79，95% 置信区间（confidence interval, CI）：1.31～5.95］。

2. 卵巢功能障碍

（1）卵巢形态和超声的作用

PCOS 患者的卵巢增大，组织学上可见边缘有较多小的窦状卵泡，中央间质增加。PCOS 的重要诊断标准是卵巢中存在 12 个或更多直径为 2～9 mm 的卵泡，和（或）卵巢体积增至大于 10 mL（没有囊肿或优势卵泡的情况下）。新的指南提出每个卵巢至少应有 20 个卵泡，且卵巢中无黄体、优势卵泡或囊肿。然而，由于年龄的变化和基于超声标准的诊断差异，仅依靠卵巢形态不足以做出诊断。因此，如果患者既有月经稀发又有 HA 的迹象，并且排除了 PCOS 以外的所有其他原因，则符合 PCOS 的诊断标准，无须进行超声检查。然而，超声检查有助于更好地理解 PCOS 的各种表型。超声也经常用于正常月经周期的 HA 症状患者，以探查多囊卵巢形态（PCOM）。在这种情况下，应尽量使用阴道超声而不是腹部超声。

Swanson 于 1981 年首次描述了 PCOM 的超声表现。值得注意的是，超声诊断中卵泡（而不是囊肿）的数量和大小很重要。鹿特丹标准被认为具有足够的特异性和敏感性来定义 PCOM，其包括任意一侧卵巢中存在 ≥ 12 个直径为 2 ~ 9 mm 的卵泡，和（或）卵巢体积增加（ > 10 mL；使用公式 "0.5 × 长 × 宽 × 厚" 计算）。PCOM 是指任何一侧卵巢符合此定义 ["2003 年修订的有关多囊卵巢综合征诊断标准和长期健康风险的共识"（2004）]。然而，根据一些报告，超过一半的正常月经周期女性符合每个卵巢中存在 ≥ 12 个小卵泡的标准，促使专家重新考虑 2003 年鹿特丹超声标准。

（2）多囊卵巢综合征的超声标准

虽然自 2003 年以来，已有许多替代标准被提出，但目前尚无关于最佳超声标准的共识。

- 基于 2014 年的系统回顾，有人提出采用更高的阈值（每侧卵巢 25 个卵泡），但前提是临床医师使用能提供最大分辨率的超声探头（如 8 MHz）。大多数临床医师并不容易掌握这项技术。
- 2018 年，一个国际循证医学组织推荐每侧卵巢的卵泡计数为 20 个。
- 在有 PCOS 或无 PCOS 的女性中，随着年龄增长，卵巢体积会减小，卵泡数量会减少。因此，有学者提出了基于年龄的多囊卵巢定义标准。

假设患者因盆腔超声或其他腹部影像学检查中偶然发现多囊卵巢而被按照 PCOS 转诊，如果没有发现其他 PCOS 的临床特征，就不需要进一步评估。因此，超声或放射性影像学检测到的多囊卵巢是一种非特异性发现。

（3）卵泡发育缺陷

在 PCOS 患者的卵巢中，卵泡的发育和功能都是紊乱的，卵泡液中的激素环境异常。有明确的证据显示卵巢中的卵泡发育存在缺陷。无排卵的 PCOS 患者比正常对照组有更高密度的窦状卵泡。总的来说，患者的初级卵泡、次级卵泡和三级卵泡的百分比明显更高，而原始（休眠）卵泡的百分比较低，并且存在闭锁卵泡数量增加的趋势。

（4）无排卵性不孕

PCOS 患者排卵不规律，这使得怀孕更加困难。许多希望怀孕的 PCOS 及稀发排卵的患者最终会接受诱导排卵治疗。由于与下丘脑性闭经相比，PCOS 患者采用枸橼酸氯米芬促排卵治疗后的妊娠率较低，所以她们可能存在其他导致不孕症的原因。最初的 PCOS 定义也包括不孕症。许多研究还报告了 PCOS 患者早期流产率增加的情况，其机制尚不清楚，但可能与肥胖有关。

3. 高雄激素血症（临床评估）

PCOS 的第二个症状是 HA。应仔细评估和解释雄激素过多的临床和生化特征以进行诊断。HA 的临床表现包括多毛症、痤疮和男性型脱发。严重者可能表现为男性化、声音嘶哑或阴蒂增大。在大多数情况下，这些发现常提示其他导致男性化的原因，如卵泡膜细胞增殖症或产生雄激素的卵巢肿瘤或肾上腺肿瘤。

（1）多毛症

雄激素过多最常见的临床表现是多毛症。它被定义为男性型分布的过多粗黑终毛，通常使用改良 Ferriman-Gallwey 评分系统进行诊断，其中包括 9 个雄激素敏感的身体部位（图 3.1）。然而，在临床实践中，这种方法有一些限制。最重要的是，不同种族群体的毛发生长表现不同。尽管所有群体的血清雄激素浓度相似，大多数东亚和美洲原住民女性的体毛很少，白种人和黑种人女性体毛中等，而地中海、南亚和中东女性的体毛明显偏多。因此，在东亚女性中，即使出现轻微的痤疮或面部毛发，也应该考虑到可能是高雄激素疾病，最常见的就是 PCOS。

一个常见的美容问题是局部性毛过度生长（"局部多毛症"）而评分在正常范围内（"即使是一根毛发也会产生阴影"）。因此，并非所有"患者认为的显著多毛症"都是异常的。成人多毛症指南还将"特发性多毛症"定义为在没有升高的循环雄激素水平或月经异常的情况下出现的多毛症。

（2）痤疮

女性的寻常痤疮可能提示 PCOS。有证据表明，寻常痤疮对 PCOS 患者的激素和代谢有影响。血清雄烯二酮浓度较高的 PCOS 患者的痤疮严重程度与其总睾酮、游离睾酮、硫酸脱氢表雄酮（DHEAS）和皮质醇水平升高相关。与之类似，血糖浓度增加与痤疮的严重程度也相关。

（3）男性化

男性化是 HA 的罕见症状。雄激素性脱发、阴蒂增大、声音变粗、肌肉增多和乳房变小都是男性化的症状。发生男性化的女性几乎都是闭经的。在男性化中，脱发通常表现为双颞部发际线后移的男性型秃发。阴蒂增大被定义为阴蒂指数（即矢状径 × 横径）大于 35 mm^2。对任何出现男性化症状的女性，特别是急性起病并迅速进展的，都应该怀疑是否存在分泌雄激素的肿瘤。然而，男性化并不一定提示严重的 HA，因为非肿瘤引起的 HA，如 PCOS 和特发性多毛症，亦可以出现任何形式或程度的雄激素过多特征。

秃发是青春期雄激素过多的罕见症状。当发生时，它可以是男性型（影响额—颞—枕部头皮）或女性型（影响头顶，通常早期表现为中线部位加宽）。皮脂溢、多汗症和化脓性汗腺炎也是雄激素过多的其他皮肤表现。化脓性汗腺炎以患者易摩擦部位的痛性炎症结节为特征，尤其常见于腋下。

（二）生化检查

基于所检测的雄激素种类和所使用的技术，50%～90% 的 PCOS 女性血清雄激素水平升高。对临床中表现为高雄的女性进行生化诊断时，血清总睾酮浓度被认为是雄激素生成总量的最佳估计值。其他雄激素也升高，但 PCOS 中雄激素过多的机制是促性腺激素依赖性的，卵泡膜细胞在长期升高的 LH 和胰岛素水平刺激下增加了雄激素的产生。尽管 PCOS 是女性多毛症最常见的原因，但必须对那些患有其他疾病的患者进行鉴别,如非经典型先天性肾上腺皮质增生症(NCCAH)或更严重的原因(分泌雄激素的肿瘤和卵巢卵泡膜细胞增殖症)。

1. 月经周期正常女性的检测

具有高雄激素症状(最常见的是多毛症)和正常月经周期的女性更可能患有PCOS或特发性多毛症,并且不太可能存在更严重的多毛症病因。对于这些患者,只检测血清总睾酮是比较恰当的第一步。

2. 月经稀发女性的检测

从生化角度来说,PCOS是一种排除性诊断。对于有月经稀发/稀发排卵的女性,应排查其月经不规律的其他可能原因。应该检查人绒毛膜促性腺激素(human chorionic gonadotropin,hCG)以排除妊娠;检查催乳素和促甲状腺激素(TSH)以排除高催乳素血症和甲状腺疾病;检查FSH以排除卵巢功能不全。在排除了这些原因之后,对于有高雄激素症状和月经稀发的女性,有必要测定其雄激素及清晨17-羟孕酮(17-OHP)的水平。

• 血清总睾酮:确定血清总睾酮浓度的最准确和特异性最强的方法是液相色谱-串联质谱法(liquid chromatography-tandem mass spectroscopy,LC-MS/MS)。血清总睾酮浓度是临床高雄女性雄激素生成量最准确的整体估计值。在使用LC-MS/MS的女性中,血清睾酮的正常范围为45~60 ng/dL(1.6~2.1 nmol/L);那些血清睾酮水平大于150 ng/dL的患者需要被评估是否存在严重HA的原因(分泌雄激素的卵巢和肾上腺肿瘤)。大多数医院实验室所提供的免疫测定法不能准确检测女性的睾酮值。

• 血清游离睾酮:在高雄激素疾病的诊断中,因目前直接检测总睾酮的结果不够准确,所以血清游离睾酮的测定可能敏感性更高。如果需要测定游离睾酮,应该使用平衡透析法。因此,总睾酮或游离睾酮水平升高是PCOS生化HA的一个关键诊断特征。

• 性激素结合球蛋白(SHBG):检测SHBG水平是间接评估游离睾酮水平的另一种选择。虽然不太准确,但实验室可通过公式,基于总睾酮和SHBG水平,估算出接近平衡透析法测定的游离睾酮结果。此外,直接检测SHBG在其他方面也是有益的。在PCOS患者中,SHBG异常降低是睾酮生物活性增加的危险因素,也就意味着会出现更严重的表型。

• DHEAS:大约25%的PCOS患者DHEAS水平升高,不过诊断时需要使用与年龄相关的截断值,因为DHEAS水平随年龄而降低。此外,只有10%的PCOS患者存在单独的DHEAS升高。因此,国际共识不推荐常规测量DHEAS。然而,当病因不太像是PCOS时,可以将其作为HA全套检查的一部分。

• 血清雄烯二酮:在PCOS患者中,血清雄烯二酮有时会升高;然而,其在评估PCOS和(或)多毛症中的作用尚不明确。18%的PCOS患者可出现血清雄烯二酮的升高;但仅有9%的病例表现为其独立的升高。

• 17-OHP:建议用晨血测定血清17-OHP以排除由21-羟化酶缺乏症引起的NCCAH。

对于那些有一定自发月经周期的女性，应该在早期卵泡期进行检查；对于那些没有自发月经周期的女性，可以在任意一天进行检查。NCCAH 的临床表现可能与 PCOS 相似甚至相同（HA、月经稀发和多囊卵巢）。NCCAH 虽比 PCOS 少见，但仍需要被排除，因存在子代发生更严重的经典型 21-羟化酶缺乏症的风险。对生活在高风险地区的女性（如阿什肯纳兹犹太人、某些高加索人和东欧女性）进行筛查尤为重要。

- LH∶FSH 的作用：升高的 LH∶FSH 不是 PCOS 诊断的标准。过去，许多临床医师会检测 LH 和 FSH，并使用升高的 LH∶FSH（≥2）作为 PCOS 诊断的证据。然而，LH∶FSH 可能具有欺骗性。例如，如果最近发生过排卵，LH 将被抑制，比例将小于或等于 2。事实上，垂体 LH 分泌的增加不一定能通过测定其血清浓度而被发现，因为约有 1/3 的患者循环 LH 水平在正常范围内。
- 血清催乳素水平：一些高雄激素女性的催乳素水平可能轻度升高，但其意义尚不明确。催乳素水平大于 40 mg/dL 时应该进一步调查其他原因。
- 抗米勒管激素（AMH）的功能：由于血清 AMH 由窦前卵泡和早期窦状卵泡产生，其血清浓度反映了原始卵泡池（卵巢储备）的大小。成年女性的 AMH 水平随着年龄的增长逐渐下降（原始卵泡池减小），到绝经期低至检测不到。与年龄匹配的对照组相比，PCOS 患者的平均 AMH 浓度较高。在纳入 10 项关于 PCOS 患者观察性研究的一项荟萃分析中，AMH 浓度大于 4.7 ng/mL 对诊断 PCOS 具有 79% 的特异性和 83% 的敏感性。尽管有关 AMH 作为 PCOS 诊断的替代标志物的证据逐渐出现，但目前尚未把升高的 AMH 作为 PCOS 的诊断标准。其中一些限制因素包括研究人群的显著异质性，青少年和成年人的截断值差异，以及在多囊卵巢形态影像学定义、检测方法和样本处理中的不一致性。

3. 接受药物治疗女性的检测

一些患者可能已经接受了药物治疗，通常是雌激素-孕激素口服避孕药（oral contraceptives，OC）。在这种情况下，检测血清雄激素是没有意义的，因为 OC 会抑制血清促性腺激素和卵巢雄激素，特别是睾酮的分泌。同样，也应避免对正在服用二甲双胍或螺内酯的女性进行雄激素测定，因为这些药物对雄激素水平的影响会使检测结果的解释变得复杂。根据建议，在检测血清雄激素前，患者应停药 4～6 周。

4. 具有其他内分泌疾病特征女性的检测

患有其他内分泌疾病的女性，如库欣综合征，偶尔会出现类似 PCOS 的症状（月经稀发、多毛症和肥胖）。然而，她们具有皮质醇过多的症状和体征，如向心性肥胖、高血压、紫纹和近端肌无力。同样，患有肢端肥大症的女性可能会出现月经稀发和多毛症，可能需要检测其血清胰岛素样生长因子-1（IGF-1）。

（三）诊断标准

1. 鹿特丹标准

大多数专家组使用鹿特丹标准来诊断 PCOS，虽然在使用这些标准时存在某些局限性，如表 9.1 所示。使用该标准时需要至少满足以下 3 项标准中的任意 2 项才能做出诊断［2003 年修订的有关多囊卵巢综合征诊断标准和长期健康风险的共识（2004）］：

- 稀发排卵和（或）无排卵。
- 临床和（或）生化 HA 的表现。
- 多囊卵巢（通过超声检查）。

表 9.1 鹿特丹标准的局限性

项目	局限性
雄激素过多	• 浓度的日间变化 • 浓度的年龄相关差异 • 检测方法在实验室之间没有统一标准化 • 临床高雄激素血症表现的种族差异 • 在量化高雄激素血症方面的主观差异
排卵功能障碍	• 排卵标准定义不清晰 • 女性一生中排卵的变化 • 对排卵功能障碍的客观检查理解不足 • 通常被理解为无排卵周期
多囊卵巢形态	• 依赖于检查者和技术 • 在月经周期和生育年龄方面缺乏规范标准 • 本质上非特异性，可能与其他疾病混淆

对于许多月经不规律和有高雄激素症状的女性，可以仅基于其病史和体格检查进行诊断。然而，只有在排除了其他导致稀发排卵/无排卵和（或）HA 的情况，如甲状腺疾病、NCCAH、高催乳素血症及分泌雄激素的肿瘤之后，才能确诊 PCOS。

2. 美国国立卫生研究院标准

1990 年，美国国立卫生研究院（NIH）制定的标准允许不使用影像学检查进行临床诊断。此外，NIH 标准要求患者存在月经不规律，而其他标准则没有这个要求。

3. 雄激素过多和多囊卵巢综合征协会标准

雄激素过多和 PCOS 协会在 2006 年提出了雄激素过多和多囊卵巢综合征协会（AE-PCOS）标准。与鹿特丹标准相比，大部分 AE-PCOS 工作组成员认为，在有排卵功能障碍和多囊卵巢但无 HA 证据的女性中，诊断 PCOS 的数据不充分。

使用多种分类系统会使临床医师和患者感到困惑。根据 2012 年 12 月美国国立卫生研究院关于 PCOS 的循证研讨会的总结报告，应暂时采用鹿特丹标准，因为它是最全面的标准（表 9.2）。他们还建议更改"PCOS"的名称，因为它侧重于 PCOM，而这一点对诊断来说既不充分也不必要，并且卵巢中充满液体的结构也并不是"囊肿"。会议提议的名称之一是"代谢性生殖综合征"，它反映了综合征的多方面性质，但与会者承认更改命名很难。

第九章 多囊卵巢综合征的诊断标准

表 9.2 多囊卵巢综合征的推荐诊断标准

1990 年 NIH 共识标准 （所有条件均需满足）	2003 年鹿特丹标准 （需要满足 3 项中的 2 项）	2008 年 AES 定义 （所有条件均需满足）
由于稀发排卵或无排卵导致的月经不规律	稀发排卵或无排卵	临床和（或）生化的高雄激素血症表现
临床和（或）生化的高雄激素血症表现	临床和（或）生化的高雄激素血症表现	卵巢功能障碍——稀发排卵/无排卵和（或）通过超声观察到多囊卵巢
排除其他疾病：NCCAH 和分泌雄激素的肿瘤	通过超声检查观察到多囊卵巢	排除其他雄激素过多或排卵障碍的疾病

注：AES，雄激素过多协会；NCCAH，非经典型先天性肾上腺皮质增生症；NIH，美国国立卫生研究院。

三、绝经后女性多囊卵巢综合征的诊断

（一）绝经后雄激素

在绝经前和绝经后的女性中，肾上腺和卵巢都会产生内源性雄激素。肾上腺雄激素，尤其是脱氢表雄酮（DHEA）及其硫酸盐（DHEAS），在成年早期会出现高峰，随着年龄的增长而显著减少。与此相比，随着年龄的增长和绝经的出现，卵巢雄激素分泌的变化并不那么剧烈。一项关于最后一次月经周期的纵向研究提示，总睾酮水平仅略微下降，而 SHBG 的下降稍微多一些。

（二）临床表现

绝经后的女性中，HA 最常见的症状是多毛症和脱发，而阴蒂增大、声音变低、肌肉力量增加及肌肉发达也与较高的雄激素水平相关。一些由肿瘤导致 HA 的绝经后患者由于雄激素在外周芳构化为雌激素，可发生子宫出血。有些患者还可能发生子宫内膜增生或子宫内膜癌。

在绝经后的女性中，新发的 HA 非常罕见。PCOS 是绝经前女性雄激素过多的最常见原因。绝经前月经周期不规则的病史结合临床 HA 表现可能提示绝经前 PCOS。在 PCOS 女性患者和健康女性中，雄激素水平通常在绝经后下降；然而，有 PCOS 病史的绝经后女性的雄激素水平仍高于健康绝经后女性。当 HA 于女性绝经后才出现或加重时，通常是由于其他原因，如卵巢卵泡膜细胞增殖症或分泌雄激素的肿瘤。

（三）诊断标准

根据 2013 年美国内分泌学会关于 PCOS 诊断和治疗的临床实践指南，对绝经前成年女性应使用鹿特丹标准诊断 PCOS。该指南承认在绝经后患者中确诊是困难的，但他们建议可以使用"有明确记载的育龄期长期月经稀发和 HA 的病史"作为推测诊断的依据。在这种情况下，盆腔超声发现 PCOS 形态将提供额外的证据。

然而，卵巢体积和卵泡数量在 PCOS 和非 PCOS 女性中均随年龄增长而减少。尽管已有学者提出了 40 岁以上女性基于年龄的 PCOS 诊断标准，但目前仍没有针对绝经

后女性而确立的诊断标准。如绝经后女性出现新发或加重的多毛症或其他严重的 HA 症状，一定要对其进行经阴道超声检查，以排除卵巢卵泡膜细胞增殖症和分泌雄激素的肿瘤等疾病。

四、青少年多囊卵巢综合征的诊断

（一）临床表现

青春期 HA 可能是成年 PCOS 的前兆，而 PCOS 的临床表现常常从青春期就开始出现。两项关于围青春期女性的研究表明，肥胖可能是雄激素增多的一个诱因，因为体重指数（BMI）增加与血清总睾酮、游离睾酮和 DHEAS 浓度增加相关。目前尚不清楚是否存在这样一种 PCOS 表型，即肥胖伴内源性卵巢 HA，但缺乏多毛症、痤疮和无排卵症状。

1. 多毛症

依据较少的正常参考数据，性毛在青春期内逐渐生长，并于月经初潮后 2 年（大约在 15 岁）达到成熟。由于特发性多毛症占轻度多毛症病例的一半，青春期 PCOS 指南认为只有中度至重度多毛症才是 HA 的临床证据。即便如此，这种证据也没有通过可靠检测确定的持续性睾酮升高那么可靠。

2. 痤疮

严重的寻常痤疮是青春期 HA 常见的异质性皮肤表现。痤疮的严重程度可以通过病变数目来确定。虽然青春期女性常见粉刺型痤疮，但在围青春期出现中度（>10 个面部病变）或严重炎性痤疮则提示 HA。

（二）诊断挑战

由于多种原因，将成人 PCOS 诊断标准应用于青少年已被证明是困难的。第一，正常的青春期女性本就具有无排卵周期和月经不规律的特点。第二，由于多毛症处于发展阶段，而寻常痤疮在青春期也很常见，所以成人 HA 的常见表现对青春期女性的适用性较差。第三，测定青春期女性的睾酮水平是困难的，因血清睾酮浓度在无排卵周期中升高，几乎没有青春期女性的雄激素水平的可靠参考范围，而青春期雄激素增多到何种程度才会对预测成年后 HA 具有意义，目前也尚不清楚。第四，按成人标准，正常的青春期女性中 PCOM 很常见。

（三）诊断标准

已有 3 个国际专家会议发表了有关青少年 PCOS 诊断的建议。这些建议在基本标准上达成了一致：除其他原因引起的持续排卵功能障碍（参照基于生理年龄而设置的标准时所表现出的月经异常）的证据，以及临床和（或）生化方面雄激素过多的证据（HA）（表 9.3）。

表 9.3　青少年多囊卵巢综合征的国际诊断标准

诊断标准	依据
1. 异常的月经模式，提示排卵功能障碍	a. 基于年龄或生理年龄而表现出的异常，并且 b. 症状持续 1～2 年
2. 临床和（或）生化证据表明存在高雄激素血症	a. 多毛症，尤其是中到重度，是高雄激素血症的临床证据 b. 通过专业的标准化测定方法检测到血清总睾酮或游离睾酮的升高，是高雄激素血症的生化证据

来源：Rosenfield RL. Perspectives on the international recommendations for the diagnosis and treatment of polycystic ovary syndrome in adolescence. *J Pediatr Adolesc Gynecol*. 2020；S1083.

注：排除其他原因后无法解释的情况下呈现表中症状的组合。

然而，在标准的临床细节方面，这些建议之间还存在一些差异。对于是否采用月经异常持续 1 年或 2 年来区分 PCOS 和正常未成熟的月经周期（"生理性青春期无排卵"），它们之间存在分歧。此外，关于何种程度的多毛症或痤疮可以等同于准确的 HA 生化证据，这两者之间仍存在分歧。然而，它们一致同意，在月经初潮后 1～2 年出现 PCOS 表现的青春期女性应被暂时诊断为"有 PCOS 风险"，并进行对症治疗。

五、多囊卵巢综合征的鉴别诊断

PCOS 是一种排除性诊断。一旦排除了其他具有类似 PCOS 特征的疾病，如 NCCAH、甲状腺疾病和高催乳素血症，就可以使用鹿特丹诊断标准进行 PCOS 的诊断。对有严重 HA 和男性化症状的女性需要进行更全面的检查，以排除雄激素过多最严重的一些原因（分泌雄激素的卵巢和肾上腺肿瘤，以及卵巢卵泡膜细胞增殖症）。表 9.4 列出了在进行 PCOS 诊断时需要排除的一些情况。

表 9.4　在诊断多囊卵巢综合征之前需要排除的情况

情况	检测
甲状腺疾病	血清促甲状腺激素
催乳素过多	血清催乳素
非经典型先天性肾上腺皮质增生症	清晨（8 点之前）血清 17-羟孕酮
妊娠	血清或尿液 hCG
下丘脑性闭经	血清 FSH 和 LH
原发性卵巢功能不全	血清 FSH 和血清雌二醇
分泌雄激素的肿瘤	血清睾酮、硫酸脱氢表雄酮、阴道超声检查卵巢、肾上腺 MRI
库欣综合征	24 小时尿皮质醇、过夜地塞米松抑制试验
肢端肥大症	血清游离型胰岛素样生长因子 -1 水平、垂体 MRI

注：hCG，人绒毛膜促性腺激素；FSH，卵泡刺激素；LH，黄体生成素；MRI，磁共振成像。

（一）非经典型先天性肾上腺皮质增生症

NCCAH 的临床表现与 PCOS 相似或相同（HA、月经稀发和多囊卵巢）。NCCAH 比 PCOS 更少见，但应该被排除，因为其后代有可能患有更严重的经典型 21-羟化酶缺乏症。对于地中海地区居民、西班牙人和德系犹太人后裔等高风险女性，这个检测尤为重要。如果早期卵泡期 17-OHP 的值小于 200 ng/dL（6 nmol/L），则不太可能诊断为 NCCAH。而早期卵泡期的 17-OHP 值超过 200 ng/dL，则强烈提示这个诊断，可以通过高剂量（250 μg）的促肾上腺皮质激素（adrenocorticotropic hormone，ACTH）1-24（替可克肽）刺激试验进行确认。大多数患者对替可克肽的反应较强烈，17-OHP 值超过 1500 ng/dL（43 nmol/L）。

（二）分泌雄激素的肿瘤 / 卵巢卵泡膜细胞增殖症

患有分泌雄激素的卵巢或肾上腺肿瘤或卵巢卵泡膜细胞增殖症的女性通常表现为新发的严重多毛症、突然进展的多毛症及男性化的症状或体征，如前额秃发、严重痤疮、阴蒂增大、肌肉量增加或声音变低。血清睾酮浓度几乎都大于 150 ng/dL（5.2 nmol/L），DHEAS 浓度通常大于 800 μg/dL（21.6 μmol/L）。尽管这些疾病在绝经后的女性中更常见，但在绝经前的女性中偶尔也会出现。

（三）其他病因

月经稀发可以出现在甲状腺功能减退、甲状腺功能亢进或高催乳素血症的情况下。然而，高雄激素症状在这些疾病中并不常见。临床特征和生化检查（高 TSH、低 TSH、高催乳素）可鉴别这些疾病。

六、青少年多囊卵巢综合征的鉴别诊断

（一）青春期生理性无排卵

青春期生理性无排卵是青春期月经不规律最常见的原因。它可能在约一半的临床上无雄激素过多表现的 HA 病例中出现，但 HA 和闭经并不持续。

（二）男性化 / 经典型先天性肾上腺皮质增生症

21- 羟化酶缺乏症导致的经典型先天性肾上腺皮质增生症（CAH）是最常见的 CAH 形式。该病几乎都在婴儿期被诊断出来，受影响的女婴因先天性男性化而导致生殖器难以辨别，并可能伴有失盐危机。如果患者未得到恰当的糖皮质激素治疗，她们可能在青春期出现类似 PCOS 的体征和症状，可能的症状包括月经不规律、多毛症和阴蒂增大。多囊卵巢可以由男性化卵巢外雄激素过多和卵巢中肾上腺残余组织（卵巢中的异位肾上腺组织）引起。在没有雄激素过多的情况下，肾上腺孕酮过多也可能通过抑制黄体生成素脉冲而引起卵巢功能障碍。

（三）肾上腺类固醇代谢或作用紊乱的先天性疾病

糖皮质激素受体信号传导缺陷导致糖皮质激素抵抗。这是一种罕见的 ACTH 依赖性的肾上腺 HA，由于来自皮质醇的负反馈作用不够充分，导致 ACTH 过度释放。在患病的青春期女性中，可能会出现高雄激素性无排卵、过早的阴毛生长及骨骼生长缺陷等。

（四）胰岛素抵抗性疾病

PCOS 与各种严重的胰岛素抵抗（IR）及高胰岛素血症状态相关，如因胰岛素受体突变引起的先天性糖尿病（如多诺霍综合征）或脂肪营养不良。IR 还与 PCOS 患者的假性库欣综合征和假性肢端肥大性巨人症相关，这些疾病在临床上类似皮质醇过多和儿童生长激素过多，但实际并没有过量产生这些激素。在这些疾病中，IR 症状通常先于 PCOS 的症状出现。此外，在 1 型和 2 型糖尿病中，轻度的 IR 与 PCOS 相关。高水平的胰岛素或可通过增加卵巢和肾上腺中类固醇合成酶的活性来促进 PCOS 发病，类似于 IGF-1。

（五）特发性高雄激素血症

约有 3.9% 的 HA 患者经过全面临床评估后未找到明确的卵巢或肾上腺雄激素来源。那些有多毛症和正常月经但没有多囊卵巢的患者通常被诊断为这种情况。肥胖可能是绝大多数特发性 HA 的原因。然而，肥胖有时也可以引起高雄激素性无排卵（"非典型 PCOS 肥胖"），体重减轻后症状可能会改善。

七、转诊至专科医师

管理 PCOS 最重要的方面是采用多学科方法。患有 PCOS 的女性可能首先咨询的是妇科医师、不孕症专家、皮肤科医师或内分泌学家。在任何情况下，专科医师都必须考虑是否将患者转诊给其他相关专科以开展综合的诊断和处理。即使在同一个领域（例如妇科学）中，对于疑似 PCOS 的患者进行诊断性检查也存在相当大的实践差异。因此，采用包括皮肤科、内分泌学、妇科、心理学和生活方式专家的多学科会诊模式可以使 PCOS 患者的大部分症状得到处理（表 9.5）。

表 9.5 各专业医师在多囊卵巢综合征评估中的作用

医师专业	作用
皮肤病学	• 多毛症：使用改良 Ferriman-Gallwey（mFG）评分系统进行评定 • 通过体格检查评估有无痤疮及其严重程度 • 通过体格检查评估有无黑棘皮症、雄激素性脱发和化脓性汗腺炎
妇科/青少年医学	• 慢性无排卵：月经不规律和记录 • 高雄激素血症的临床和（或）生化表现：总/游离睾酮、硫酸脱氢表雄酮 • 多囊卵巢形态：盆腔超声检查 • 子宫内膜增生：子宫内膜活检 • 讨论未来可能出现的不孕症问题
内分泌学	• 肥胖：体重指数测量 • 激素紊乱：总/游离睾酮、硫酸脱氢表雄酮（催乳素、17-羟孕酮、雄烯二酮、促甲状腺激素） • 葡萄糖耐受不良/糖尿病：葡萄糖耐量试验，血红蛋白 A1c • 血脂异常：血脂全套检查（最好是空腹） • 脂肪肝：肝功能检查 • 高血压：测量血压 • 对于患有 PCOS 的超重/肥胖青少年，筛查阻塞性睡眠呼吸暂停症状

续表

医师专业	作用
心理学	• 心理健康症状（如焦虑、抑郁） • 饮食自我管理 • 情绪性进食 • 为改变生活方式设定目标 • 优化睡眠健康
运动	• 阐述运动的目标 • 每次门诊设定活动和锻炼目标
营养	• 管理从基线到每次随访的体重变化趋势 • 提供关于饮食习惯的健康教育

来源：Torres-Zegarra C, Sundararajan D Benson J, et al. Care for adolescents with polycystic ovary syndrome: development and prescribing patterns of a multidisciplinary clinic. J Ped Adolesc Gynecol. 2021；34[5]: 617–625.

八、随访

PCOS 有 2 个主要后果：代谢风险和生育能力下降。关于这 2 种影响的信息非常有限。大多数研究样本很小，并缺乏共识建议的统一标准。不过，从这些数据中可以预测出几方面长期的影响，因此在这种"代谢生殖综合征"的每个领域中都需要进行仔细的监测和随访。

随访将根据个体症状和体征的组合确定，并可分为 2 类：心血管代谢评估和生殖结局评估。

（一）心血管代谢评估

在没有 PCOS 的患者中，应根据各个指南和建议定期评估冠心病、CVD、糖尿病、高血压、血脂异常、肥胖和非酒精性脂肪性肝病的风险。然而，具有高危因素的女性至少应参照以下指标进行随访：

• 检查体重、BMI、腰围。

• 监测血压。

• 检测空腹血糖，必要时进行标准口服葡萄糖耐量试验（oral glucose tolerance test，OGTT）和空腹血脂检测。

• 测定骨密度。

（二）生殖结局评估

许多患有 PCOS 的女性以不孕症、低生育力或流产为首发症状。这些症状可以轻松评估以确定原因（是否存在 PCOS），然后通过包括生活方式干预和人工生殖技术的多学科管理来实现她们的受孕目标。此外，由于患者可能存在子宫内膜癌的风险，必须对其进行全面评估和定期随访（请参见前文），以便预防和治疗。最后，在这些 PCOS 患者中，相关的妊娠并发症更常见，如妊娠期糖尿病（gestational diabetes mellitus，GDM）、妊娠高血压、子痫前期和早产，以及一些新生儿并发症，因此在为这些患者提供产科治疗时应注意到这些方面。监测和随访 PCOS 患者的生殖方面时，应牢记以下要点：

- 注意对子宫内膜增生和子宫内膜癌的预防，这些疾病可能是由慢性排卵障碍引起的。无排卵性功能失调性子宫出血（尤其是伴有子宫内膜增生）需要口服或宫腔内使用孕激素治疗（最初每 3～6 个月进行 1 次）。
- 对于不希望怀孕的患者来说，需要采取避孕措施，因为月经稀发女性的排卵具有间歇性，可能会发生计划外怀孕。
- 对于希望怀孕的患者来说，需要进行促排卵治疗，并进行与妊娠相关的并发症随访，如前所述。
- 抗雄激素治疗监测（最初每 3～6 个月进行 1 次）。
- 对所有女性常规进行乳房检查、宫颈涂片和乳腺 X 线检查。

九、结论

PCOS 是一种复杂的代谢生殖综合征，临床评估需要对其体征和症状有全面的了解。每个临床特征都有它自己的标准和定义，这些标准和定义是根据各种临床和生化评分系统确定的。鹿特丹标准是一套被全世界广泛接受的成年女性 PCOS 的诊断标准，但需在排除重要的鉴别诊断后才能使用。对于青少年和一些可能存在分泌雄激素的恶性肿瘤的绝经后女性来说，诊断更加困难。由于患者可能就诊于多个临床专科，大多数诊断可能较迟或不完整。因此，临床医师需要在必要时将患者转诊给相关专家，制定多学科管理方案，并进行长期随访和监测。

参考文献

1. Wolf WM, Wattick RA, Kinkade ON, Olfert MD. Geographical prevalence of polycystic ovary syndrome as determined by region and race/ethnicity. Int J Environ Res Public Health. 2018;15(11):2589.
2. Stein I, Leventhal M. Amenorrhea associated with bilateral polycystic ovaries. Am J Obstet Gynecol. 1935;29:181-191.
3. Bahadur A, Mundhra R, Kashibhatla J, Rajput R, Verma N, Kumawat M. Prevalence of metabolic syndrome among women with different PCOS phenotypes - a prospective study. Gynecol Endocrinol. 2021;37(1):21-25. doi:10.1080/09513590.2020.1775193.
4. Zaeemzadeh N, Sadatmahalleh SJ, Ziaei S, et al. Prevalence of metabolic syndrome in four phenotypes of PCOS and its relationship with androgenic components among Iranian women: a cross-sectional study. Int J Reprod Biomed. 2020;18(4):253-264. doi:10.18502/ijrm.v13i4.6888.
5. Johnson T, Kaplan L, Ouyang P, Rizza PJ. National Institutes of Health Evidence-Based Methodology Workshop on Polycystic Ovary Syndrome. NIH EbMW Reports. Bethesda, MD: National Institutes of Health; 2019:1-14.
6. Witchel SF, Burghard AC, Tao RH, Oberfield SE. The diagnosis and treatment of PCOS in adolescents: an update. Curr Opin Pediatr. 2019;31(4):562-569. doi:10.1097/MOP.0000000000000778.
7. Legro RS, Arslanian SA, Ehrmann DA, et al. Diagnosis and treatment of polycystic ovary syndrome: an Endocrine Society clinical practice guideline. J Clin Endocrinol Metab. 2013;98(12):4565-4592. doi:10.1210/jc.2013-2350.

8. Teede HJ, Misso ML, Costello MF, et al. Recommendations from the international evidence-based guideline for the assessment and management of polycystic ovary syndrome. Fertil Steril. 2018;110(3):364-379. doi:10.1016/j.fertnstert.2018.05.004.
9. Strowitzki T, Capp E, von Eye Corleta H. The degree of cycle irregularity correlates with the grade of endocrine and metabolic disorders in PCOS patients. Eur J Obstet Gynecol Reprod Biol. 2010;149(2):178-181.
10. Hull MG, Savage PE, Bromham DR, Ismail AA, Morris AF. The value of a single serum progesterone measurement in the midluteal phase as a criterion of a potentially fertile cycle ("ovulation") derived from treated and untreated conception cycles. Fertil Steril. 1982;37(3):355-360.
11. Sheehan MT. Polycystic ovarian syndrome: diagnosis and management. Clin Med Res. 2004;2(1):13-27.
12. Taylor AE, McCourt B, Martin KA, et al. Determinants of abnormal gonadotropin secretion in clinically defined women with polycystic ovary syndrome. J Clin Endocrinol Metab. 1997;82(7):2248-2256. doi:10.1210/jcem.82.7.4105.
13. Speert H. Carcinoma of the endometrium in young women. Surg Gynecol Obstet. 1949;88(3):332-336.
14. Haoula Z, Salman M, Atiomo W. Evaluating the association between endometrial cancer and polycystic ovary syndrome. Hum Reprod. 2012;27(5):1327-1331. doi:10.1093/humrep/des042.
15. Hardiman P, Pillay OS, Atiomo W. Polycystic ovary syndrome and endometrial carcinoma. Lancet. 2003;361(9371):1810-1812.
16. Furberg A, Thune I. Metabolic abnormalities, lifestyle and endometrial cancer risk in a Norwegian cohort. Int J Cancer. 2003;104:669-676.
17. Ignatov A, Ortmann O. Endocrine risk factors of endometrial cancer: polycystic ovary syndrome, oral contraceptives, infertility, tamoxifen. Cancers (Basel). 2020;12(7):1766.
18. Barry JA, Azizia MM, Hardiman PJ. Risk of endometrial, ovarian and breast cancer in women with polycystic ovary syndrome: a systematic review and meta-analysis. Hum Reprod Update. 2014;20(5):748-758. doi:10.1093/humupd/dmu012.
19. Broekmans FJ, Knauff EA, Valkenburg O, Laven JS, Eijkemans MJ, Fauser BC. PCOS according to the Rotterdam consensus criteria: change in prevalence among WHO-II anovulation and association with metabolic factors. BJOG. 2006;113(10):1210-1217. doi:10.1111/j.1471-0528.2006.01008.x.
20. Adams JM, Taylor AE, Crowley Jr WF, Hall JE. Polycystic ovarian morphology with regular ovulatory cycles: insights into the pathophysiology of polycystic ovarian syndrome. J Clin Endocrinol Metab. 2004;89(9):4343-4350. doi:10.1210/jc.2003-031600.
21. Welt CK, Arason G, Gudmundsson JA, et al. Defining constant versus variable phenotypic features of women with polycystic ovary syndrome using different ethnic groups and populations. J Clin Endocrinol Metab. 2006;91(11):4361-4368. doi:10.1210/jc.2006-1191.
22. Swanson M, Sauerbrei EE, Cooperberg PL. Medical implications of ultrasonically detected polycystic ovaries. J Clin Ultrasound. 1981;9(5):219-222. doi:10.1002/jcu.1870090504.
23. Rotterdam ESHRE/ASRM-Sponsored PCOS Consensus Workshop Group. Revised 2003 consensus on diagnostic criteria and long-term health risks related to polycystic ovary syndrome (PCOS). Hum Reprod. 2004;19(1):41-47. doi:10.1093/humrep/deh098.
24. Johnstone EB, Rosen MP, Neril R, et al. The polycystic ovary post-Rotterdam: a common, age-dependent finding in ovulatory women without metabolic significance. J Clin Endocrinol Metab. 2010;95(11):4965-4972. doi:10.1210/jc.2010-0202.
25. Dewailly D, Lujan ME, Carmina E, et al. Definition and significance of polycystic ovarian morphology: a task force report from the Androgen Excess and Polycystic Ovary Syndrome Society. Hum Reprod Update. 2014;20(3):334-352. doi:10.1093/humupd/dmt061.
26. Ahmad AK, Quinn M, Kao CN, Greenwood E, Cedars MI, Huddleston HG. Improved diagnostic performance for the diagnosis of polycystic ovary syndrome using age-stratified criteria. Fertil Steril. 2019;111(4):787-793. e2. doi:10.1016/j.fertnstert.2018.11.044.

27. Alsamarai S, Adams JM, Murphy MK, et al. Criteria for polycystic ovarian morphology in polycystic ovary syndrome as a function of age. J Clin Endocrinol Metab. 2009;94(12):4961-4970. doi:10.1210/jc.2009-0839.
28. Mason HD, Willis DS, Beard RW, Winston RM, Margara R, Franks S. Estradiol production by granulosa cells of normal and polycystic ovaries: relationship to menstrual cycle history and concentrations of gonadotropins and sex steroids in follicular fluid. J Clin Endocrinol Metab. 1994;79(5):1355-1360. doi:10.1210/jcem.79.5.7962330.
29. Hughesdon P. Morphology and morphogenesis of the Stein-Leventhal ovary and of so-called "hyperthecosis". Obstet Gynecol Surv. 1982;37(2):59-77.
30. Webber LJ, Stubbs S, Stark J, et al. Formation and early development of follicles in the polycystic ovary. Lancet. 2003;362(9389):1017-1021. doi:10.1016/s0140-6736(03)14410-8.
31. Abbott DH, Dumesic DA, Franks S. Developmental origin of polycystic ovary syndrome - a hypothesis. J Endocrinol. 2002;174(1):1-5. doi:10.1677/joe.0.1740001.
32. Maciel GA, Baracat EC, Benda JA, et al. Stockpiling of transitional and classic primary follicles in ovaries of women with polycystic ovary syndrome. J Clin Endocrinol Metab. 2004;89(11):5321-5327. doi:10.1210/jc.2004-0643.
33. Franks S, McCarthy MI, Hardy K. Development of polycystic ovary syndrome: involvement of genetic and environmental factors. Int J Androl. 2006;29(1):278-285.
34. Balen AH, Tan SL, MacDougall J, Jacobs HS. Miscarriage rates following in-vitro fertilization are increased in women with polycystic ovaries and reduced by pituitary desensitization with buserelin. Hum Reprod. 1993;8(6):959-964. doi:10.1093/oxfordjournals.humrep.a138174.
35. Makrantonaki E, Zouboulis CC. [Hyperandrogenism, adrenal dysfunction, and hirsutism]. Hautarzt. 2020;71(10):752-761. doi:10.1007/s00105-020-04677-1.
36. Meczekalski B, Szeliga A, Maciejewska-Jeske M, et al. Hyperthecosis: an underestimated nontumorous cause of hyperandrogenism. Gynecol Endocrinol. 2021;37(8):677-682. doi:10.1080/09513590.2021.1903419.
37. Fanta M. [Hirsutism]. Ceska Gynekol. 2017;82(3):237-242.
38. Ferriman D, Gallwey JD. Clinical assessment of body hair growth in women. J Clin Endocrinol Metab. 1961;21(11):1440-1447.
39. Hatch R, Rosenfield RL, Kim MH, Tredway D. Hirsutism: implications, etiology, and management. Am J Obstet Gynecol. 1981;140(7):815-830.
40. Wijeyaratne CN, Balen AH, Barth JH, Belchetz PE. Clinical manifestations and insulin resistance (IR) in polycystic ovary syndrome (PCOS) among South Asians and Caucasians: is there a difference? Clin Endocrinol (Oxf). 2002;57(3):343-350. doi:10.1046/j.1365-2265.2002.01603.x.
41. Mangelsdorf S, Otberg N, Maibach HI, Sinkgraven R, Sterry W, Lademann J. Ethnic variation in vellus hair follicle size and distribution. Skin Pharmacol Physiol. 2006;19(3):159-167. doi:10.1159/000093050.
42. Cheewadhanaraks S, Peeyananjarassri K, Choksuchat C. Clinical diagnosis of hirsutism in Thai women. J Med Assoc Thai. 2004;87(5):459-463.
43. Zhao X, Ni R, Li L, et al. Defining hirsutism in Chinese women: a cross-sectional study. Fertil Steril. 2011;96(3):792-796. doi:10.1016/j.fertnstert.2011.06.040.
44. Martin KA, Anderson RR, Chang RJ, et al. Evaluation and treatment of hirsutism in premenopausal women: an endocrine society clinical practice guideline. J Clin Endocrinol Metab. 2018;103(4):1233-1257. doi:10.1210/jc.2018-00241.
45. Franik G, Bizoń A, Włoch S, Kowalczyk K, Biernacka-Bartnik A, Madej P. Hormonal and metabolic aspects of acne vulgaris in women with polycystic ovary syndrome. Eur Rev Med Pharmacol Sci. 2018;22(14):4411-4418. doi:10.26355/eurrev_201807_15491.
46. Ludwig E. Classification of the types of androgenetic alopecia (common baldness) occurring in the female sex. Br J Dermatol. 1977;97(3):247-254. doi:10.1111/j.1365-2133.1977.tb15179.x.
47. Tagatz GE, Kopher RA, Nagel TC, Okagaki T. The clitoral index: a bioassay of androgenic stimulation. Obstet Gynecol. 1979;54(5):562-564.

48. Fraser IS, Kovacs G. Current recommendations for the diagnostic evaluation and follow-up of patients presenting with symptomatic polycystic ovary syndrome. Best Pract Res Clin Obstet Gynaecol. 2004;18(5):813-823.
49. Carmina E, Azziz R, Bergfeld W, et al. Female pattern hair loss and androgen excess: a report from the multidisciplinary androgen excess and PCOS committee. J Clin Endocrinol Metab. 2019;104(7):2875-2891. doi:10.1210/jc.2018-02548.
50. Karagiannidis I, Nikolakis G, Sabat R, Zouboulis CC. Hidradenitis suppurativa/Acne inversa: an endocrine skin disorder? Rev Endocr Metab Disord. 2016;17(3):335-341. doi:10.1007/s11154-016-9366-z.
51. DeVane GW, Czekala NM, Judd HL, Yen SS. Circulating gonadotropins, estrogens, and androgens in polycystic ovarian disease. Am J Obstet Gynecol. 1975;121(4):496-500. doi:10.1016/0002-9378(75)90081-2.
52. Ehrmann DA, Barnes RB, Rosenfield RL. Polycystic ovary syndrome as a form of functional ovarian hyperandrogenism due to dysregulation of androgen secretion. Endocr Rev. 1995;16(3):322-353. doi:10.1210/edrv-16-3-322.
53. Lizneva D, Gavrilova-Jordan L, Walker W, Azziz R. Androgen excess: investigations and management. Best Pract Res Clin Obstet Gynaecol. 2016;37:98-118. doi:10.1016/j.bpobgyn.2016.05.003.
54. Rosner W, Auchus RJ, Azziz R, Sluss PM, Raff H. Position statement: utility, limitations, and pitfalls in measuring testosterone: an Endocrine Society position statement. J Clin Endocrinol Metab. 2007;92(2):405-413. doi:10.1210/jc.2006-1864.
55. Rosner W, Vesper H. Toward excellence in testosterone testing: a consensus statement. J Clin Endocrinol Metab. 2010;95(10):4542-4548. doi:10.1210/jc.2010-1314.
56. Azziz R, Carmina E, Dewailly D, et al. The Androgen Excess and PCOS Society criteria for the polycystic ovary syndrome: the complete task force report. Fertil Steril. 2009;91(2):456-488. doi:10.1016/j.fertnstert.2008.06.035.
57. Goodman NF, Cobin RH, Futterweit W, et al. American Association of Clinical Endocrinologists, American College of Endocrinology, and androgen excess and PCOS society disease state clinical review: guide to the best practices in the evaluation and treatment of polycystic ovary syndrome-part 1. Endocr Pract. 2015;21(11):1291-1300.
58. Ly LP, Handelsman DJ. Empirical estimation of free testosterone from testosterone and sex hormone-binding globulin immunoassays. Eur J Endocrinol. 2005;152(3):471-478. doi:10.1530/eje.1.01844.
59. Sartorius G, Ly LP, Sikaris K, McLachlan R, Handelsman DJ. Predictive accuracy and sources of variability in calculated free testosterone estimates. Ann Clin Biochem. 2009;46(Pt 2):137-143. doi:10.1258/acb.2008.008171.
60. Lim SS, Norman RJ, Davies MJ, Moran LJ. The effect of obesity on polycystic ovary syndrome: a systematic review and meta-analysis. Obes Rev. 2013;14(2):95-109. doi:10.1111/j.1467-789X.2012.01053.x.
61. Huang A, Landay M, Azziz R. O-26: The association of androgen levels with the severity of hirsutism in the polycystic ovary syndrome (PCOS). Fertil Steril. 2006;86(3):S12.
62. Pinola P, Piltonen TT, Puurunen J, et al. Androgen profile through life in women with polycystic ovary syndrome: a Nordic multicenter collaboration study. J Clin Endocrinol Metab. 2015;100(9):3400-3407. doi:10.1210/jc.2015-2123.
63. Azziz R, Sanchez LA, Knochenhauer ES, et al. Androgen excess in women: experience with over 1000 consecutive patients. J Clin Endocrinol Metab. 2004;89(2):453-462. doi:10.1210/jc.2003-031122.
64. Nordenström A, Falhammar H. Management of endocrine disease: diagnosis and management of the patient with non-classic CAH due to 21-hydroxylase deficiency. Eur J Endocrinol. 2019;180(3):R127-R145. doi:10.1530/eje-18-0712.
65. Carmina E, Dewailly D, Escobar-Morreale HF, et al. Non-classic congenital adrenal hyperplasia due to 21-hydroxylase deficiency revisited: an update with a special focus on adolescent and adult women. Hum Reprod Update. 2017;23(5):580-599. doi:10.1093/humupd/dmx014.
66. Saucedo de la Llata E, Moraga-Sánchez MR, Romeu-Sarrió A, Carmona-Ruiz IO. [LH-FSH ratio and polycystic ovary syndrome: a forgotten test?]. Ginecol Obstet Mex. 2016;84(2):84-94.
67. Cho LW, Jayagopal V, Kilpatrick ES, Holding S, Atkin SL. The LH/FSH ratio has little use in diagnosing polycystic ovarian syndrome. Ann Clin Biochem. 2006;43(Pt 3):217-219. doi:10.1258/000456306776865188.

68. Banaszewska B, Spaczyński RZ, Pelesz M, Pawelczyk L. Incidence of elevated LH/FSH ratio in polycystic ovary syndrome women with normo- and hyperinsulinemia. Rocz Akad Med Bialymst. 2003;48:131-134.
69. Baskind NE, Balen AH. Hypothalamic-pituitary, ovarian and adrenal contributions to polycystic ovary syndrome. Best Pract Res Clin Obstet Gynaecol. 2016;37:80-97. doi:10.1016/j.bpobgyn.2016.03.005.
70. Delcour C, Robin G, Young J, Dewailly D. PCOS and hyperprolactinemia: what do we know in 2019? Clin Med Insights Reprod Health. 2019;13:1179558119871921. doi:10.1177/1179558119871921.
71. Seifer DB, Baker VL, Leader B. Age-specific serum anti-Müllerian hormone values for 17,120 women presenting to fertility centers within the United States. Fertil Steril. 2011;95(2):747-750. doi:10.1016/j.fertnstert.2010.10.011.
72. Casadei L, Madrigale A, Puca F, et al. The role of serum anti-Müllerian hormone (AMH) in the hormonal diagnosis of polycystic ovary syndrome. Gynecol Endocrinol. 2013;29(6):545-550.
73. Saxena U, Ramani M, Singh P. Role of AMH as diagnostic tool for polycystic ovarian syndrome. J Obstet Gynaecol India. 2018;68(2):117-122.
74. Wiweko B, Maidarti M, Priangga MD, et al. Anti-mullerian hormone as a diagnostic and prognostic tool for PCOS patients. J Assist Reprod Genet. 2014;31(10):1311-1316.
75. Iliodromiti S, Kelsey TW, Anderson RA, Nelson SM. Can anti-Mullerian hormone predict the diagnosis of polycystic ovary syndrome? A systematic review and meta-analysis of extracted data. J Clin Endocrinol Metab. 2013;98(8):3332-3340. doi:10.1210/jc.2013-1393.
76. Teede H, Misso M, Tassone EC, et al. Anti-Müllerian hormone in PCOS: a review informing international guidelines. Trends Endocrinol Metab. 2019;30(7):467-478.
77. Hahn S, Quadbeck B, Elsenbruch S, et al. [Metformin, an efficacious drug in the treatment of polycystic ovary syndrome]. Dtsch Med Wochenschr. 2004;129(19):1059-1064. doi:10.1055/s-2004-824847.
78. Sánchez LA, Pérez M, Centeno I, David M, Kahi D, Gutierrez E. Determining the time androgens and sex hormone-binding globulin take to return to baseline after discontinuation of oral contraceptives in women with polycystic ovary syndrome: a prospective study. Fertil Steril. 2007;87(3):712-714. doi:10.1016/j.fertnstert.2006.07.1507.
79. Kyritsi EM, Dimitriadis GK, Kyrou I, Kaltsas G, Randeva HS. PCOS remains a diagnosis of exclusion: a concise review of key endocrinopathies to exclude. Clin Endocrinol (Oxf). 2017;86(1):1-6. doi:10.1111/cen.13245.
80. Rachoń D. Differential diagnosis of hyperandrogenism in women with polycystic ovary syndrome. Exp Clin Endocrinol Diabetes. 2012;120(4):205-209. doi:10.1055/s-0031-1299765.
81. Zawadski JK, Dunaif A. Diagnostic Criteria for Polycystic Ovary Syndrome: Towards a Rational Approach. In: Dunaif A, Givens JR, Haseltine F, eds. Polycystic Ovary Syndrome. Boston: Blackwell Scientific; 1992:377-384.
82. National Institute of Health. Evidence-Based Methodology Workshop on Polycystic Ovary Syndrome. 2013. Available at: https://prevention.nih.gov/sites/default/files/2018-06/FinalReport.pdf.
83. Burger HG. Androgen production in women. Fertil Steril. 2002;77(suppl 4):S3-S5. doi:10.1016/s0015-0282(02)02985-0.
84. Burger HG, Dudley EC, Cui J, Dennerstein L, Hopper JL. A prospective longitudinal study of serum testosterone, dehydroepiandrosterone sulfate, and sex hormone-binding globulin levels through the menopause transition. J Clin Endocrinol Metab. 2000;85(8):2832-2838. doi:10.1210/jcem.85.8.6740.
85. Rannevik G, Jeppsson S, Johnell O, Bjerre B, Laurell-Borulf Y, Svanberg L. A longitudinal study of the perimenopausal transition: altered profiles of steroid and pituitary hormones, SHBG and bone mineral density. Maturitas. 1995;21(2):103-113. doi:10.1016/0378-5122(94)00869-9.
86. Kaltsas GA, Isidori AM, Kola BP, et al. The value of the low-dose dexamethasone suppression test in the differential diagnosis of hyperandrogenism in women. J Clin Endocrinol Metab. 2003;88(6):2634-2643. doi:10.1210/jc.2002-020922.
87. Kaltsas GA, Mukherjee JJ, Kola B, et al. Is ovarian and adrenal venous catheterization and sampling helpful in the investigation of hyperandrogenic women? Clin Endocrinol (Oxf). 2003;59(1):34-43. doi:10.1046/j.1365-2265.2003.01792.x.

88. Outwater EK, Marchetto B, Wagner BJ. Virilizing tumors of the ovary: imaging features. Ultrasound Obstet Gynecol. 2000;15(5):365-371. doi:10.1046/j.1469-0705.2000.00123.x.
89. Daniilidis A, Dinas K. Long term health consequences of polycystic ovarian syndrome: a review analysis. Hippokratia. 2009;13(2):90-92.
90. Markopoulos MC, Rizos D, Valsamakis G, et al. Hyperandrogenism in women with polycystic ovary syndrome persists after menopause. J Clin Endocrinol Metab. 2011;96(3):623-631. doi:10.1210/jc.2010-0130.
91. McCartney CR, Prendergast KA, Chhabra S, et al. The association of obesity and hyperandrogenemia during the pubertal transition in girls: obesity as a potential factor in the genesis of postpubertal hyperandrogenism. J Clin Endocrinol Metab. 2006;91(5):1714-1722. doi:10.1210/jc.2005-1852.
92. Reinehr T, de Sousa G, Roth CL, Andler W. Androgens before and after weight loss in obese children. J Clin Endocrinol Metab. 2005;90(10):5588-5595. doi:10.1210/jc.2005-0438.
93. Zore T, Lizneva D, Brakta S, Walker W, Suturina L, Azziz R. Minimal difference in phenotype between adolescents and young adults with polycystic ovary syndrome. Fertil Steril. 2019;111(2):389-396. doi:10.1016/j.fertnstert.2018.10.020.
94. Lucky AW, Biro FM, Daniels SR, Cedars MI, Khoury PR, Morrison JA. The prevalence of upper lip hair in black and white girls during puberty: a new standard. J Pediatr. 2001;138(1):134-136. doi:10.1067/mpd.2001.109790.
95. Ibáñez L, Oberfield SE, Witchel S, et al. An international consortium update: pathophysiology, diagnosis, and treatment of polycystic ovarian syndrome in adolescence. Horm Res Paediatr. 2017;88(6):371-395. doi:10.1159/000479371.
96. Deplewski D, Rosenfield RL. Role of hormones in pilosebaceous unit development. Endocr Rev. 2000;21(4):363-392. doi:10.1210/edrv.21.4.0404.
97. Rosenfield RL. The diagnosis of polycystic ovary syndrome in adolescents. Pediatrics. 2015;136(6):1154-1165. doi:10.1542/peds.2015-1430.
98. Lucky AW, Biro FM, Simbartl LA, Morrison JA, Sorg NW. Predictors of severity of acne vulgaris in young adolescent girls: results of a five-year longitudinal study. J Pediatr. 1997;130(1):30-39. doi:10.1016/s0022-3476(97)70307-x.
99. Rothenberg SS, Beverley R, Barnard E, Baradaran-Shoraka M, Sanfilippo JS. Polycystic ovary syndrome in adolescents. Best Pract Res Clin Obstet Gynaecol. 2018;48:103-114. doi:10.1016/j.bpobgyn.2017.08.008.
100. Witchel SF, Oberfield S, Rosenfield RL, et al. The diagnosis of polycystic ovary syndrome during adolescence. Horm Res Paediatr. 2015. doi:10.1159/000375530.
101. Rosenfield RL. Perspectives on the international recommendations for the diagnosis and treatment of polycystic ovary syndrome in adolescence. J Pediatr Adolesc Gynecol. 2020;33(5):445-447. doi:10.1016/j.jpag.2020.06.017.
102. Rosenfield RL. Clinical review: adolescent anovulation: maturational mechanisms and implications. J Clin Endocrinol Metab. 2013;98(9):3572-3583. doi:10.1210/jc.2013-1770.
103. Van Hooff MH, Voorhorst FJ, Kaptein MB, Hirasing RA, Koppenaal C, Schoemaker J. Predictive value of menstrual cycle pattern, body mass index, hormone levels and polycystic ovaries at age 15 years for oligo-amenorrhoea at age 18 years. Hum Reprod. 2004;19(2):383-392. doi:10.1093/humrep/deh079.
104. Venturoli S, Porcu E, Fabbri R, et al. Menstrual irregularities in adolescents: hormonal pattern and ovarian morphology. Horm Res. 1986;24(4):269-279. doi:10.1159/000180567.
105. Wiksten-Almströmer M, Hirschberg AL, Hagenfeldt K. Prospective follow-up of menstrual disorders in adolescence and prognostic factors. Acta Obstet Gynecol Scand. 2008;87(11):1162-1168. doi:10.1080/00016340802478166.
106. Barnes RB, Rosenfield RL, Ehrmann DA, et al. Ovarian hyperandrogynism as a result of congenital adrenal virilizing disorders: evidence for perinatal masculinization of neuroendocrine function in women. J Clin Endocrinol Metab. 1994;79(5):1328-1333. doi:10.1210/jcem.79.5.7962325.

107. Bachelot A, Chakhtoura Z, Plu-Bureau G, et al. Influence of hormonal control on LH pulsatility and secretion in women with classical congenital adrenal hyperplasia. Eur J Endocrinol. 2012;167(4):499-505. doi:10.1530/eje-12-0454.
108. Charmandari E, Kino T, Ichijo T, Chrousos GP. Generalized glucocorticoid resistance: clinical aspects, molecular mechanisms, and implications of a rare genetic disorder. J Clin Endocrinol Metab. 2008;93(5):1563-1572. doi:10.1210/jc.2008-0040.
109. Lungu AO, Zadeh ES, Goodling A, Cochran E, Gorden P. Insulin resistance is a sufficient basis for hyperandrogenism in lipodystrophic women with polycystic ovarian syndrome. J Clin Endocrinol Metab. 2012;97(2):563-567. doi:10.1210/jc.2011-1896.
110. Littlejohn EE, Weiss RE, Deplewski D, Edidin DV, Rosenfield R. Intractable early childhood obesity as the initial sign of insulin resistant hyperinsulinism and precursor of polycystic ovary syndrome. J Pediatr Endocrinol Metab. 2007;20(1):41-51. doi:10.1515/jpem.2007.20.1.41.
111. Codner E, Escobar-Morreale HF. Clinical review: hyperandrogenism and polycystic ovary syndrome in women with type 1 diabetes mellitus. J Clin Endocrinol Metab. 2007;92(4):1209-1216. doi:10.1210/jc.2006-2641.
112. Peppard HR, Marfori J, Iuorno MJ, Nestler JE. Prevalence of polycystic ovary syndrome among premenopausal women with type 2 diabetes. Diabetes Care. 2001;24(6):1050-1052. doi:10.2337/diacare.24.6.1050.
113. Sanchón R, Gambineri A, Alpañés M, Martínez-García M, Pasquali R, Escobar-Morreale HF. Prevalence of functional disorders of androgen excess in unselected premenopausal women: a study in blood donors. Hum Reprod. 2012;27(4):1209-1216. doi:10.1093/humrep/des028.
114. Carmina E. Mild androgen phenotypes. Best Pract Res Clin Endocrinol Metab. 2006;20(2):207-220. doi:10.1016/j.beem.2006.02.001.
115. Rosenfield RL. Evidence that idiopathic functional adrenal hyperandrogenism is caused by dysregulation of adrenal steroidogenesis and that hyperinsulinemia may be involved. J Clin Endocrinol Metab. 1996;81(3):878-880. doi:10.1210/jcem.81.3.8772543.
116. Rosenfield RL, Mortensen M, Wroblewski K, Littlejohn E, Ehrmann DA. Determination of the source of androgen excess in functionally atypical polycystic ovary syndrome by a short dexamethasone androgen-suppression test and a low-dose ACTH test. Hum Reprod. 2011;26(11):3138-3146. doi:10.1093/humrep/der291.
117. Escobar-Morreale HF, Santacruz E, Luque-Ramírez M, Botella Carretero JI. Prevalence of 'obesity-associated gonadal dysfunction' in severely obese men and women and its resolution after bariatric surgery: a systematic review and meta-analysis. Hum Reprod Update. 2017;23(4):390-408. doi:10.1093/humupd/dmx012.
118. Sivayoganathan D, Maruthini D, Glanville JM, Balen AH. Full investigation of patients with polycystic ovary syndrome (PCOS) presenting to four different clinical specialties reveals significant differences and undiagnosed morbidity. Hum Fertil (Camb). 2011;14(4):261-265. doi:10.3109/14647273.2011.632058.
119. Bonny AE, Appelbaum H, Connor EL, et al. Clinical variability in approaches to polycystic ovary syndrome. J Pediatr Adolesc Gynecol. 2012;25(4):259-261. doi:10.1016/j.jpag.2012.03.004.
120. Torres-Zegarra C, Sundararajan D, Benson J, et al. Care for adolescents with polycystic ovary syndrome: development and prescribing patterns of a multidisciplinary clinic. J Pediate Adolesc Gynecol. 2021;34(5):617-625.
121. Hudecova M, Holte J, Olovsson M, Sundström Poromaa I. Long-term follow-up of patients with polycystic ovary syndrome: reproductive outcome and ovarian reserve. Hum Reprod. 2009;24(5):1176-1183.
122. Wekker V, van Dammen L, Koning A, et al. Long-term cardiometabolic disease risk in women with PCOS: a systematic review and meta-analysis. Hum Reprod Update. 2020;26(6):942-960. doi:10.1093/humupd/dmaa029.
123. Sha T, Wang X, Cheng W, Yan Y. A meta-analysis of pregnancy-related outcomes and complications in women with polycystic ovary syndrome undergoing IVF. Reprod Biomed Online. 2019;39(2):281-293. doi:10.1016/j.rbmo.2019.03.203.
124. Qin JZ, Pang LH, Li MJ, Fan XJ, Huang RD, Chen HY. Obstetric complications in women with polycystic ovary syndrome: a systematic review and meta-analysis. Reprod Biol Endocrinol. 2013;11:56. doi:10.1186/1477-7827-11-56.

第十章 多囊卵巢综合征和代谢综合征：后期生活中的风险

一、引言

多囊卵巢综合征（PCOS）是影响育龄女性最常见的内分泌-代谢-生殖疾病。PCOS 与代谢紊乱密切相关，如肥胖和胰岛素抵抗（IR），而这些代谢紊乱也在其发病机制中起着核心作用。大部分患有 PCOS 的女性都有超重或肥胖，并表现出伴随的代偿性高胰岛素血症，这在 PCOS 的一些表型特征的发展中起着重要作用，同时，与 β 细胞功能障碍一起增加了患其他代谢异常的风险，如 2 型糖尿病（T2DM）、高血压、血脂异常和心血管疾病（CVD）。此外，一部分体形偏瘦的 PCOS 女性也表现出 IR。

代谢综合征（MetS）是一组葡萄糖和脂肪代谢障碍，包括向心性肥胖、葡萄糖耐受不良、血脂异常和高血压。它已经被证实是 T2DM 和 CVD 的危险因素。IR 和向心性肥胖被证明在 MetS 和 PCOS 的发病机制中起着重要作用。基于个体中存在各种 CVD 风险因素，MetS 的几种定义正在全球范围内被使用（表 10.1）。有关 PCOS 患者 MetS 的研究使用了这些标准中的一种或几种，以获得其研究对象中 MetS 的患病率。

表 10.1 基于不同标准的常用代谢综合征定义

项目	NCEP-ATP Ⅲ	IDF	联合标准
要求	—	WC（女性≥ 80 cm） （南亚、中国女性≥ 80 cm，日本女性≥ 90 cm）	—
异常数目	≥ 3 项以下内容：	≥ 2 项以下内容：	≥ 3 项以下内容：
肥胖	女性 WC ≥ 88 cm	—	WC：不同人群和国家定义不同
甘油三酯	≥ 150 mg/dL	≥ 150 mg/dL	≥ 150 mg/dL
HDL 胆固醇	女性＜ 50 mg/dL	女性＜ 50 mg/dL	女性＜ 50 mg/dL
高血压	≥ 130/85 mmHg	≥ 130/85 mmHg	≥ 130/85 mmHg
葡萄糖	≥ 110 mg/dL	≥ 100 mg/dL	≥ 100 mg/dL

注：HDL，高密度脂蛋白；IDF，国际糖尿病联合会；NCEP-ATP Ⅲ，美国国家胆固醇教育计划成人治疗组第三版（ATP Ⅲ）；WC，腰围。

二、多囊卵巢综合征和肥胖

PCOS 是一种与肥胖、IR 和心脑血管代谢风险相关的疾病，但这些特征并不属于 PCOS 的诊断标准。PCOS 女性患者患有超重或肥胖的风险更高，并且与健康女性相比，她们的向心性肥胖患病率更高（危险比 1.73）。但到底是 PCOS 导致了体重增加和肥胖，还是肥胖与 PCOS 的发展有关，目前尚不清楚。作为病理生理机制之一，体重增加和肥胖通过加重 IR 促进了 PCOS 的发展，导致糖耐量减低（impaired glucose tolerance，IGT），并存在发生 T2DM 的风险。事实上，具有遗传易感性的女性在其一生中体重增加后发生 PCOS 的风险更高。流行病学研究显示，大多数（38%～88%）患有 PCOS 的患者出现了超重或肥胖。无论体重指数（BMI）如何，PCOS 患者主要出现向心性肥胖或腹型肥胖。肥胖加重了激素紊乱和代谢后果，不仅恶化了 PCOS 的临床特征，还导致生育结局不理想，并增加了 MetS、T2DM 和 CVD 的风险。此外，即使只有 5% 的体重减少和胰岛素敏感性的改善，通常也会在雄激素过多、生殖和代谢特征方面产生明显的临床效益。然而，很清楚的一点是，PCOS 本质上与 IR、血脂异常和非酒精性脂肪性肝病（NAFLD）等代谢异常相关，而与肥胖和脂肪量无关。

三、多囊卵巢综合征和胰岛素抵抗

除遗传和环境因素外，IR 在 PCOS 中的致病作用最早于 20 世纪 80 年代被认识到。随后，学者们逐渐认识到，IR 引起的代偿性高胰岛素血症会通过一系列机制导致卵巢源性雄激素生成的增加，包括刺激下丘脑促性腺激素释放激素（GnRH）的基因转录和随后垂体黄体生成素（LH）的脉冲频率升高。因此，胰岛素作用于下丘脑 – 垂体 – 卵巢轴的各个水平，并且卵巢组织中的 IR 引起了一系列代谢信号紊乱，导致在有丝分裂和类固醇合成未受影响的情况下出现高雄激素血症（HA）。增加的雄激素又通过升高游离脂肪酸和改变肌肉组织结构和功能进一步加重了 IR，从而进一步形成"IR—高胰岛素血症—HA"的恶性循环。HA 进一步恶化 IR，从而使恶性循环继续。此外，肥胖不仅增加了卵巢中雄激素的产生，同时也增加了皮下脂肪组织和肾上腺雄激素的生成，从而使得这个恶性循环中所有的环节都更加严重。瘦素可以扰乱卵巢生理功能并诱导慢性全身性炎症状态。最终，IR 和慢性炎症使与 PCOS 相关的所有内分泌代谢紊乱越发严重，进而导致女性患者面临患 T2DM 和 CVD 的风险（图 10.1）。

IR 是 PCOS 患者中常见的病理改变，但并非所有患者都存在 IR。一组关于 526 名生育年龄女性的数据显示，PCOS 女性中 112 名（42.6%）存在 IR，而对照组中的 45 名（17.1%）存在 IR（$P < 0.001$）。伊朗的一项研究显示，PCOS 患者中 36.5% 存在 IR。IR 和胰岛素敏感性（insulin sensitive，IS）PCOS 患者的 MetS 患病率之间有显著差异（43.5% vs. 20.0%；$P = 0.034$）。

另一项有趣的研究比较了伴 MetS 的 PCOS 女性 IR 标志物和循环中的雄激素水平。该研究纳入了 1223 名患 PCOS 的白种人女性和 277 名没有患 PCOS 的女性，对其进行 BMI 匹配。结果显示，伴 MetS 的 PCOS 女性 IR 显著高于不伴 MetS 的 PCOS 女性。有意思的是，作者发现，伴 MetS 的对照组比不伴 MetS 的 PCOS 女性有更严重的 IR（在所有 IR 标志物的比较中，$P < 0.001$）。而无论是否患有 MetS，PCOS 女性都具有较高的循环雄激素水平。

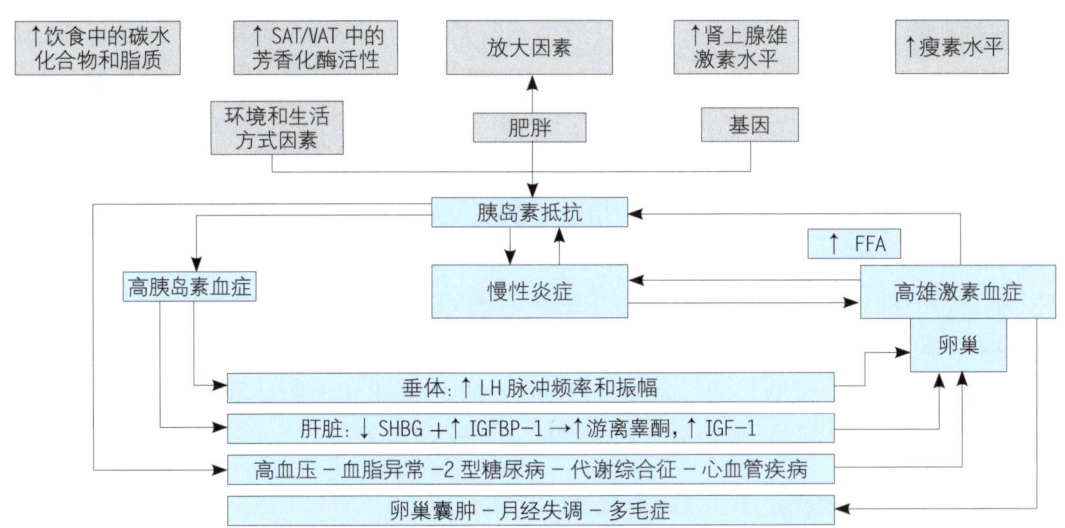

FFA，游离脂肪酸；IGF-1，胰岛素样生长因子 -1；IGFBP-1，胰岛素样生长因子结合蛋白 -1；LH，黄体生成素；SAT，皮下脂肪组织；SHBG，性激素结合球蛋白；VAT，内脏脂肪组织。

图 10.1　多囊卵巢综合征及其相关合并症的发病机制和进展

1. 高胰岛素 - 正常血糖钳夹术

测定 IS 的金标准是通过高胰岛素 - 正常血糖钳夹（M- 钳）术实现的。该过程基于恒定的胰岛素输注，导致新的稳态胰岛素水平高于空腹水平，最终一方面增加骨骼肌和脂肪组织对葡萄糖的摄取，另一方面减缓肝糖异生。同时输注 20% 葡萄糖将血糖水平"钳夹"在正常范围内。该技术可直接测量恒定胰岛素条件下全身葡萄糖代谢总量，但这项技术繁琐、费力、昂贵且具有专业挑战性。

2. 胰岛素抵抗的替代标志物

由于 M- 钳的临床应用存在困难，基于空腹或给予糖负荷后的血糖和胰岛素水平的数学公式计算结果，研究人员开发了各种替代标志物来评估 IS/IR（表 10.2）。这些替代指标已经与 M- 钳进行了比较，同时被广泛用于临床研究。这些 IR 的替代指标与 M- 钳的相关性是合理的。Moghetti 等研究了 375 名 PCOS 患者，其中 74.9% 的患者通过 M- 钳识别为 IR。肥胖的 PCOS 中 IR 更为普遍（PCOS 患者肥胖组 vs. 超重组 vs. 正常体重组 = 93.9% vs. 77.5% vs. 59.3%）。研究人员进一步将替代指标与 M- 钳进行了比较，发现两者高度相关。然而，作者指出这些标记对于识别 IR 的敏感性较低，特别是在正常体重的 PCOS 患者中，这导致正常体重的 PCOS 患者被错误地判断为 IS。基于此，作者建议这些指数可用于确定而非排除 PCOS 中的 IR。许多研究人员尝试使用这些替代指标来评估 PCOS 中的 IR，并提前预测 MetS 和心血管疾病的结局。由此，这些研究也进一步证实了，应用这些指标有益于改进医疗资源利用、节约成本和降低副作用。

表 10.2　胰岛素抵抗替代指标

指标	计算方法
HOMA（稳态模型评估）	空腹血糖^a× 空腹胰岛素^b/22.5
G：I（血糖：胰岛素）	空腹血糖^c/空腹胰岛素^b
QUICKI（胰岛素敏感性定量检查指数）	1/Log（空腹胰岛素^b）+ log（空腹血糖^c）
Gutt 指数	{[75 000 +（空腹血糖^c — 血糖$_{120'}$）×0.19× 体重, kg/120]/[（空腹血糖^c + 血糖$_{120'}$）/2]}/log[（空腹胰岛素^b + 胰岛素$_{120'}$）/2]
Stumvoll	0.156 — 0.000 045 9× 胰岛素$_{120'}$, pmol/L — 0.000 321× 空腹胰岛素^b — 0.005 41× 血糖$_{120'}$^{a}
Matsuda	10 000/[（空腹血糖^c× 空腹胰岛素^b）×（血糖$_{30'}$ + 血糖$_{60'}$ + 血糖$_{90'}$ + 血糖$_{120'}$）/4×（胰岛素$_{30'}$ + 胰岛素$_{60'}$ + 胰岛素$_{90'}$ + 胰岛素$_{120'}$）/4]$^{0.5}$

注：^{a} mmol/L；^{b} mU/L；^{c} mg/dL。

3. 新型生物标志物

近年来，许多蛋白质被发现可能是 PCOS 中 IR 的潜在生物标志物。脂肪细胞因子（如脂连蛋白、内脂素、内脏脂肪特异性丝氨酸蛋白酶抑制剂和爱帕琳肽）、和肽素、鸢尾素、纤溶酶原激活物抑制物 -1（plasminogen activator inhibitor，PAI-1）和连蛋白与 IR 及 PCOS 的病理生理学之间存在强关联。

四、多囊卵巢综合征和代谢综合征

PCOS 患者面临患 MetS 的风险。大量研究报告显示，与无 PCOS 的女性相比，患有 PCOS 女性的 MetS 发病率更高，并且肥胖的 PCOS 女性与非肥胖的 PCOS 女性相比风险更高。表 10.3 列出了一些已发表的研究。

表 10.3　关于多囊卵巢综合征女性中代谢综合征发病率的几篇新近研究

研究	n	对照组	使用的 Met 标准	IR 标志物	MetS 的百分比	其他 CVD 风险报告	评论
Jamil 等，2015	526	有	NCEP-ATP Ⅲ	空腹血糖：胰岛素、HOMA-IR、HOMA-B、QUICKI、Metsuda 指数	53.6% vs. 32.7%（$P < 0.001$）	TG：HDL，（3.17±3.03）vs.（2.28±1.61）（$P < 0.001$）	女性接受生育治疗。PCOS 组的 BMI 和 WC 较高
Abdelazim & Elsawah, 2015	220	无	NCEP-ATP Ⅲ	未报道	30.5%	未报道	患有 PCOS 的不孕女性，>35 岁女性中 MetS 的患病率为 100%
Montazerifar, Ghasemi, Arabpour, Karajibani, & Keikhah, 2020	240	有	NCEP-ATP Ⅲ	—	29.2% vs. 7.5%（$P < 0.000\ 1$）	HDL 低，TG 高，TG：HDL 高，WC 增加	不孕女性

续表

研究	n	对照组	使用的Met标准	IR标志物	MetS的百分比	其他CVD风险报告	评论
N. Anjum, Zohra, Arif, Azhar, & Qureshi, 2013	425	有	NCEP-ATP Ⅲ	空腹血糖：胰岛素	35.6% vs. 9.5% ($P < 0.000\ 1$)	BMI、WC、收缩压、舒张压、TG均升高，HDL低，TG：HDL高	—
Panidis 等，2013	1500	有	所有MetS标准	G：I、HOMA-IR、QUICKI	31～39年龄组：联合标准：39.1% vs. 28.5%（$P = 0.045$）NCEP-ATP Ⅲ标准：27.1% vs. 12.1%（$P = 0.001$）	校正BMI后，WC、WHR、BP及血脂在PCOS和对照组间无显著性差异	如果根据BMI进行校正，则在31岁以下的年龄组与其他年龄组之间MetS没有差异。在所有BMI组中，患有PCOS的女性比对照组更容易出现IR
Moghetti 等，2013	137	无	IDF/NCEP-ATP Ⅲ	M-钳	32.8%（IDF）31.3%（NCEP-ATP Ⅲ）	WC增加（73.7%）且HDL胆固醇低（54.1%）	71.4%为IR
Meyer 等，2020	1427	有	联合	未报道	19.3%（联合）	腹型肥胖（> 66%），HDL胆固醇低（> 42%），BP升高（20.6%）	用OC进行月经调节或治疗痤疮与MetS之间没有显著关联，BMI ≥ 30 kg/m² 的交互作用在统计学上不显著（$P > 0.26$）
Liang 等，2012	290	有	NCEP-ATP Ⅲ	HOMA-IR	30% vs. 18%（$P = 0.008$）	与对照组相比，PCOS组的BMI、WC、WHR和TG均升高	肥胖是唯一一个显著增加MetS风险的变量（OR: 54）
Le 等，2018	441	无	NCEP-ATP Ⅲ	改良的ACE标准	10.4%	伴有MetS的PCOS女性BMI高，腹型肥胖（84.8%），收缩压高（18.2%），TG高（78.8%）和HDL低（93.9%）	不孕女性IRS 27%
Kyrkou 等，2016	385	有	IDF	—	12.6% vs. 1.9%	BMI、BP、TG均高	—
Karee, Gundabattula, Sashi, Boorugu, & Chowdhury, 2020	382	无	NCEP-ATP Ⅲ	—	38.5%	HDL低，WC升高	BMI和年龄之间存在显著关联
Hosseinpanah, Barzin, Tehrani, & Azizi, 2011	559	有	联合临时声明	HOMA-IR	18.5% vs. 18.3%（$P = NS$）	腹型肥胖，血脂异常，BP无显著性差异	IR: 27.2% vs. 24.2%（$P < 0.01$）
S. Anjum, Askari, Riaz, & Basit, 2020	153	无	AHA/NHLBI	HOMA-IR	46.4%	肥胖82.4%，血脂异常56.2%	在PCOS女性中，是否伴有MetS对IR没有影响

注：ACE，美国内分泌学院；AHA/NHLBI，美国心脏协会/美国国家心脏、肺部和血液研究所；BMI，体重指数；BP，血压；CVD，心血管疾病；HDL，高密度脂蛋白；HOMA，稳态模型评估；IDF，国际糖尿病联合会；IR，胰岛素抵抗；IRS，胰岛素受体底物；MetS，代谢综合征；NCEP-ATP Ⅲ，美国国家胆固醇教育计划成人治疗组第三版；NS，不显著；OC，口服避孕药；OR，优势比；PCOS，多囊卵巢综合征；TG，甘油三酯；WC，腰围；WHR，腰臀比。

第十章 多囊卵巢综合征和代谢综合征：后期生活中的风险

一项对 35 项研究进行的荟萃分析报道，患有 PCOS 的女性 MetS 的患病率高于无 PCOS 的女性（OR：2.88）。作者给出了患有 PCOS 的女性中 MetS 不同组成部分的发病率：腰围或 BMI 增加（11%～98%）、高密度脂蛋白（HDL）胆固醇降低（28.6%～95.0%）、甘油三酯增加（5.5%～56.0%）、血压升高（7.3%～70.0%）和空腹血糖升高（0～43.5%）。另一项系统综述和荟萃分析报道，PCOS 女性中 MetS 的汇总患病率为 26.3%，但具体数值在 7.1%～37.5%，具体取决于所使用的诊断标准。降低的 HDL 和增加的腰围是报告中 PCOS 女性里 MetS 最常见的组成部分，分别占 61.87% 和 52.23%。与健康对照组相比，PCOS 患者中 MetS 的整体汇总 OR 为 2.09，但具体数值在 0.31～4.69，具体取决于所使用的诊断标准。

（一）代谢综合征风险的种族差异

许多研究对不同种族的 MetS 风险进行了调查，无论是居住在同一地理位置还是不同地理位置的种族。与白种人 PCOS 患者相比，黑种人青少年［危险比（risk ratio，RR）：2.65］和成年女性（RR：1.44）的 MetS 风险增加。另一项研究报告指出，与非西班牙裔黑种人和白种人女性相比，患有 PCOS 的西班牙裔女性具有更明显的雄激素过多和更高的 MetS 风险。与非西班牙裔白种人和亚裔美国人相比，患有 PCOS 的西班牙裔白种人和黑种人女性具有更高的基础状态 IR、升高的 β 细胞反应和餐后高胰岛素血症。然而，亚裔美国女性的胰岛素反应较低。PCOS 女性发生 MetS 的构成比是不同的，如与来自美国的白种人女性（28.3%）相比，患有 PCOS 的美国黑种人女性的 MetS 患病率最高（52%），而印度（38.2%）和挪威（41.1%）女性的 MetS 患病率较高且独立于肥胖（OR 分别为 6.53 和 2.16）。在同一地理位置生活的白种人、南亚裔和东亚裔女性 PCOS 患者，其代谢特征相似，而亚洲女性的 2 小时胰岛素水平较高，特别是东亚女性。

这些发现表明，在筛查 PCOS 女性患者的代谢紊乱时，应考虑种族和民族因素。需要进行纵向对比，以研究 PCOS 和种族对这些患者发生 CVD 风险的独立影响。

（二）非肥胖多囊卵巢综合征女性患者的代谢紊乱

一些作者报道，在使用美国国家胆固醇教育计划成人治疗组第三版（NCEP-ATP Ⅲ）定义时，即使是非肥胖的 PCOS 患者也会出现较高的代谢紊乱率。非肥胖 PCOS 患者出现的代谢紊乱包括 IR、IGT、高甘油三酯（triglycerides，TG）、低 HDL 和 MetS。

有学者对 100 名瘦型 PCOS 患者进行了研究，探讨稳态模型评估 - 胰岛素抵抗指数（HOMA-IR）（截断值 2.5）对代谢参数的影响。结果显示 47% 伴有 IR 患者的 IR 程度与腰臀比（waist-hip ratio，WHR）、收缩压、舒张压、雌二醇水平、Ferriman-Gallwey 评分和总睾酮水平呈正相关。对 22 项研究进行的一项荟萃分析比较了非肥胖 PCOS 患者与非肥胖对照组（白种人患者 BMI < 30 kg/m²，亚洲患者 BMI < 25 kg/m²）之间的 MetS 患病率，结果显示非肥胖 PCOS 患者的高胰岛素血症（OR：36.27）、IR（OR：5.70）、IGT（OR：3.42）、T2DM（OR：1.47）、高甘油三酯血症（OR：10.46）、低 HDL（OR：

4.03）和 MetS（*OR*：2.57）患病率更高。在这项荟萃分析中，对于两组之间的空腹血糖受损（impaired fasting glucose，IFG）、糖尿病前期、血脂异常、高胆固醇血症和高血压未观察到显著差异。在亚组分析中，白种人患者的 IR、IGT、IFG、T2DM、高血压和 MetS 的患病风险增加，而亚洲患者的代谢变化不显著。目前没有研究对非肥胖 PCOS 患者心肌梗死、脑卒中、脑血管意外、动脉闭塞性疾病或冠心病的发生率进行专门报道。

（三）复方口服避孕药的使用与多囊卵巢综合征的代谢综合征风险

复方口服避孕药（COC）经常用于治疗 PCOS 患者，以实现调整月经周期和改善雄激素过多的症状，因为它们可以显著增加性激素结合球蛋白（SHBG）和降低雄激素水平。关于在 PCOS 患者中使用 COC 的小型观察性研究引发了对代谢状况恶化、激发炎症反应和凝血参数的担忧，而这些又进一步增加了 T2DM、心血管疾病和静脉血栓栓塞的风险。然而，一项荟萃分析指出，关于 COC 对葡萄糖耐受状况影响的数据结论并不一致。至于血脂方面，COC 可提高 HDL、总胆固醇和甘油三酯水平，但需要进行更多的纵向研究来评估这些血脂异常的临床影响。另一项研究表明，使用 COC 调节月经周期或治疗痤疮的患者，其 MetS 患病率与不使用口服避孕药的人类似（20.1% *vs.* 21.0%）。根据现有证据，对于有 PCOS 的患者，个体化使用口服避孕药需要考虑患者个人的心血管风险和使用这些药物的风险 – 收益比。

（四）维生素 D 缺乏与多囊卵巢综合征患者的代谢标志物的关联

全球人群普遍存在维生素 D 缺乏，但与对照组相比，PCOS 患者更容易出现严重维生素 D 缺乏（44.0% *vs.* 11.2%），这与多种 MetS 风险因素相关。肥胖的 PCOS 患者伴有 IR 时维生素 D 缺乏更为明显。研究发现 25（OH）D 水平与 BMI、WHR、空腹胰岛素、HOMA-IR、总胆固醇、低密度脂蛋白胆固醇（low-density lipoprotein cholesterol，LDL-C）和高敏 C 反应蛋白（high-sensitivity CPR，hs-CRP）呈显著负相关（$P < 0.05$）。相反，血清 25（OH）D 浓度与高密度脂蛋白胆固醇（high-density lipoprotein cholesterol，HDL-C）呈正相关（$P < 0.05$），因此可能具有保护作用。

（五）高雄激素血症与代谢综合征风险

PCOS 患者的雄激素过多会增加肝脏疾病和 IR 等代谢后果的风险。在 PCOS 患者中，雄激素过多是导致 MetS 高发的独立因素。

一项研究评估了 275 名 PCOS 女性与 35 名按 BMI 匹配的健康对照组中睾酮：双氢睾酮（TT：DHT）作为不良代谢状况生物标志物的价值。在 PCOS 患者中，肥胖女性和合并 MetS、IGT 或 IR 的患者 TT：DHT 显著升高（$P < 0.001$）。TT：DHT 与不良人体测量、激素，以及肝功能、血脂和糖代谢的各种参数显著相关。另有研究报告称，SHBG（而非睾酮）与超重 PCOS 女性的 MetS 独立相关，并与 IR 和 PCOS 诊断标准相关。因此，在不考虑雄激素水平的情况下，SHBG 可能是指示 MetS 的独立标志物。文献报道了在 PCOS 患者中 SHBG 与 HDL 水平呈正相关。此外，SHBG 与 BMI、收缩压、

第十章 多囊卵巢综合征和代谢综合征：后期生活中的风险

舒张压、甘油三酯、空腹胰岛素、HOMA-IR 和给予葡萄糖负荷后 2 小时的血浆葡萄糖水平呈显著负相关。在预测 PCOS 中的 MetS 方面，SHBG 的截断值为 21.3 nmol/L（敏感性为 100%，特异性为 85%）。

对于不同的 PCOS 表型，无论是经典型还是排卵型，患者的胰岛素作用都明显受损，而在雄激素正常的表型中却没有明显受损。其他研究发现 SHBG 与腰围、收缩压、甘油三酯、低密度脂蛋白、载脂蛋白 B、丙氨酸氨基转移酶（alanine transaminase，ALT）、天冬氨酸氨基转移酶（aspartate transaminase，AST）和血尿素氮呈负相关，但与高密度脂蛋白和载脂蛋白 A1 呈正相关。逻辑回归发现 SHBG 是 MetS 的保护性预测因子，OR 为 0.96。

（六）代谢综合征和多囊卵巢综合征表型

鹿特丹分类将 PCOS 分为 4 种不同的表型，根据稀发排卵/无排卵（OA）、临床和（或）生化的高雄激素血症（HA）及多囊卵巢（PCO）形态，分为表型 A（HA + OA + PCO）、表型 B（HA + OA）、表型 C（HA + PCO）和表型 D（OA + PCO）。研究人员估计了不同 PCOS 表型之间的 MetS 风险（表 10.4）。正如前面讨论的，与对照组相比，所有 PCOS 表型中的 MetS 发生率均显著升高，但非雄激素过多的 PCOS 表型（表型 OA + PCO）在所有 PCOS 表型中具有最低的 MetS 发生率。表型 A 组除了患 MetS 的风险增加外，抗米勒管激素（AMH）的水平也是最高的。

表 10.4 各种族中不同表型的代谢综合征患病率的比较

作者	种族	PCO+OA+HA	OA+HA	PCO+HA	OA+PCO	对照
Wiweko 等，2020	南亚	36.1%	8.3%	6.2%	17.8%	—
Moghetti 等，2013	高加索	39.1%	28.6%	未报道	9.5%	—
Krentowska 等，2021	高加索	19.05%	20%	0	4.35%	—
Bahadur 2020	南亚	9.9%	8.0%	0	14.9%	—
Zaeemzadeh 等，2020	中东	17.1%	13.5%	3.0%	2.5%	0
Zhang 等，2018	东亚	30.6%	36.4%	21.1%	15.0%	—
Jamil 等，2015	中东	58.3%	80.0%	47.2%	44.9%	32.7%
Borzan 等，2021	澳大利亚	14.5%	14.7%	9.6%	5.3%	4.3%
Yildirim 等，2017	土耳其	19.5%	20.0%	16.0%	7.4%	3.8%

注：HA，高雄激素血症；OA，稀发排卵/无排卵；PCO，多囊卵巢形态。

因此，很明显，具有 HA 表型的 PCOS 患者比非 HA 表型的患者面临更高的代谢风险。同样，经典表型、排卵表型和非 HA 表型亚组中 IR 的发生率分别为 80.4%、65.0% 和 38.1%（$P < 0.001$）。根据鹿特丹标准提出的正常雄激素表型与基于美国国立卫生研究院（NIH）共识标准的表型相比，MetS 风险较低。一项荟萃分析指出，经典表型（A 型）的代谢风险最高。一般来说，正常雄激素表型的 PCOS 患者具有相对最好的代谢状态，类似于健康对照组女性。然而，在东亚人群中进行的研究表明，即使是正常雄激素表型也与增加的代谢风险相关。

五、多囊卵巢综合征中的糖耐量异常和糖尿病

IR 和 MetS 使 PCOS 患者出现糖耐量异常的风险更高。一项对 35 项研究进行的荟萃分析报告称，与 BMI 匹配的未患 PCOS 的女性相比，PCOS 女性的 IGT（*OR*：2.48）、T2DM（*OR*：4.43）和 MetS（*OR*：2.88）患病率增加。即使是体重较轻的 PCOS 女性也有较高的 IGT 患病率（*OR*：3.22）。患有 PCOS 的女性与非 PCOS 的女性相比，IFG 的患病率更高（32.5% *vs.* 17.4%）。通常情况下，PCOS 女性出现 IGT，主要反映了骨骼肌水平的 IR。IR 的女性中，59.3% 患有 IGT，而没有 IR 的女性中只有 10.3% 患有 IGT。与对照组相比，PCOS 患者罹患 T2DM 的可能性更大（分别为 4.6% 和 2.3%）。PCOS 患者在四五十岁时出现糖耐量异常，比一般人群更早。

（一）体重指数与血糖异常的关联

血糖异常［空腹血糖 ≥ 100 mg/dL 和（或）75 g 葡萄糖负荷后 2 小时血糖 ≥ 140 mg/dL］主要表现在葡萄糖负荷后血糖水平的升高，其风险随着体重增加而增加，在 BMI > 30 kg/m² 的人群中最高。然而，即使是体重较轻的 PCOS 女性也有较高的 IGT 和 T2DM 发病率。Liang 等对 220 名 PCOS 女性和 70 名对照女性进行的研究表明，肥胖是预测 IGT 和 MetS 的唯一因素（*OR*：8）。肥胖的 PCOS 患者伴有 IGT 的概率为 43%，肥胖的非 PCOS 女性伴有 IGT 的概率为 25%，非肥胖的 PCOS 患者 IGT 的发生率为 10%，非肥胖、非 PCOS 的女性则未观察到 IGT 的发生。因此，肥胖应被视为决定 PCOS 相关的长期健康后果的主要因素。

（二）纵向研究中发生血糖异常的风险

关于代谢异常和 IGT/T2DM 进展的长期纵向研究资料较少。一项对 PCOS 患者进行的意大利队列研究在超过 10 年的随访中证实了 PCOS 患者患 T2DM 的风险增加。具体而言，随访结束时，PCOS 组 T2DM 的年龄标准化患病率为 39.3%，而一般同龄女性的患病率则为 5.8%。一项针对小规模 PCOS 患者队列的澳大利亚研究表明，在起始时血糖正常的 PCOS 患者中，约有 9% 在不到 10 年的随访中发展为 IGT，进而有 8% 发展为 T2DM。此外，在起始时患有 IGT 的 PCOS 患者中，54% 在随访期间发展为 T2DM。基线 BMI 被发现是后期不良血糖状况的独立预测因素。

（三）血糖异常的测定

与其他血糖异常相比，PCOS 患者更容易发生 IGT；因此，口服葡萄糖耐量试验（OGTT）（葡萄糖负荷后 2 小时血糖）是确定血糖异常（即 IGT 和 T2DM）的理想测试。与 OGTT 相比，糖化血红蛋白（HbA1c）在检测 PCOS 的血糖异常方面具有较低的敏感性。来自雄激素过多学会和英国皇家妇产科学院的立场声明和指南建议对所有 PCOS 患者进行 OGTT 筛查。如果 OGTT 正常，至少每 2 年进行再筛查，或者如果存在其他风险因素（如年龄增长、超重或肥胖、既往有妊娠期糖尿病史或家族中有 T2DM 患者），则需提前进行再筛查。伴有 IGT 的 PCOS 患者应每年进行再筛查。

六、晚年风险

由 MetS 各方面表现的聚集性可以看出，PCOS 患者从较小的年龄就开始暴露于多种心血管风险因素。向心性肥胖或内脏型肥胖、IR、T2DM、高血压和血脂异常的存在使得这些患者将来发生心血管事件的风险比非 PCOS 女性更高。总的来说，女性在围绝经期体重增加的趋势使其更易患心血管疾病；然而，在围绝经期 PCOS 女性中这种风险是否进一步加重仍不确定。PCOS 女性的生化 HA 随着年龄增长而改善，而血糖异常和血脂异常在 PCOS 和非 PCOS 女性中均随时间加重。与此发现相反，其他报告称，随着年龄的增长，患有 PCOS 的女性心血管疾病的患病率低于预期。

Livadas 等研究了 1345 名患有 PCOS 的女性及 302 名非 PCOS 女性的年龄对其 IR 和 MetS 的影响。作者指出，在肥胖的 PCOS 患者中，IR 随着年龄增长而增加。而在 30 岁以上的 PCOS 患者和对照的亚组中，无论是消瘦还是肥胖，PCOS 女性的 HOMA-IR 都显著高于非 PCOS 女性。研究还报道了 IR 与 BMI 和雄激素水平呈正相关。众所周知，随着年龄的增长，雄激素水平下降，非肥胖的 PCOS 可能随着时间推移呈现出稍好一些的代谢特征，PCOS 甚至可能成为一个隐性的疾病。这一观察结果强烈证实了实施生活方式干预以防止体重增加的必要性，这可能会改善 PCOS 女性的不良心脏代谢特征。

在一项纵向研究中，117 名患有 PCOS 的女性（平均年龄 45.8 岁）与对照女性相比，IGT 的患病率更高（25.0% vs. 9.2%；$P < 0.001$）。那些同时具有 HA 和 OA 的患者出现更差的代谢和激素参数的发生率最高。

一些研究观察到，在被推测患有 PCOS 的高龄患者中，MetS 的患病率较对照组更高。其中一部分研究还指出，PCOS 的 HA 表型与正常雄激素表型相比，MetS 的患病率更高。一项 12 年的随访研究报告称，在初始没有 MetS 的人群中，PCOS 患者 MetS 的发生率更高［发生率：3.57%（PCOS 组）vs. 2.26%（对照组）］。然而，在校正 BMI 后，差异变得不显著，这也许提示着，在生育期没有 MetS 的 PCOS 患者可能代表着在长期内进展为 MetS 风险较低。一项针对 PCOS 患者（平均年龄 43 岁）长期随访的瑞典研究报告，PCOS 患者 MetS 的患病率为 23.8%，而对照组为 8%。该研究未能显示 PCOS 表型与 MetS 患病率之间的任何关联，无论是在初始阶段还是在长期随访中。此外，研究还发现，与对照组相比，PCOS 组中腰围增加、高甘油三酯血症和使用降糖药物的概率更高，而高血压或使用降压药物的概率则较低。

其他研究还评估了年龄超过 45 岁的中年女性（$n = 200$）PCOS 患者的心脏代谢表型和 CVD 患病率，与年龄匹配的对照组（$n = 200$）进行了比较，并评估了心血管健康和 10 年 CVD 风险。与对照组相比，PCOS 患者更有可能出现腰围增加、BMI 升高、高血压和葡萄糖耐受不良，但在 PCOS 患者中 T2DM、MetS 和血脂异常的患病率并无升高。PCOS 患者的颈动脉内膜中层厚度较小（$P < 0.001$）。经计算，PCOS 女性和对照组的心血管健康和 10 年 CVD 风险相似。PCOS 患者的 10 年 CVD 风险中位数为 5.79%，

而对照组为 7.38%（$P = 0.214$）。

尽管存在争议，但数据显示，多囊卵巢综合征患者即便年轻时状况不理想，其远期心血管健康似乎与一般人群相似。这是不是因为大多数 PCOS 患者在年轻时调整为更健康的生活方式并接受了适当的预防性治疗，从而获得了更好的 DNA 修复和基因保护，这一点尚有待确认。

七、代谢综合征的筛查

（一）病史

对于 PCOS 患者，详细了解其病史非常重要，其中必须包括年龄、种族、吸烟史、妊娠期糖尿病或糖尿病前期、体重变化、对生活方式干预或减肥药物的反应/依从性、胰岛素增敏剂的使用及其过去的反应，以及对阻塞性睡眠呼吸暂停的评估。相关特征应在临床随访中重新评估。此外，还应记录家族史中是否有 MetS、糖尿病前期、T2DM、高血压或动脉粥样硬化性心血管疾病（atherosclerotic cardiovascular disease，ASCVD）的情况，并在随访时进行回顾。

（二）体格检查和实验室评估

PCOS 患者需要进行糖耐量、血脂和肝功能的评估。因此，应该为每个 PCOS 患者进行基线 OGTT、血脂全套检查和肝功能检查（liver function test，LFT）。如果这些检查在基线时正常，那么应该定期监测这些检测指标，可以每 2 年进行一次复查，或在体重增加或发现其他风险因素时提前复查（图 10.2）。

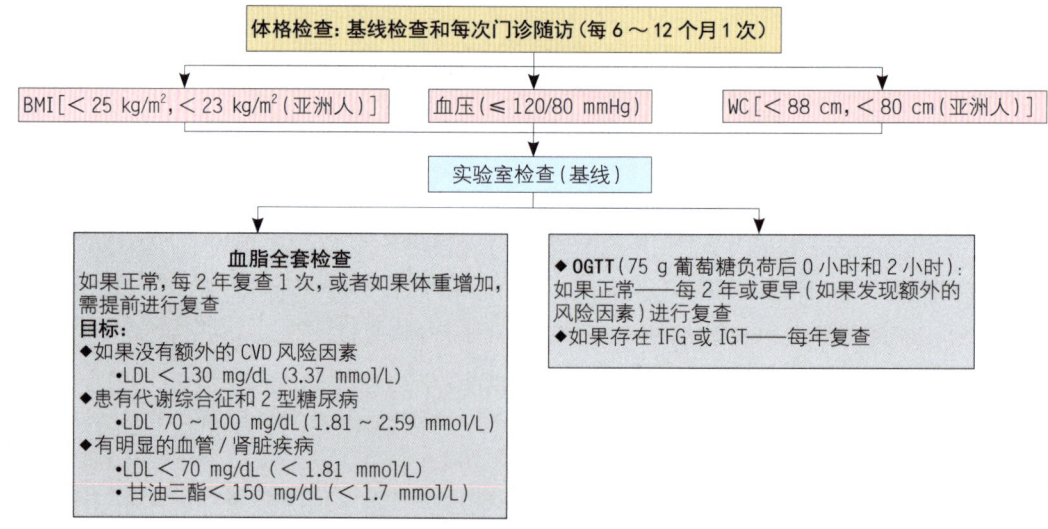

BMI，体重指数；CVD，心血管疾病；IFG，空腹血糖受损；IGT，糖耐量减低；LDL，低密度脂蛋白；OGTT，口服葡萄糖耐量试验；WC，腰围。

图 10.2　多囊卵巢综合征的体格检查（基线检查和门诊随访）

八、临床意义

PCOS 患者存在潜在的 IR 风险,并且其中相当一部分患者患 MetS,而这将会增加其未来发生心血管疾病的风险。

4 种不同表型之间 MetS 患病率的差异突出了对 PCOS 患者进行个体化筛查和干预的必要性。

PCOS 患者需要进行 MetS 的评估,包括向心性肥胖的标志物、体重、血压、OGTT 及基线时的血脂全套,并进行定期复查。

生活方式干预(包括医学营养治疗和运动)和作为胰岛素增敏剂的二甲双胍,仍然是 PCOS 管理的基石,重点是降低 T2DM 和 ASCVD 的风险。

九、未来研究需求

未来的研究需要集中于阐明 PCOS 患者及其表型中 IR 和 MetS 的机制。同时也有必要阐明不同种族之间 MetS 患病率差异的原因。

目前缺乏对 PCOS 患者的纵向研究,需要对 PCOS 女性群体开展有良好对照和适当设计的长期纵向研究,以找出 MetS 及相关心血管风险筛查的理想时间点,以及预防措施的最佳干预时机。此外,这些纵向研究可以回答 PCOS 患者发展成 T2DM、高血压、MetS 和 CVD 的确切风险。

此外,世界各地和不同种族的 PCOS 登记数据库也可以帮助研究人员解答许多对个人生活具有重大影响但尚未得到解答的问题。

参考文献

1. Diamanti-Kandarakis E, Dunaif A. Insulin resistance and the polycystic ovary syndrome revisited: an update on mechanisms and implications. Endocr Rev. 2012;33(6):981-1030. doi:10.1210/er.2011-1034.
2. Rojas J, Chavez M, Olivar L, et al. Polycystic ovary syndrome, insulin resistance, and obesity: navigating the pathophysiologic labyrinth. Int J Reprod Med. 2014;2014:719050. doi:10.1155/2014/719050.
3. Samson SL, Garber AJ. Metabolic syndrome. Endocrinol Metab Clin North Am. 2014;43(1):1-23. doi:10.1016/j.ecl.2013.09.009.
4. National Institute of Health. National Institutes of Health Third Report of the National Cholesterol Education Program Expert Panel on Detection, Evaluation, and Treatment of High Blood Cholesterol in Adults (Adult Treatment Panel III). Executive Summary. Bethesda, MD: National Institutes of Health, National Heart, Lung, and Blood; 2001.
5. Alberti KGM, Zimmet P, Shaw J. The metabolic syndrome—a new worldwide definition. Lancet. 2005;366(9491):1059-1062.
6. Alberti KG, Eckel RH, Grundy SM, et al. Harmonizing the metabolic syndrome: a joint interim statement of the International Diabetes Federation Task Force on Epidemiology and Prevention; National Heart, Lung, and Blood Institute; American Heart Association; World Heart Federation; International Atherosclerosis Society; and International Association for the Study of Obesity. Circulation. 2009;120(16):1640-1645.
7. Lim SS, Kakoly NS, Tan JWJ, et al. Metabolic syndrome in polycystic ovary syndrome: a systematic review, meta-analysis and meta-regression. Obes Rev. 2019;20(2):339-352. doi:10.1111/obr.12762.

8. Jeanes YM, Reeves S. Metabolic consequences of obesity and insulin resistance in polycystic ovary syndrome: diagnostic and methodological challenges. Nutr Res Rev. 2017;30(1):97-105. doi:10.1017/S0954422416000287.
9. Dadachanji R, Patil A, Joshi B, Mukherjee S. Elucidating the impact of obesity on hormonal and metabolic perturbations in polycystic ovary syndrome phenotypes in Indian women. PLoS One. 2021;16(2):e0246862. doi:10.1371/journal.pone.0246862.
10. Legro RS. Obesity and PCOS: implications for diagnosis and treatment. Paper presented at the Seminars in reproductive medicine; 2012.
11. Alves AC, Valcarcel B, Mäkinen VP, et al. Metabolic profiling of polycystic ovary syndrome reveals interactions with abdominal obesity. Int J Obes (Lond). 2017;41(9):1331-1340.
12. Jamil AS, Alalaf SK, Al-Tawil NG, Al-Shawaf T. A case–control observational study of insulin resistance and metabolic syndrome among the four phenotypes of polycystic ovary syndrome based on Rotterdam criteria. Reprod Health. 2015;12:7.
13. Ebrahimi-Mamaghani M, Saghafi-Asl M, Pirouzpanah S, et al. Association of insulin resistance with lipid profile, metabolic syndrome, and hormonal aberrations in overweight or obese women with polycystic ovary syndrome. J Health Popul Nutr. 2015;33(1):157-167.
14. Tziomalos K, Katsikis I, Papadakis E, Kandaraki EA, Macut D, Panidis D. Comparison of markers of insulin resistance and circulating androgens between women with polycystic ovary syndrome and women with metabolic syndrome. Hum Reprod. 2013;28(3):785-793. doi:10.1093/humrep/des456.
15. DeFronzo RA, Tobin JD, Andres RJ. Glucose clamp technique: a method for quantifying insulin secretion and resistance. Am J Physiol. 1979;237(3):E214-E223.
16. Tosi F, Bonora E, Moghetti P. Insulin resistance in a large cohort of women with polycystic ovary syndrome: a comparison between euglycaemic-hyperinsulinaemic clamp and surrogate indexes. Hum Reprod. 2017;32(12):2515-2521. doi:10.1093/humrep/dex308.
17. Matthews DR, Hosker J, Rudenski A, Naylor B, Treacher D, Turner RC. Homeostasis model assessment: insulin resistance and β-cell function from fasting plasma glucose and insulin concentrations in man. Diabetologia. 1985;28(7):412-419.
18. Legro RS, Finegood D, Dunaif A. A fasting glucose to insulin ratio is a useful measure of insulin sensitivity in women with polycystic ovary syndrome. J Clin Endocrinol Metab. 1998;83(8):2694-2698.
19. Katz A, Nambi SS, Mather K, et al. Quantitative insulin sensitivity check index: a simple, accurate method for assessing insulin sensitivity in humans. J Clin Endocrinol Metab. 2000;85(7):2402-2410.
20. Gutt M, Davis CL, Spitzer SB, et al. Validation of the insulin sensitivity index (ISI0, 120): comparison with other measures. Diabetes Res Clin Pract. 2000;47(3):177-184.
21. Stumvoll M, Van Haeften T, Fritsche A, Gerich J. Oral glucose tolerance test indexes for insulin sensitivity and secretion based on various availabilities of sampling times. Diabetes Care. 2001;24(4):796-797.
22. Matsuda M, DeFronzo RA. Insulin sensitivity indices obtained from oral glucose tolerance testing: comparison with the euglycemic insulin clamp. Diabetes Care. 1999;22(9):1462-1470.
23. Polak K, Czyzyk A, Simoncini T, Meczekalski B. New markers of insulin resistance in polycystic ovary syndrome. J Endocrinol Invest. 2017;40(1):1-8. doi:10.1007/s40618-016-0523-8.
24. Abdelazim IA, Elsawah WF. Metabolic syndrome among infertile women with polycystic ovary syndrome. Asian Pac J Reprod. 2015;4(1):44-48. doi:10.1016/s2305-0500(14)60057-9.
25. Montazerifar F, Ghasemi M, Arabpour N, Karajibani M, Keikhah NJ. Metabolic syndrome in women with and without polycystic syndrome, a case control study in Iran. Caspian J Reprod Med. 2020;6(1):9-15.
26. Anjum N, Zohra S, Arif A, Azhar A, Qureshi M. Prevalence of metabolic syndrome in Pakistani women with polycystic ovarian syndrome. Pak J Biochem Mol Biol. 2013;46(3):97-100.
27. Panidis D, Tziomalos K, Macut D, et al. Age- and body mass index-related differences in the prevalence of

metabolic syndrome in women with polycystic ovary syndrome. Gynecol Endocrinol. 2013;29(10):926-930. doi:10.3109/09513590.2013.819079.
28. Moghetti P, Tosi F, Bonin C, et al. Divergences in insulin resistance between the different phenotypes of the polycystic ovary syndrome. J Clin Endocrinol Metab. 2013;98(4):E628-E637. doi:10.1210/jc.2012-3908.
29. Meyer ML, Sotres-Alvarez D, Steiner AZ, et al. Polycystic ovary syndrome signs and metabolic syndrome in premenopausal hispanic/latina women: the HCHS/SOL study. J Clin Endocrinol Metab. 2020;105(3):e447-e456. doi:10.1210/clinem/dgaa012.
30. Liang SJ, Liou TH, Lin HW, Hsu CS, Tzeng CR, Hsu MI. Obesity is the predominant predictor of impaired glucose tolerance and metabolic disturbance in polycystic ovary syndrome. Acta Obstet Gynecol Scand. 2012;91(10):1167-1172. doi:10.1111/j.1600-0412.2012.01417.x.
31. Le MT, Nguyen VQH, Truong QV, Le DD, Le VNS, Cao NT. Metabolic syndrome and insulin resistance syndrome among infertile women with polycystic ovary syndrome: a cross-sectional study from central Vietnam. Endocrinol Metab (Seoul). 2018;33(4):447-458. doi:10.3803/EnM.2018.33.4.447.
32. Einhorn DJ, Reaven GM, Cobin RH, et al. American College of Endocrinology position statement on the insulin resistance syndrome. Endocr Pract. 2003;9:237-252.
33. Kyrkou G, Trakakis E, Attilakos A, et al. Metabolic syndrome in Greek women with polycystic ovary syndrome: prevalence, characteristics and associations with body mass index. A prospective controlled study. Arch Gynecol Obstet. 2016;293(4):915-923. doi:10.1007/s00404-015-3964-y.
34. Karee M, Gundabattula SR, Sashi L, Boorugu H, Chowdhury A. Prevalence of metabolic syndrome in women with polycystic ovary syndrome and the factors associated: a cross sectional study at a tertiary care center in Hyderabad, south-eastern India. Diabetes Metab Syndr. 2020;14(4):583-587. doi:10.1016/j.dsx.2020.05.006.
35. Hosseinpanah F, Barzin M, Tehrani FR, Azizi F. The lack of association between polycystic ovary syndrome and metabolic syndrome: Iranian PCOS prevalence study. Clin Endocrinol (Oxf). 2011;75(5):692-697. doi:10.1111/j.1365-2265.2011.04113.x.
36. Anjum S, Askari S, Riaz M, Basit A. Clinical presentation and frequency of metabolic syndrome in women with polycystic ovary syndrome: an experience from a tertiary care hospital in Pakistan. Cureus. 2020;12(12):e11860. doi:10.7759/cureus.11860.
37. Moran LJ, Misso ML, Wild RA, Norman RJ. Impaired glucose tolerance, type 2 diabetes and metabolic syndrome in polycystic ovary syndrome: a systematic review and meta-analysis. Hum Reprod Update. 2010;16(4):347-363. doi:10.1093/humupd/dmq001.
38. Hallajzadeh J, Khoramdad M, Karamzad N, et al. Metabolic syndrome and its components among women with polycystic ovary syndrome: a systematic review and meta-analysis. J Cardiovasc Thorac Res. 2018;10(2):56-69. doi:10.15171/jcvtr.2018.10.
39. Hillman JK, Johnson LN, Limaye M, Feldman RA, Sammel M, Dokras A. Black women with polycystic ovary syndrome (PCOS) have increased risk for metabolic syndrome and cardiovascular disease compared with white women with PCOS. Fertil Steril. 2014;101(2):530-535. doi:10.1016/j.fertnstert.2013.10.055.
40. Engmann L, Jin S, Sun F, et al. Racial and ethnic differences in the polycystic ovary syndrome metabolic phenotype. Am J Obstet Gynecol. 2017;216(5):493.e1-493.e13. doi:10.1016/j.ajog.2017.01.003.
41. Ezeh U, Ida Chen YD, Azziz R. Racial and ethnic differences in the metabolic response of polycystic ovary syndrome. Clin Endocrinol (Oxf). 2020;93(2):163-172. doi:10.1111/cen.14193.
42. Chan JL, Kar S, Vanky E, et al. Racial and ethnic differences in the prevalence of metabolic syndrome and its components of metabolic syndrome in women with polycystic ovary syndrome: a regional cross-sectional study. Am J Obstet Gynecol. 2017;217(2):189.e1-e189.e8. doi:10.1016/j.ajog.2017.04.007.
43. Chahal N, Quinn M, Jaswa EA, Kao CN, Cedars MI, Huddleston HG. Comparison of metabolic syndrome elements in White and Asian women with polycystic ovary syndrome: results of a regional, American cross-sectional study. F S Rep. 2020;1(3):305-313. doi:10.1016/j.xfre.2020.09.008.

44. Yildizhan B, Anik Ilhan G, Pekin T. The impact of insulin resistance on clinical, hormonal and metabolic parameters in lean women with polycystic ovary syndrome. J Obstet Gynaecol. 2016;36(7):893-896. doi:10.3109/01443615.2016.1168376.
45. Zhu S, Zhang B, Jiang X, et al. Metabolic disturbances in non-obese women with polycystic ovary syndrome: a systematic review and meta-analysis. Fertil Steril. 2019;111(1):168-177. doi:10.1016/j.fertnstert.2018.09.013.
46. Manzoor S, Ganie MA, Amin S, et al. Oral contraceptive use increases risk of inflammatory and coagulatory disorders in women with polycystic ovarian syndrome: an observational study. Sci Rep. 2019;9(1):10182.
47. De Medeiros SF. Risks, benefits size and clinical implications of combined oral contraceptive use in women with polycystic ovary syndrome. Reprod Biol Endocrinol. 2017;15(1):93.
48. Li HW, Brereton RE, Anderson RA, Wallace AM, Ho CK. Vitamin D deficiency is common and associated with metabolic risk factors in patients with polycystic ovary syndrome. Metabolism. 2011;60(10):1475-1481. doi:10.1016/j.metabol.2011.03.002.
49. Joham AE, Teede HJ, Cassar S, et al. Vitamin D in polycystic ovary syndrome: relationship to obesity and insulin resistance. Mol Nutr Food Res. 2016;60(1):110-118. doi:10.1002/mnfr.201500259.
50. Wang L, Lv S, Li F, Yu X, Bai E, Yang X. Vitamin D deficiency is associated with metabolic risk factors in women with polycystic ovary syndrome: a cross-sectional study in Shaanxi China. Front Endocrinol (Lausanne). 2020;11:171. doi:10.3389/fendo.2020.00171.
51. Albu A, Radian S, Fica S, Barbu CG. Biochemical hyperandrogenism is associated with metabolic syndrome independently of adiposity and insulin resistance in Romanian polycystic ovary syndrome patients. Endocrine. 2015;48(2):696-704. doi:10.1007/s12020-014-0340-9.
52. Munzker J, Hofer D, Trummer C, et al. Testosterone to dihydrotestosterone ratio as a new biomarker for an adverse metabolic phenotype in the polycystic ovary syndrome. J Clin Endocrinol Metab. 2015;100(2):653-660. doi:10.1210/jc.2014-2523.
53. Moran LJ, Teede HJ, Noakes M, Clifton PM, Norman RJ, Wittert GA. Sex hormone binding globulin, but not testosterone, is associated with the metabolic syndrome in overweight and obese women with polycystic ovary syndrome. J Endocrinol Invest. 2013;36(11):1004-1010. doi:10.3275/9023.
54. Fu C, Minjie C, Weichun Z, et al. Efficacy of sex hormone-binding globulin on predicting metabolic syndrome in newly diagnosed and untreated patients with polycystic ovary syndrome. Hormones (Athens). 2020;19(3):439-445. doi:10.1007/s42000-020-00219-5.
55. Luo X, Yang XM, Cai WY, et al. Decreased sex hormone-binding globulin indicated worse biometric, lipid, liver, and renal function parameters in women with polycystic ovary syndrome. Int J Endocrinol. 2020;2020:7580218. doi:10.1155/2020/7580218.
56. Lizneva D, Suturina L, Walker W, Brakta S, Gavrilova-Jordan L, Azziz R. Criteria, prevalence, and phenotypes of polycystic ovary syndrome. Fertil Steril. 2016;106(1):6-15.
57. Zaeemzadeh N, Sadatmahalleh SJ, Ziaei S, et al. Prevalence of metabolic syndrome in four phenotypes of PCOS and its relationship with androgenic components among Iranian women: a cross-sectional study. Int J Reprod Biomed. 2020;18(4):253-264. doi:10.18502/ijrm.v13i4.6888.
58. Wiweko B, Handayani LK, Harzif AK, et al. Correlation of anti-Mullerian hormone levels with metabolic syndrome events in polycystic ovary syndrome: a cross-sectional study. Int J Reprod Biomed. 2020;18(3):187-192. doi:10.18502/ijrm.v18i3.6716.
59. Krentowska A, Lebkowska A, Jacewicz-Swiecka M, et al. Metabolic syndrome and the risk of cardiovascular complications in young patients with different phenotypes of polycystic ovary syndrome. Endocrine. 2021;72(2):400-410. doi:10.1007/s12020-020-02596-8.
60. Zhang L, Fang X, Li L, et al. The association between circulating irisin levels and different phenotypes of polycystic ovary syndrome. J Endocrinol Invest. 2018;41(12):1401-1407. doi:10.1007/s40618-018-0902-4.
61. Borzan V, Lerchbaum E, Missbrenner C, et al. Risk of insulin resistance and metabolic syndrome in women with hyperandrogenemia: a comparison between PCOS phenotypes and beyond. J Clin Med. 2021;10(4):829.

doi:10.3390/jcm10040829.

62. Yildirim E, Karabulut O, Yuksel UC, et al. Echocardiographic evaluation of diastolic functions in patients with polycystic ovary syndrome: a comperative study of diastolic functions in subphenotypes of polycystic ovary syndrome. Cardiol J. 2017;24(4):364-373. doi:10.5603/CJ.a2017.0032.

63. Krentowska A, Kowalska I. Metabolic syndrome and its components in different phenotypes of polycystic ovary syndrome. Diabetes Metab Res Rev. 2021;38:e3464. doi:10.1002/dmrr.3464.

64. Gambineri A, Patton L, Altieri P, et al. Polycystic ovary syndrome is a risk factor for type 2 diabetes: results from a long-term prospective study. Diabetes. 2012;61(9):2369-2374. doi:10.2337/db11-1360.

65. Norman RJ, Masters L, Milner CR, Wang JX, Davies MJ. Relative risk of conversion from normoglycaemia to impaired glucose tolerance or non-insulin dependent diabetes mellitus in polycystic ovarian syndrome. Hum Reprod. 2001;16(9):1995-1998.

66. Goodman NF, Cobin RH, Futterweit W, et al. American Association of Clinical Endocrinologists, American College of Endocrinology, and Androgen Excess and PCOS Society disease state clinical review: guide to the best practices in the evaluation and treatment of polycystic ovary syndrome-part 1. Endocr Pract. 2015;21(11):1291-1300.

67. Goodman NF, Cobin RH, Futterweit W, et al. American Association of Clinical Endocrinologists, American College of Endocrinology, and Androgen Excess and PCOS Society disease state clinical review: guide to the best practices in the evaluation and treatment of polycystic ovary syndrome-part 2. Endocr Pract. 2015;21(12):1415-1426.

68. American College of Obstetricians and Gynecologists' Committee on Practice Bulletins—Gynecology. ACOG Practice Bulletin No. 194: Polycystic Ovary Syndrome [published correction appears in Obstet Gynecol. 2020 Sep;136(3):638]. Obstet Gynecol. 2018;131(6):e157-e171. doi:10.1097/AOG.0000000000002656.

69. Wild RA, Carmina E, Diamanti-Kandarakis E, et al. Assessment of cardiovascular risk and prevention of cardiovascular disease in women with the polycystic ovary syndrome: a consensus statement by the Androgen Excess and Polycystic Ovary Syndrome (AE-PCOS) Society. J Clin Endocrinol Metab. 2010;95(5):2038-2049.

70. Lobo RA. Metabolic syndrome after menopause and the role of hormones. Maturitas. 2008;60(1):10-18. doi:10.1016/j.maturitas.2008.02.008.

71. De Medeiros SF, Yamamoto MMW, Souto de Medeiros MA, Barbosa BB, Soares JM, Baracat EC. Changes in clinical and biochemical characteristics of polycystic ovary syndrome with advancing age. Endocr Connect. 2020;9(2):74-89. doi:10.1530/EC-19-0496.

72. Livadas S, Kollias A, Panidis D, Diamanti-Kandarakis E. Diverse impacts of aging on insulin resistance in lean and obese women with polycystic ovary syndrome: evidence from 1345 women with the syndrome. Eur J Endocrinol. 2014;171(3):301-309. doi:10.1530/EJE-13-1007.

73. Polotsky AJ, Allshouse A, Crawford SL, et al. Relative contributions of oligomenorrhea and hyperandrogenemia to the risk of metabolic syndrome in midlife women. J Clin Endocrinol Metab. 2012;97(6):E868-E877. doi:10.1210/jc.2011-3357.

74. Louwers YV, Laven JSE. Characteristics of polycystic ovary syndrome throughout life. Ther Adv Reprod Health. 2020;14:2633494120911038. doi:10.1177/2633494120911038.

75. Hudecova M, Holte J, Olovsson M, Larsson A, Berne C, Sundstrom-Poromaa I. Prevalence of the metabolic syndrome in women with a previous diagnosis of polycystic ovary syndrome: long-term follow-up. Fertil Steril. 2011;96(5):1271-1274. doi:10.1016/j.fertnstert.2011.08.006.

76. Meun C, Gunning MN, Louwers YV, et al. The cardiovascular risk profile of middle-aged women with polycystic ovary syndrome. Clin Endocrinol (Oxf). 2020;92(2):150-158. doi:10.1111/cen.14117.

77. Al Wattar BH, Fisher M, Bevington L, et al. Clinical practice guidelines on the diagnosis and management of polycystic ovary syndrome: a systematic review and quality assessment study. J Clin Endocrinol Metab. 2021;106(8):2436-2446. doi:10.1210/clinem/dgab232.

第十一章 多囊卵巢综合征和心理健康

一、引言

多囊卵巢综合征（PCOS）是影响育龄女性最常见的内分泌紊乱之一，不同研究使用不同的PCOS诊断标准，报道了不同的患病率。

这种疾病的临床症状包括月经不规律、多毛症、痤疮、肥胖和不孕症。这些不仅对患者的身体产生负面影响，还对患者的心理健康产生长期的巨大影响。

二、抑郁症和焦虑症

大量研究表明，被诊断为PCOS的女性存在不同程度的焦虑症和抑郁症。女性的抑郁症和焦虑症有生物心理社会的原因。下丘脑－垂体－肾上腺轴功能失调已被认为与PCOS患者的这两种疾病的发病机制有关。神经影像学研究还证明了PCOS患者前额叶皮质活动增加，这可能与焦虑症有关。一项研究的结果显示，高体重指数（BMI）、更多子女和较低教育水平的患者更容易患抑郁症。

焦虑症在PCOS患者中很常见，症状从轻微、中度到严重不等。焦虑可能来自多种因素，如无法生育的可能性，以及对建立家庭的担忧，这些可能对其未来产生威胁并使她们容易产生恐惧。由于外貌发生明显变化，社会对个人的负面态度可能导致患者产生高度社交焦虑。

三、身体形象

身体形象是一个复杂而多维的概念，它描述了一个人对自己身体的想象、思考和感受。它由多个组成部分构成，如体重、体形和整体外貌。健康的身体形象意味着对自己的外貌感到满意，而很多PCOS患者则有消极体象。对自己体形不满和身材的走样可能导致自信心下降，并严重影响社交活动。

四、文化、病耻感

文化倾向于通过整体外貌来判断一个人。符合这些美的标准对女性来说已成为一种责任，而无法达到这些标准则会产生很深的影响。女性的女性化特征有多种表现形式，其中之一是规律的月经，它代表着生育力，以及光滑的面部和无体毛的躯体。一旦这些特征因PCOS的部分表现而丧失，女性就会遭受来自公众的羞辱和周围人的歧视。随后，这些负面的态度和信念会被患者内化为病耻感。在种族、精神疾病和人类免疫缺陷病毒（human immunodeficiency virus，HIV）/获得性免疫缺陷综合征（acquired immunodeficiency syndrome，AIDS）等领域，病耻感已经得到了广泛研究。然而，与 PCOS 相关的病耻感问题尚未得到充分研究。一项有趣的定性研究发现，1/3 的女性患者使用"怪异"这个词来描述自己与其他非 PCOS 女性间不同的主观体验。来自社会的病耻态度可能导致患者自尊心下降，随之影响其社交人际关系。

世界卫生组织（World Health Organization，WHO）依据个体所处文化而定义的生活质量（quality of life，QoL）在 PCOS 患者中也明显受损。它包括身体健康、情感状态和社会关系等多个领域。患有 PCOS 这种身体疾病的女性亦会遭受情感困扰。这种困扰最终会导致社会和人际功能的受损。此外，在传统地域文化的背景下，外貌和体重被认为是新郎家庭用来寻找完美儿媳的重要特征。生育子女是女性生命中的一个重要里程碑，如果女性无法实现这一点，将对她们的 QoL 产生影响。社会羞辱、文化期望、社会压力和履行社会预期的女性角色的强烈使命感，使 PCOS 患者面临着一系列心理问题。

五、性与婚姻生活

性对一个人的情感幸福有着重要的影响。在育龄期，找到性伴侣、发展亲密关系、建立恋爱关系及渴望生育孩子都是重要的里程碑，而 PCOS 恰恰在此时期表现出来。无法生育可能对婚姻关系和性功能产生长期的重大影响。性功能障碍有各种表现，包括性欲减退和性兴奋度降低。患有 PCOS 的女性反映，她们对自己的性生活不够满意，并认为自己不够有吸引力。这可能是由于配偶觉得妻子的吸引力减弱，或者可能是由于低自尊和对身体不满而产生的认知扭曲。抑郁在 PCOS 患者中非常常见，它与性欲减退有关。性行为不足也与多毛症相关。

六、生活质量

PCOS 的身体和心理症状共同导致 QoL 的显著下降。QoL 可能受到各种因素的影响，最重要的因素包括肥胖和不孕症。此外，即使在非 PCOS 患者中，痤疮也会影响 QoL。有力的证据显示，多毛症也是影响 QoL 的症状之一。不仅是多毛症本身，还有为了掩盖症状而采取的化妆步骤，这些都可能增加负面情绪压力。

七、应对策略

应对策略主要可以分为问题解决和情绪调节两类。问题解决策略包括应对压力情况的各种实用方法，而情绪调节策略则指调节对压力源的情绪反应。文献表明，PCOS 患者更倾向于使用情绪应对策略，这些策略通常被归类为消极应对，并且在很多情况下是不适用的。这些措施可以在短期内抑制情绪反应，但长期来看会带来更大的困难。"回避"在任何身体疾病的早期阶段都不适用，因为它会延误早期治疗，从而使预后变差。

八、进食障碍

许多 PCOS 患者存在临床和亚临床的进食障碍。这可能与试图减肥有关,从而导致暴食和催吐行为。进食障碍可能对 PCOS 本身的结局产生负面影响。

九、双相情感障碍

用于双相情感障碍发作的紧急处理和维持治疗的情绪稳定剂丙戊酸,可能会引起月经不规律、代谢综合征和高雄激素血症(HA),但没有证据证明它可以直接引起 PCOS。

十、肥胖、多囊卵巢综合征和心理问题之间的复杂关系

PCOS 和肥胖之间的关系是复杂的。肥胖是 PCOS 的一个危险因素,同时也是疾病本身通过复杂的病理生理机制引起的一种症状。任何心理障碍或情绪问题都可能显著干扰生活方式干预,进而使 PCOS 预后变差。肥胖也是阻塞性睡眠呼吸暂停的一个危险因素,后者在 PCOS 患者中很常见。

请参见表 11.1,了解常见的心理障碍及它们与 PCOS 的关联程度。

表 11.1 多囊卵巢综合征患者的心理障碍

序号	精神疾病	预计患病率/频率[a]
1	抑郁症	23.1%
2	焦虑症	11.5%
3	双相情感障碍	3.2%
4	性功能障碍	57.7%[b]
5	进食障碍 神经性贪食症 暴食症 夜间进食障碍	6.1% 17.6% 12.9%
6	阻塞性睡眠呼吸暂停综合征	0.22%

注:[a] 这些估计值可能因使用不同方法而在不同研究中有所不同。
[b] 此处指频率,而不是患病率。

十一、多囊卵巢综合征患者的心理健康管理

考虑到 PCOS 患者心理疾病的沉重负担,必须对患有 PCOS 的女性进行精神障碍筛查,然后进行恰当的干预。根据个人需求量身定制的个体化治疗计划对于特定的精神障碍是必要的。

(一)心理教育

根据循证文献,针对疾病进行心理教育是非常重要的。

第十一章 多囊卵巢综合征和心理健康

（二）原发病的治疗对疾病的结局至关重要

了解PCOS患者情绪和其他精神障碍风险增加背后的病因非常重要。PCOS患者的心理问题不仅来自该诊断带来的心理社会压力，还来自PCOS的激素失衡。因此，在考虑治疗策略时，首先必须更好地控制原发病。帮助患者改善不孕症、肥胖和多毛症将从整体上改善患者的心理健康。

（三）精神障碍筛查

所有接受PCOS治疗的女性应定期进行抑郁症和焦虑症的筛查，也可以同时进行进食障碍和性功能障碍的筛查。根据疾病的严重程度，可以将患者转诊至精神科门诊进行干预。

（四）生活方式干预

作息规律、定期锻炼和有计划的正念活动或放松技巧等健康的生活方式可以帮助改善心境障碍和PCOS。

（五）心理治疗

医疗保健专业人员乐观、谦逊和富有同理心的态度将有助于他们去理解许多患者在被诊断为PCOS时所感受到的痛苦。在非药物干预中，心理治疗是一个重要的治疗选择。

（六）认知行为疗法

目前已经证明认知行为疗法（cognitive behavioral therapy，CBT）有助于治疗心理问题。治疗重点在于对疾病的接纳，认识它如何影响个人的思维和感受，并学习如何限制消极思维并应对难以承受的情绪。CBT强调动机和建立良好的身体形象，这有助于提高自尊。因为许多患有PCOS的女性使用了不恰当的处理策略，教会她们适当的应对策略是有益处的。群体咨询也被证明是有效的。

十二、抑郁症和焦虑症的特殊管理

如前所述，无论PCOS是否伴随焦虑症或抑郁症，治疗基础的身体疾病（PCOS）都是必要的。英国国家卫生与临床优化研究所描述的广泛性焦虑症分层护理模型，根据疾病严重程度，为量身定制最有效的干预措施提供了指南。治疗的方式涵盖了从疾病的心理教育和治疗及初期的积极监测开始，到自我帮助（非指导/指导）和心理教育小组。对于症状更严重或对低强度治疗没有反应的患者，推荐进行CBT和（或）药物干预。在药物干预中，选择性5-羟色胺再摄取抑制药（selective serotonin reuptake inhibitors，SSRI）在焦虑谱系障碍的管理中显示出疗效。对于轻度抑郁症的治疗，不推荐使用抗抑郁药物；相反，建议进行自我帮助、定期锻炼和保持充足的睡眠。然而，中度至重度抑郁症可以采用药物治疗和（或）心理干预联合治疗。大多数权威机构推荐使用SSRI，如果需要镇静作用，则推荐使用米氮平。

请参见图 11.1，了解 PCOS 女性复杂的心理后遗症。

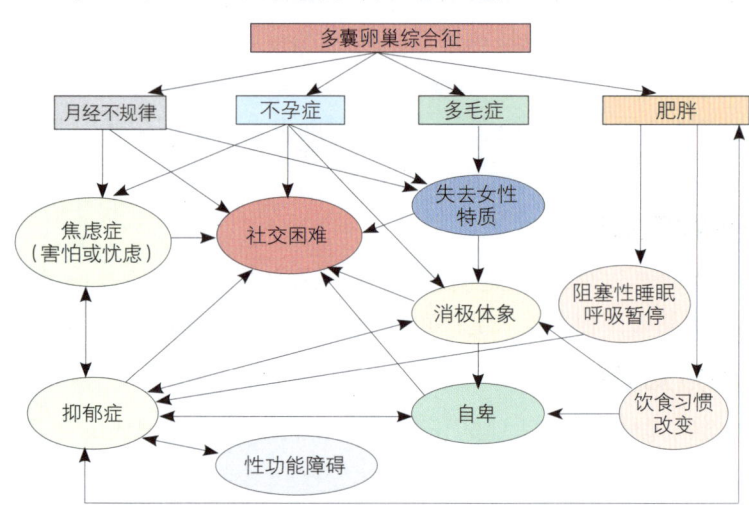

图 11.1　多囊卵巢综合征在女性中产生的复杂心理后遗症

十三、多囊卵巢综合征心境障碍的药物治疗

最终，如果心境障碍症状非常严重或在进行了 3 个月的 PCOS 治疗后没有改善，则应考虑药物治疗。螺内酯等药物的抗雄激素作用也可以减轻抑郁症状。

十四、转诊至精神专科

转诊决策在很大程度上取决于治疗医师的专业水平及精神健康服务的可及性。焦虑和抑郁症状不复杂的病例可以在初级医疗机构中处理，需要更深入地评估和干预的复杂病例则需要专科转诊。

十五、结论

总之，患有 PCOS 的女性经历了"诊断—长期治疗—不同结果"这一系列创伤性生活事件。并非某一个单一因素使她们易受情绪困扰，而是在疾病本身的过程中，她们出现了严重影响其女性特质的症状，这可能使她们容易患上心理障碍。采用综合的生物心理社会多学科方法管理 PCOS 患者将提高她们的整体结局。

请参见图 11.2，了解广泛性焦虑症的分级护理方法。

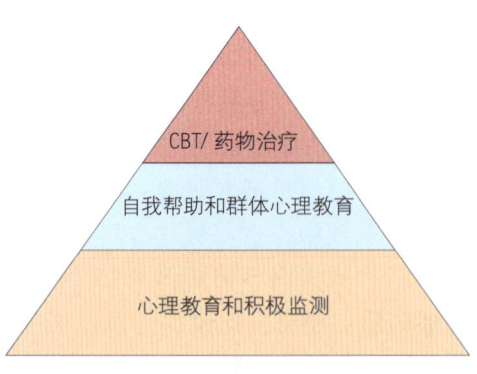

CBT，认知行为疗法。
图 11.2　广泛性焦虑症的分级护理方法

参考文献

1. March WA, Moore VM, Willson KJ, Phillips DI, Norman RJ, Davies MJ. The prevalence of polycystic ovary syndrome in a community sample assessed under contrasting diagnostic criteria. Hum Reprod. 2010;25(2):544-551.
2. Jones GL, Hall JM, Lashen HL, Balen AH, Ledger WL. Health-related quality of life among adolescents with polycystic ovary syndrome. J Obstet Gynecol Neonatal Nurs. 2011;40(5):577-588.
3. Sayyah-Melli M, Alizadeh M, Pourafkary N, et al. Psychosocial factors associated with polycystic ovary syndrome: a case control study. J Caring Sci. 2015;4(3):225.
4. Mueller SC, Ng P, Sinaii N, et al. Psychiatric characterization of children with genetic causes of hyperandrogenism. Eur J Endocrinol. 2010;163(5):801.
5. Marsh CA, Berent-Spillson A, Love T, et al. Functional neuroimaging of emotional processing in women with polycystic ovary syndrome: a case-control pilot study. Fertil Steril. 2013;100(1):200-207.
6. Cipkala-Gaffin J, Talbott EO, Song MK, Bromberger J, Wilson J. Associations between psychologic symptoms and life satisfaction in women with polycystic ovary syndrome. J Womens Health. 2012;21(2):179-187.
7. Brutocao C, Zaiem F, Alsawas M, Morrow AS, Murad MH, Javed A. Psychiatric disorders in women with polycystic ovary syndrome: a systematic review and meta-analysis. Endocrine. 2018;62(2):318-325.
8. Kamathenu UK, Velayudhan A, Krishna KV, Nithya R. Social anxiety and interpersonal relationship of women with PCOD. Med Leg Update. 2021;21(3):523-528.
9. Deeks AA, Gibson-Helm ME, Paul E, Teede HJ. Is having polycystic ovary syndrome a predictor of poor psychological function including anxiety and depression? Hum Reprod. 2011;26(6):1399-1407.
10. Bazarganipour F, Ziaei S, Montazeri A, Foroozanfard F, Kazemnejad A, Faghihzadeh S. Body image satisfaction and self-esteem status among the patients with polycystic ovary syndrome. Iran J Reprod Med. 2013;11(10):829.
11. Fredrickson BL, Roberts TA. Objectification theory: toward understanding women's lived experiences and mental health risks. Psychol Women Q. 1997;21(2):173-206.
12. Feagin JR, McKinney KD. The Many Costs of Racism. Lanham Maryland, United States: Rowman & Littlefield Publishers; 2005.
13. Corrigan PW, Rao D. On the self-stigma of mental illness: stages, disclosure, and strategies for change. Can J Psychiatry. 2012;57(8):464-469.
14. Parker R, Aggleton P. HIV and AIDS-related stigma and discrimination: a conceptual framework and implications for action. Soc Sci Med. 2003;57(1):13-24.
15. Kitzinger C, Willmott J. 'The thief of womanhood': women's experience of polycystic ovarian syndrome. Soc Sci Med. 2002;54(3):349-361.
16. WHO Division of Mental Health. WHO-QOL Study Protocol: The Development of the World Health Organization Quality-of-Life Assessment Instrument. Geneva: United Nations; 1993.
17. Eftekhar T, Sohrabvand F, Zabandan N, Shariat M, Haghollahi F, Ghahghaei-Nezamabadi A. Sexual dysfunction in patients with polycystic ovary syndrome and its affected domains. Iran J Reprod Med. 2014;12(8):539.
18. Elsenbruch S, Hahn S, Kowalsky D, et al. Quality of life, psychosocial well-being, and sexual satisfaction in women with polycystic ovary syndrome. J Clin Endocrinol Metab. 2003;88(12):5801-5807.
19. Fliegner M, Richter-Appelt H, Krupp K, Brunner F. Sexual function and socio-sexual difficulties in women with polycystic ovary syndrome (PCOS). Geburtshilfe Frauenheilkd. 2019;79(5):498-509.
20. Krępuła K, Bidzińska-Speichert B, Lenarcik A, Tworowska-Bardzińska U. Psychiatric disorders related to polycystic ovary syndrome. Endokrynol Pol. 2012;63(6):488-491.
21. Yazici K, Baz K, Yazici AE, et al. Disease-specific quality of life is associated with anxiety and depression in patients with acne. J Eur Acad Dermatol Venereol. 2004;18(4):435-439.
22. Khomami MB, Tehrani FR, Hashemi S, Farahmand M, Azizi F. Of PCOS symptoms, hirsutism has the most

significant impact on the quality of life of Iranian women. PLoS One. 2015;10(4):e0123608.
23. Morshedi T, Salehi M, Farzad V, Hassani F, Shakibazadeh E. The status of relationship between coping strategies and quality of life in women with polycystic ovary syndrome. J Educ Health Promot. 2021;10(1):185.
24. Benson S, Hahn S, Tan S, Janssen OE, Schedlowski M, Elsenbruch S. Maladaptive coping with illness in women with polycystic ovary syndrome. J Obstet Gynecol Neonatal Nurs. 2010;39(1):37-45.
25. Bernadett M. Prevalence of eating disorders among women with polycystic ovary syndrome. Psychiatr Hung. 2016;31(2):136-145.
26. McIntyre RS, Mancini DA, McCann S, Srinivasan J, Kennedy SH. Valproate, bipolar disorder and polycystic ovarian syndrome. Bipolar Disord. 2003;5(1):28-35.
27. Barber TM, Franks S. Obesity and polycystic ovary syndrome. Clin Endocrinol. 2021;95(4):531-541.
28. Berni TR, Morgan CL, Berni ER, Rees DA. Polycystic ovary syndrome is associated with adverse mental health and neurodevelopmental outcomes. J Clin Endocrinol Metab. 2018;103(6):2116-2125.
29. Lee I, Cooney LG, Saini S, et al. Increased risk of disordered eating in polycystic ovary syndrome. Fertil Steril. 2017;107(3):796-802.
30. Helvaci N, Karabulut E, Demir AU, Yildiz BO. Polycystic ovary syndrome and the risk of obstructive sleep apnea: a meta-analysis and review of the literature. Endocr Connect. 2017;6(7):437-445.
31. Brutocao C, Zaiem F, Alsawas M, Morrow AS, Murad MH, Javed A. Psychiatric disorders in women with polycystic ovary syndrome: a systematic review and meta-analysis. Endocrine. 2018;62(2):318-325.
32. Kaur I, Suri V, Rana SV, Singh A. Treatment pathways traversed by polycystic ovary syndrome (PCOS) patients: a mixed-method study. PLoS One. 2021;16(8):e0255830.
33. Harmancı H, Hergüner S, Toy H. Psychiatric symptoms in women with polycystic ovary syndrome. Düşünen Adam J Psychiatry Neurol Sci. 2013;26:157-163.
34. Lamb JD, Johnstone EB, Rousseau JA, et al. Physical activity in women with polycystic ovary syndrome: prevalence, predictors, and positive health associations. Am J Obstet Gynecol. 2011;204(4):352.e1-352.e6.
35. Sharma TR. Polycystic ovarian syndrome and borderline personality disorder: 3 case reports and scientific review of literature. J Psychiatry. 2015;18(6):1-4.
36. Elizabeth M, Leslie NS, Critch EA. Managing polycystic ovary syndrome: a cognitive behavioral strategy. Nurs Womens Health. 2009;13(4):292-300.
37. Roessler KK, Glintborg D, Ravn P, Birkebaek C, Andersen M. Supportive relationships-psychological effects of group counselling in women with polycystic ovary syndrome (PCOS). Commun Med. 2012;9(2):125.
38. National Institute for Health and Clinical Excellence. Generalized Anxiety Disorder and Panic Disorder in Adults: Management. Clinical Guideline [CG113]. 2011. Last updated July 2019. Available at: http://guidance.nice.org.uk/CG113.
39. Baldwin D, Woods R, Lawson R, Taylor D. Efficacy of drug treatments for generalised anxiety disorder: systematic review and meta-analysis. BMJ. 2011;342:d1199.
40. Batelaan NM, Van Balkom AJ, Stein DJ. Evidence-based pharmacotherapy of panic disorder: an update. Int J Neuropsychopharmacol. 2012;15:403-415.
41. National Institute for Health and Clinical Excellence. Depression: The Treatment and Management of Depression in Adults. Clinical Guideline 90. London: National Institute for Health and Clinical Excellence; 2009.
42. Rasgon N, Elman S. When not to treat depression in PCOS with antidepressants. Curr Psychiatry. 2005;4:47-60.
43. Baldwin DS, Anderson IM, Nutt DJ, et al. Evidence-based pharmacological treatment of anxiety disorders, post-traumatic stress disorder and obsessive-compulsive disorder: a revision of the 2005 guidelines from the British Association for Psychopharmacology. J Psychopharmacol. 2014;28:403-439.

第十二章 多囊卵巢综合征和非酒精性脂肪性肝病

一、多囊卵巢综合征与非酒精性脂肪性肝病之间是否存在关联

非酒精性脂肪性肝病（nonalcoholic fatty liver disease，NAFLD）是全球慢性肝病（chronic liver disease，CLD）最常见的原因之一，影响着大约30%的普通人群。它不仅是年轻成人肝移植需求增长最快的原因，在女性群体中也已成为肝移植的主要驱动因素之一，但在不同种族间存在差异。NAFLD包括从单纯的脂肪变性到非酒精性脂肪性肝炎（nonalcoholic steatohepatitis，NASH）的一系列肝脏疾病，可能会进展为肝纤维化、肝硬化和肝细胞癌（hepatocellular carcinoma，HCC）。鉴于NAFLD惊人的增长趋势，我们需要建立有效的筛查策略，并识别高危人群，以便在较早阶段降低与NAFLD进展相关的发病率和死亡率。

多囊卵巢综合征（PCOS）是最常见的内分泌和代谢功能障碍之一，影响着6%～20%的绝经前女性，具体比例取决于使用的诊断标准和特定种族人群。早期PCOS被称为Stein-Leventhal综合征，根据在1935年首次描述该疾病的Stein和Leventhal医师命名。根据鹿特丹标准，该综合征以临床和（或）生物学上的高雄激素血症（HA）、稀发排卵/无排卵和B超下的多囊卵巢形态（PCOM）为特征。PCOS不仅会影响生殖系统（是无排卵性不孕的主要原因之一），而且还与机体的代谢紊乱有关。

有报道称NAFLD与PCOS之间存在相关性。这可能是因为NAFLD和PCOS都与代谢综合征（MetS）的组成部分［即内脏型肥胖、高血压、血脂异常和胰岛素抵抗（IR）］具有强相关性。PCOS患者中NAFLD的高患病率也支持这一关联。Macut等指出，51%的PCOS女性患有NAFLD，而非PCOS女性仅34%患有NAFLD。与之类似，另一文献报道50%的PCOS女性患有NAFLD，这与其体重指数（BMI）无关。此外，各种不同的研究表明，PCOS女性中NAFLD的患病率为34%～70%，高于普通人群。

二、多囊卵巢综合征与非酒精性脂肪性肝病之间可能存在的关联是什么

PCOS和NAFLD之间确切的病理生理联系、驱动因素和机制仍需进一步探索。尽管如此，内脏型肥胖和IR与这两种疾病均存在强烈相关性。据报道，40%～70%的PCOS患者有肥胖或超重，并伴有IR和代偿性高胰岛素血症。这增加了其他代谢紊乱，

如高血压、2型糖尿病（T2DM）、血脂异常和心血管疾病等发生的可能性。HA也被认为是独立于IR和肥胖而与NAFLD和PCOS都相关的因素。

IR被认为是这两种疾病发病机制的主要驱动因素，因为IR的发生率随着糖尿病（DM）、肥胖和MetS的发病率增加而增加。IR和NAFLD之间存在双向关联，这增强了IR在PCOS患者中的作用。靶组织对胰岛素变化（由IR导致的高胰岛素血症）做出反应，激活了从NAFLD到NASH的进展途径。在细胞水平上发生的各种改变可以解释这种关联；例如，IR通过增强内脏脂肪组织的脂肪分解和增加脂肪在肝脏中的沉积来产生游离脂肪酸，而由于脂肪毒素增加、线粒体功能障碍和脂肪分解产生的活性氧化物，胰岛素信号传导受阻。最终，它激活肝星状细胞释放胶原和纤维蛋白原，在肝脏中形成纤维化。

IR通过促进卵巢内雄激素的产生和抑制性激素结合球蛋白（SHBG）的产生，导致游离雄激素水平升高，从而在PCOS患者中引起HA。IR和HA反映了PCOS和NAFLD之间的病理生理联系。一项研究表明，出现HA的PCOS患者比正常雄激素水平的PCOS患者和没有PCOS的女性更容易患肝脂肪变性（hepatic steatosis，HS）。此外，许多研究表明，只有HA可以导致PCOS女性出现NAFLD。相反，Macut等显示HA和NAFLD之间并非独立相关，而是通过IR实现的。在细胞和分子水平上，线粒体发挥着调节代谢和能量生产的生理学作用。在PCOS中，由于IR和HA导致线粒体功能障碍，引起甘油三酯和胆固醇的产生增加，以及脂肪酸β-氧化的降低，从而加速了HS，并促进了NAFLD的发展。另外，肝细胞中脂质沉积引起的炎症反应会进展为NASH。

虽然遗传关联尚不清楚，但可能同时影响NAFLD和PCOS的基因可以分为3类：① *CYP17*、*CYP11A*和*SHBG*这些帮助合成雄激素的基因；② *IL-6*、肿瘤坏死因子-α（*TNF-α*）和*TNF-R*这些参与细胞因子分泌和作用的基因；③胰岛素和胰岛素受体这些参与胰岛素分泌和作用的基因。与NAFLD高发生率相关的种族和民族差异可归因于遗传因素：含patatin样磷脂酶域蛋白3（patatin-like phospholipase domain containing 3，PNPLA3）的多态性。

微生物组学在PCOS和NAFLD的病理生理学研究中处于新兴地位。一项研究表明，患PCOS的女性具有与未患这种综合征的女性不同的肠道微生物群。因此，有必要更深入地探索肠道微生物群的改变，以探求潜在的治疗靶点。

（一）何时开始怀疑及对谁进行筛查

大多数NAFLD患者在诊断时无症状，但有些人可能有非特异性症状，如右上腹（right upper quadrant，RUQ）隐痛、疲劳和不适感。在体格检查中，肝大很常见，但由于肥胖而难以评估；而慢性肝病的色斑可以发现，但主要见于NASH肝硬化期。因此，如果患者出现与NAFLD强相关的病情（如DM或MetS），可合理怀疑患者患有NAFLD。2005年Brown等首次报道了一位PCOS女性患NAFLD的病例。由于目前对早期诊断的长期益处和成本效益的认识非常欠缺，暂不建议对 PCOS 患者进行 NAFLD 的常规筛查。然而，女性中 PCOS 患病率更高的事实引起了关注，需要研究筛查和早期治疗 NAFLD 的有效性，至少针对高风险的 PCOS 患者群体应进行筛查和早期治疗。因此，在处理与 PCOS 或 NAFLD 有关的问题时，医疗保健专业人员要注意在育龄女性中进行识别和相应检查。

（二）如何诊断非酒精性脂肪性肝病

目前，NAFLD 是一种排除性诊断。在诊断之前需要排除饮酒量过大（表 12.1）、其他引起 HS 的病因，以及共存的 CLD 的诱因，如药物、毒素、病毒感染、营养和代谢因素、自身免疫/代谢/遗传性 CLD 诱因、减重术和快速减重等。

表 12.1　各指南中大量饮酒的酒精摄入量

协会	男性	女性
亚太地区肝病研究协会	每周＞14 标准杯（140 g 酒精）	每周＞7 标准杯（70 g 酒精）
美国肝病研究协会	平均每周＞21 标准杯	平均每周＞14 标准杯
欧洲肝病研究协会	每天＞30 g	每天＞20 g

来源：Paul, J. Recent advances in non-invasive diagnosis and medical management of non-alcoholic fatty liver disease in adult. Egypt Liver J. 2020; 10[1]: 37.

注：亚洲和欧洲的标准杯含有大约 10 g 纯酒精，而在美国则为 14 g。

以下实验室检查可用于诊断 NAFLD：

• NAFLD 通常是由于肝功能检查（LFT）结果异常、脂肪肝或其他原因而进行影像学检查时偶然被发现的。在 LFT 中，血清氨基转移酶水平通常升高，可达正常上限的 1.5～4.0 倍，很少超过正常上限的 10 倍。与酒精性肝病相比，NAFLD 中血清 ALT 水平通常高于 AST 碱性磷酸酶和 γ-谷氨酰转移酶（gamma-glutamyltransferase，GGTP）水平可能会升高，但发生率较低。除了需要排除其他导致 HS 的原因外，还建议评估和早期识别可能导致 NAFLD 的因素，如肥胖、血脂异常、IR、糖尿病前期或 DM、甲状腺功能减退、PCOS 和睡眠呼吸暂停等。

• 常规超声检查是诊断 NAFLD 的首选影像学检查项目。它不仅可及性高、接受程度好、成本效益高，而且在识别中度到重度 HS 时的敏感性可达 85%（80%～89%），特异性可达 93%（87%～97%）。然而，超声检查也存在一些局限性，包括无法评估肝纤维化的严重程度，对肥胖患者的敏感性有限，以及当脂肪变性程度低于 20% 时敏感性有限。

• 对比增强和非对比计算机体层成像（computed tomography，CT）都可以通过检测肝实质相对于肝内血管、脾脏和肾脏的衰减来识别 NAFLD，且对中度到重度脂肪肝识别的特异性为 100%。其限制包括高昂的成本、缺乏广泛的可及性、辐射暴露和检测轻度脂肪肝时准确性有限。

• 磁共振成像（MRI）能提供最明确的 HS 定性和定量评估，其敏感性为 76.7%～

90.0%，特异性为 87.1%～91.0%。MRI 有几个优点：能够识别低至 5%～10% 的脂肪变性；不会受到人口统计学、组织学活动或并发肝脏疾病的显著影响。然而，它成本高、耗时长，因此主要用于临床试验。

- 瞬时弹性成像（也称振动控制瞬时弹性成像或 Fibroscan）是一种基于超声的成像模式，通过受控衰减参数（controlled attenuation parameter，CAP）和硬度（纤维化）测量肝脏中的脂肪含量。一项关于 CAP 的诊断准确性的荟萃分析显示截断值为 248 dB/m。CAP 在使用 241 dB/m 的截断值时对 NAFLD 是否存在 HS 具有优异的诊断表现，但在评估脂肪肝程度方面，尤其是在 BMI 较高（> 30 kg/m²）的患者中价值有限。

- ALT 升高虽然常见，但对于评估 NAFLD 的严重程度来说并不具有特异性。因此，研究人员提出了各种非侵入性生物标志物，如透明质酸、骨桥蛋白、Ⅳ型胶原和基质金属蛋白酶。此外，另一个日益普及的生物标志物是细胞角蛋白-18（cytokeratin-18，CK-18）；胱天蛋白酶生成的片段可提示肝细胞的凋亡，提示 NASH 的存在。此外，其成本较高，这些新型生物标志物目前尚没有广泛应用于临床。

- 有一些非侵入性评分系统可用于评估肝纤维化的严重程度，包括 FibroTest（FibroSure）、FibroMeter、NAFLD 纤维化评分、Fibrosis-4（FIB-4）、AST 与血小板比值（AST-to-platelet ratio，APRI）、BARD[BMI、(AST：ALT)、DM]、增强肝纤维化（ELF）评分[TIMP-1、Ⅲ型前胶原氨基末端前体（PⅢNP）、透明质酸]、NashTest 和 AST：ALT。其中，NAFLD 纤维化评分、FIB-4 和 APRI 是常用的评估工具。

- 肝组织活检是诊断 NAFLD 并评估其严重程度和预后的金标准。然而，由于它是一种侵入性的过程，费用高昂，并且在 30% 的活检中存在评估的差异性，这些相关风险限制了其应用。建议可在特定情况下使用这种检查，例如：当患者有较高的 SH 和（或）晚期纤维化风险时；不经过肝活检就无法排除其他病因和评估 NAFLD 严重程度时；临床试验中结局的客观评估。

导致 NAFLD 和 PCOS 的常见因素是肥胖和 IR。因此，BMI 和腰围是评估 NAFLD 风险的预测因素，但现在引入了结合血脂和人体测量指标的新代谢指数，可以准确预测 IR、糖尿病前期和 T2DM。这些指标包括脂质蓄积产物（lipid accumulation product，LAP）指数、内脏脂肪指数（visceral adiposity index，VAI）和甘油三酯葡萄糖乘积（triglycerides and glucose，TyG）指数。LAP 指数反映腹型肥胖，与无疾病的对照组相比，患有 PCOS 和 MetS 的女性 LAP 指数较高；另一项研究表明，它是检测 PCOS 女性是否患有 NAFLD 的一个重要预测因子。

（三）可采用的治疗选择

我们目前在治疗与 PCOS 相关的代谢紊乱，包括 NAFLD 方面，并没有太多可选择的办法。因此，就像没有 PCOS 的女性一样，NAFLD 的治疗包括治疗相关疾病（如肥胖、DM、MetS）、改变生活方式、药物治疗，以及减重术或减重内镜手术。

1. 生活方式干预

如前所述，50% 的 PCOS 患者存在肥胖和 IR，导致代偿性高胰岛素血症，并且更容易患上 T2DM。内脏型肥胖往往与血清性激素水平升高和 SHBG 降低有关。与非肥胖的 PCOS 女性和没有 PCOS 的女性相比，肥胖的 PCOS 女性更容易出现代谢和心血管异常。因此，对肥胖患者来说，减重治疗应该是被优先推荐的一线治疗。可通过生活方式干预、体育活动和饮食管理减重，如有必要可以采用药物治疗。减重带来的好处是巨大的，可以降低体脂率、性激素和胰岛素水平，改善排卵和生育力，并降低心血管疾病（CVD）的整体风险。一项系统综述显示，饮食调节辅以中等程度有氧运动对改善内分泌和代谢症状有巨大影响。对于不同类型的饮食也有很多研究，如生酮饮食、低碳水化合物饮食，都显示出明显的改善效果。一项荟萃分析表明，单不饱和脂肪酸的摄入可导致减重明显，低糖饮食可改善月经周期并降低 IR。要改善 HS，需要减重 3%～5%，而要改善 NASH 的组织病理学特征，需要减重 7%～10%。因此，低热量饮食（每日减少 500～1000 kcal）结合中等强度的运动是长期保持体重的关键。高强度间歇训练（high-intensity interval training，HIIT）与降低内脏脂肪、改善肝脂肪变性和纤维化相关联，尤其适用于没有时间锻炼的人群。总体而言，每周 150 分钟中等强度有氧运动，以及每周 2～3 次力量训练非常有效。不能开展系统性运动计划的人可以通过每天减少久坐时间或多次中断久坐，并重复几分钟的步行来改善身体状况。无论如何，在任何情况下，遵守饮食改变和定期进行体育锻炼对于目标的实现起着关键作用。

2. 胰岛素增敏剂

高胰岛素血症和 IR 都会促进 T2DM、CVD 和 NAFLD 的发展；因此，管理 PCOS 代谢谱的药物治疗也应考虑对抗胰岛素的作用。

• 噻唑烷二酮类药物：吡格列酮是一种过氧化物酶体增殖物激活受体 -γ（peroxisome proliferator-activated receptor-gamma，PPAR-γ）激动剂，可调节葡萄糖摄取、脂肪生成和胰岛素功能。在随机试验、荟萃分析和随机开放标签研究中，吡格列酮对 PCOS 患者代谢状况的改善显示出有潜力的效果。然而，它有液体潴留和让肥胖者的体重进一步增加的副作用，这是在应用该药物时最主要的担心和阻碍。

• 二甲双胍：它属于双胍家族，其作用机制是抑制葡萄糖产生、增强胰岛素敏感性和葡萄糖摄取，并改善 PCOS 中因高胰岛素血症而常见的脂质异常。初始剂量为每天 500～800 mg，最大可达 2000 mg（如果耐受）。常见的不良反应是腹泻、腹胀及恶心和呕吐。长期使用还会导致维生素 B_{12} 缺乏。一项比较二甲双胍和生活方式干预的研究显示，两者对降低 BMI 的效果相似，但二甲双胍组降低了雄激素水平。该药物降低 BMI 的效果也独立于生活方式干预。

• 胰高血糖素样肽 -1 受体类似物：这是一类具有肠促胰岛素模拟活性的物质，可释放葡萄糖依赖性胰岛素，尤其是在餐后。它们包括胰高血糖素样肽 -1（glucagon-like peptide-1，GLP-1）和葡萄糖依赖性促胰岛素多肽（glucose-dependent insulinotropic polypeptide，GIP）。利拉鲁肽和司美格鲁肽在肥胖患者（即使不伴有 T2DM）中已经明确有持续的减重效果。使用这两种药物治疗 NAFLD 的组织学缓解率在 40%～60%。因此，GLP-1 受体激动剂预计在管理肥胖和 NAFLD 方面将发挥至关重要的作用。

- 减重术和内镜手术：有助于在病态肥胖的患者中实现减重，并提高胰岛素敏感性，从而改善 DM、降低 HS 和心血管发病率和缓解其他 PCOS 症状。目前推荐无法通过其他措施减轻体重的重度肥胖患者考虑手术治疗。

（四）并发症和预后

1. 与肝脏相关的并发症

在具有晚期肝纤维化的 NAFLD 患者中，肝脏相关死亡率和全因死亡率均增加，在这些患者中有 20% 的人甚至在没有肝硬化的情况下就发展为 HCC。因此，由于和 MetS 的强相关性，患有 PCOS 的 NAFLD 患者如果早期治疗 NAFLD，可能会获得益处。

2. 其他并发症

NAFLD 被认为是 MetS 的肝脏表现，DM 和 NAFLD 之间存在双向关系。NAFLD 是疾病进展的独立预测因子，也与高血压有关。血脂异常是并发症之一，它增加了动脉粥样硬化的风险，并可能导致心肌梗死（发生率为每 1000 人每年 4.8 次）和脑血管意外事件。正如前面提到的，IR 和肥胖是 NAFLD 的主要驱动因素，也可能导致 CVD 进展及更高的死亡率。一项荟萃分析报告了抑郁症和神经认知功能障碍与 NAFLD 的关联。其他并发症包括胆囊结石、阻塞性睡眠呼吸暂停、骨质疏松症及甲状腺功能异常。最常见的死因是 CVD，其次是肝外癌症。

PCOS 可以引起许多并发症（如月经失调、低生育力、子宫内膜腺癌和潜在的血管性疾病），并增加了代谢紊乱（如 T2DM 和 NAFLD）的风险。它是一种终身性疾病，从婴儿期到绝经后期的女性都会受到影响。而且患有 PCOS 母亲的女性后代患病风险增加 5 倍。此外，研究表明，在啮齿动物模型中，产前性激素暴露（而非肥胖）导致了肝脏代谢和生殖系统的跨代功能障碍。PCOS 女性的后代可能较早发生心血管代谢紊乱和 NAFLD，因此，在怀孕前达到正常的 BMI 应该是避免发生 NAFLD 的关键目标。这就是为什么早期预防 DM 和肥胖至关重要，它们会威胁患有 PCOS 女性的整体健康，并可能在怀孕和分娩期间引起并发症。

三、结论

NAFLD 和 PCOS 有相似的风险因素，并且与 MetS 的组成部分，尤其是肥胖和 IR 有着密切关联。关于对所有 PCOS 患者进行筛查的有效性的数据尚有限。然而，对于具有多个风险因素（包括 IR 和 HA）的 PCOS 女性，如果能早期识别 NAFLD，可能有助于预防疾病进展和避免肝硬化并发症。

参考文献

1. Younossi Z, Tacke F, Arrese M, et al. Global perspectives on nonalcoholic fatty liver disease and nonalcoholic steatohepatitis. Hepatology. 2019;69(6):2672-2682.
2. Doycheva I, Issa D, Watt KD, Lopez R, Rifai G, Alkhouri N. Nonalcoholic steatohepatitis is the most rapidly increasing indication for liver transplantation in young adults in the United States. J Clin Gastroenterol. 2018;52(4):339-346.
3. Noureddin M, Vipani A, Bresee C, et al. NASH leading cause of liver transplant in women: updated analysis of indications for liver transplant and ethnic and gender variances. Am J Gastroenterol. 2018;113(11):1649-1659.
4. Sayiner M, Koenig A, Henry L, Younossi ZM. Epidemiology of nonalcoholic fatty liver disease and nonalcoholic steatohepatitis in the United States and the rest of the world. Clin Liver Dis. 2016;20(2):205-214.
5. Ding T, Hardiman PJ, Petersen I, Wang FF, Qu F, Baio G. The prevalence of polycystic ovary syndrome in reproductive-aged women of different ethnicity: a systematic review and meta-analysis. Oncotarget. 2017;8(56):96351.
6. Lim SS, Davies M, Norman RJ, Moran L. Overweight, obesity and central obesity in women with polycystic ovary syndrome: a systematic review and meta-analysis. Hum Reprod Update. 2012;18(6):618-637.
7. Rotterdam ESHRE/ASRM-Sponsored PCOS Consensus Workshop Group. Revised 2003 consensus on diagnostic criteria and long-term health risks related to polycystic ovary syndrome (PCOS). Hum Reprod. 2004;19(1):41-47.
8. Franks S. Assessment and management of anovulatory infertility in polycystic ovary syndrome. Endocrinol Metab Clin North Am. 2003;32(3):639-651.
9. Cerda C, Pérez-Ayuso RM, Riquelme A, Soza A, et al. Nonalcoholic fatty liver disease in women with polycystic ovary syndrome. J Hepatol. 2007;47(3):412-417.
10. Chalasani N, Younossi Z, Lavine JE, et al. The diagnosis and management of non-alcoholic fatty liver disease: practice guideline by the American Gastroenterological Association, American Association for the Study of Liver Diseases, and American College of Gastroenterology. Gastroenterology. 2012;142(7):1592-1609.
11. Gambarin-Gelwan M, Kinkhabwala SV, Schiano TD, Bodian C, Yeh HC, Futterweit W. Prevalence of nonalcoholic fatty liver disease in women with polycystic ovary syndrome. Clin Gastroenterol Hepatol. 2007;5(4):496-501.
12. Setji TL, Holland ND, Sanders LL, Pereira KC, Diehl AM, Brown AJ. Nonalcoholic steatohepatitis and nonalcoholic fatty liver disease in young women with polycystic ovary syndrome. J Clin Endocrinol Metab. 2006;91(5):1741-1747.
13. Jeanes YM, Reeves S. Metabolic consequences of obesity and insulin resistance in polycystic ovary syndrome: diagnostic and methodological challenges. Nutr Res Rev. 2017;30(1):97.
14. Jensen T, Wieland A, Cree-Green M, Nadeau K, Sullivan S. Clinical workup of fatty liver for the primary care provider. Postgrad Med. 2019;131(1):19-30.
15. Cai J, Wu C, Zhang Y, Wang Y, et al. High-free androgen index is associated with increased risk of non-alcoholic fatty liver disease in women with polycystic ovary syndrome, independent of obesity and insulin resistance. Int J Obes. 2017;41(9):1341-1347.
16. Carreau AM, Pyle L, Garcia-Reyes Y, et al. Clinical prediction score of nonalcoholic fatty liver disease in adolescent girls with polycystic ovary syndrome (PCOS-HS index). Clin Endocrinol. 2019;91(4):544-552.
17. Rocha A, Faria L, Guimarães T, et al. Non-alcoholic fatty liver disease in women with polycystic ovary syndrome: systematic review and meta-analysis. J Endocrinol Invest. 2017;40(12):1279-1288.
18. Wu J, Yao XY, Shi RX, Liu SF, Wang XY. A potential link between polycystic ovary syndrome and non-alcoholic fatty liver disease: an update meta-analysis. Reprod Health. 2018;15(1):1-9.
19. Macut D, Tziomalos K, Božić-Antić I, et al. Non-alcoholic fatty liver disease is associated with insulin

resistance and lipid accumulation product in women with polycystic ovary syndrome. Hum Reprod. 2016;31(6):1347-1353.
20. Salva-Pastor N, Chavez-Tapia NC, Uribe M, Nuno-Lambarri N. Understanding the association of polycystic ovary syndrome and non-alcoholic fatty liver disease. J Steroid Biochem Mol Biol. 2019;194:105445.
21. Cussons AJ, Watts GF, Mori TA, Stuckey BG. Omega-3 fatty acid supplementation decreases liver fat content in polycystic ovary syndrome: a randomized controlled trial employing proton magnetic resonance spectroscopy. Obstet Gynecol Surv. 2010;65(3):175-176.
22. Jones H, Sprung VS, Pugh CJ, et al. Polycystic ovary syndrome with hyperandrogenism is characterized by an increased risk of hepatic steatosis compared to nonhyperandrogenic PCOS phenotypes and healthy controls, independent of obesity and insulin resistance. J Clin Endocrinol Metab. 2012;97(10):3709-3716.
23. Petta S, Ciresi A, Bianco J, et al. Insulin resistance and hyperandrogenism drive steatosis and fibrosis risk in young females with PCOS. PLoS One. 2017;12(11):e0186136.
24. Ramezani-Binabaj M, Motalebi M, Karimi-Sari H, Rezaee-Zavareh MS, Alavian SM. Are women with polycystic ovarian syndrome at a high risk of non-alcoholic fatty liver disease; a meta-analysis. Hepat Mon. 2014;14(11):e23235.
25. Vassilatou E. Nonalcoholic fatty liver disease and polycystic ovary syndrome. World J Gastroenterol. 2014;20(26):8351.
26. Vassilatou E, Lafoyianni S, Vryonidou A, et al. Increased androgen bioavailability is associated with non-alcoholic fatty liver disease in women with polycystic ovary syndrome. Hum Reprod. 2010;25(1):212-220.
27. Vassilatou E, Vassiliadi D, Salambasis K, et al. Increased prevalence of polycystic ovary syndrome in premenopausal women with nonalcoholic fatty liver disease. Eur J Endocrinol. 2015;173(6):739-747.
28. Gastaldelli A. Insulin resistance and reduced metabolic flexibility: cause or consequence of NAFLD? Clin Sci. 2017;131(22):2701-2704.
29. Kumarendran B, O'Reilly MW, Manolopoulos KN, et al. Polycystic ovary syndrome, androgen excess, and the risk of nonalcoholic fatty liver disease in women: a longitudinal study based on a United Kingdom primary care database. PLoS Med. 2018;15(3):e1002542.
30. Macut D, Bjekić-Macut J, Livadas S, et al. Nonalcoholic fatty liver disease in patients with polycystic ovary syndrome. Curr Pharm Des. 2018;24(38):4593-4597.
31. Minato S, Sakane N, Kotani K, et al. Prevalence and risk factors of elevated liver enzymes in Japanese women with polycystic ovary syndrome. J Clin Med Res. 2018;10(12):904.
32. Vassilatou E, Lafoyianni S, Vassiliadi DA, et al. Visceral adiposity index for the diagnosis of nonalcoholic fatty liver disease in premenopausal women with and without polycystic ovary syndrome. Maturitas. 2018;116:1-7.
33. Gilbert EW, Tay CT, Hiam DS, Teede HJ, Moran LJ. Comorbidities and complications of polycystic ovary syndrome: an overview of systematic reviews. Clin Endocrinol. 2018;89(6):683-699.
34. Moran C, Arriaga M, Rodriguez G, Moran S. Obesity differentially affects phenotypes of polycystic ovary syndrome. Int J Endocrinol. 2012;2012:317241.
35. Panidis D, Macut D, Tziomalos K, et al. Prevalence of metabolic syndrome in women with polycystic ovary syndrome. Clin Endocrinol. 2013;78(4):586-592.
36. Yildiz BO, Knochenhauer ES, Azziz R. Impact of obesity on the risk for polycystic ovary syndrome. J Clin Endocrinol Metab. 2008;93(1):162-168.
37. Legro RS, Castracane VD, Kauffman RP. Detecting insulin resistance in polycystic ovary syndrome: purposes and pitfalls. Obstet Gynecol Surv. 2004;59(2):141-154.
38. Marshall JC, Dunaif A. Should all women with PCOS be treated for insulin resistance? Fertil Steril. 2012;97(1):18-22.
39. Won YB, Seo SK, Yun BH, Cho S, Choi YS, Lee BS. Non-alcoholic fatty liver disease in polycystic ovary syndrome women. Sci Rep. 2021;11(1):1-11.
40. Polyzos SA, Mantzoros CS. Nonalcoholic fatty future disease. Metabolism. 2016;65(8):1007-1016.

41. Vernon G, Baranova A, Younossi Z. Systematic review: the epidemiology and natural history of non-alcoholic fatty liver disease and non-alcoholic steatohepatitis in adults. Aliment Pharmacol Ther. 2011;34(3):274-285.
42. Williams CD, Stengel J, Asike MI, et al. Prevalence of nonalcoholic fatty liver disease and nonalcoholic steatohepatitis among a largely middle-aged population utilizing ultrasound and liver biopsy: a prospective study. Gastroenterology. 2011;140(1):124-131.
43. Pearson T, Wattis JA, King JR, MacDonald IA, Mazzatti DJ. The effects of insulin resistance on individual tissues: an application of a mathematical model of metabolism in humans. Bull Math Biol. 2016;78(6):1189-1217.
44. Lee HY, Birkenfeld AL, Jornayvaz FR, et al. Apolipoprotein CIII overexpressing mice are predisposed to diet-induced hepatic steatosis and hepatic insulin resistance. Hepatology. 2011;54(5):1650-1660.
45. Magkos F, Su X, Bradley D, et al. Intrahepatic diacylglycerol content is associated with hepatic insulin resistance in obese subjects. Gastroenterology. 2012;142(7):1444-1446.e2.
46. Jelenik T, Kaul K, Séquaris G, et al. Mechanisms of insulin resistance in primary and secondary nonalcoholic fatty liver. Diabetes. 2017;66(8):2241-2253.
47. Chalasani N, Deeg MA, Crabb DW. Systemic levels of lipid peroxidation and its metabolic and dietary correlates in patients with nonalcoholic steatohepatitis. Am J Gastroenterol. 2004;99(8):1497-1502.
48. Staehr P, Hother-Nielsen O, Landau BR, Chandramouli V, Holst JJ, Beck-Nielsen H. Effects of free fatty acids per se on glucose production, gluconeogenesis, and glycogenolysis. Diabetes. 2003;52(2):260-267.
49. Diamanti-Kandarakis E, Dunaif A. Insulin resistance and the polycystic ovary syndrome revisited: an update on mechanisms and implications. Endocr Rev. 2012;33(6):981-1030.
50. Yildiz BO, Azziz R. The adrenal and polycystic ovary syndrome. Rev Endocr Metab Disord. 2007;8(4):331-342.
51. Birkenfeld AL, Shulman GI. Nonalcoholic fatty liver disease, hepatic insulin resistance, and type 2 diabetes. Hepatology. 2014;59(2):713-723.
52. Kim J, Kim D, Yim J, et al. Polycystic ovary syndrome with hyperandrogenism as a risk factor for non-obese non-alcoholic fatty liver disease. Aliment Pharmacol Ther. 2017;45(11):1403-1412.
53. Rocha AL, Oliveira FR, Azevedo RC, et al. Recent advances in the understanding and management of polycystic ovary syndrome. F1000Res. 2019;8:F1000.
54. Friedman JR, Nunnari J. Mitochondrial form and function. Nature. 2014;505(7483):335-343.
55. Whigham LD, Butz DE, Dashti H, et al. Metabolic evidence of diminished lipid oxidation in women with polycystic ovary syndrome. Curr Metabolomics. 2013;1(4):269-278.
56. Garcimartín A, López-Oliva ME, Sántos-López JA, et al. Silicon alleviates nonalcoholic steatohepatitis by reducing apoptosis in aged Wistar rats fed a high-saturated fat, high-cholesterol diet. J Nutr. 2017;147(6):1104-1112.
57. Ju J, Huang Q, Sun J, et al. Correlation between PPAR-α methylation level in peripheral blood and atherosclerosis of NAFLD patients with DM. Exp Ther Med. 2018;15(3):2727-2730.
58. Kanda T, Matsuoka S, Yamazaki M, et al. Apoptosis and non-alcoholic fatty liver diseases. World J Gastroenterol. 2018;24(25):2661.
59. Khambu B, Yan S, Huda N, Liu G, Yin XM. Autophagy in nonalcoholic fatty liver disease and alcoholic liver disease. Liver Res. 2018;2(3):112-119.
60. Lee S, Kim S, Hwang S, Cherrington NJ, Ryu DY. Dysregulated expression of proteins associated with ER stress, autophagy and apoptosis in tissues from nonalcoholic fatty liver disease. Oncotarget. 2017;8(38):63370.
61. Shimano H, Sato R. SREBP-regulated lipid metabolism: convergent physiology—divergent pathophysiology. Nat Rev Endocrinol. 2017;13(12):710.
62. Stankov MV, Panayotova-Dimitrova D, Leverkus M, et al. Autophagy inhibition due to thymidine analogues as novel mechanism leading to hepatocyte dysfunction and lipid accumulation. AIDS. 2012;26(16):1995-2006.

63. Gao B, Tsukamoto H. Inflammation in alcoholic and nonalcoholic fatty liver disease: friend or foe? Gastroenterology. 2016;150(8):1704-1709.
64. Michael MD, Kulkarni RN, Postic C, et al. Loss of insulin signaling in hepatocytes leads to severe insulin resistance and progressive hepatic dysfunction. Mol Cell. 2000;6(1):87-97.
65. Wang J, Wu D, Guo H, Li M. Hyperandrogenemia and insulin resistance: the chief culprit of polycystic ovary syndrome. Life Sci. 2019;236:116940.
66. Sarkar M, Terrault N, Duwaerts CC, Tien P, Cedars MI, Huddleston H. The association of Hispanic ethnicity with nonalcoholic fatty liver disease in polycystic ovary syndrome. Curr Opin Gynecol Obstet. 2018;1(1):24.
67. Zhang J, Hu J, Zhang C, et al. Analyses of risk factors for polycystic ovary syndrome complicated with non-alcoholic fatty liver disease. Exp Ther Med. 2018;15(5):4259-4264.
68. Thackray VG. Sex, microbes, and polycystic ovary syndrome. Trends Endocrinol Metab. 2019;30(1):54-65.
69. Wieland A, Frank D, Harnke B, Bambha K. Systematic review: microbial dysbiosis and nonalcoholic fatty liver disease. Aliment Pharmacol Ther. 2015;42(9):1051-1063.
70. Jobira B, Frank DN, Pyle L, et al. Obese adolescents with PCOS have altered biodiversity and relative abundance in gastrointestinal microbiota. J Clin Endocrinol Metab. 2020;105(6):e2134-e2144.
71. Angulo P. Nonalcoholic fatty liver disease. N Engl J Med. 2002;346(16):1221-1231.
72. Matteoni CA, Younossi ZM, Gramlich T, Boparai N, Liu YC, McCullough AJ. Nonalcoholic fatty liver disease: a spectrum of clinical and pathological severity. Gastroenterology. 1999;116(6):1413-1419.
73. Brown AJ, Tendler DA, McMurray RG, Setji TL. Polycystic ovary syndrome and severe nonalcoholic steatohepatitis: beneficial effect of modest weight loss and exercise on liver biopsy findings. Endocr Pract. 2005;11(5):319-324.
74. Chalasani N, Younossi Z, Lavine JE, et al. The diagnosis and management of nonalcoholic fatty liver disease: practice guidance from the American Association for the Study of Liver Diseases. Hepatology. 2018;67(1):328-357. doi:10.1002/hep.29367.
75. Clark JM. The epidemiology of nonalcoholic fatty liver disease in adults. J Clin Gastroenterol. 2006;40:S5-S10.
76. Castera L, Friedrich-Rust M, Loomba R. Noninvasive assessment of liver disease in patients with nonalcoholic fatty liver disease. Gastroenterology. 2019;156(5):1264-1281.e4. doi:10.1053/j.gastro.2018.12.036.
77. Paul J. Recent advances in non-invasive diagnosis and medical management of non-alcoholic fatty liver disease in adult. Egypt Liver J. 2020;10(1):37. doi:10.1186/s43066-020-00043-x.
78. Ratziu V, Charlotte F, Heurtier A, et al. Sampling variability of liver biopsy in nonalcoholic fatty liver disease. Gastroenterology. 2005;128(7):1898-1906.
79. Sberna A, Bouillet B, Rouland A, et al. European Association for the Study of the Liver (EASL), European Association for the Study of Diabetes (EASD) and European Association for the Study of Obesity (EASO) clinical practice recommendations for the management of non-alcoholic fatty liver disease: evaluation of their application in people with Type 2 diabetes. Diabet Med. 2018;35(3):368-375.
80. Amato MC, Giordano C, Galia M, et al. Visceral Adiposity Index: a reliable indicator of visceral fat function associated with cardiometabolic risk. Diabetes Care. 2010;33(4):920-922.
81. Angulo P, Hui JM, Marchesini G, et al. The NAFLD fibrosis score: a noninvasive system that identifies liver fibrosis in patients with NAFLD. Hepatology. 2007;45(4):846-854.
82. Demir M, Lang S, Nierhoff D, et al. Stepwise combination of simple noninvasive fibrosis scoring systems increases diagnostic accuracy in nonalcoholic fatty liver disease. J Clin Gastroenterol. 2013;47(8):719-726.
83. Harrison SA, Oliver D, Arnold HL, Gogia S, Neuschwander-Tetri BA. Development and validation of a simple NAFLD clinical scoring system for identifying patients without advanced disease. Gut. 2008;57(10):1441-1447.
84. Kotronen A, Peltonen M, Hakkarainen A, et al. Prediction of non-alcoholic fatty liver disease and liver fat using metabolic and genetic factors. Gastroenterology. 2009;137(3):865-872.
85. Sumida Y, Yoneda M, Hyogo H, et al. A simple clinical scoring system using ferritin, fasting insulin, and type

IV collagen 7S for predicting steatohepatitis in nonalcoholic fatty liver disease. J Gastroenterol. 2011;46(2):257-268.
86. Muthiah MD, Han NC, Sanyal AJ. A clinical overview of NAFLD: a guide to diagnosis, the clinical features, and complications–What the non-specialist needs to know. Diabetes Obes Metab. 2022;24(suppl 2):3-14.
87. Loomis AK, Kabadi S, Preiss D, et al. Body mass index and risk of nonalcoholic fatty liver disease: two electronic health record prospective studies. J Clin Endocrinol Metab. 2016;101(3):945-952.
88. Motamed N, Sohrabi M, Ajdarkosh H, et al. Fatty liver index vs waist circumference for predicting non-alcoholic fatty liver disease. World J Gastroenterol. 2016;22(10):3023.
89. Wakabayashi I, Daimon T. A strong association between lipid accumulation product and diabetes mellitus in Japanese women and men. J Atheroscler Thromb. 2014;21(3):282-288.
90. Ahn N, Baumeister SE, Amann U, et al. Visceral adiposity index (VAI), lipid accumulation product (LAP), and product of triglycerides and glucose (TyG) to discriminate prediabetes and diabetes. Sci Rep. 2019;9(1):1-11.
91. Nusrianto R, Ayundini G, Kristanti M, et al. Visceral adiposity index and lipid accumulation product as a predictor of type 2 diabetes mellitus: the Bogor cohort study of non-communicable diseases risk factors. Diabetes Res Clin Pract. 2019;155:107798.
92. Roriz AKC, Passos LCS, de Oliveira CC, Eickemberg M, de Almeida Moreira P, Sampaio LR. Evaluation of the accuracy of anthropometric clinical indicators of visceral fat in adults and elderly. PLoS One. 2014;9(7):e103499.
93. Domecq JP, Prutsky G, Mullan RJ, et al. Lifestyle modification programs in polycystic ovary syndrome: systematic review and meta-analysis. J Clin Endocrinol Metab. 2013;98(12):4655-4663.
94. Kiddy D, Sharp P, White D, et al. Differences in clinical and endocrine features between obese and non-obese subjects with polycystic ovary syndrome: an analysis of 263 consecutive cases. Clin Endocrinol. 1990;32(2):213-220.
95. Yildirim B, Sabir N, Kaleli B. Relation of intra-abdominal fat distribution to metabolic disorders in nonobese patients with polycystic ovary syndrome. Fertil Steril. 2003;79(6):1358-1364.
96. Kiddy DS, Hamilton-Fairley D, Bush A, et al. Improvement in endocrine and ovarian function during dietary treatment of obese women with polycystic ovary syndrome. Clin Endocrinol. 1992;36(1):105-111.
97. Moran LJ, Hutchison SK, Norman RJ, Teede HJ. Lifestyle changes in women with polycystic ovary syndrome. Cochrane Database Syst Rev. 2011;(2):CD007506.
98. Moran LJ, Pasquali R, Teede HJ, Hoeger KM, Norman RJ. Treatment of obesity in polycystic ovary syndrome: a position statement of the Androgen Excess and Polycystic Ovary Syndrome Society. Fertil Steril. 2009;92(6):1966-1982.
99. Ndefo UA, Eaton A, Green MR. Polycystic ovary syndrome: a review of treatment options with a focus on pharmacological approaches. Pharm Ther. 2013;38(6):336-355.
100. Harrison CL, Lombard CB, Moran LJ, Teede HJ. Exercise therapy in polycystic ovary syndrome: a systematic review. Hum Reprod Update. 2011;17(2):171-183.
101. Mavropoulos JC, Yancy WS, Hepburn J, Westman EC. The effects of a low-carbohydrate, ketogenic diet on the polycystic ovary syndrome: a pilot study. Nutr Metab. 2005;2(1):1-5.
102. Moran LJ, Ko H, Misso M, et al. Dietary composition in the treatment of polycystic ovary syndrome: a systematic review to inform evidence-based guidelines. J Acad Nutr Diet. 2013;113(4):520-545.
103. Hamasaki H. Perspectives on interval exercise interventions for non-alcoholic fatty liver disease. Medicines. 2019;6(3):83. doi:10.3390/medicines6030083.
104. Carels RA, Darby LA, Rydin S, Douglass OM, Cacciapaglia HM, O'Brien WH. The relationship between self-monitoring, outcome expectancies, difficulties with eating and exercise, and physical activity and weight loss treatment outcomes. Ann Behav Med. 2005;30(3):182-190. doi:10.1207/s15324796abm3003_2.
105. Guzick D. Polycystic ovary syndrome: symptomatology, pathophysiology, and epidemiology. Am J Obstet

Gynecol. 1998;179(6):S89-S93.

106. Brettenthaler N, De Geyter C, Huber PR, Keller U. Effect of the insulin sensitizer pioglitazone on insulin resistance, hyperandrogenism, and ovulatory dysfunction in women with polycystic ovary syndrome. J Clin Endocrinol Metab. 2004;89(8):3835-3840.
107. Xu Y, Wu Y, Huang Q. Comparison of the effect between pioglitazone and metformin in treating patients with PCOS: a meta-analysis. Arch Gynecol Obstet. 2017;296(4):661-677.
108. Jearath V, Vashisht R, Rustagi V, Raina S, Sharma R. Pioglitazone-induced congestive heart failure and pulmonary edema in a patient with preserved ejection fraction. J Pharmacol Pharmacother. 2016;7(1):41.
109. Jensterle M, Kravos NA, Ferjan S, Goricar K, Dolzan V, Janez A. Long-term efficacy of metformin in overweight-obese PCOS: longitudinal follow-up of retrospective cohort. Endocr Connect. 2020;9(1):44-54.
110. Duleba AJ. Medical management of metabolic dysfunction in PCOS. Steroids. 2012;77(4):306-311.
111. Pasquali R. Metformin in women with PCOS, pros. Endocrine. 2014;48(2):422-426.
112. Harborne LR, Sattar N, Norman JE, Fleming R. Metformin and weight loss in obese women with polycystic ovary syndrome: comparison of doses. J Clin Endocrinol Metab. 2005;90(8):4593-4598.
113. Cefalu WT. The physiologic role of incretin hormones: clinical applications. J Am Osteopath Med. 2010;110(suppl 32):8-14.
114. Barritt AS 4th, Marshman E, Noureddin M: Review article: role of glucagon-like peptide-1 receptor agonists in non-alcoholic steatohepatitis, obesity and diabetes-what hepatologists need to know. Aliment Pharmacol Ther. 2022;55(8):944-959. doi:10.1111/apt.16794.
115. Batterham RL, Cummings DE. Mechanisms of diabetes improvement following bariatric/metabolic surgery. Diabetes Care. 2016;39(6):893-901.
116. Maggard MA, Yermilov I, Li Z, et al. Pregnancy and fertility following bariatric surgery: a systematic review. JAMA. 2008;300(19):2286-2296.
117. Priyadarshini P, Singh VP, Aggarwal S, Garg H, Sinha S, Guleria R. Impact of bariatric surgery on obstructive sleep apnoea–hypopnea syndrome in morbidly obese patients. J Minim Access Surg. 2017;13(4):291.
118. Sacks J, Mulya A, Fealy CE, et al. Effect of Roux-en-Y gastric bypass on liver mitochondrial dynamics in a rat model of obesity. Physiol Rep. 2018;6(4):e13600.
119. D'Amico G, Garcia-Tsaog G, Pagliaro L. Natural history and prognostic indicators in cirrhosis: a systematic review of 118 studies. J Hepatol. 2006;44(1):217-231.
120. Garcia-Tsao G, Abraldes JG, Berzigotti A, Bosch J. Portal hypertensive bleeding in cirrhosis: risk stratification, diagnosis, and management: 2016 practice guidance by the American Association for the study of liver diseases. Hepatology. 2017;65(1):310-335.
121. Stepanova M, Rafiq N, Makhlouf H, et al. Predictors of allcause mortality and liver-related mortality in patients with nonalcoholic fatty liver disease (NAFLD). Dig Dis Sci. 2013;58(10):3017-3023.
122. Younossi ZM, Stepanova M, Ong J, et al. Nonalcoholic steatohepatitis is the most rapidly increasing indication for liver transplantation in the United States. Clin Gastroenterol Hepatol. 2021;19(3):580-589.e5.
123. Lonardo A, Nascimbeni F, Mantovani A, Targher G. Hypertension, diabetes, atherosclerosis and NASH: cause or consequence? J Hepatol. 2018;68(2):335-352.
124. McPherson S, Hardy T, Henderson E, Burt AD, Day CP, Anstee QM. Evidence of NAFLD progression from steatosis to fibrosing-steatohepatitis using paired biopsies: implications for prognosis and clinical management. J Hepatol. 2015;62(5):1148-1155.
125. Bril F, Sninsky JJ, Baca AM, et al. Hepatic steatosis and insulin resistance, but not steatohepatitis, promote atherogenic dyslipidemia in NAFLD. J Clin Endocrinol Metab. 2016;101(2):644-652.
126. Siddiqui MS, Fuchs M, Idowu MO, et al. Severity of nonalcoholic fatty liver disease and progression to cirrhosis are associated with atherogenic lipoprotein profile. Clin Gastroenterol Hepatol. 2015;13(5):1000-1008.e3.
127. Targher G, Byrne CD, Tilg H. NAFLD and increased risk of cardiovascular disease: clinical associations,

pathophysiological mechanisms and pharmacological implications. Gut. 2020;69(9):1691-1705.
128. Younossi ZM, Koenig AB, Abdelatif D, Fazel Y, Henry L, Wymer M. Global epidemiology of nonalcoholic fatty liver disease—meta-analytic assessment of prevalence, incidence, and outcomes. Hepatology. 2016;64(1):73-84.
129. Park H, Dawwas GK, Liu X, Nguyen MH. Nonalcoholic fatty liver disease increases risk of incident advanced chronic kidney disease: a propensity-matched cohort study. J Intern Med. 2019;286(6):711-722.
130. Wilechansky RM, Pedley A, Massaro JM, Hoffmann U, Benjamin EJ, Long MT. Relations of liver fat with prevalent and incident chronic kidney disease in the Framingham heart study: a secondary analysis. Liver Int. 2019;39(8):1535-1544.
131. Colognesi M, Gabbia D, De Martin S. Depression and cognitive impairment—extrahepatic manifestations of NAFLD and NASH. Biomedicines. 2020;8(7):229.
132. Xiao J, Lim LKE, Ng CH, et al. Is fatty liver associated with depression? A meta-analysis and systematic review on the prevalence, risk factors, and outcomes of depression and non-alcoholic fatty liver disease. Front Med. 2021;8:912.
133. Loria P, Lonardo A, Lombardini S, et al. Gallstone disease in non-alcoholic fatty liver: prevalence and associated factors. J Gastroenterol Hepatol. 2005;20(8):1176-1184.
134. Asfari MM, Niyazi F, Lopez R, Dasarathy S, McCullough AJ. The association of nonalcoholic steatohepatitis and obstructive sleep apnea. Eur J Gastroenterol Hepatol. 2017;29(12):1380.
135. Chen HJ, Yang HY, Hsueh KC, et al. Increased risk of osteoporosis in patients with nonalcoholic fatty liver disease: a population-based retrospective cohort study. Medicine. 2018;97(42):e12835.
136. Guo Z, Li M, Han B, Qi X. Association of non-alcoholic fatty liver disease with thyroid function: a systematic review and meta-analysis. Dig Liver Dis. 2018;50(11):1153-1162.
137. Rafiq N, Bai C, Fang Y, et al. Long-term follow-up of patients with nonalcoholic fatty liver. Clin Gastroenterol Hepatol. 2009;7(2):234-238.
138. Li J, Wu Q, Wu XK, et al. Effect of exposure to second-hand smoke from husbands on biochemical hyperandrogenism, metabolic syndrome and conception rates in women with polycystic ovary syndrome undergoing ovulation induction. Hum Reprod. 2018;33(4):617-625.
139. Mykhalchenko K, Lizneva D, Trofimova T, et al. Genetics of polycystic ovary syndrome. Expert Rev Mol Diagn. 2017;17(7):723-733.
140. Risal S, Pei Y, Lu H, et al. Prenatal androgen exposure and transgenerational susceptibility to polycystic ovary syndrome. Nat Med. 2019;25(12):1894-1904.
141. Hogg K, Wood C, McNeilly AS, Duncan WC. The in utero programming effect of increased maternal androgens and a direct fetal intervention on liver and metabolic function in adult sheep. PLoS One. 2011;6(9):e24877.
142. Yan X, Dai X, Wang J, Zhao N, Cui Y, Liu J. Prenatal androgen excess programs metabolic derangements in pubertal female rats. J Endocrinol. 2013;217(1):119-129.
143. Ayonrinde OT, Oddy WH, Adams LA, et al. Infant nutrition and maternal obesity influence the risk of non-alcoholic fatty liver disease in adolescents. J Hepatol. 2017;67(3):568-576.
144. de Wilde MA, Eising JB, Gunning MN, et al. Cardiovascular and metabolic health of 74 children from women previously diagnosed with polycystic ovary syndrome in comparison with a population-based reference cohort. Reprod Sci. 2018;25(10):1492-1500.
145. Gunning MN, Sir Petermann T, Crisosto N, et al. Cardiometabolic health in offspring of women with PCOS compared to healthy controls: a systematic review and individual participant data meta-analysis. Hum Reprod Update. 2020;26(1):104-118.
146. Grieger JA, Bianco-Miotto T, Grzeskowiak LE, et al. Metabolic syndrome in pregnancy and risk for adverse pregnancy outcomes: a prospective cohort of nulliparous women. PLoS Med. 2018;15(12):e1002710.

第十三章 男性类多囊卵巢综合征

一、引言

多囊卵巢综合征（PCOS）是育龄期女性中最常见和研究最多的代谢和内分泌紊乱之一。据估计，生育年龄组中高达13%的女性可能受到该疾病的影响，然而其中很大一部分患者未被诊断出来（70%）。与该疾病相关的不适和并发症通常是患者寻求医疗帮助的原因，包括但不限于月经周期紊乱、不孕症、多毛症、痤疮、代谢并发症［如体重增加、糖尿病（DM）、代谢综合征（MetS）］及进食障碍和心境障碍。

该疾病的研究始于1935年，当时它被称为Stein-Leventhal综合征，多囊卵巢是该综合征的一个重要组成部分。多年来，其潜在的病理生理学和代谢紊乱背景已得到很大程度上的阐明，并且在许多特征上已达成共识［即胰岛素不敏感、高雄激素血症（HA）和促性腺激素调节异常］。据推测，大多数病例都具有相似的上游异常（如类固醇生成或胰岛素异常），但在下游表现上可能有所不同；多囊卵巢（PCO）形态是一个明显的例子，因为它仅在80%的PCOS患者中出现，并且也可能在正常人中发现。实际上，由于临床表现的广泛性，并为避免混淆，许多组织试图提出可帮助临床医师做出正确诊断的标准［如美国国立卫生研究院（NIH）、雄激素过多协会和欧洲人类生殖与胚胎学协会/美国生殖医学协会（ESHRE/ASRM）或鹿特丹共识］，最终版本是基于鹿特丹标准提出的2018年国际PCOS指南（表13.1）。NIH在2012年的方法学研讨会上发布了循证建议，概述了在研究中报告PCOS表型的必要性，并详细说明了4种表型（表13.2）。值得注意的是，PCOS的诊断是一种排除性诊断，因为许多特征与其他疾病重叠（如甲状腺疾病、高催乳素血症、非经典型先天性肾上腺皮质增生症）。

多年来，逐渐有证据表明男性中存在类似PCOS的情况，尤其是PCOS女性的男性亲属。事实上，在男性中亦可观察到类似PCOS的上游异常，且女性PCOS表现具有多样性，许多作者认为"PCOS"这个名称具有误导性（如"Stein-Leventhal综合征"是一个相对不容易引起困惑的术语），由此，人们提出男性中存在类PCOS这个假设就并不奇怪了。

本章的目的是回顾目前关于男性类PCOS表现的研究文献，总结PCOS女性患者亲属的观察结果、男性类PCOS的风险、性别差异及有关该主题的共识声明，并提供临床指导，将这些内容转化为有利于筛查和诊断的建议。

表 13.1　多囊卵巢综合征诊断标准的演变历程

诊断项目	1990 年 NIH 标准	2003 年鹿特丹标准（ESHRE/ASRM）	2006 年 AE-PCOS 标准	2018 年国际 PCOS 循证指南
项目	1. 慢性无排卵/月经失调 2. 临床和（或）生化证据表明高雄激素血症	1. 稀发排卵或无排卵 2. 临床和（或）生化证据表明高雄激素血症 3. 多囊卵巢形态	1. 临床和（或）生化证据表明高雄激素血症 2. 卵巢功能障碍和（或）多囊卵巢形态	1. 认可 2003 年鹿特丹标准，并强调在月经初潮后 8 年内无须关注卵巢形态 对于有风险的女性，需要随访监测其是否符合诊断标准 2. 更加注重临床评估，而非实验室/超声检查
诊断所需项目	两项均有	3 项中至少满足 2 项	两项均有	与 2003 年鹿特丹标准相同，但在青少年中不包括多囊卵巢形态

改编自：Aversa A, la Vignera S, Rago R, et al. Fundamental concepts and novel aspects of polycystic ovarian syndrome: expert consensus resolutions. Front Endocrinol (Lausanne). 2020; 11(516); Teede H, Misso M, Costello M, et al. International evidence-based guideline for the assessment and management of polycystic ovary syndrome. Monash University. 2018. Monash.edu/medicine/sphpm/mchri/pcos; and NIH Evidence-Based Workshop Panel. NIH evidence-based workshop on polycystic ovary syndrome. 2012. http: //prevention.nih.gov/workshops/2012/pcos/resources.aspx.

注：AE-PCOS，雄激素过多和多囊卵巢综合征协会；ESHRE/ASRM，欧洲人类生殖与胚胎学协会/美国生殖医学协会；NIH，美国国立卫生研究院；PCOS，多囊卵巢综合征。

表 13.2　按 NIH 循证方法学研讨会分类的多囊卵巢综合征各种表型

表型 A	表型 B	表型 C	表型 D
• 高雄激素血症 • 排卵功能障碍 • 多囊卵巢形态	• 高雄激素血症 • 排卵功能障碍	• 高雄激素血症 • 多囊卵巢形态	• 排卵功能障碍 • 多囊卵巢形态

注：表型包括肥胖和非肥胖的亚型。

二、有关多囊卵巢综合征女性患者的男性亲属的研究发现

有关 PCOS 女性患者的男性亲属（尤其是一级亲属）的研究结果支持男性类 PCOS 的假设。从 1989 年的遗传学研究开始，PCOS 的聚集和遗传被认为主要是常染色体显性遗传，并与男性的早期秃发特征相关，提示可能与某个单基因有关。不过值得注意的是，卵泡刺激素 B（*FSHB*）基因启动子的遗传多态性与男性中 PCOS 类似的激素模式相关，即较高的黄体生成素（LH）和较低的卵泡刺激素（FSH）；*FSHB* 是位于染色体 11p14.1 的易感位点，后来通过全基因组关联分析（genome-wide association study，GWAS）证实了它与女性 PCOS 和 LH 水平的强相关，这种关联强烈支持了 PCOS 样异常在女性患者亲属中的遗传性假设。

关于 PCOS 患者男性亲属激素差异的问题越来越受到关注，学者们对此开展了一系列研究，虽然数量较少，但仍发现在男性一级亲属中存在 PCOS 患者与男性发生相似异常之间的强相关。与对照组相比，PCOS 患者的兄弟似乎表现出以下特点：较高的硫酸脱氢表雄酮（DHEAS）水平（而她们未患 PCOS 的姐妹似乎也有较高的 DHEAS 和睾酮）；较高的抗米勒管激素（AMH）、LH 和 FSH 基础水平（父亲似乎也有相同的异

常）；促性腺激素释放激素（GnRH）刺激测试的 LH 和 FSH 反应过度增强（即进一步加剧了上游缺陷，如促性腺激素释放缺陷的假设）。PCOS 女性患者的儿子在青春期前的 AMH 水平似乎更高。许多研究由于样本量限制而不能进一步推广结果（特别是涉及 PCOS 患者亲属的早期秃发的发现）。

关于 PCOS 患者亲属的心血管疾病和其他风险的证据越来越多。Taylor 等将女性心血管疾病（CVD）风险不增加的原因归结为两个可能性：她们风险因素的异常不足以升高 10 年 CVD 风险［即她们的研究是根据 Framingham 冠心病（coronary heart disease，CHD）评分计算的，参考美国国家健康和营养调查（National Health and Nutrition Examination Survey，NHANES）人群］和（或）女性患者具有 PCOS 赋予的某些保护性因素（即卵巢储备较高）。

有人认为，PCOS 患者的男性亲属患代谢紊乱（如肥胖、DM、高血压和血脂异常）的风险增加，然而 MetS 风险的增加被归因于该人群中升高的肥胖率，这与 Coviello 等在他们的 NHANES 对照横断面研究中发现的结果（雄激素对女性 MetS 风险的独立影响）相反。Yilmaz 等进行的一项荟萃分析得出结论，一级亲属患有 MetS、高血压和血脂异常的风险增加，不过他们指出了采用的方法和包含研究的几个局限性（即都是横断面研究，只限于 PubMed 来源的英文文献，抽样来自内分泌科/妇科门诊，并且可能使用了不同的诊断标准）。

PCOS 患者的兄弟表现出内皮功能受损［通过血流介导的血管舒张（flow-mediated dilatation，FMD）测量］，尤其是他们有 DM 家族史的情况下；他们的血压和血脂水平也比对照组高。Kaushal 等未能在没有 DM 家族史的 PCOS 女性中找到相同的 FMD 降低（即与男性群体中的结果相反）。

只有少数几项研究探讨了胰岛素抵抗（IR）与拥有 PCOS 一级亲属之间的关系。在他们的研究中，Kaushal 等还证明了男性和女性亲属的胰岛素敏感性下降（通过胰岛素耐受试验进行检测），而 DM 家族史仅在女性中显著降低了胰岛素敏感性。这个结果与 Norman 等先前的研究结果一致，后者显示在将近 70% 的样本中存在高胰岛素血症（早发性秃发似乎是男性中重要且普遍的发现，尽管为小样本研究）。Yilmaz 等使用年龄和体重指数（BMI）匹配的对照组数据，证明了 PCOS 患者的一级亲属具有显著更高的 IR 指数［即稳态模型评估 – 胰岛素抵抗指数（HOMA-IR），口服葡萄糖耐量试验期间胰岛素曲线下面积（AUCI、AUCG）等］，同时具有显著更低的胰岛素敏感性指数［即胰岛素敏感性指数（insulin sensitivity index，ISI），定量胰岛素敏感性定量检查指数（QUICKI）］和更低的血清脂连蛋白水平。

因此，鉴于代谢和心血管并发症的风险增加，PCOS 一级亲属家族史提示临床医师应对全部现有代谢紊乱的患者进行筛查/评估。然而，目前尚不清楚生育力下降是否与 PCOS 一级亲属有关。

三、早发性雄激素性脱发：可能是男性类多囊卵巢综合征的标志吗

（一）背景和研究对象的特点

早发性雄激素性脱发（androgenic alopecia，AGA）[也称为早发性男性型秃发（premature male-pattern baldness，PMB）]可以定义为在35岁之前（一些作者主张以30岁为截断值；值得注意的是，这两个分界线是随意选择的）在雄激素依赖的区域［即头顶和（或）发线中间］出现脱发，根据Hamilton-Norwood评分标准至少达到Ⅲ级或更高的程度（图13.1），这可能是因为较长的休止期、较短的生长期，以及每个毛发生长周期中的毛发生长长度变短（最终导致秃发）。

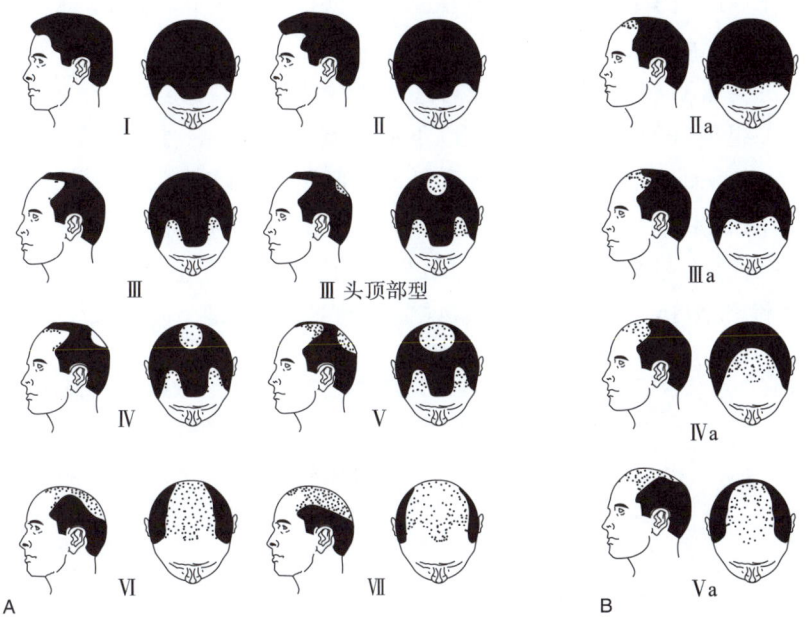

左侧（A）为早发性男性型秃发Ⅰ～Ⅶ级最常见的表现，右侧（B）为Ⅱa～Ⅴa级的变异形式。Ⅲ级被一些学者视为早发性雄激素性脱发（AGA）的最低级别，其特征是双侧额颞部后退超过两侧外耳道冠状连接线前2cm处（还有头顶部型和a型变异型）。有关其他类型的详细描述，尤其是与早发性AGA定义相关的类型（即Ⅳ～Ⅶ级），请查看主要参考文献。

图13.1　Hamilton-Norwood评分标准（常见类型和变异类型）

来源：Norwood OT. Male pattern baldness: Classification and incidence. South Med J. 1975; 68(11): 1359–1365; Figures 1 & 2.

如先前提到的，PCOS和早发性AGA共享同一可遗传单基因突变的研究结果表明，后者的征象也许可以作为男性类PCOS的标志物，特别是因为一些作者观察到PCOS患者一级亲属中的早发性AGA的患病率显著升高。然而，值得注意的是，随后的研究未能发现相同显著性的观察结果，并将与样本中早发性AGA之间的关系归因于偶然；他们研究样本中的早发性AGA男性亲属样本很小，但作者仍然认为基于先前美国的脱发调查，这个结论应该是可靠的，但也有学者提出，在英国，早发性秃发不是男性类

PCOS 表型的可靠标志。

Stárka 等首次研究了这种特定的男性类 PCOS 表型，后来他们的发现［即较低的性激素结合球蛋白（SHBG）和类似的性激素水平］得到了证实，并由 Duskovà 等进一步研究。在后一项研究中，他们发现 SHBG 较低、FSH 较低、LH 较高、游离雄激素指数（free androgen index，FAI）较高的亚组与那些没有生化异常的、年龄（即所有人都低于 30 岁）和 BMI 相似的亚组相比，其 IR 显著升高（使用胰岛素耐受性试验）。有趣的是，在 PCOS 激素模式亚组中，SHBG 明显降低，IR 明显升高。此外，胰岛素基因多态性频率在亚组之间无显著差异，与以前尝试研究早发性 AGA 和胰岛素多态性之间关系的结果相符——考虑到 SHBG 与胰岛素水平之间的强关联，以及胰岛素被认为在毛囊生长中具有局部作用——因此可能涉及其他基因（如前所述）。

事实上，一项包括共计 1009 名无亲缘关系男性的多项研究的荟萃分析证实，具有早发性 AGA 的男性具有明显较差的激素和糖脂代谢特征，类似于患有 PCOS 的女性，而早发性 AGA 组与其他男性群体存在以下显著差异：SHBG 水平较低；LH 和 DHEAS 水平高；胰岛素、总胆固醇、甘油三酯和低密度脂蛋白（LDL）水平高；HOMA 指数较高（即使在使用 BMI 匹配对照组的研究中也是如此）。这些结果与作者（即 Cannarella 等）后来的研究结果及其他系统性综述的结果一致。表 13.3 很好地总结了关于有 PCOS 女性亲属的男性和 AGA（早发性和老年型）男性的研究发现［临床和（或）生化］。

表 13.3 多囊卵巢综合征患者的男性亲属、无亲属关系的早发性 AGA 男性及老年 AGA 男性之间各项研究结果［临床和（或）生化］的差异

参数	多囊卵巢综合征患者的男性亲属	早发性 AGA 男性	老年 AGA 男性
血清游离睾酮水平	—	↑	—
血清 SHBG 水平	—	↓	—
游离睾酮指数	—	↑	—
血清 LH 水平	—	↑	—
血清 FSH 水平	—	↓	—
LH：FSH	—	↑	—
LH 和 FSH 对 GnRH 类似物的反应	↑		
血清 AMH 水平	↑		
血清 DHEAS 水平	↑	↑	
血清 17α-羟孕酮（17α-OHP）水平		↑	
血清脂连蛋白水平	↑	—	
血清葡萄糖水平			
血清胰岛素水平	↑	↑	↑
胰岛素抵抗风险	↑	↑	
血清胆固醇水平		↑	
代谢综合征风险	—	↑	↑

续表

参数	多囊卵巢综合征患者的男性亲属	早发性 AGA 男性	老年 AGA 男性
2 型糖尿病风险	—	—	↑
内皮功能障碍风险	↑	—	—
血压	↑	↑	↑
血清醛固酮水平	—	—	↑
血清纤维蛋白原水平	—	—	↑
动脉粥样硬化斑块风险	—	—	↑
缺血性心脏病风险	—	—	↑
前列腺增生风险	—	—	↑
前列腺癌风险	—	—	↑

改编自：Cannarella R, Condorelli RA, Barbagallo F, la Vignera S, Calogero AE. Endocrinology of the aging prostate: current concepts. Front Endocrinol. 2021; 12: 554078; Table 1.

注：此表基于先前发表的工作。↑表示增加；↓表示减少；—表示未报告。AGA，雄激素性脱发；AMH，抗米勒管激素；DHEAS，硫酸脱氢表雄酮；FSH，卵泡刺激素；GnRH，促性腺激素释放激素；LH，黄体生成素；SHBG，性激素结合球蛋白。

1. 性激素结合球蛋白——重要标志物

如前所述，低水平的 SHBG 似乎是早发性 AGA 患者中常见的情况。此外，它似乎与更高的胰岛素水平和葡萄糖耐受不良有关。虽然目前 IR 在 AGA 发病机制中的作用还没有被广泛接受，但 IR 仍然可以通过增加游离雄激素并进一步降低 SHBG 来加重病情。因此，SHBG 水平的正常化仍然是一个重要的治疗目标（即希望通过减重或营养／生活方式干预使其正常化）。尽管样本较小，Arias-Santiago 等仍指出，低水平的 SHBG 也许可以作为早发性 AGA 患者 IR 的标志物（即与较高的葡萄糖水平密切相关，无论性别、BMI 或 FAI 如何）；而 Narad 等报告，早发性 AGA 组与年龄匹配的对照组相比，SHBG 水平显著降低，但代谢特征相似。前一项病例对照研究的对象年龄较大（45～60 岁），而后者的对象年龄较小（30 岁以下），由此可以引发一个假设，即 SHBG 水平低下的 AGA 患者可能有晚年发展至 IR 的风险，故值得考虑进行 SHBG 检查以预测风险。这一假设与其他作者的结论相吻合，他们提出早发性 AGA 可以作为 IR 的标志物，无论 BMI 如何。

2. 循环雄激素水平和性别差异

在对男性进行的研究中，HA 的性质可能是类 PCOS 表现的性别差异之一。与女性不同的是，高睾酮血症似乎不是男性类 PCOS 综合征的一部分症状（即使增加，通常仍在正常范围内），并且关于 FAI 的报道也存在争议。实际上，临床 HA 的水平通常与游离睾酮的水平不成比例。因此，我们必须怀疑其他雄激素（尤其是肾上腺激素，如 DHEAS 或甚至较少研究的 11-氧合 C19 类固醇）的作用，以及它们在外周转化为更强雄激素的作用。有关性别之间睾酮水平差异的一种有趣的解释是，胰岛素对卵泡膜细胞和睾丸间质细胞可能存在不同的作用，它在前者中刺激类固醇产生，从而增加女性的睾酮产生，但在后者中抑制类固醇产生，这使得男性的睾酮水平低于正常水平。此外，与 HA 无关，IR 似乎对痤疮存在独立的影响。更有趣的是，雄激素、脂肪组织和非脂肪组织之间的相互作用在性别间似乎稍有不同。较高的循环雄激素水平似乎会导致脂肪细胞肥大，促进男性向心性肥胖形成（即腹型肥胖），但这一效应通常被非脂肪组织的协同性增生所平衡，因其有利于代谢状态的改善（尽管随着衰老过程，保护作用可能会丧失，导致肌肉萎缩/肌肉萎缩性肥胖）。环境中内分泌干扰物的暴露和其在肥胖和 PCOS 中可能的作用似乎是一个有趣的研究目标。

正如前面提到的，BMI 似乎对 PCOS 并不具有特异性诊断意义，尽管其存在可能加剧已有的代谢和激素紊乱。因此，即使是非肥胖表型的男性仍然有可能出现此综合征，并且这与苗条女性中亦可发现 PCOS 的结果一致。一个非肥胖的男性如患有早发性 AGA 和类似 PCOS 的激素改变，则其将来患腹型肥胖的风险增加，因此早期采取更健康的生活方式仍然对他们有益。

Cannarella 等设法提供了一份所有可能的病因机制的总结，以及它们之间是如何相互作用并促进男性类 PCOS 发生的，如图 13.2 所示。

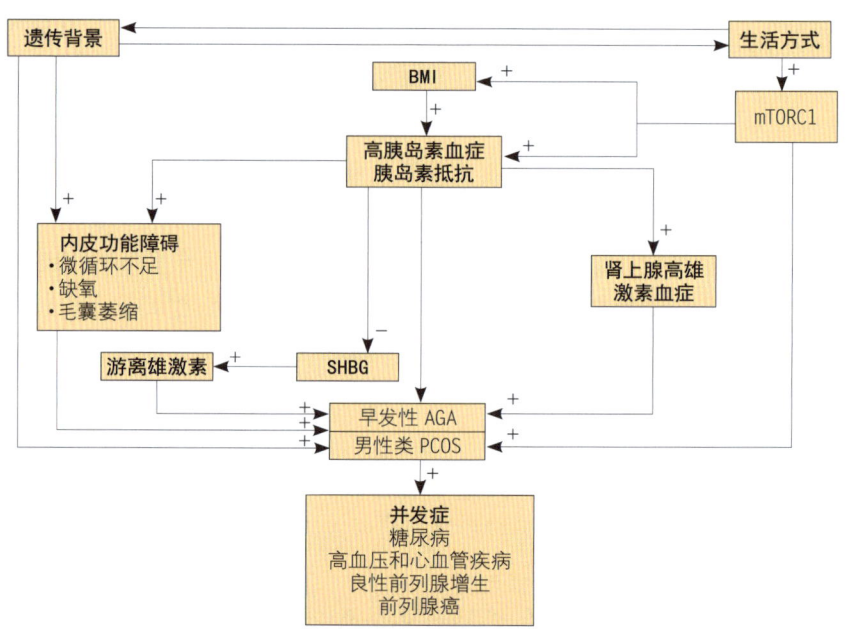

该图描绘了导致男性类 PCOS 的多种可能机制。西罗莫司激酶（mTORC）信号传导机制性靶点过度活跃，可能是由于饮食过量和（或）高血糖，易于发生肥胖、胰岛素抵抗（IR）、2 型糖尿病、高血压和癌症，并可以加速毛发生长 [这与高胰岛素血症和伴随的内皮功能障碍一起，导致雄激素性脱发（AGA）的发生]。此外，较低的性激素结合球蛋白（SHBG）水平会导致糖代谢受损，而高胰岛素血症会导致肾上腺高雄激素血症，这在早发性 AGA 的男性中更为常见（即雄激素受体超活化也与代谢紊乱有关）。BMI，体重指数。

图 13.2　男性类多囊卵巢综合征及其并发症的可能病因机制

来源：Cannarella R, Condorelli RA, Mongioì LM, la Vignera S, Calogero AE. Does a male polycystic ovarian syndrome equivalent exist? *J Endocrinol Invest*. 2018; 41(1): 49-57; Figure 1.

（二）与雄激素性脱发相关的风险

1. 心血管疾病和代谢综合征风险

早发性 AGA 与心血管和代谢风险密切相关。从与 MetS 的关联开始，有关男性 AGA 与 MetS 之间关系的研究结果就存在矛盾。然而，Wu 等进行的一项荟萃分析证实，AGA 在两性和不同人群（即欧洲人和亚洲人）中都与 MetS 有很好的相关性。鉴于低睾酮水平在早发性 AGA 患者中常见，他们的结果进一步证实了观察性研究的荟萃分析结果，表明 MetS 是男性性腺功能减退的独立危险因素，并使 CVD 风险增加。

关于 AGA 患者 CVD 风险的研究加强了之前对 PCOS 患者亲属的描述。特别是头顶部变异型的 AGA，似乎与冠状动脉疾病风险最相关（心肌梗死风险可能增加 3.4 倍），而且在高血压或高胆固醇水平的患者中，关联性更强。在一项以 22 071 名男性医师为对象的研究中，调整混杂因素并未改变头顶部 AGA 与心血管疾病风险的关联。NHANES-Ⅰ 和 Framingham 研究数据曾经提示，秃发迅速进展和严重类型的 AGA 与冠状动脉疾病、心血管死亡率和全因死亡率密切相关。之后，一项基于人群的前瞻性队列研究纳入 2429 名男性，研究指出 AGA 与高 CVD 死亡风险相关，且独立于 MetS。事实上，Trieu 等发表的一项纳入 29 254 名脱发患者的荟萃分析发现，AGA 与冠心病风险呈正相关，并存在剂量 – 反应关系，此外还增加了 MetS、高血压、IR 和血脂异常的风险。

2. 危害男性生育力的风险

有必要进一步研究 AGA 对男性不育的影响（如低 FSH 水平的发现就提供了一个线索），因为关于这方面的研究很少且结果令人困惑。此前，Recabarren 等对 PCOS 女性的儿子进行了研究，发现他们的睾丸体积和 AMH 水平明显较高，但仍在正常范围内，同时精液分析也正常（这可能是由于睾丸支持细胞数量增加而代偿性减少了精子产量）。至于 IR 对男性生育力的影响，Verit 等的研究未发现睾丸体积或精液分析方面的差异。近期，Güngor 等发现 Hamilton-Norwood 评分为 Ⅲ 或 Ⅳ 的患者精液参数（体积、计数、活动力和形态）明显较差。Cannarella 等随后的研究只发现 AGA 患者精子凋亡的频率显著增加，此外在存在 IR、较低的 SHBG 水平或较高的 BMI 等其他危险因素时，睾丸体积较小的风险也显著增加（该研究中左侧睾丸的体积明显较小）。他们的结论是，AGA 男性未来存在性腺功能障碍的风险，在进一步的研究结果出来之前，这在目前阶段似乎是一个合理的担心。

3. 前列腺相关风险

现有证据强烈表明，AGA 与前列腺疾病存在关联。AGA 男性（特别是早发性和严重型）被发现患较大前列腺、良性前列腺增生（benign prostatic hyperplasia，BPH）、前列腺炎，以及前列腺特异性抗原（prostate-specific antigen，PSA）水平升高、出现雄激素受体基因多态性（SNP rs6152）、国际前列腺症状评分（international prostate symptom scores，IPSS）较高和年龄较大时的最大尿流率降低的概率较高。一些作者甚至得出结论，AGA 可以作为 BPH 的早期标志，但其他学者不同意，因为 BPH 的易感性在本质上是多因素的（其他因素与 AGA 和 BPH 具有共同的关联）。有趣的是，一项荟萃分析显示，女性 PCOS 患者的 PSA 水平显著升高，但这一发现的意义尚待进一步研究。在前列腺癌（prostate cancer，PCa）风险方面，Amoretti 等的一项荟萃分析表明，头顶部 AGA 的患者患癌的风险显著增加，不过它所纳入的研究存在方法学缺陷，包括没有关于发病年龄的信息，其中一些研究并没有评估头顶部脱发。

老化的前列腺及其相关异常似乎受多种激素相互作用（以及肥胖、MetS、IR 和甲状腺功能异常等合并症的存在）的影响，Cannarella 等最近撰写的一篇非常全面的综述对此进行了详细报道。图 13.3 很好地总结了各种激素的作用。睾酮介导的效应非常有趣。目前普遍认为，它在转化为更强效的双氢睾酮（DHT）后作用于雄激素受体，可促进前列腺在胎儿期的发育。在生命后期，与普遍看法相反，睾酮对前列腺细胞增殖的影响似乎遵循一个 S 形曲线的饱和模型，在血清值上升到 8 nmol/L 的水平时，可以引起细胞增殖和 PSA 的快速上升。考虑到有 PCa 病史的患者接受睾酮替代治疗的争议性，对 PCa 及其去势抵抗亚型的研究提供了更多细节。有人提出，其他弱雄激素（如 DHEAS 或雄烯二酮）在前列腺组织内代谢为更强效的 DHT，Storbeck 等则指出较少研究的 11- 氧合 C19 类固醇（即 11 酮 DHT 和 11β- 羟基 DHT）可能具有与 DHT 类似的雄激素受体和浓度效应。然而，雌激素的效应根据其类型和激活的受体类型而有所不同：雌酮（E1）和雌三醇（E3）的浓度很低，对前列腺影响很小；17β- 雌二醇（E2）由脂肪细胞芳构化产生，对前列腺细胞具有强的促增殖作用。雌激素受体 α 刺激增殖，而雌激素受体 β 则抑制该过程，前者的激活超过后者可引起增殖。甲状腺激素对前列腺增殖具有刺激作用，但随着年龄的增长而下降，使它们不太可能成为 BPH 和其他疾病发病机制的促进因素。关于胰岛素样生长因子 -1（IGF-1）及其对前列腺细胞增殖的影响也有类似的争论，因为它亦随着年龄的增长而下降；但是，IGF-1 在 DM 和肢端肥大症中升高，且患有非活动性肢端肥大症超过 2 年的患者，其前列腺体积与之前增大的状态相比有所缩小。MetS 及其组成部分（特别是 IR）与 BPH 相关，有证据表明抗糖尿病药物，如二甲双胍，在降低前列腺癌发病率和改善生存率方面起到一定作用。

四、结论和结语

男性类 PCOS 确实存在，有关它的研究已经进行了十余年，大多数特征现在已经被广泛认可。PCOS 女性患者的男性一级亲属会遗传该病或某些特征，并且具有相似（如果不是更严重的话）的心血管和代谢风险。早发性 AGA 是一个独特的临床特征，它伴随着其他 PCOS 样特征并且与类似的风险相关。然而，男性类 PCOS 表现的范围相当广泛（表 13.4）；并非所有早发性 AGA 的男性都有类似 PCOS 的异常，即使是那些迟发性 AGA 的男性也可以出现类似 PCOS 的一些情况，因此即使在这种人群中开展筛查也是值得的。考虑到在一般人群中早发性 AGA 的患病率为 30%，而 PCOS 的患病率为 4%～7%，假设两性 PCOS 的患病率相同，则预计 15%～25% 的早发性脱发男性可能患有类 PCOS。值得注意的是，该病的名称（即 PCOS）会使公众和医疗界对其真正构成的理解产生偏差（即使在谈论女性综合征时也是如此），因此更名为更能描述对两性综合征现有理解的名称（如 Stein-Leventhal）将是最好的选择。

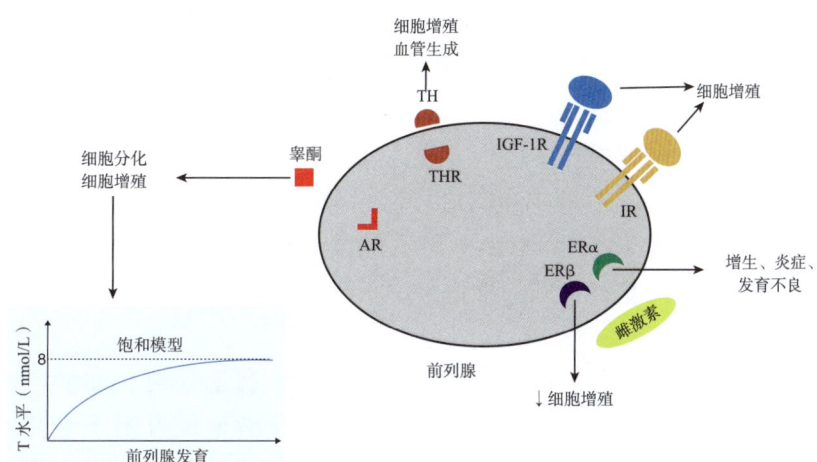

尽管睾酮在胎儿期前列腺的发育过程中至关重要，但在出生后的生命阶段，它似乎遵循一种饱和模型。在这一模型中，血清睾酮水平在达到一定程度（即，当睾酮水平约为 8 nmol/L 时，受体达到饱和状态）之前，与细胞增殖密切相关。甲状腺激素通过其在前列腺细胞上的受体，对细胞增殖和血管生成起到促进作用。IR 与 IGF-1 之间的相互作用会诱导细胞增殖。内源性雌激素因类型和所作用的受体不同，作用有所差异：17β-雌二醇（E2，芳香化作用的产物）通过作用于 ERα 来刺激细胞增殖，而作用于 ERβ 时则会抑制细胞增殖。

AR：雄激素受体；ERα：雌激素受体 α；ERβ：雌激素受体 β；IGF-1：胰岛素样生长因子 -1；IGF-1R：胰岛素样生长因子 -1 受体；IR：胰岛素抵抗；T：睾酮；TH：甲状腺激素；THR：甲状腺激素受体。

图 13.3　激素在前列腺组织中的作用概述

改编自：Cannarella R, Condorelli RA, Barbagallo F, la Vignera S, and Calogero AE. Endocrinology of the aging prostate: current concepts. Front Endocrinol. 2021; 12: 554078.

表 13.4　各年龄段男性类多囊卵巢综合征的特征

年龄	男性类多囊卵巢综合征的特征
<35 岁	1. 高雄激素血症的临床征象［早发性 AGA 和（或）痤疮和（或）毛发过多症］ 2. 类似 PCOS 的激素模式（DHEAS、AMH、17α-OHP、FAI 增加，FSH 减少） 3. 代谢异常（胰岛素抵抗、SHBG 水平降低、高血糖、高胰岛素血症）和（或）BMI 值偏高的趋势 4. 家族中有 PCOS 病史
≥35 岁	糖尿病、心血管疾病、良性前列腺增生、前列腺炎、前列腺癌

来源：Cannarella R, Condorelli RA, Mongioì LM, la Vignera S, Calogero AE. Does a male polycystic ovarian syndrome equivalent exist? J Endocrinol Invest. 2018; 41(1): 49-57; Table 3.

注：上述条件有助于专家在生命早期怀疑该综合征。与女性的 PCOS 类似，男性的特征似乎也随着年龄而变化。该综合征也会使男性易患长期并发症，因此早期诊断非常重要。

17α-OHP，血清 17α-羟孕酮；AGA，雄激素性脱发；AMH，抗米勒管激素；BMI，体重指数；DHEAS，硫酸脱氢表雄酮；FAI，游离雄激素指数；FSH，卵泡刺激素；PCOS，多囊卵巢综合征；SHBG，性激素结合球蛋白。

人们对该综合征的临床表现存在一种性别特异的认知，这在一定程度上可以解释对男性类 PCOS 识别的延迟。男性不太可能寻求医疗照护和内分泌咨询，例如，早发性 AGA 可能被视为男性的正常现象；然而，女性通常会因月经异常和 HA 症状而寻求咨询。由于患有该综合征的男性也面临着风险，可以尝试对这一人群采取以下处理策略：

- 首先对 PCOS 女性患者的一级亲属进行代谢、心血管和激素方面异常的筛查。
- 对出现早发性 AGA（即 Hamilton-Norwood 分级为Ⅲ级或更严重）（从十几岁到二十岁）的男性进行体重和糖脂代谢指标监测；对于严重 AGA 和头顶部变异型 AGA，无论年龄多大，都可以建议进行监测。
- 在表 13.4 中列出的对应年龄段中寻找该综合征及其相关并发症和风险。

根据最近的专家共识，在具有 PCOS 样激素异常、代谢异常和（或）较高的 BMI，临床表现出 HA（特别是早发性 AGA）且有家族史的年轻患者中，可以诊断该综合征。需对男性类 PCOS 的精确诊断标准进行深入研究，以得出像女性标准那样的综合性标准。

最后，应在男性中早期且适当地识别该综合征，启动针对代谢异常的治疗，以防止并发症。与女性 PCOS 患者类似的生活方式干预措施也可用于男性（对于 BMI 较高者，至少应将体重降低 5% 作为目标之一）；这些措施包括低卡高蛋白饮食、代餐、间歇性禁食和运动计划。保健营养品，如肌醇、特别是植酸（Myo-inositol，MI）、D- 手性肌醇（D-chiro-inositol，DCI）及 α- 硫辛酸具有胰岛素增敏的作用，并且结合维生素 D 补充（对于缺乏者）可作为治疗选择。未来的研究需要比较不同的生活方式干预措施及潜在的药物治疗（即二甲双胍和非那雄胺），并了解哪种方式对该男性综合征不同方面的治疗更有效。

参考文献

1. Aversa A, la Vignera S, Rago R, et al. Fundamental concepts and novel aspects of polycystic ovarian syndrome: expert consensus resolutions. Front Endocrinol (Lausanne). 2020;11:516. doi:10.3389/fendo.2020.00516.
2. Teede H, Misso M, Costello M, et al. International Evidence-Based Guideline for the Assessment and Management of Polycystic Ovary Syndrome. Melbourne Australia; Monash University. 2018. Available at: monash.edu/medicine/sphpm/mchri/pcos.
3. Kurzrock R, Cohen PR. Polycystic ovary syndrome in men: Stein–Leventhal syndrome revisited. Med Hypotheses. 2007;68(3):480-483.
4. NIH Evidence Based Workshop Panel. NIH Evidence Based Workshop on Polycystic Ovary Syndrome. 2012. Available at: https://prevention.nih.gov/sites/default/files/2018-06/FinalReport.pdf
5. Carey AH, Chan KL, Short F, White D, Williamson R, Franks S. Evidence for a single gene effect causing polycystic ovaries and male pattern baldness. Clin Endocrinol. 1993;38(1993):653-658.
6. Carey AH, Waterworth D, Patel K, et al. Polycystic ovaries and premature male pattern baldness are associated with one allele of the steroid metabolism gene CYP17. Hum Mol Genet. 1994;3(10):1873-1876.
7. Lunde O, Magnus P, Sandvik L, Heglo S. Familial clustering in the polycystic ovarian syndrome. Gynecol Obstet Invest. 1989;28(1):23-30. doi:10.1159/000293493.

8. Govind A, Obhrai S, Clayton RN. Polycystic ovaries are inherited as an autosomal dominant trait: analysis of 29 polycystic ovary syndrome and 10 control families. J Clin Endocrinol Metab. 1999;84(1):38-43. doi:10.1210/jcem.84.1.5382.
9. Tüttelmann F, Laan M, Grigorova M, Punab M, Sõber S, Gromoll J. Combined effects of the variants FSHB-211G T and FSHR 2039A G on male reproductive parameters. J Clin Endocrinol Metab. 2012;97(10):3639-3647. doi:10.1210/jc.2012-1761.
10. Hayes MG, Urbanek M, Ehrmann DA, et al. Genome-wide association of polycystic ovary syndrome implicates alterations in gonadotropin secretion in European ancestry populations. Nat Commun. 2015;6(1):7502. doi:10.1038/ncomms8502.
11. Legro RS, Kunselman AR, Demers L, Wang SC, Bentley-Lewis R, Dunaif A. Elevated dehydroepiandrosterone sulfate levels as the reproductive phenotype in the brothers of women with polycystic ovary syndrome. J Clin Endocrinol Metab. 2002;87(5):2134-2138. doi:10.1210/jcem.87.5.8387.
12. Lenarcik A, Bidzińska-Speichert B, Tworowska-Bardzińska U, Krępuła K. Hormonal abnormalities in first-degree relatives of women with polycystic ovary syndrome (PCOS). Endokrynol Pol. 2011;62(2):129-133.
13. Torchen LC, Kumar A, Kalra B, et al. Increased antimüllerian hormone levels and other reproductive endocrine changes in adult male relatives of women with polycystic ovary syndrome. Fertil Steril. 2016;106(1):50-55. doi:10.1016/j.fertnstert.2016.03.029.
14. Liu DM, Torchen LC, Sung Y, et al. Evidence for gonadotrophin secretory and steroidogenic abnormalities in brothers of women with polycystic ovary syndrome. Hum Reprod. 2014;29(12):2764-2772.
15. Recabarren SE, Sir-Petermann T, Rios R, et al. Pituitary and testicular function in sons of women with polycystic ovary syndrome from infancy to adulthood. J Clin Endocrinol Metab. 2008;93(9):3318-3324. doi:10.1210/jc.2008-0255.
16. Hunter A, Vimplis S, Sharma A, Eid N, Atiomo W. To determine whether first-degree male relatives of women with polycystic ovary syndrome are at higher risk of developing cardiovascular disease and type II diabetes mellitus. J Obstet Gynaecol. 2007;27(6):591-596. doi:10.1080/01443610701497520.
17. Taylor MC, Kar AR, Kunselman AR, Stetter CM, Dunaif A, legro RS. Evidence for increased cardiovascular events in the fathers but not mothers of women with polycystic ovary syndrome. Hum Reprod. 2011;26(8):2226-2231. doi:10.1093/humrep/der101.
18. Benítez R, Sir-Petermann T, Palomino A, et al. Prevalence of metabolic disorders among family members of patients with polycystic ovary syndrome. Rev Med Chil. 2001;129(7):707-712. doi:10.4067/S0034-98872001000700001.
19. Coviello AD, Sam S, legro RS, Dunaif A. High prevalence of metabolic syndrome in first-degree male relatives of women with polycystic ovary syndrome is related to high rates of obesity. J Clin Endocrinol Metab. 2009;94(11):4361-4366. doi:10.1210/jc.2009-1333.
20. Yilmaz B, Vellanki P, Ata B, Yildiz BO. Metabolic syndrome, hypertension, and hyperlipidemia in mothers, fathers, sisters, and brothers of women with polycystic ovary syndrome: a systematic review and meta-analysis. Fertil Steril. 2018;109(2):356-364.e32. doi:10.1016/j.fertnstert.2017.10.018.
21. Kaushal R, Parchure N, Bano G, Kaski JC, Nussey SS. Insulin resistance and endothelial dysfunction in the brothers of Indian subcontinent Asian women with polycystic ovaries. Clin Endocrinol (Oxf). 2004;60(3):322-328. doi:10.1111/j.1365-2265.2003.01981.x.
22. Norman RJ, Masters S, Hague W. Hyperinsulinemia is common in family members of women with polycystic ovary syndrome. Fertil Steril. 1996;66(6):942-947. doi:10.1016/s0015-0282(16)58687-7.
23. Yilmaz M, Bukan N, Ersoy R, et al. Glucose intolerance, insulin resistance and cardiovascular risk factors in first degree relatives of women with polycystic ovary syndrome. Hum Reprod. 2005;20(9):2414-2420. doi:10.1093/humrep/dei070.
24. Hamilton JB. Patterned loss of hair in man: types and incidence. Ann N Y Acad Sci. 1951;53(3):708-728. doi:10.1111/j.1749-6632.1951.tb31971.x.

25. Norwood OT. Male pattern baldness: classification and incidence. South Med J. 1975;68(11):1359-1365. doi:10.1097/00007611-197511000-00009.
26. Stárka L, Dušková M. Remarks on the hormonal background of the male equivalent of polycystic ovary syndrome. Prague Med Rep. 2021;122(2):73-79. doi:10.14712/23362936.2021.8.
27. Ellis JA, Stebbing M, Harrap SB. Insulin gene polymorphism and premature male pattern baldness in the general population. Clin Sci. 1999;96(6):659-662.
28. Di Guardo F, Ciotta L, Monteleone M, Palumbo M. Male equivalent polycystic ovarian syndrome: hormonal, metabolic and clinical aspects. Int J Fertil Steril. 2020;14(2):79-83. doi:10.22074/ijfs.2020.6092.
29. Stárka L, Hill M, Poláček V. Hormonal profile in men with premature androgenic alopecia. Sb Lek. 2000;101(1):17-22.
30. Dusková M, Cermáková I, Hill M, Vanková M, Sámalíková P, Stárka L. What may be the markers of the male equivalent of polycystic ovary syndrome? Physiol Res. 2004;53(3):287-294.
31. Golden SH, Dobs AS, Vaidya D, et al. Endogenous sex hormones and glucose tolerance status in postmenopausal women. J Clin Endocrinol Metab. 2007;92(4):1289-1295. doi:10.1210/jc.2006-1895.
32. Cannarella R, la Vignera S, Condorelli RA, Calogero AE. Glycolipid and hormonal profiles in young men with early-onset androgenetic alopecia: a meta-analysis. Sci Rep. 2017;7:7801. doi:10.1038/s41598-017-08528-3.
33. Cannarella R, Condorelli RA, Mongioì LM, la Vignera S, Calogero AE. Does a male polycystic ovarian syndrome equivalent exist? J Endocrinol Invest. 2018;41(1):49-57. doi:10.1007/s40618-017-0728-5.
34. Cannarella R, Condorelli RA, Dall'Oglio F, et al. Increased DHEAS and decreased total testosterone serum levels in a subset of men with early-onset androgenetic alopecia: does a male PCOS-equivalent exist? Int J Endocrinol. 2020;2020:1942126. doi:10.1155/2020/1942126.
35. Di Guardo F, Cerana MC, D'urso G, Genovese F, Palumbo M. Male PCOS equivalent and nutritional restriction: are we stepping forward? Med Hypotheses. 2019;126:1-3. doi:10.1016/j.mehy.2019.03.003.
36. Arias-Santiago S, Gutiérrez-Salmerón MT, Buendía-Eisman A, Girón-Prieto MS. Sex hormone-binding globulin and risk of hyperglycemia in patients with androgenetic alopecia. Am Acad Dermatol. 2011;65(1):48-53. doi:10.1016/j.jaad.2010.05.002.
37. Narad S, Pande S, Gupta M, Chari S. Hormonal profile in Indian men with premature androgenetic alopecia. Int J Trichol. 2013;5(2):69-72. doi:10.4103/0974-7753.122961.
38. Matilainen V, Koskela P, Keinänen-Kiukaanniemi S. Early androgenetic alopecia as a marker of insulin resistance. Lancet. 2000;356(9236):1165-1166. doi:10.1016/s0140-6736(00)02763-x.
39. Stárka L, Čermáková I, Dušková M, Hill M, Doležal M, Poláček V. Hormonal profile of men with premature balding. Exp Clin Endocrinol Diabetes. 2004;112(1):24-28. doi:10.1055/s-2004-815723.
40. Ahn SW, Gang G-T, Kim YD, et al. Insulin directly regulates steroidogenesis via induction of the orphan nuclear receptor DAX-1 in testicular Leydig cells. J Biol Chem. 2013;288(22):15937-15946. doi:10.1074/jbc.M113.451773.
41. Cadagan D, Khan R, Amer S. Thecal cell sensitivity to luteinizing hormone and insulin in polycystic ovarian syndrome. Reprod Biol. 2016;16(1):53-60. doi:10.1016/j.repbio.2015.12.006.
42. Del Prete M, Mauriello M, Faggiano A, et al. Insulin resistance and acne: a new risk factor for men? Endocrine. 2012;42(3):555-560. doi:10.1007/s12020-012-9647-6.
43. Nagpal M, De D, Handa S, Pal A, Sachdeva N. Insulin resistance and metabolic syndrome in young men with acne. JAMA Dermatol. 2016;152(4):399-404. doi:10.1001/jamadermatol.2015.4499.
44. Dimitriadis GK, Kyrou I, Randeva HS. Polycystic ovary syndrome as a proinflammatory state: the role of adipokines. Curr Pharm Des. 2016;22(36):5535-5546. doi:10.2174/1381612822666160726103133.
45. Escobar-Morreale HF, Alvarez-Blasco F, Botella-Carretero JI, Luque-Ramírez M. The striking similarities in the metabolic associations of female androgen excess and male androgen deficiency. Hum Reprod. 2014;29(10):2083-2091. doi:10.1093/humrep/deu198.

46. Šimková M, Vítků J, Kolátorová L, et al. Endocrine disruptors, obesity and cytokines – How relevant are they to PCOS? Physiol Res. 2020;69:S279-S293. doi:10.33549/physiolres.934521.
47. Ozbas Gok S, Akin Belli A, Dervis E. Is there really relationship between androgenetic alopecia and metabolic syndrome? Dermatol Res Pract. 2015;2015:980310. doi:10.1155/2015/980310.
48. Su LH, Chen THH. Association of androgenetic alopecia with metabolic syndrome in men: a community-based survey. Br J Dermatol. 2010;163(2):371-377. doi:10.1111/j.1365-2133.2010.09816.x.
49. Yi SM, Son SW, Lee KG, et al. Gender-specific association of androgenetic alopecia with metabolic syndrome in a middle-aged Korean population. Br J Dermatol. 2012;167(2):306-313. doi:10.1111/j.1365-2133.2012.10978.x.
50. Mumcuoglu C, Ekmekci TR, Ucak S. The investigation of insulin resistance and metabolic syndrome in male patients with early-onset androgenetic alopecia. Eur J Dermatol. 2011;21(1):79-82. doi:10.1684/ejd.2010.1193.
51. Pengsalae N, Tanglertsampan C, Phichawong T, Lee S. Association of early-onset androgenetic alopecia and metabolic syndrome in Thai men: a case-control study. J Med Assoc Thai. 2013;96(8):947-951.
52. Banger HS, Malhotra SK, Singh S, Mahajan M. Is early onset androgenic alopecia a marker of metabolic syndrome and carotid artery atherosclerosis in young Indian male patients? Int J Trichology. 2015;7(4):141-147. doi:10.4103/0974-7753.171566.
53. Wu DX, Wu LF, Yang ZX. Association between androgenetic alopecia and metabolic syndrome: a meta-analysis. Zhejiang Da Xue Xue Bao Yi Xue Ban. 2014;43(5):597-601. doi:10.3785/j.issn.1008-9292.2014.09.016.
54. Corona G, Maseroli E, Rastrelli G, et al. Cardiovascular risk associated with testosterone-boosting medications: a systematic review and meta-analysis. Expert Opin Drug Saf. 2014;13(10):1327-1351.
55. Corona G, Rastrelli G, Di Pasquale G, Sforza A, Mannucci E, Maggi M. Endogenous testosterone levels and cardiovascular risk: meta-analysis of observational studies. J Sex Med. 2018;15(9):1260-1271. doi:10.1016/j.jsxm.2018.06.012.
56. Lesko SM, Rosenberg L, Shapiro S. A case-control study of baldness in relation to myocardial infarction in men. JAMA. 1993;269(8):998-1003. doi:10.1001/jama.1993.03500080046030.
57. Lotufo PA, Chae CU, Ajani UA, Hennekens CH, Manson JE. Male pattern baldness and coronary heart disease: the physicians' health study. Arch Intern Med. 2000;160(2):165-171. doi:10.1001/archinte.160.2.165.
58. Herrera CR, D'Agostino R, Gerstman BB, Bosco LA, Belanger AJ. Baldness and coronary heart disease rates in men from the Framingham study. Am J Epidemiol. 1995;142(8):828-833. doi:10.1093/oxfordjournals.aje.a117722.
59. Ford ES, Freedman DS, Byers T. Baldness and ischemic heart disease in a national sample of men. Am J Epidemiol. 1996;143(7):651-657. doi:10.1093/oxfordjournals.aje.a008797.
60. Su LH, Chen LS, Lin SC, Chen HH. Association of androgenetic alopecia with mortality from diabetes mellitus and heart disease. JAMA Dermatol. 2013;149(5):601-606. doi:10.1001/jamadermatol.2013.130.
61. Verit A, Verit FF, Oncel H, Ciftci H. Is there any effect of insulin resistance on male reproductive system? Arch Ital Urol Androl. 2013;86(1):5-8. doi:10.4081/aiua.2014.1.5.
62. Güngör ES, Güngör Ş, Zebitay AG. Assessment of semen quality in patients with androgenetic alopecia in an infertility clinic. Dermatol Sin. 2016;34(1):10-13. doi:10.1016/j.dsi.2015.06.003.
63. Oh BR, Kim SJ, Moon JD, et al. Association of benign prostatic hyperplasia with male pattern baldness. Urology. 1998;51(5):744-748. doi:10.1016/s0090-4295(98)00108-3.
64. Chen W, Yang CC, Chen GY, Wu MC, Sheu HM, Tzai TS. Patients with a large prostate show a higher prevalence of androgenetic alopecia. Arch Dermatol Res. 2004;296(6):245-249. doi:10.1007/s00403-004-0514-z.
65. Kucerova R, Bienova M, Kral M, et al. Androgenetic alopecia and polymorphism of the androgen receptor gene (SNP rs6152) in patients with benign prostate hyperplasia or prostate cancer. J Eur Acad Dermatol Venereol. 2015;29(1):91-96. doi:10.1111/jdv.12468.
66. Arias-Santiago S, Arrabal-Polo M, Buendıa-Eisman A, et al. Androgenetic alopecia as an early marker of benign

prostatic hyperplasia. J Am Acad Dermatol. 2012;66(3):401-408. doi:10.1016/j.jaad.2010.12.023.
67. Kaplan SA. Re: androgenetic alopecia as an early marker of benign prostatic hyperplasia. J Urol. 2012;188(5):1846-1847. doi:10.1016/j.juro.2012.07.079.
68. Maleki-Hajiagha A, Razavi M, Razaeinejad M, et al. Serum prostate-specific antigen level in women with polycystic ovary syndrome: a systematic review and meta-analysis. Horm Metab Res. 2019;51:230-242. doi:10.1055/a-0863-5779.
69. Amoretti A, Laydner H, Bergfeld W. Androgenetic alopecia and risk of prostate cancer: a systematic review and meta-analysis. J Am Acad Dermatol. 2013;68(6):937-943. doi:10.1016/j.jaad.2012.11.034.
70. Cannarella R, Condorelli RA, Barbagallo F, la Vignera S, Calogero AE. Endocrinology of the aging prostate: current concepts. Front Endocrinol (Lausanne). 2021;12:554078. doi:10.3389/fendo.2021.554078.
71. Storbeck KH, Bloem LM, Africander D, Schloms L, Swart P, Swart AC. 11 -hydroxydihydrotestosterone and 11-ketodihydrotestosterone, novel C19 steroids with androgenic activity: a putative role in castration resistant prostate cancer? Mol Cell Endocrinol. 2013;377(1-2):135-146. doi:10.1016/j.mce.2013.07.006.
72. Sanke S, Chander R, Jain A, Garg T, Yadav P. A comparison of the hormonal profile of early androgenetic alopecia in men with the phenotypic equivalent of polycystic ovarian syndrome in women. JAMA Dermatol. 2016;152(9):986-991. doi:10.1001/jamadermatol.2016.1776.
73. Azziz R, Woods KS, Reyna R, Key TJ, Knochenhauer ES, Yildiz BO. The prevalence and features of the polycystic ovary syndrome in an unselected population. J Clin Endocrinol Metab. 2004;89(6):2745-2749. doi:10.1210/jc.2003-032046.
74. Di Tucci C, Galati G, Mattei G, et al. The role of alpha lipoic acid in female and male infertility: a systematic review. Gynecol Endocrinol. 2020;37(6):497-505. doi:10.1080/09513590.2020.1843619.

第三篇

多囊卵巢综合征及其相关并发症的管理

第十四章 多囊卵巢综合征的药物治疗：月经不规律

一、定义

成年女性的月经周期少于每年 8 次，或者周期短于 21 天或长于 35 天时，被认为是月经不规律或月经稀发。需要进一步评估这些女性是否符合鹿特丹标准的其他特征。在多囊卵巢综合征（PCOS）中，月经失调通常表现为月经不规则、月经稀发和（或）闭经。

PCOS 应与高催乳素血症和功能性下丘脑性闭经等其他引起月经稀发的原因区分开来。在这些患者中，体重指数（BMI）正常或偏低，黄体生成素（LH）：卵泡刺激素（FSH）正常，雌激素水平正常或偏低。

PCOS 在一般人群中的患病率为 2%～13%。PCOS 最常见的表现是 60%～85% 的女性出现月经不规律，37% 的女性出现继发性闭经。

二、病理生理学

PCOS 的月经失调影响各个年龄组的女性。有关 PCOS 的病理生理学在第四章中已进行了详细讨论。为了从月经不规律的角度总结并对图 14.1 进行补充，以下几点值得关注。许多影响年轻女性生理发育的因素可能导致内分泌和代谢紊乱，从而引起月经不规律。此外，下丘脑-垂体-卵巢轴的功能失调也可能导致这些异常。因此，这些紊乱取决于血雄激素水平升高、LH∶FSH 增加和胰岛素水平升高，以及卵泡数量增加，这将影响排卵并导致月经失调。据观察，随着年龄的增长，窦状卵泡池减少，因此抗米勒管激素（AMH）水平降低，导致周期缩短。

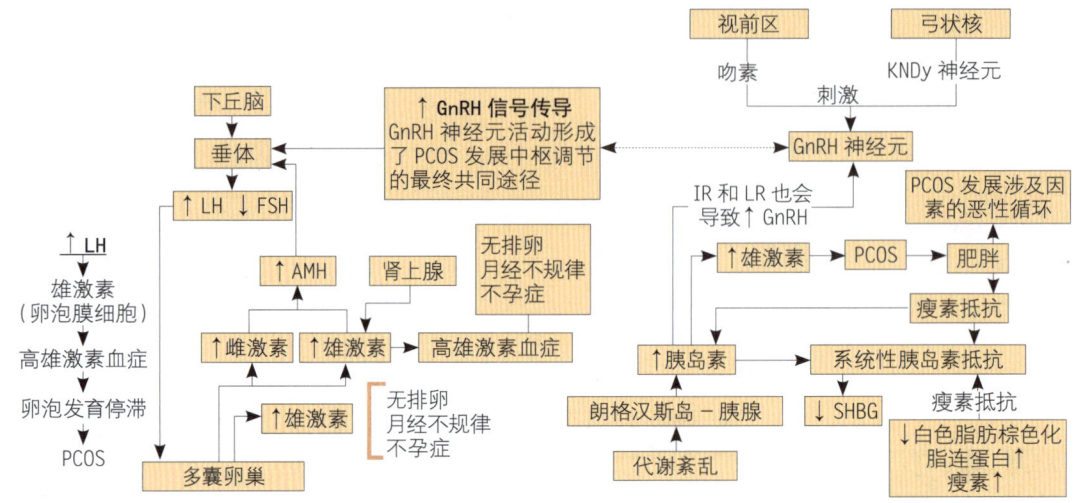

AMH，抗米勒管激素；FSH，卵泡刺激素；GnRH，促性腺激素释放激素；IR，胰岛素抵抗；KNDy，吻素、神经激肽 B 和强啡肽；LH，黄体生成素；LR，瘦素抵抗；PCOS，多囊卵巢综合征；SCFA，短链脂肪酸；SHBG，性激素结合球蛋白。

图 14.1　多囊卵巢综合征患者体内导致月经不规律的各种机制间的相互作用

（一）促性腺激素释放激素的影响

研究表明，增加促性腺激素释放激素（GnRH）脉冲频率可以刺激 PCOS 患者合成 LH，导致 LH∶FSH 升高。高水平的 LH 可引起生殖和代谢紊乱，并在卵泡膜细胞中产生雄激素，最终导致高雄激素血症（HA）和卵泡发育停滞。外周性激素可以通过反馈作用调节 GnRH 神经元的作用，该反馈作用在 PCOS 患者中受损，因此形成了恶性循环。

吻素位于下丘脑，是 GnRH 脉冲形成的重要上游调节因子。吻素和神经激肽 B（neurokinin B，NKB）、强啡肽作为 KNDy 系统共同表达，这些神经元调节 GnRH 脉冲和 LH 分泌，其中吻素可以刺激 GnRH 神经元，NKB 可以作为协同刺激因子，而强啡肽抑制吻素的产生，从而调节下游的 GnRH 分泌。

（二）调节促性腺激素释放激素神经元作用的卵巢激素

PCOS 患者表现出异常的性激素水平，如 HA、雌激素水平异常和 AMH 水平升高，这些变化会引起卵巢功能障碍并导致 PCOS 患者生殖障碍。

1. 雄激素

雄激素在 PCOS 发展的卵巢内和卵巢外机制中都起到一定作用。它可能在下丘脑、卵巢、骨骼肌和脂肪细胞中被过度激活，从而介导 PCOS 的发展。

2. 抗米勒管激素

AMH 影响下丘脑-垂体-卵巢（HPO）轴并影响卵巢。PCOS 患者由于卵巢中小窦状卵泡积累而导致 AMH 水平升高。AMH 可以降低颗粒细胞中 FSH 受体和芳香化酶的表达，从而形成恶性循环，影响卵泡生长并导致卵泡闭锁。

（三）促性腺激素释放激素生成的代谢调节

1. 胰岛素抵抗

胰岛素抵抗（IR）导致胰岛素水平异常升高，可以促进人类卵巢卵泡膜细胞中的睾酮生物合成，并减少性激素结合球蛋白（SHBG）的产生。最终使 PCOS 患者出现 HA。胰岛素对 LH 分泌有直接刺激作用并改变生殖功能。

在下丘脑中，瘦素受体与吻素和 NKB 共定位，显示了其在食物摄入和能量消耗的中枢调控及糖代谢中的作用。提高瘦素水平对 KNDy 神经元和黄体生成素分泌产生的刺激作用，促进了 PCOS 的发病。瘦素对胰岛素抵抗产生的中枢和外周效应导致了肥胖和代谢变化。

2. 肥胖

图 14.1 显示了肥胖和胰岛素抵抗、瘦素抵抗之间相互关系的恶性循环，突显了它们在 PCOS 发病机制中的复杂作用。下丘脑水平的瘦素抵抗导致体重增加。脂肪细胞中瘦素分泌的增加加剧了瘦素抵抗并促进了 PCOS 的发展。肥胖或肥胖相关的交感神经激活在 PCOS 的发展中的具体作用有待确定。

三、多囊卵巢综合征患者月经不规律的含义

慢性排卵障碍导致无拮抗的雌激素作用和孕酮生成障碍。这会导致子宫内膜细胞增殖和子宫内膜增生，可能进展为子宫内膜癌。据估计，患有 PCOS 的患者发生生殖系统癌症的风险增加 2.7～3.0 倍，其中 85% 的子宫内膜癌是由雌激素主导。对于月经后期的患者，子宫内膜厚度超过 10 mm 者需要进行子宫内膜活检。然而，由于排卵障碍和长期使用避孕药，PCOS 患者患卵巢癌的风险降低。肥胖可能导致其患乳腺癌的风险增加。然而，没有证据表明 PCOS 与其他生殖道癌症之间存在任何关联。

四、多囊卵巢综合征患者月经不规律的管理

（一）一线治疗

除药物治疗外，应考虑包括生活方式干预在内的整体处理方法，如节食和运动减重。

雄激素过多和多囊卵巢综合征协会（AE-PCOS）指出，体重减轻 5～10 kg 或超过 5%，可缓解生化紊乱，从而改善月经不规律。摄入低热量饮食，无论是通过减少脂肪

还是碳水化合物都同样有效。每天进行 30 分钟有计划的锻炼对减轻体重和降低体脂率具有协同作用,同时也能改善月经不规律和提高生育力。

Dileep 等在平均 BMI 为 34.7 ± 4.3 kg/m^2 的患者中,给予其 750～1000 mg 的二甲双胍,并进行生活方式干预,共 9 个月。他们发现 BMI 显著降低,并且 PCOS 的临床症状得到改善。

对于减重失败的女性,可以使用奥利司他和西布曲明等减肥药物。通过使用这些药物及生活方式干预,可以额外减轻 30%～50% 的体重。

如果女性无法减轻体重,尤其是 BMI > 40 kg/m^2 并伴有合并症的患者,可以考虑进行减重术。

(二)内分泌治疗

1. 口服避孕药

口服避孕药(oral contraceptive,OC)是月经周期长于 90 天的患者调节月经周期的主要治疗方法。治疗还取决于患者的意愿,以及(除月经不规律以外的)PCOS 相关特征/表型,如 HA 和 IR。然而,对于计划怀孕的夫妇来说,OC 不是首选药物。

共轭马雌激素、炔雌醇和戊雌醇都是强效合成雌激素,其中,戊酸雌二醇更有优势,因为它的代谢副作用较少。复方口服避孕药(combined oral contraceptive,COC)中最常见的雌激素是炔雌醇。它通过向促性腺激素发送负反馈,抑制肝脏释放 SHBG。因此,它可以将 LH 水平和游离雄激素指数降低 40%～60%。

此外,COC 增加了静脉血栓栓塞的风险,并且需考虑到 PCOS 是雌激素主导的环境。但雌激素对避孕和调节月经周期至关重要。

因此,为了平衡利弊,需要选择最接近天然雌二醇且有效剂量最低的雌激素。最佳雌激素剂量应小于 35 μg。更高剂量的药物会增加血栓栓塞的风险,而小于 20 μg 的剂量则对月经周期的控制性较差。

在 35 岁以上的女性、BMI > 29 kg/m^2 的女性和吸烟者中使用 COC 时应小心。有活动性肝病、雌激素依赖性肿瘤、已知伴有先兆偏头痛,以及个人或家族有血栓栓塞病史或易栓症阳性是 COC 的绝对禁忌证。

2. 孕酮

口服避孕药中的孕酮成分可以抑制 LH 峰值(从而抑制排卵)。此外,它可以使宫颈黏液变得黏稠从而抑制精子穿过。孕酮通常根据年代和其逐渐降低的雄激素副作用而分为几代。含有第二代(如左炔诺孕酮)和第三代(如孕二烯酮)孕酮的 COC 的可选择范围很广。具有抗雄激素作用的孕激素包括屈螺酮和地诺孕素衍生物,如 19-去甲睾酮和 17α-螺内酯。此外,环丙孕酮是一种有较强抗雄激素作用的 17-羟孕酮衍生物。在具有月经不规律和 HA 特征的患者中,屈螺酮和环丙孕酮被认为是首选的孕酮。屈螺酮与醋酸环丙孕酮相比,前者的抗雄激素效力仅有后者的 30%。而屈螺酮的使用频率超过了醋酸环丙孕酮是因为它获得了美国食品药品监督管理局（Food and Drug Administration，FDA）的批准。澳大利亚和欧洲人类生殖与胚胎学协会（ESHRE）PCO 工作组有一个具体的建议，即不应将含 35 μg 炔雌醇和醋酸环丙孕酮的达英 -35 作为一线治疗药物，因为存在增加静脉血栓栓塞的风险。

孕酮组分可使子宫内膜产生分泌性改变和撤药性出血。子宫内膜的脱落可以预防子宫内膜增生和子宫内膜癌。

对于有 COC 禁忌证或不能耐受的患者，也可以提供单用孕酮治疗。可以以 21 天为周期给药，或在月经周期的最后 14 天间断给药。在一些病例研究中，每晚口服 300 mg 微粒化孕酮可以缩短周期，并显著改善经前期症状。但目前没有强有力的证据，仍需要进一步研究。此外，应告知患者该药没有避孕效果。对于那些不想怀孕的患者，单一孕酮避孕药（每日 0.35 mg 炔诺酮）、注射型甲羟孕酮、含依托孕烯的埋植剂和含左炔诺孕酮的宫内节育系统（levonorgestrel-containing intrauterine system，LNG IUS）被视为具有避孕和预防子宫内膜增生和癌症的双重作用。尽管如此，孕酮的代谢效应仍应被考虑在内。

（三）二线药物治疗

生活方式干预和 COC 应和其他药物联合使用，并考虑到个体需求和风险因素，如肥胖、高脂血症、高血压和 HA 特征（图 14.2）。

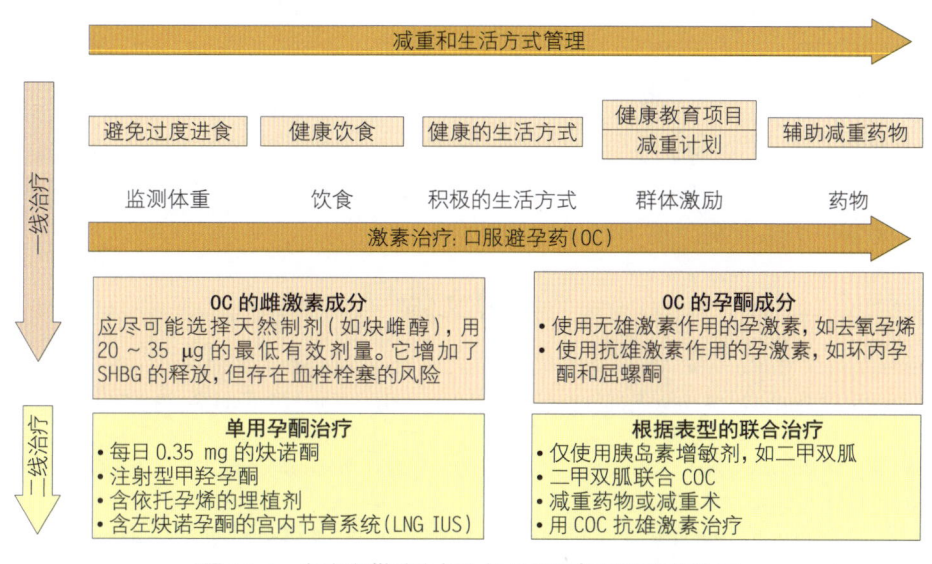

图 14.2　多囊卵巢综合征女性月经不规律的药物治疗

1. 二甲双胍

二甲双胍是一种常用于空腹胰岛素水平升高患者的胰岛素增敏药物。然而，国际 PCOS 学会建议在 BMI > 25 kg/m² 的女性中使用二甲双胍。一项回顾性研究显示，使用二甲双胍后月经周期频率显著增加。二甲双胍连续使用 1 年可导致 11 次月经出血。

2017 年 Cochrane 的综述表明，月经频率有所提高（OR：1.72，95%CI：1.14～2.61）。两项随机对照试验（randomized controlled trials，RCT）比较了 COC 与二甲双胍在肥胖和非肥胖患者中的应用，结果显示总体上两组的胆固醇、睾酮和空腹血糖均有所改善。由于样本量较小，需要进行大型研究以支持这些发现。然而，二甲双胍普遍引起胃肠不适，因此较难耐受。其他胰岛素增敏药物，如罗格列酮和吡格列酮，由于副作用和结果不一而未被常规使用。

2. 肌醇

Unfer V 等进行的 12 项 RCT 系统综述证明，以 40 : 1 比例组合的 Myo-ins 和 D-chiro-ins 可以改善激素失衡和 IR。此组合进一步调整了排卵，某种程度上也调整了月经，但与 COC 相比其效果略差。然而，肌醇的使用仅限于实验目的。

3. 二甲双胍联合生活方式干预和 COC

BMI > 25 kg/m^2、血清胰岛素高或葡萄糖耐受不良的患者对二甲双胍治疗的反应更佳。Wei Feng 进行的一项 RCT 将单用 COC 与 COC 与二甲双胍联合治疗进行了比较。联合治疗在减少体脂、改善血脂和空腹胰岛素方面表现出更优的结果。

4. COC 与抗雄激素治疗

这种治疗方法适用于连续服用含醋酸环丙孕酮的 COC 及美容治疗 6 个月后 HA 没有改善的患者。未避孕的情况下不可单独使用抗雄激素治疗。

五、总结

综上所述，月经不规律的药物治疗取决于个人特征、表型和偏好。此外，虽然大多数治疗未被临床试验认可，但也都是基于证据的。医师应在符合所在执业国家的法律规定的前提下，给患者提供恰当的咨询和治疗。

参考文献

1. Teede H, Misso M, Costello M, et al. International Evidence-Based Guideline for the Assessment and Management of Polycystic Ovary Syndrome 2018. National Health and Medical Research Council (NHMRC), Monash University; 2018:1-198.
2. Walker K, Decherney AH, Saunders R. Menstrual dysfunction in PCOS. Clin Obstet Gynecol. 2021;64(1):119-125.
3. Sherif SA, Newman R, Haboosh S, et al. Investigating the potential of clinical and biochemical markers to differentiate between functional hypothalamic amenorrhoea and polycystic ovarian syndrome: a retrospective observational study. Clin Endocrinol. 2021;95(4):618-627.
4. Phylactou M, Clarke SA, Patel B, et al. Clinical and biochemical discriminants between functional hypothalamic amenorrhoea (FHA) and polycystic ovary syndrome (PCOS). Clin Endocrinol. 2021;95(2):239-252.
5. Jalilian A, Kiani F, Sayehmiri F, Sayehmiri K, Khodaee Z, Akbari M. Prevalence of polycystic ovary syndrome and its associated complications in Iranian women: a meta-analysis. Iran J Reprod Med. 2015;13(10):591.
6. Dewhurst J. Dewhurst's textbook of obstetrics and gynaecology. In: Edmonds K, Lees H, Bourne T, eds. Dewhurst's Textbook of Obstetrics and Gynaecology. 9th ed. Hoboken, NJ: John Wiley & Sons; 2012:645.

7. Taylor HS, Pal L, Sell E. Speroff's Clinical Gynecologic Endocrinology and Infertility. 9th ed. Philadelphia, PA: Wolters Kluwer Health/Lippincott Williams & Wilkins; 2019.
8. Zhang Y, Guo X, Ma S, et al. The treatment with complementary and alternative traditional Chinese medicine for menstrual disorders with polycystic ovary syndrome. Evid-Based Complement Alternat Med. 2021;2021:6678398.
9. Rajiwade SR, Sagili H, Soundravally R, Subitha L. Endocrine abnormalities in adolescents with menstrual disorders. J Obstet Gynecol India. 2018;68(1):58-64.
10. Rostami Dovom M, Ramezani Tehrani F, Djalalinia S, Cheraghi L, Behboudi Gandavani S, Azizi F. Menstrual cycle irregularity and metabolic disorders: a population-based prospective study. PLoS One. 2016;11(12):e0168402.
10a. Zhang Y, Chua Jr S. Leptin function and regulation. Comprehensive physiology. 2011 Jan 17;8(1):351-69.
11. Tokmak A, Kokanali MK, Guzel AI, Kara A, Topcu HO, Cavkaytar S. Polycystic ovary syndrome and risk of endometrial cancer: a mini-review. Asian Pac J Cancer Prev. 2014;15(17):7011-7014.
12. Harris H, Titus L, Cramer D, Terry K. Long and irregular menstrual cycles, polycystic ovary syndrome, and ovarian cancer risk in a population-based case-control study. Int J Cancer. 2017;140(2):285-291.
13. Dumesic DA, Lobo RA. Cancer risk and PCOS. Steroids. 2013;78(8):782-785. doi:10.1016/j.steroids.2013.04.004.
14. Moran LJ, Pasquali R, Teede HJ, Hoeger KM, Norman RJ. Treatment of obesity in polycystic ovary syndrome: a position statement of the Androgen Excess and Polycystic Ovary Syndrome Society. Fertil Steril. 2009;92(6):1966-1982.
15. Dileep A, Samy MAF, Hussain N, Alabdind SZ. Effect of weight loss on symptoms of polycystic ovarian syndrome among women of reproductive age. Dubai Med J. 2021;l4(1):64-69.
16. Yasmin E, Balen AH. Management of polycystic ovary syndrome. Womens Health. 2007;3(3):355-367.
17. Dewhurst J. Dewhurst's textbook of obstetrics and gynaecology. In: Edmonds K, Lees H, Bourne T, eds. Dewhurst's Textbook of Obstetrics and Gynaecology. 9th ed. Hoboken, NJ: John Wiley & Sons; 2012:946.
18. Unfer V, Nestler JE, Kamenov ZA, Prapas N, Facchinetti F. Effects of inositol (s) in women with PCOS: a systematic review of randomized controlled trials. Int J Endocrinol. 2016;2016;1849162.
19. Yildiz BO. Oral contraceptives in polycystic ovary syndrome: risk-benefit assessment. Paper presented at the Semin Reprod Med. 2008;26(1):111-120.
20. Schwingl PJ, Ory HW, Visness CM. Estimates of the risk of cardiovascular death attributable to low-dose oral contraceptives in the United States. Am J Obstet Gynecol. 1999;180(1):241-249.
21. IARC Working Group on the Evaluation of Carcinogenic Risks to Humans, World Health Organization, International Agency for Research on Cancer. Combined Estrogen-Progestogen Contraceptives and Combined Estrogen-Progestogen Menopausal Therapy. Vol 91. World Health Organization; 2007.
22. Elger W, Beier S, Pollow K, Garfield R, Shi SQ, Hillisch A. Conception and pharmacodynamic profile of drospirenone. Steroids. 2003;68(10-13):891-905.
23. Teede HJ, Misso ML, Boyle JA, et al. Translation and implementation of the Australian-led PCOS guideline: clinical summary and translation resources from the International Evidence-based Guideline for the Assessment and Management of Polycystic Ovary Syndrome. Med J Aust. 2018;209:S3-S8.
24. Teede HJ, Misso ML, Costello MF, et al. Recommendations from the international evidence-based guideline for the assessment and management of polycystic ovary syndrome. Hum Reprod. 2018;33(9):1602-1618.
25. Briden L, Shirin S, Prior JC. The central role of ovulatory disturbances in the etiology of androgenic polycystic ovary syndrome (PCOS)—Evidence for treatment with cyclic progesterone. Drug Discov Today Dis Models. 2020;32:71-82.
26. Shirin S, Murray F, Hajjaran M, Goshtasebi A, Kalidasan D, Prior JC. MON-LB9 cyclic progesterone therapy in androgenic polycystic ovary syndrome (PCOS) - person-related 6-month experience changes. J Endoc Soc.

2020;4(suppl 1). doi:10.1210/jendso/bvaa046.2332.
27. American College of Obstetricians and Gynecologists' Committee on Practice Bulletins—Gynecology. ACOG practice bulletin No. 194: polycystic ovary syndrome. Obstet Gynecol. 2018;131(6):e157-e171.
28. Palshetkar N, Gudi SN. Tackling PCOS with Hormonal Contraceptives. FOGSI Focus Benefits Beyond Contraception. 25. https://fogsi.org/wp-content/uploads/fogsi-focus/FOGSI-Focus-Benefit-Beyond-Contraception.pdf#page=35.
29. da Silva AV, de Melo AS, Barboza RP, de Paula Martins W, Ferriani RA, Vieira CS. Levonorgestrel-releasing intrauterine system for women with polycystic ovary syndrome: metabolic and clinical effects. Reprod Sci. 2016;23(7):877-884. doi:10.1177/1933719115623648.
30. Jensterle M, Kravos NA, Ferjan S, Goricar K, Dolzan V, Janez A. Long-term efficacy of metformin in overweight-obese PCOS: longitudinal follow-up of retrospective cohort. Endocr Connect. 2020;9(1):44-54.
31. Morley LC, Tang T, Yasmin E, Norman RJ, Balen AH. Insulin-sensitising drugs (metformin, rosiglitazone, pioglitazone, D-chiro-inositol) for women with polycystic ovary syndrome, oligo amenorrhoea and subfertility. Cochrane Database Syst Rev. 2017;11:CD003053.
32. Morin-Papunen L, Vauhkonen I, Koivunen R, Ruokonen A, Martikainen H, Tapanainen JS. Metformin versus ethinyl estradiol-cyproterone acetate in the treatment of nonobese women with polycystic ovary syndrome: a randomized study. J Clin Endocrinol Metab. 2003;88(1):148-156.
33. Morin-Papunen LC, Vauhkonen I, Koivunen RM, et al. Endocrine and metabolic effects of metformin versus ethinyl estradiol-cyproterone acetate in obese women with polycystic ovary syndrome: a randomized study. J Clin Endocrinol Metab. 2000;85(9):3161-3168.
34. Feng W, Jia YY, Zhang DY, Shi HR. Management of polycystic ovarian syndrome with Diane-35 or Diane-35 plus metformin. Gynecol Endocrinol. 2016;32(2):147-150.

第十五章 多囊卵巢综合征的药物治疗：多毛症和痤疮

一、引言

寻常痤疮和多毛症是多囊卵巢综合征（PCOS）女性常见的问题，给患者带来了很大的困扰。这两种情况都有多种治疗选择。对于多毛症，药物对终毛不完全有效，需要通过物理方法去除不需要的毛发。治疗多毛症需要使用药物以减少雄激素分泌，并去除已经存在的终毛。电解和光热疗法是非常有效的物理脱毛方法。治疗多毛症的有效药物是抗雄激素类药。痤疮可以通过不同的局部和全身用药方法进行治疗。治疗的选择取决于痤疮的严重程度及其对患者生活质量的影响。不同的治疗方法包括局部和全身应用抗生素、维A酸、抗雄激素类药和具有雄激素抑制作用的口服避孕药。

二、多毛症的治疗

毛发生长是一个缓慢的周期性过程。多毛症是一个常见的问题，其影响往往被低估。使用药物治疗多毛症需要数月时间才能看到临床效果，可能需要一年以上才能观察到完全的效果。此外，治疗多毛症是对症的；停止治疗后，毛发生长的变化会逆转，特别是在高雄激素的人群中。尽管如此，治疗应该持续较长时间，并注意患者的安全。毛发向终毛转化是一个不可逆的过程，药物对终毛不完全有效，通常需要去除毛发。有多种治疗方法可选择，根据个体临床特点进行调整，可获得良好的效果。治疗多毛症应采用非药物治疗技术与药物治疗相结合的方法。

（一）美容和直接去除毛发措施

可以通过非永久性方法直接去除毛发。这些措施包括剃须、脱毛剂脱毛、蜜蜡脱毛和线脱毛。在受影响的区域将毛发漂成与皮肤颜色相似的颜色是一种掩饰的方法。这些措施只能起到暂时的作用，可以随时根据需要重复使用。它们可能会刺激皮肤，但相对廉价、有效且安全。

光疗脱毛包括激光和强脉冲光疗法，通过光热裂解作用选择性破坏毛囊色素区来快速去除深色毛发。这种方法需要多次治疗，治疗间隔取决于治疗的身体区域。激光治疗比电解治疗要舒适得多，并且显效更快。

电解是轻度色素化毛发的推荐治疗方法，因为激光的光源仅破坏具有深色球部的生长期毛囊。激光和强脉冲光疗法的主要不良反应包括炎症后色素沉着、毛囊炎、单纯疱疹病毒再活化和反常的毛发过多症。通过使用长波长激光及合适的皮肤冷却装置可以避免这些并发症。

电解是一种可以永久去除毛发的方法，它通过损伤真皮乳头最终导致毛囊完全破坏。电解的过程是使用细针插入单个毛囊，通过电流（电流电解）、高频交流电（热溶解）或两者的组合来破坏毛囊。该技术的主要缺点是容易出现瘢痕、毛囊炎和过度色素沉着。由于该方法会使人产生不适感且费用较高，通常只用于局部身体区域的治疗。

（二）医学疗法

1. 局部治疗

依氟鸟氨酸是美国食品药品监督管理局（FDA）批准的局部用药，用于减少女性面部的多余毛发。它是一种不可逆的鸟氨酸脱羧酶抑制剂，这种酶可以催化毛囊聚胺合成的限速步骤，这一步骤对毛发的生长至关重要。这种治疗需要6～8周才能看到临床效果，并且应经常使用以防止毛发生长。它是光疗脱毛的有效辅助治疗方法，可快速看到疗效。

2. 全身治疗

（1）复方口服避孕药

雌激素和孕激素联合治疗方式，即复方口服避孕药（COC），是治疗痤疮和多毛症的一线内分泌疗法。雌激素-孕激素的组合会抑制下丘脑-垂体-卵巢轴，有助于减少卵巢过量分泌雄激素。它有助于调节月经周期并减少痤疮和多毛症的发生。COC是按照连续21天每天服用一次来进行包装的。COC的选择取决于具体患者的临床特征和费用考量。

（2）雄激素受体拮抗剂

抗雄激素治疗与COC联合使用可减轻多毛症，但有效率因个体而异。抗雄激素类药抑制雄激素诱导的毳毛向终毛的转化，从而减少毛发生长。然而，由于毛囊的生长周期较长，这类药物最明显的效果需要9～12个月才能观察到。在接受抗雄激素治疗时应同时采取避孕措施，而在这种情况下，最佳的避孕选择是COC，因为它是治疗月经不规律的最佳方法，而抗雄激素类药常常引起月经不规律。抗雄激素类药对与PCOS相关的代谢异常影响较小。有以下几种不同的抗雄激素类药可供选择：

1）螺内酯

螺内酯是一种醛固酮拮抗剂，具有抗雄激素作用，可用于治疗多毛症。传统上，它作为利尿剂来治疗高血压。它通过与雄激素受体竞争并在细胞质和细胞核受体上取代双氢睾酮来影响毛囊。它是最安全且最有效的抗雄激素类药，与COC联合使用可以降低多毛症的严重程度。

使用螺内酯时以低剂量起始，逐渐增加至最大治疗剂量。毛发生长周期较长，需要9～12个月的治疗才能达到预期效果。治疗1年后可以逐渐减少剂量。治疗开始后应监测电解质和肝功能。副作用包括暂时性利尿、疲劳、多饮、月经过多、乳房胀痛和胃肠道出血；不过没有发现长期不良事件。

2）醋酸环丙孕酮

醋酸环丙孕酮是最早用于治疗多毛症的雄激素受体拮抗剂。其抗雄激素作用是通过与双氢睾酮竞争与其受体的结合，并减少皮肤中 5α- 还原酶的活性而产生的。

孕激素活性可以抑制促性腺激素，也可以抑制卵巢睾酮分泌。醋酸环丙孕酮是一种具有抗雄激素活性的孕激素，可用于治疗多毛症。长期使用可能会因其孕激素特性导致闭经。因为存在肝毒性风险，欧洲的药品监管机构已经将其限制为二线疗法。

3）氟他胺

氟他胺是一种选择性抗雄激素药，其疗效类似于环丙孕酮。它可能会诱导 PCOS 患者排卵，但由于存在男性胎儿女性化的风险，该药对希望怀孕的患者使用受限。闭经、性欲减退、食欲减退和皮肤干燥是常见的不良反应。肝毒性反应不常见，但曾有患者出现该不良反应的记录。因此，氟他胺通常被用于顽固性多毛症病例的治疗，并且使用该药物的人应定期检查肝功能。

4）非那雄胺

非那雄胺通过竞争性抑制 5α- 还原酶来阻断睾酮向双氢睾酮的转化，从而起到干扰雄激素的作用。它对治疗女性多毛症的效果略逊于螺内酯。暂时性的胃肠不适、头痛和总睾酮意外升高是该药的常见副作用。

三、寻常痤疮的治疗

对痤疮进行早期和有效的治疗非常重要，因为瘢痕和炎症可能导致长期的社会心理和身体并发症。大多数痤疮患者受到面部瘢痕的影响，瘢痕的严重程度与痤疮的类型和持续时间相关。治疗痤疮的目标包括：

- 减少皮脂产生。
- 控制角质过度生成。
- 减少痤疮丙酸杆菌的生成。
- 控制炎性痤疮。

可用局部和全身药物来治疗痤疮，根据皮肤状况的类型和严重程度来进行选择。除了皮脂产生之外，局部治疗通常会对导致痤疮发展的所有关键因素进行干预，而全身疗法则对引起痤疮的所有环节进行干预。

（一）局部治疗

1. 局部维 A 酸类药物

局部维 A 酸类药物包括异维 A 酸（他扎罗汀）、全反式维 A 酸（维 A 酸）和阿达帕林。维 A 酸类药物可减少毛囊皮脂腺单位角质细胞的异常增生。毛囊管内超角化的逆转和毛囊上皮的诱导使毛囊得到疏通。阿达帕林和他扎罗汀比维 A 酸更有效，且很少引起皮肤刺激。局部使用维A酸可能引起皮肤刺激和光敏感。可以从使用最低浓度的乳膏（0.025%乳膏）开始来控制。此外，强烈建议使用防晒霜。

2. 局部抗生素

在治疗炎症性痤疮方面，包括克林霉素和过氧化苯甲酰（benzyl peroxide，BPO）在内的局部抗生素比安慰剂更有效。但是，由于存在细菌耐药的风险，不建议将其作为单一疗法用于治疗痤疮。BPO是一种强效的抗微生物药物，可以破坏腺管内和皮肤表面的痤疮丙酸杆菌和酵母菌。涂抹在皮肤上后，它在皮脂腺中分解，并释放出具有抗炎和杀菌活性的游离氧。BPO可能会引起过敏性接触性皮炎，而其他局部药物则很少引起此类反应。该药可以与局部抗生素交替使用或与局部维A酸联合使用，这些组合疗法比单一疗法更好。

3. 局部氨苯砜

在两个安慰剂对照试验中，使用5%的局部氨苯砜凝胶可改善痤疮的严重程度，但尚未进行它与其他活性药物的比较试验，以确定这种独特制剂的潜在益处。

4. 壬二酸

壬二酸通过使毛囊漏斗内的角质细胞分化正常化来减少粉刺的产生。目前市面上常见的是壬二酸含量为20%的外用乳膏。它不具有抑制皮脂的作用，但可以减少痤疮丙酸杆菌的数量并破坏其功能。推荐其用于轻度到中度的丘疹脓疱性痤疮。

（二）全身治疗

1. 全身性抗生素

口服抗生素通常是处方药，常用于广泛的躯干和面部痤疮，以及对局部治疗无效的中度面部痤疮。口服抗生素比局部治疗更快地产生临床反应，但可能会引起胃肠紊乱。四环素类（土霉素、四环素、多西环素、米诺环素、赖甲环素）是首选的抗生素。由于有潜在严重的不良反应报道，包括药物超敏综合征（drug hypersensitivity syndrome，DHS）、弥漫性皮疹、肺嗜酸性粒细胞浸润症、药物性狼疮和肝炎，因此不推荐将米诺环素作为一线治疗。大环内酯类（红霉素、阿奇霉素或克林霉素）也可用于治疗痤疮，但由于会产生耐药的痤疮丙酸杆菌菌株而失去了使用的优势。阿奇霉素可以在间歇剂量方案中使用（250 mg，每周3次），因为其半衰期较长，在痤疮治疗中是有效的。在痤疮患者中，抗生素耐药性是常见问题，因此应添加局部药物，仅在必要时开具抗生素，并缩短治疗时间。

2. 内分泌治疗

（1）雌激素和孕激素

COC可能会改善痤疮。COC通常含有雌激素（最常见的是炔雌醇）和孕激素。雌激素增加了性激素结合球蛋白（SHBG）的合成，增强了睾酮的结合并降低了游离循环睾酮的水平。

（2）雄激素受体拮抗剂

雄激素受体拮抗剂可抑制皮脂分泌，对痤疮治疗有潜在益处。炔雌醇环丙孕酮复合片（Estelle-35 和达英）是一种口服避孕药，可改善痤疮。它与口服四环素 6 个月的疗效相同。它有深静脉血栓栓塞的风险，并且最近的研究表明，在痤疮得到改善后，环丙孕酮炔雌醇复合片应更换为含有较低剂量雌激素的 COC。

螺内酯在治疗痤疮方面非常有效。常见的副作用包括体液潴留、乳房胀痛、月经不规律，罕见情况下可能出现黄褐斑。怀孕期间应避免使用该药，因为会增加男婴发育异常的风险。

3. 口服异维 A 酸

口服异维 A 酸（13-顺式-维 A 酸）是一种合成的维生素 A 类似物。它是最常见和最有效的痤疮治疗药物，能够使痤疮患者得到长期缓解和改善。它可以减少皮脂分泌，抑制痤疮丙酸杆菌的增殖，阻止粉刺的形成，并具有抗炎特性。异维 A 酸是传统疗法无效的严重痤疮的首选药物。异维 A 酸的常规剂量为每日 1 mg/kg，对大多数痤疮病例有效。然而，由于其副作用，建议将异维 A 酸用于对其他治疗无效的严重病例。需要与患者详细沟通该药的致畸性和避孕建议。常见的不良反应包括黏膜干燥、结膜炎、头痛、疲劳、浅表掌跖剥落、血清甘油三酯升高及肝功能检查暂时异常。常见的皮肤不良反应与剂量相关，可以通过调整剂量和定期使用良好的润肤剂来改善。此外，定期监测肝功能和甘油三酯水平也很重要。

4. 口服锌

两项双盲试验发现，葡萄糖酸锌对炎症性痤疮病变有显著改善作用。与每日 100 mg 米诺环素相比，米诺环素治疗痤疮的改善率可达到 63%，而每日 30 mg 元素锌只有 32% 的改善率。

四、活动性痤疮的治疗设备和物理疗法

轻度烧灼或电灼已被证明对具有多处巨型粉刺的患者有益。为了避免任何不适，电灼或烧灼应尽量采用最低强度。处理每个皮肤病损只需几秒钟，但会留下炎症后色素沉着或轻度瘢痕。对于巨型粉刺，这种治疗方式比局部维 A 酸疗法更有效。

可见光疗法是另一种有效的治疗方式。一项比较红蓝光光疗和 BPO 治疗轻至中度丘疹脓疱型痤疮的研究发现，光疗法优于 BPO。建议低剂量光疗法用于治疗轻度至重度丘疹脓疱型痤疮。

激光和光动力疗法通过靶向痤疮丙酸杆菌产生的卟啉来破坏痤疮丙酸杆菌。它还能抑制不同的促炎细胞因子。一项综合分析对 16 项随机对照试验和 3 项对照试验中光动力治疗和激光光源对痤疮的疗效进行了评价，大多数光源可以在短期内帮助治疗炎症性痤疮病变，而光动力疗法提供了最一致的效果（改善率高达 68%，甲基氨基酮戊酸盐、氨基酮戊酸和红光）。光疗可能导致疼痛、红斑、结痂、水肿、色素改变和脓疱性皮疹。

五、结论

痤疮和多毛症是 PCOS 的常见症状,给患者带来困扰。显然,抗雄激素类药可以减缓多数高雄激素个体的毛发生长。这些药物对终毛无效,因此需要使用美容手段来去除这些毛发。在处理现有多毛症时,口服避孕药的效果不太明显。醋酸环丙孕酮和螺内酯是一线的抗雄激素类药,用于治疗多毛症。多毛症的治疗是长期的,选择治疗方式时应优先考虑患者的安全性。根据痤疮的严重程度,可以使用局部治疗或全身治疗。局部治疗是一线疗法。然而,对于严重痤疮或对局部治疗未产生反应的患者,应该开具全身性抗生素和维 A 酸。全身性维 A 酸被认为是治疗中度至重度痤疮最有效的疗法。抗雄激素类药和口服避孕药可能是这些治疗的有益辅助措施。

参考文献

1. Teede HJ, Misso ML, Costello MF, et al. Recommendations from the international evidence-based guideline for the assessment and management of polycystic ovary syndrome. Hum Reprod. 2018;33(9):1602-1618.
2. Zaenglein A.L., Pathy A.L., Schlosser B.J., Alikhan, A., et al. Guidelines of care for the management of acne vulgaris. J Am Acad Dermatol. 2016;74(5):945-973.
3. Lookingbill, D. P., Chalker, D. K., Lindholm, J. S., Katz, H. I., et al. Treatment of acne with a combination clindamycin/benzoyl peroxide gel compared with clindamycin gel, benzoyl peroxide gel and vehicle gel: combined results of two double-blind investigations. J Am Acad Dermatol. 1997;37(4):590-595
4. Aktar R, Gunes Bilgili S, Yavuz IH, et al. Evaluation of hirsutism and hormonal parameters in acne vulgaris patients treated with isotretinoin. Int J Clin Pract. 2021;75(3):e13791.
5. Yoost J, Savage A. Screening and management of the hyperandrogenic adolescent. Obstet Gynecol. 2019;134(4):E106-E114.
6. DeUgarte CM, Woods KS, Bartolucci AA, Azziz R. Degree of facial and body terminal hair growth in unselected black and white women: toward a populational definition of hirsutism. J Clin Endocrinol Metab. 2006;91(4):1345-1350.
7. Haedersdal M, Wulf H. Evidence-based review of hair removal using lasers and light sources. J Eur Acad Dermatol Venereol. 2006;20(1):9-20.
8. Wolf Jr JE, Shander D, Huber F, et al. Randomized, double-blind clinical evaluation of the efficacy and safety of topical eflornithine HCl 13.9% cream in the treatment of women with facial hair. Int J Dermatol. 2007;46(1):94-98.
9. Adeniji AA, Essah PA, Nestler JE, Cheang KI. Metabolic effects of a commonly used combined hormonal oral contraceptive in women with and without polycystic ovary syndrome. J Womens Health. 2016;25(6):638-645.
10. Stegeman BH, de Bastos M, Rosendaal FR, et al. Different combined oral contraceptives and the risk of venous thrombosis: systematic review and network meta-analysis. BMJ. 2013;347:f5298.
11. Brown J, Farquhar C, Lee O, Toomath R, Jepson RG. Spironolactone versus placebo or in combination with steroids for hirsutism and/or acne. Cochrane Database Syst Rev. 2009;(2):CD00194.
12. van der Spuy ZM, Le Roux PA. Matjila MJ. Cyproterone acetate for hirsutism. Cochrane Database Syst Rev. 2003;2003(4):CD001125.
13. De Zegher F, Ibáñez L. Therapy: low-dose flutamide for hirsutism: into the limelight, at last. Nat Rev Endocrinol. 2010;6(8):421-422.
14. Manso G, Thole Z, Salgueiro E, Revuelta P, Hidalgo A. Spontaneous reporting of hepatotoxicity associated with antiandrogens: data from the Spanish pharmacovigilance system. Pharmacoepidemiol Drug Saf. 2006;15(4):253-259.

15. Barth JH, Cherry CA, Wojnarowska F, Dawber RP. Cyproterone acetate for severe hirsutism: results of a double-blind dose-ranging study. Clin Endocrinol. 1991;35(1):5-10.
16. Hart R, Doherty DA. The potential implications of a PCOS diagnosis on a woman's long-term health using data linkage. J Clin Endocrinol Metab. 2015;100(3):911-919.
17. Katsambas, A.D., Stefanaki, C., Cunliffe, W. J., et al. Guidelines for treating acne. Clinics in dermatology. 2004; 22(5):439-444.
18. Worret WI, Fluhr JW. Acne therapy with topical benzoyl peroxide, antibiotics and azelaic acid. J Dtsch Dermatolo Ges. 2006;4(4):293-300.
19. Draelos ZD, Carter E, Maloney JM, et al. Two randomized studies demonstrate the efficacy and safety of dapsone gel, 5% for the treatment of acne vulgaris. J Am Acad Dermatol. 2007;56(3):439.e1-439.e10.
20. Graupe K, Cunliffe WJ, Gollnick HP, Zaumseil RP. Efficacy and safety of topical azelaic acid (20 percent cream): an overview of results from European clinical trials and experimental reports. Cutis. 1996;57(suppl 1):20-35.
21. Leyden J, Thiboutot DM, Shalita AR, et al. Comparison of tazarotene and minocycline maintenance therapies in acne vulgaris: a multicenter, double-blind, randomized, parallel-group study. Arch Dermatol. 2006;142(5):605-612.
22. Acmaz G, Cınar L, Acmaz B, et al. The effects of oral isotretinoin in women with acne and polycystic ovary syndrome. Biomed Res Int. 2019;2019:2513067.
23. Mathew ML, Karthik R, Mallikarjun M, Bhute S, Varghese A. Intense pulsed light therapy for acne-induced post-inflammatory erythema. Indian Dermatol Online J. 2018;9(3):159-164.
24. Franik G, Bizoń A, Włoch S, Kowalczyk K, Biernacka-Bartnik, Madej P. Hormonal and metabolic aspects of acne vulgaris in women with polycystic ovary syndrome. Eur Rev Med Pharmacol Sci. 2018;22(14):4411-4418.

第十六章 多囊卵巢综合征的药物治疗：减重

一、体重的重要性

多囊卵巢综合征（PCOS）是一种以月经周期不规律和高雄激素血症（HA）为主要表现的综合征。2003年的鹿特丹共识会议修改了以前关于PCOS诊断的指南。根据鹿特丹标准，排除继发性诊断后，如果女性符合以下3项标准中的任意2项，就可以诊断为PCOS：

- 月经稀发/无排卵。
- HA［HA的临床和（或）生化证据］：
  - 临床：多毛症、痤疮和（或）黑棘皮症。
  - 生化：睾酮水平升高（游离睾酮比总睾酮水平更敏感）和（或）雄烯二酮升高和（或）硫酸脱氢表雄酮（DHEAS）水平升高。
- 超声检查发现多囊卵巢（一个卵巢内直径2～9 mm的卵泡≥12个或卵巢体积＞10 cm^3），并排除其他病因（先天性肾上腺皮质增生症、分泌雄激素的肿瘤、库欣综合征）。

临床上，被诊断为PCOS的患者中，大多数（50%～80%）都超重［体重指数（BMI）为25～30 kg/m^2］或肥胖（BMI＞30 kg/m^2）。对于所有25～35岁的女性，包括那些患有PCOS的女性，理想体重为BMI＜24 kg/m^2。在一项荟萃分析中，对于超过35岁的PCOS患者，当BMI截断值在18～20 kg/m^2时妊娠率显著降低（OR：0.6969，95%CI：0.4947～0.9817）。超过35岁的非PCOS患者，BMI和妊娠率之间没有明显的截断值。全球范围内，随着肥胖患病率的增加，PCOS患者肥胖的患病率也急剧增加，从20世纪90年代的51%增加到现在的74%。然而，需要注意的是，仍存在一小部分BMI≤25 kg/m^2的女性符合PCOS的诊断标准。这种现象被称为"瘦型PCOS"，在不同的族群中总体患病率为1.5%～6.6%。患有"瘦型PCOS"的患者患上胰岛素抵抗（IR）、2型糖尿病（T2DM）和其他合并症的风险较低。

多种机制导致了PCOS患者体重逐渐增加（图16.1）。由此产生的肥胖增加了相关并发症的风险，如糖尿病前期、T2DM、高血压和阻塞性睡眠呼吸暂停。PCOS最普遍的特征仍然是IR，它可引起多种表现。高胰岛素血症导致PCOS患者发展至代谢综合征、胰岛素受体下调、游离脂肪酸和细胞内脂质浓度增加，并通过肿瘤坏死因子-α（TNF-α）和白细胞介素-6（IL-6）的循环改变其自身作用。

第十六章 多囊卵巢综合征的药物治疗：减重

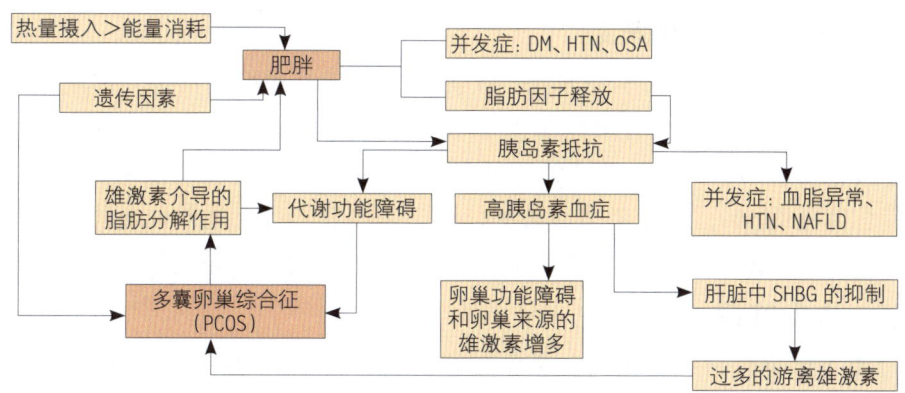

DM，糖尿病；HTN，高血压；NAFLD，非酒精性脂肪性肝病；OSA，阻塞性睡眠呼吸暂停；SHBG，性激素结合球蛋白。

图 16.1 多囊卵巢综合征和肥胖的发病机制

达到并保持适宜的健康体重是 PCOS 管理的重要组成部分，可以改善胰岛素敏感性，并减轻 HA 和无排卵的症状。

二、体重管理

体重管理包括减重、防止体重进一步增加和保持体重平衡的整个过程。已有研究表明，在被诊断为 PCOS 的患者中，体重减轻 5%～10% 可以在心理、生殖和代谢方面产生益处。减重的方式有很多种，包括饮食和生活方式干预、药物干预和手术（表 16.1 和表 16.2）。

表 16.1 多囊卵巢综合征患者减重的药物干预方法

序号	药物类型	药物名称
1	胰高血糖素样肽-1（GLP-1）激动剂	利拉鲁肽：美国食品药品监督管理局（FDA）批准 司美格鲁肽：FDA 批准
2	拟交感神经药/抗惊厥药	苯丁胺/托吡酯缓释剂：FDA 批准
3	阿片受体拮抗剂/抗抑郁药	纳曲酮缓释剂/安非他酮缓释剂：FDA 批准
4	脂肪酶抑制剂	奥利司他：FDA 批准
5	5-羟色胺 2c 受体激动剂	氯卡色林：不推荐使用，已下市，因为存在恶性肿瘤风险

表 16.2 多囊卵巢综合征患者减重的手术干预方法

序号	减重术类型	减重术名称
1	限制性：减少胃的自然容量，从而限制食物摄入并减轻体重	• 水平胃成形术 • 垂直带状胃成形术 • 硅胶环垂直胃成形术 • 可调节胃束带术
2	吸收不良：改变肠道走向，绕过一大部分小肠，导致养分吸收减少，从而降低体重	• 空肠回肠旁路术 • 胆胰分流术 • 十二指肠转位术 • 长肢胃旁路术
3	混合型：限制型和吸收不良（减小胃的大小，并绕过大部分小肠）	• Roux-en-Y 胃旁路术（RYGB）

（一）生活方式干预策略

生活方式干预主要包括3个方面：饮食、体育活动和行为指导。多项纵向研究已经证明，这3项干预措施联合可以实现10%的减重并至少维持1年，其中热量限制对减重起着最主要作用，而通过持续的活动/运动计划可以维持减重效果。通过生活方式干预减轻总体重的5%，可以带来显著的代谢、生殖和心理上的益处。长期维持减重的主要挑战是缺乏预先规划的目标和持续的行为指导，因此在减重过程中需要更多关注。

（二）饮食管理

减重主要通过制造热量摄入缺口来实现。对于包括PCOS患者在内的所有人来说都是如此。目前尚无关于PCOS特殊饮食的科学数据，但任何引起热量缺乏的饮食计划都将带来减重效果。

在启动特定的饮食计划之前，设定目标对于饮食计划的个性化和可实现性至关重要。如果向着每周减重0.5～1.0 kg的目标努力，可以从患者正常饮食中减少500～1000 kcal/d的热量。需要进行缓慢但持续的饮食调整，包括减小餐量、用水代替含糖饮料、增加全谷物麦片的摄入量，以及减少饮食中饱和脂肪或复杂碳水化合物。

采用极低能量饮食的女性（每天提供800 cal或更少的热量，每周平均减重1.0～2.5 kg），初期减重效果比其他形式的热量限制更好，但需要由医疗保健专业人员监测以防止微量元素缺乏。为了达到最大的减重效果和更好的长期结果，需要在热量限制的基础上结合体育锻炼。

（三）体育活动

体育活动在减重中的作用主要集中在维持体重减轻上。为了减少普通人群的肥胖，《美国体育活动指南》推荐进行中等强度有氧运动150～300分钟/周，或高强度有氧运动75～150分钟/周。英国国家卫生服务信托的考文垂营养师建议成年人每周5天进行30分钟的中等强度体育锻炼。类似的指南可以扩展到PCOS患者身上，他们可以通过中等强度到高强度的体育锻炼和饮食限制来实现规定的减重目标。

PCOS患者存在脂解作用障碍，这导致体重增加。一些研究表明，有氧运动可以部分逆转脂肪分解障碍，从而减轻体重。此外，有氧运动对IR和心血管疾病（CVD）风险具有有利影响。对于PCOS患者来说，力量训练也非常有益，包括瑜伽、普拉提，以及渐进式抗阻训练（progressive resistance training，PRT），这是一种旨在通过增加负荷来促进肌肉质量适应性增加的力量训练方法。有学者针对PCOS患者进行了PRT的研究，结果显示PRT可以促进总体脂率降低，腰围缩小，肌肉力量提高，以及HA减轻。研究显示，PCOS患者练习瑜伽和普拉提，可使腹围和臀围显著减小。

随机对照试验（RCT）显示，对于PCOS患者，将饮食疗法（如低碳水化合物饮食）与定期运动相结合，比单独进行运动，在持续减重方面效果更好。这些干预措施的结合还显示出更明显的减轻IR和HA症状的效果。

（四）行为改变

行为改变治疗旨在帮助患有 PCOS 的肥胖患者认识、理解并相应地改变他们的饮食和活动习惯，以取得良好的效果。纳入了为数不多的有关行为改变干预措施的文献的一篇系统综述强调了结合多种干预措施的益处。从这个综述中提取出来的关键建议包括：

- 自我监测，定期测量体重和记录饮食情况。
- 使用 SMART（specific, measurable, achievable, realistic, and timely）模型（具体、可衡量、可实现、现实和及时）设定切实可行的目标和结果。
- 理解和区分减重和体重管理的组成部分。
- 通过鼓励积极的态度来重构认知。
- 识别健康行为的障碍，然后深入分析可能的解决方案。
- 要与鼓励你的人在一起。
- 在需要时寻求专业人士的帮助［如认知行为疗法（CBT）和其他行为改变疗法的专家］。

三、药物干预

在肥胖（BMI＞30.0 kg/m^2）或超重（BMI 为 25～30 kg/m^2）且存在与体重相关的合并症（如高血压、T2DM、血脂异常、睡眠呼吸暂停、关节炎或高尿酸血症）的 PCOS 患者中，应首先考虑药物干预治疗。在过去几十年里，通过不同机制发挥作用的新型药物已经上市，可用于肥胖和超重人群的减重，这些药物也可用于满足减重适应证的 PCOS 患者。

目前 FDA 批准用于慢性减重管理的 5 种药物治疗方式是：利拉鲁肽皮下注射、司美格鲁肽皮下注射、口服苯丁胺和托吡酯、口服奥利司他、口服纳曲酮和安非他酮。不推荐使用二甲双胍和氯卡色林。

（一）二甲双胍

根据科学数据，不推荐将二甲双胍用作 PCOS 患者减重的药物治疗。它适用于具有临床表现或生化证据的胰岛素抵抗、糖尿病前期和（或）糖尿病的患者。传统上，二甲双胍被用于 PCOS 患者的症状管理，其主要作用是增加胰岛素敏感性和预防 T2DM 的发展，其对体重的影响存在争议。其副作用虽然轻微，但存在胃肠不耐受和维生素 B$_{12}$ 缺乏的风险。

（二）氯卡色林

不应使用氯卡色林减重，虽然它曾经用于减重，但现在由于服药患者患胰腺癌、结肠直肠癌和肺癌的风险较高而不再获得批准。

经证实的 PCOS 患者减重药物的选择将在下面的部分详细讨论。

（三）胰高血糖素样肽 –1 激动剂（利拉鲁肽和司美格鲁肽）

胰高血糖素样肽 -1（GLP-1）是调节食物摄入的主要肽类激素之一。它通过增加葡萄糖依赖性胰岛素分泌、减少胰高血糖素释放，以及抑制食欲和延缓胃排空来发挥作用。艾塞那肽是 2005 年在美国首次被临床使用的 GLP-1 类似物，被批准为具有降低心血管风险的葡萄糖调节药物。自 2014 年以来，GLP-1 激动剂也被批准用作减重药物，其通过外周和中枢神经系统途径对食欲进行调节。在外周方面，它减慢胃排空，导致胃窦运动减少和幽门张力增加，从而刺激迷走神经，将信号传导至延髓和下丘脑，诱导产生饱腹感。在中枢方面，这些类似物，特别是利拉鲁肽，已被证明可以直接刺激阿黑皮素原（proopiomelanocortin，POMC）神经元，并抑制弓状核内的神经肽 Y 和 Agouti 相关肽神经元，从而抑制食欲。除了改善葡萄糖稳态，GLP-1 激动剂还可以增加饱腹感，减少肠道运动，并减轻体重。

利拉鲁肽是首个被批准用于非糖尿病患者减重的 GLP-1 类似物，剂量为每天 1 次皮下注射 3 mg。确凿的证据表明，在生活方式干预的基础上，利拉鲁肽可使体重平均减少 4.9% ~ 7.4%。与二甲双胍和奥利司他相比，它已被证明具有较少的副作用，并有明显的与剂量相关的减重效果。

司美格鲁肽是一种长效 GLP-1 类似物，于 2017 年被 FDA 批准用于每周 1 次皮下注射治疗糖尿病。口服司美格鲁肽于 2019 年 9 月获得批准，用于辅助饮食和运动以改善成人 T2DM 患者的血糖。2021 年 6 月，司美格鲁肽（2.4 mg 每周 1 次皮下注射）获批用于治疗肥胖或超重且至少存在一种与体重相关疾病（如高血压、T2DM 或高胆固醇）的成人，同时需配合减少热量摄入和增加体育活动。研究表明，采用所有干预措施的组合可使体重平均减轻 9.6% ~ 16.0%。

评估司美格鲁肽在 PCOS 中疗效的试验显示，该药可导致明显的体重减轻，并具有减少 CVD 风险的益处。在一项试验中，连续皮下注射 0.5 mg 和 1.0 mg 司美格鲁肽 104 周后，平均体重分别减轻了 3.6 kg 和 4.9 kg。与之类似，在另一项为期 26 周的试验中，受试者还被给予了最大可耐受剂量的口服二甲双胍。结果显示，口服司美格鲁肽在减重方面优于皮下注射利拉鲁肽。PIONEER 2 试验还表明，持续 52 周后，每天口服 14 mg 的司美格鲁肽较每天口服 25 mg 的恩格列净（钠 – 葡萄糖共转运体 2 抑制剂）更具优势，前者体重减轻了 4.8 kg，而后者只减轻了 3.8 kg。

利拉鲁肽和司美格鲁肽最常见的副作用包括恶心和呕吐。使用利拉鲁肽的缺点是需要皮下注射，因此更推荐使用口服司美格鲁肽。但后者目前尚未被批准用于非糖尿病患者，并且有严格的用法指导，即必须在清晨空腹时，在进食或饮水前至少 30 分钟给药。其他罕见不良反应包括利拉鲁肽引起的胰腺炎，以及司美格鲁肽与甲状腺素一起应用可能导致甲状腺素水平过高。所有 GLP-1 激动剂在啮齿动物中均增加了甲状腺 C 细胞瘤的风险；尚未发现人类病例，但一般应避免在甲状腺 C 细胞瘤风险较高的患者中使用 GLP-1 激动剂。

（四）盐酸苯丁胺与托吡酯联合应用

苯丁胺与托吡酯联合应用已经获得FDA批准用于减重。虽然其中每种药物的单药治疗也是可行的，但联合使用缓释（extended release，ER）制剂显示出副作用减少的特点。苯丁胺与苯丙胺有药理学上的关联，可能通过在下丘脑释放儿茶酚胺来起到抑制食欲的作用。托吡酯是一种磺酸酰基取代的单糖，常用作抗癫痫药物，现在的研究显示它对体重有减轻效果，56周减重10.2～10.8 kg。关于托吡酯减重的作用机制有几种推测，认为它具有中枢和全身分布的活性。在大鼠的减重研究中，它显示出对神经肽Y及其Y1和Y5受体、促肾上腺皮质激素释放激素和Ⅱ型糖皮质激素受体有影响，从而抑制食欲、增加饱腹感，导致减重。

使用苯丁胺/托吡酯ER时于每天早上口服一次。有4种不同剂量的苯丁胺和托吡酯ER可供选择：①起始剂量（3.75 mg/23 mg）；②推荐剂量（7.5 mg/46 mg）；③过渡剂量（11.25 mg/69 mg）；④最大剂量（15 mg/92 mg）。在治疗后，应在12周后评估体重；如果体重减轻不到3%，则可以停止治疗，或者使用过渡剂量治疗14天后转换为最大剂量。然而，如果使用最大剂量后体重减轻不到5%，则应在连续1周内每隔一天服用一次后停药，因为突然停药可能会引发癫痫。经过苯丁胺/托吡酯与生活方式干预等综合治疗后，患者的平均体重减轻率为9.8%～10.9%。EQUIP试验是一项为期56周的RCT，比较了苯丁胺/托吡酯控释（controlled release，CR）制剂与安慰剂的效果，包括4周的随机化后滴定期和随后52周的随机治疗期。3.75 mg/23 mg和15 mg/92 mg的剂量在52周内比安慰剂更有效，并且相对于其他市售药物，体重减少百分比更高。CONQUER是另一项为期56周的RCT，使用7.5 mg/46 mg和15 mg/92 mg的苯丁胺/托吡酯控释制剂，也显示出比安慰剂更明显的减重效果。作为后续随访，SEQUEL试验用于评估该药物的长期疗效，持续时间为52周。在第108周，参与者中观察到剂量相关的体重减轻（安慰剂组体重减轻率为1.8%，7.5 mg/46 mg剂量组为9.3%，15 mg/92 mg剂量组为10.7%），该药物导致甘油三酯、高密度脂蛋白胆固醇和低密度脂蛋白胆固醇水平显著降低，使其成为PCOS减重最有效的药物之一。

最常报告的副作用包括感觉异常、口干和便秘。此药物对怀孕期的女性、青光眼患者、甲状腺功能亢进患者、接受单胺氧化酶抑制剂治疗或治疗后14天内的患者，以及对拟交感胺类药物、托吡酯或药物中的任何非活性成分过敏或不耐受的患者禁用。

（五）纳曲酮与安非他酮联合应用

2014年9月，FDA批准了纳曲酮与安非他酮的联合应用。该药物以每日2次16 mg/180 mg的联合剂量可有效辅助生活方式干预，使患者平均体重下降3.7%～8.1%。

纳曲酮是一种阿片受体拮抗剂，对μ、δ和κ阿片受体产生作用，其中对μ阿片受体的拮抗效果最强。它能够阻断β-内啡肽对下丘脑POMC细胞负反馈机制的影响，从而促使其分泌黑素细胞刺激激素（melanocyte-stimulating hormone，MSH）。由于

MSH 通过向大脑传递饱腹感来调节食欲，连续的 MSH 分泌可导致食欲下降。安非他酮是一种多巴胺和去甲肾上腺素再摄取抑制剂，类似于苯丙胺，通过对下丘脑的作用来抑制食欲。

在首个基于上文提到剂量的临床试验中，两种药物联合应用结合均衡饮食和每周 180 分钟的运动，结果显示在 56 周后，与对照组相比达到总体减重 5% 目标的参与者数量存在显著差异，平均体重减轻了 4.2%。另一项具有相似人群、相同干预持续时间及基线生活方式干预的试验显示，纳曲酮 ER/ 安非他酮 ER 16 mg/360 mg 和 32 mg/360 mg 减重幅度分别为 3.7% 和 4.8%，减重效果呈剂量依赖性。在糖尿病人群中，该联合应用加控制饮食和体育活动可导致体重减轻 3.2%。

纳曲酮 ER/ 安非他酮 ER 最常见的副作用包括恶心、便秘、头痛、头晕和口干。由于安非他酮具有抗抑郁作用，可能引发自杀念头和行为。该药物绝对禁用于滥用阿片类药物的患者，相对禁用于未得到控制的高血压和缺血性心脏病患者（因为安非他酮可能进一步加重这些症状），以及因药物可能引起的肝功能和肾功能障碍的患者。

（六）奥利司他

奥利司他 120 mg 于 1999 年获得 FDA 批准作为处方药物，需配合饮食管理用于肥胖症治疗，并降低减重后体重反弹的风险。它通过与胰腺和胃脂肪酶不可逆地结合改变脂质的消化，从而导致食物中脂质的吸收减少。通过这种机制，奥利司他显示出对减少体重、改善血脂和糖代谢指标具有持久的维持效应。使用奥利司他与生活方式干预相结合的平均体重减轻范围为 4.6%～10.2%。对于一般肥胖人群，推荐剂量是口服 120 mg，每天 3 次，在进食 1 小时内服用。然而，如果有任何一餐未进食，该餐后用药可以省略。

一项荟萃分析评估了奥利司他对多个 PCOS 参数的影响，结果显示在超重 / 肥胖的 PCOS 女性中，BMI/ 体重显著降低。此外，类似于二甲双胍，它还对睾酮水平、IR 和血脂谱具有有利影响，副作用较轻且易耐受，如恶心和上腹痛等。另一项 RCT 的回顾性研究显示，相对于安慰剂，在使用 52 周后，奥利司他可实现至少 5% 的总体重减轻。奥利司他的副作用包括增加胃肠胀气、脂肪 / 油质大便及可能的大便失禁，严重限制了患者的依从性。由于这些副作用，孕妇、慢性吸收不良综合征患者和胆汁淤积患者禁用该药物。

四、减重术

减重术是肥胖患者实现减重最有效的方法。根据美国国立卫生研究院（NIH）国立糖尿病和消化、肾脏疾病研究所（National Institute of Diabetes and Digestive and Kidney Diseases，NIDDK）的建议，体重减轻手术适用于以下情况的患者：BMI > 40 kg/m^2，BMI > 35 kg/m^2 并伴有 T2DM、睡眠呼吸暂停或心脏疾病等合并症，或者 BMI > 30 kg/m^2 并伴有无法通过生活方式干预和药物有效治疗的 T2DM。胃减重术主要分为 3 类：限制性手术(水平胃成形术、垂直带状胃成形术、硅胶环垂直胃成形术和可调节胃束带术)、吸收不良手术(空肠回肠旁路术、胆胰分流术、十二指肠转位术和长肢胃旁路术),以及这两种类型的组合手术[Roux-en-Y 胃旁路术(Roux-en-Y gastric bypass procedure,RYGB)]。减重术后体重减轻的假设与神经内分泌机制和肠道化学物质(胃饥饿素)的激素调节有关,其增加了饱腹感并降低了饥饿感。

近年来,胃减重术的进展使其变得侵入性更低,减重效果明显,并常常对代谢并发症有继发治疗效果。正如国际肥胖和代谢障碍外科联合会(International Federation for the Surgery of Obesity and Metabolic Disorders,IFSO)在 2019 年全球登记报告中所指出的,这使得手术减重的选择越来越受欢迎。该报告评论称,2018—2019 年,根据 61 个国家的记录,胃减重术数量增加了 439 256 例,几乎增加了一倍,其中最常见的手术包括 RYGB、袖状胃切除术(垂直胃切除术)、一次吻合胃旁路术和胃束带术(图 16.2)。

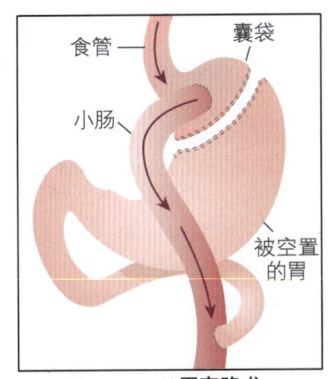
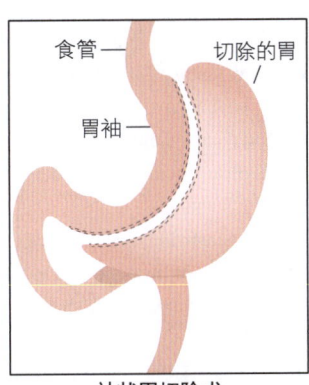
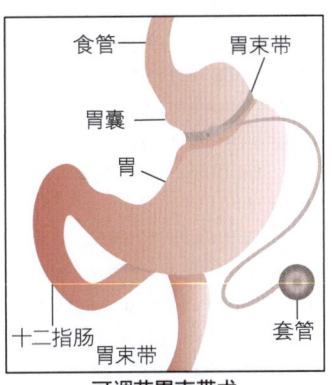

图 16.2 常见的减重术

来源:Gandhi D., Boregowda U, Sharma P, et al., A review of commonly performed bariatric surgeries: Imaging features and its complications. Clinical Imaging. 2021; 72: 122-135.

一些研究评估了减重术对 PCOS 代谢方面的影响。证据显示 Roux-en-Y 胃旁路术在体重减轻方面优于袖状胃切除术;然而,尚未进行 RCT 来确立这种关系。在一项评估经胆胰旁路或腹腔镜 Roux-en-Y 胃旁路术后的 PCOS 患者体重减轻的研究中,平均减重达 41 kg,同时改善了多毛症、降低了睾酮水平并调节了月经周期。另一项回顾性研究得出结论,PCOS 患者在接受 Roux-en-Y 胃旁路术后的 12 个月内体重减轻了约 56.7%,HbA1c 在 3 个月内降低了 3%。最近的研究支持减重术对 PCOS 患者体重减轻和其他雄激素特征的疗效;在 6 个月的随访中,体重减轻了至少 25 kg,而在 1 年内体重减轻范围从 34.0 kg 到 93.6 kg 不等,可能实现 100% 的规律性月经周期,有不到 50% 的患者术后至少 1 年内多毛症减轻。

除了减重术外，FDA 还批准了使用一些非侵入性减重 / 管理装置，如临时放置胃内气囊系统（通过占据空间增加饱腹感）、胃排空系统（用于餐后排出一部分胃内容物以防止吸收）、口服可拆卸腭上空间占据装置（帮助限制口腔容量），暂时性摄入性空间占据装置（摄入材料旨在占据胃内空间）。每种装置都有其自身的风险和益处，因此对于这些干预措施来说，选择适宜的患者对获得最佳效果非常重要。

参考文献

1. Rotterdam ESHRE/ASRM-Sponsored PCOS Consensus Workshop Group. Revised 2003 consensus on diagnostic criteria and long-term health risks related to polycystic ovary syndrome (PCOS). Hum Reprod. 2004;19(1):41-47.
2. Anagnostis P, Paparodis R, Bosdou J, et al. The major impact of obesity on the development of Type 2 Diabetes (T2D) in women with PCOS: a systematic review and meta-analysis of observational studies [Abstract]. J Endocr Soc. 2021;5(suppl 1):A746-A747.
3. Obesity Raises Type 2 Diabetes Risk in Women with PCOS. Endocrine.org. 2021. Available at: https://www.endocrine.org/news-and-advocacy/news-room/featured-science-from-endo-2021/obesity-raises-type-2-diabetes-risk-in-women-with-pcos, in press.
4. Wang F, Dai W, Yang X, Guo Y, Sun Y. Analyses of optimal body mass index for infertile patients with either polycystic or non-polycystic ovary syndrome during assisted reproductive treatment in China. Sci Rep. 2016;6(1):34538.
5. Teede H, Misso M, Costello M, et al. Recommendations from the international evidence-based guideline for the assessment and management of polycystic ovary syndrome. Clin Endocrinol. 2018;89(3):251-268.
6. Pourmatroud E. Lean women with polycystic ovary syndrome. In: Agrawal NK, Singh K, eds. Debatable Topics in PCOS Patients. London: IntechOpen; 2017.
7. Brennan L, Teede H, Skouteris H, Linardon J, Hill B, Moran L. Lifestyle and behavioral management of polycystic ovary syndrome. J Womens Health. 2017;26(8):836-848.
8. Jameson J. Harrison's Endocrinology. 4th ed. New York: McGraw-Hill Education; 2017.
9. Gardner D, Shoback D, Greenspan F. Greenspan's Basic & Clinical Endocrinology. 10th ed. Cenveo Publisher Services; 2018.
10. Melmed S, Polonsky K, Larson P, Kronenberg H. Williams Textbook of Endocrinology. 13th ed. New Delhi: Elsevier; 2016.
11. Piercy K, Troiano R. Physical activity guidelines for Americans from the US department of health and human services. Circ Cardiovasc Qual Outcomes. 2018;11(11):e005263.
12. NHS. Weight Management: Advice for Asian People. England: NHS Trust; 2017.
13. Abazar E, Mardanian F, Forozandeh D, Taghian F. Effects of aerobic exercise on plasma lipoproteins in overweight and obese women with polycystic ovary syndrome. Adv Biomed Res. 2015;4(1):68.
14. Kogure G, Miranda-Furtado C, Pedroso D, et al. Effects of progressive resistance training on obesity indices in polycystic ovary syndrome and the relationship with telomere length. J Phys Act Health. 2019;16(8):601-607.
15. Mohseni M, Eghbali M, Bahrami H, Dastaran F, Amini L. Yoga effects on anthropometric indices and polycystic ovary syndrome symptoms in women undergoing infertility treatment: a randomized controlled clinical trial. Evid Based Complement Alternat Med. 2021;2021:5564824.
16. Karam N, Nathan J. A Review of FDA-Approved Medications for Chronic Weight Management. Drug Topics; 2021. Available from: https://www.drugtopics.com/view/a-review-of-fda-approved-medications-for-chronic-weight-management.
17. Lashen H. Review: Role of metformin in the management of polycystic ovary syndrome. Ther Adv Endocrinol

Metab. 2010;1(3):117-128.
18. Abdalla M, Deshmukh H, Atkin S, Sathyapalan T. A review of therapeutic options for managing the metabolic aspects of polycystic ovary syndrome. Ther Adv Endocrinol Metab. 2020;11:204201882093830.
19. NIH. LiverTox: Clinical and Research Information on Drug-Induced Liver Injury. Bethesda (MD): National Institute of Diabetes and Digestive and Kidney Diseases; 2012. Available from: https://www.ncbi.nlm.nih.gov/books/NBK548834/.
20. Rodbard H. The clinical impact of GLP-1 receptor agonists in type 2 diabetes: focus on the long-acting analogs. Diabetes Technol Ther. 2018;20(suppl 2):S233-S241.
21. Crane J, McGowan B. The GLP-1 agonist, liraglutide, as a pharmacotherapy for obesity. Ther Adv Chronic Dis. 2016;7(2):92-107.
22. Marso SP, Bain SC, Consoli A, et al. Semaglutide and cardiovascular outcomes in patients with type 2 diabetes. N Engl J Med. 2016;375(19):1834-1844.
23. Pratley R, Amod A, Hoff S, et al. Oral semaglutide versus subcutaneous liraglutide and placebo in type 2 diabetes (PIONEER 4): a randomised, double-blind, phase 3a trial. Lancet. 2019;394(10192):39-50.
24. Rodbard H, Rosenstock J, Canani L, et al. Oral Semaglutide versus empagliflozin in patients with type 2 diabetes uncontrolled on metformin: the PIONEER 2 trial. Diabetes Care. 2019;42(12):2272-2281.
25. Hughes S, Neumiller JJ. Oral semaglutide. Clin Diabetes. 2020;38(1):109-111.
26. Chiu W, Shih S, Tseng C. A review on the association between glucagon-like peptide-1 receptor agonists and thyroid cancer. Exp Diabetes Res. 2012;2012:924168.
27. Cosentino G, Conrad AO, Uwaifo GI. Phentermine and topiramate for the management of obesity: a review. Drug Des Devel Ther. 2011;7:267-278.
28. Allison DB, Gadde KM, Garvey WT, et al. Controlled-release phentermine/topiramate in severely obese adults: a randomized controlled trial (EQUIP). Obesity (Silver Spring). 2012;20(2):330-342.
29. Gadde KM, Allison DB, Ryan DH, et al. Effects of low-dose, controlled-release, phentermine plus topiramate combination on weight and associated comorbidities in overweight and obese adults (CONQUER): a randomised, placebo-controlled, phase 3 trial. Lancet. 2011;377(9774):1341-1352.
30. Garvey WT, Ryan DH, Look M, et al. Two-year sustained weight loss and metabolic benefits with controlled-release phentermine/topiramate in obese and overweight adults (SEQUEL): a randomised, placebo-controlled, phase 3 extension study. Am J Clin Nutr. 2012;95(2):297-308.
31. Tek C. Naltrexone HCl/bupropion HCl for chronic weight management in obese adults: patient selection and perspectives. Patient Prefer Adherence. 2016;10:751-759.
32. Wadden TA, Foreyt JP, Foster GD, et al. Weight loss with naltrexone SR/bupropion SR combination therapy as an adjunct to behavior modification: the COR-BMOD trial. Obesity (Silver Spring). 2011;19(1):110-120.
33. Greenway FL, Fujioka K, Plodkowski RA, et al. Effect of naltrexone plus bupropion on weight loss in overweight and obese adults (COR-I): a multicentre, randomised, double-blind, placebo-controlled, phase 3. Lancet. 2010;376(9741):595-605.
34. Hollander P, Gupta AK, Plodkowski R, et al. Effects of naltrexone sustained-release/bupropion sustained-release combination therapy on body weight and glycemic parameters in overweight and obese patients with type 2 diabetes. Diabetes Care. 2013;36(12):4022-4029.
35. Ornellas T, Chavez B. Naltrexone SR/Bupropion SR (Contrave): a new approach to weight loss in obese adults. P T. 2011;36(5):255-262.
36. Graff SK, Mario FM, Ziegelmann P, Spritzer PM. Effects of orlistat vs. metformin on weight loss-related clinical variables in women with PCOS: systematic review and meta-analysis. Int J Clin Pract. 2016;70(6):450-461.
37. Khera R, Murad MH, Chandar AK, et al. Association of pharmacological treatments for obesity with weight loss and adverse events: a systematic review and meta-analysis. JAMA. 2016;315(22):2424-2434.
38. NIH. Potential Candidates for Weight-Loss Surgery | NIDDK. National Institute of Diabetes and Digestive

and Kidney Diseases; 2021. Available at: https://www.niddk.nih.gov/health-information/weight-management/bariatric-surgery/potential-candidates.
39. IFSO. IFSO Registry | International Federation for the Surgery of Obesity and Metabolic Disorders. Ifso.com; 2021. Available at: https://www.ifso.com/ifso-registry.php.
40. Escobar-Morreale HF, Botella-Carretero JI, Alvarez-Blasco F, Sancho J, San Millán JL. The polycystic ovary syndrome associated with morbid obesity may resolve after weight loss induced by bariatric surgery. J Clin Endocrinol Metab. 2005;90(12):6364-6369.
41. Eid GM, Cottam DR, Velcu LM, et al. Effective treatment of polycystic ovarian syndrome with Roux-en-Y gastric bypass. Surg Obes Relat Dis. 2005;1(2):77-80.
42. Christ JP, Falcone T. Bariatric surgery improves hyperandrogenism, menstrual irregularities, and metabolic dysfunction among women with polycystic ovary syndrome (PCOS). Obes Surg. 2018;28(8):2171-2177.
43. Singh D, Arumalla K, Aggarwal S, Singla V, Ganie A, Malhotra N. Impact of bariatric surgery on clinical, biochemical, and hormonal parameters in women with polycystic ovary syndrome (PCOS). Obes Surg. 2020;30(6):2294-2300.
44. Weight-Loss and Weight-Management Devices. U.S. Food and Drug Administration; 2021. Available at: https://www.fda.gov/medical-devices/products-and-medical-procedures/weight-loss-and-weight-management-devices#loss.

第十七章 胰岛素增敏剂在多囊卵巢综合征管理中的作用

一、引言

高胰岛素血症和胰岛素抵抗（IR）被认为是多囊卵巢综合征（PCOS）的病理生理学机制。高胰岛素血症和 IR 通过多种途径影响内分泌腺体（卵巢、肾上腺、垂体）和外周组织（脂肪、肝脏和肌肉），导致慢性无排卵、高雄激素血症（HA）、代谢功能障碍及其相关的合并症。基于这些推断，研究人员对各种胰岛素增敏剂进行了研究，以观察其是否可以成为 PCOS 患者的治疗选择。结合生活方式干预，胰岛素增敏剂可降低胰岛素水平和改善 IR，最终改善与 PCOS 相关的内分泌和代谢问题。

在大多数 PCOS 患者中使用胰岛素增敏剂的前提是，几乎所有肥胖的 PCOS 女性和超过一半正常体重的 PCOS 患者都存在 IR，并且在某种程度上表现出空腹或刺激后高胰岛素血症。

二、胰岛素增敏剂在多囊卵巢综合征中的作用机制

胰岛素增敏剂的益处源于其可以降低胰岛素水平，增加性激素结合球蛋白（SHBG）的含量，从而降低作用于外周组织的游离雄激素水平及循环中的雄激素水平。改善胰岛素敏感性和降低胰岛素浓度可以增加不孕和低生育力 PCOS 女性的生育机会。胰岛素水平的下降会减少与雄激素的结合和降低游离雄激素水平，从而改善大部分患者的 HA。通过胰岛素增敏剂改善胰岛素抵抗和降低胰岛素水平，可以改善葡萄糖耐受不良，延缓 2 型糖尿病（T2DM）的发生和代谢综合征的进展，以及降低相关的心血管疾病（CVD）风险。

三、治疗多囊卵巢综合征的胰岛素增敏剂

PCOS 的管理中主要用以下药物作为胰岛素增敏剂：
- 二甲双胍。
- 噻唑烷二酮类药物。
- 胰高血糖素样肽 -1 受体激动剂。
- 肌醇。
- α - 硫辛酸。

（一）二甲双胍

1994年，二甲双胍成为首个用于PCOS患者的抗糖尿病药物，以探索IR在该综合征发病机制中的作用。

二甲双胍在过去40年中改变了多种代谢紊乱的治疗方法。与其他降糖药物相比，二甲双胍是短期和长期治疗方案中被研究最多的药物。然而，目前仍缺乏强有力的证据，迫切需要进一步探索这种传统药物对PCOS患者的多种治疗方式。

1. 作用机制

二甲双胍在PCOS中对多种组织发挥作用，这些组织和器官引起了生殖和代谢异常，如肝脏、脂肪组织、骨骼肌和卵巢。该药可以降低肝糖异生、减少脂肪生成，并增强肝脏、脂肪组织、骨骼肌和卵巢对葡萄糖的摄取。

二甲双胍被认为可以直接或间接影响卵巢的雄激素产生。在PCOS患者中使用二甲双胍治疗可导致细胞色素P450 17A1（CYP17A1）活性降低、血清胰岛素水平下降。此外，二甲双胍可以直接抑制卵巢类固醇合成，其中线粒体复合物I的抑制可能是其中一个潜在的作用机制。二甲双胍也可以通过抑制3β-羟基类固醇脱氢酶/Δ^5-Δ^4异构酶2型来降低雄激素水平。

二甲双胍治疗的临床反应在不同的PCOS表型之间有时差异很大，许多遗传因素被认为是可能的原因。然而，需要进行大规模的基因组研究来确定这些差异表现的标记物。

2. 临床效果

（1）对雄激素的影响

二甲双胍通过降低胰岛素水平，在20%～25%的PCOS女性中引起睾酮水平下降，而在非肥胖的PCOS患者中，这种睾酮水平下降更明显。然而，也有研究报道了二甲双胍降低睾酮水平的其他潜在机制。一些研究指出，在开始二甲双胍治疗后的48小时内睾酮水平立即降低，甚至在出现实质性的胰岛素敏感性改善和产生其他代谢成分之前。二甲双胍可以对游离雄激素指数、总睾酮和SHBG水平产生显著影响。一些研究显示，即使通过常规静脉采样的葡萄糖耐受试验评估胰岛素敏感性没有改善，二甲双胍仍可以降低PCOS女性的睾酮水平。二甲双胍的这些效果可能因不同的PCOS表型而异。

（2）对月经不规律和临床高雄激素血症的影响

尽管二甲双胍可以降低睾酮水平，但其在PCOS中的使用并不一定能改善月经不规律或临床HA。证据显示，二甲双胍治疗只能略微改善月经模式，且具有相当大的异质性。此外，二甲双胍并没有成为改善临床HA症状（如痤疮或多毛症）的有效疗法。因此，在PCOS中治疗月经不规律和临床HA的首选药物并不是二甲双胍。

（3）对生育力和活产率的影响

二甲双胍在PCOS中的使用可以改善排卵率、妊娠率和生育率；但是，它并不会改善每次妊娠的流产率和活产率。与枸橼酸氯米芬相比，二甲双胍在诱导排卵、多胎妊娠或活产方面没有显著差异。因此，并不推荐其作为PCOS无排卵性不孕的治疗方法。

（4）对胰岛素不敏感和高胰岛素血症的影响

Burghan最早描述了PCOS和高胰岛素血症之间的关系。在口服葡萄糖耐量试验（OGTT）中，他比较了患有PCOS和未患有PCOS的女性对胰岛素的反应。他发现两组女性的葡萄糖反应相似，而PCOS患者的胰岛素反应明显更高。后来，使用黄金标准的高胰岛素-正常血糖钳夹术的各种研究表明，与年龄和体重指数（BMI）相匹配的正常生育能力女性组相比，PCOS女性患者的胰岛素介导的葡萄糖处理能力下降。基于以上证据，二甲双胍成为一种用于PCOS患者的胰岛素增敏剂。

二甲双胍似乎可以降低PCOS患者的空腹胰岛素水平，但存在显著异质性。这种作用在非肥胖女性中更为显著。没有证据表明二甲双胍和口服避孕药联合使用对PCOS患者的胰岛素水平产生影响。因此，二甲双胍治疗PCOS改善胰岛素敏感性的临床显著性具有较高的变异度，它取决于代谢特征和PCOS表型。

（5）对葡萄糖耐受不良的影响

PCOS管理指南推荐二甲双胍作为治疗T2DM或糖耐量减低且无法从生活方式干预中受益患者的首选药物。目前尚没有研究探讨二甲双胍对糖尿病风险的影响，特别是对PCOS患者的影响。然而，考虑到这些患者发展成为糖尿病的风险非常高，有学者认为二甲双胍可能为具有更高代谢风险的个体带来更大的益处，包括那些具有糖尿病风险因素、糖耐量减低或高风险种族的人。

（6）对体重和身体成分的影响

关于二甲双胍对身体成分和减重的影响存在争议。每天使用1500 mg二甲双胍治疗6个月对BMI没有影响，只轻微地降低了腰臀比（WHR），但当二甲双胍与生活方式干预相结合时，对BMI和向心性肥胖产生了有益效果。单独使用二甲双胍与BMI的降低无关。二甲双胍对内脏与皮下脂肪的影响尚未得到很好的研究。有证据表明，在PCOS患者中，当二甲双胍与低热量饮食结合使用时，对体重和向心性肥胖会产生适度影响。然而，为了确定二甲双胍在这方面的应用，还需要进一步的研究。

（7）对血脂异常和心血管疾病的影响

由于IR及其相关的代谢后果，即T2DM、代谢综合征和血脂异常，PCOS患者患心血管疾病的风险很高。然而，PCOS中心血管疾病的确切患病率尚不清楚。关于二甲双胍治疗是否能改善PCOS患者的血脂异常和降低心血管疾病风险的证据可靠性较低，未来需要进行设计良好、大规模的前瞻性随机临床试验来解决这些不确定性。

3. 剂量和副作用

一般建议每天使用500～1000 mg的二甲双胍以减少副作用并增加依从性。缓释制剂有助于减少副作用。

胃肠道不适（如腹泻、消化不良、胀气、恶心）是二甲双胍最常见的不良反应。10%～50%的患者会出现这些副作用，但通常是暂时的，在几天到一周内会缓解。为了减少副作用，建议从每天500 mg的低剂量开始治疗，并在1～2周内逐渐增加剂量，或者在进食期间服用二甲双胍。

由二甲双胍治疗引起的维生素B_{12}吸收不良很少见。它主要与剂量、年龄和治疗时间有关。与二甲双胍相关的乳酸酸中毒和巨幼红细胞性贫血极为罕见。在估算的肾小球滤过率降低至30 mL/min之前，都可以安全地使用二甲双胍。然而，当肾小球滤过率低于45 mL/min时建议减少剂量。禁忌证包括酗酒，因为如果同时摄入二甲双胍和酒精会导致低血糖和乳酸酸中毒。

在大多数国家，二甲双胍被认为是治疗PCOS的超说明书用药，但如果医护人员告知患者并讨论其效果，其使用并没有受到严格限制。

（二）噻唑烷二酮类药物

曲格列酮是噻唑烷二酮类药物（thiazolidinedione，TZD）中首个且最重要的药物，它于1997年被批准作为降糖药物。然而，该药物在2000年因其对肝脏的毒性作用而从市场撤回。目前有两种TZD可供使用：吡格列酮和罗格列酮。因心脏毒性作用，国际机构限制了罗格列酮的使用，尽管它被认为具有肝脏保护作用。

1. 作用机制

TZD可以选择性地结合到过氧化物酶体增殖物激活受体。后者是一类核转录因子，主要表达于胰岛细胞、血管内皮细胞、脂肪细胞和巨噬细胞中，在心脏和骨骼肌组织中表达较少。TZD的作用机制包括刺激脂肪酸的摄取和在皮下脂肪组织中沉积，以及促进脂肪组织分泌脂连蛋白。因此，TZD特异性地提高了肝脏的胰岛素敏感性。TZD还可以抑制肝糖异生，改善血脂异常，增强抗动脉硬化能力，具有抗炎效果。

2. 代谢效应和内分泌效应

吡格列酮和罗格列酮是在PCOS患者中得到最广泛研究的TZD。TZD在降低空腹和餐后血糖水平方面发挥着重要作用。吡格列酮可以积极调节卵巢雄激素合成，在培养的卵巢颗粒细胞中，通过多种方式影响类固醇激素代谢，如：①促进孕酮的生物合成；②抑制睾酮；③通过胰岛素依赖和非胰岛素依赖途径产生雌二醇（E2）。

有证据表明，在PCOS中，吡格列酮改善了月经周期，但对内分泌（睾酮、SHBG）、代谢（空腹胰岛素）和人体测量（BMI、WHR）结果没有产生任何影响。与二甲双胍相比，罗格列酮在调节总睾酮、硫酸脱氢表雄酮（DHEAS）、卵泡刺激素和黄体生成素水平方面表现出潜在优势，而二甲双胍则在调节游离睾酮、雌二醇和雄烯二酮水平方面疗效更优。就空腹葡萄糖、胰岛素或IR的稳态模型评估结果来看，二甲双胍和罗格列酮的治疗效果没有显著差异。

3. 副作用

TZD 会导致体重增加、疲劳、腹泻、水肿、贫血和充血性心力衰竭，具体而言，吡格列酮会增加膀胱癌和骨质疏松的风险。此外，吡格列酮和罗格列酮都被归类为妊娠期的 C 类药物。这两种药物也有导致体重增加、液体潴留和骨折的风险。

此外，当期望的效果是减重时，不建议使用 TZD 和二甲双胍联合治疗，如果计划怀孕，则此联合疗法是禁忌。

（三）胰高血糖素样肽 –1 激动剂

1. 作用机制

胰高血糖素样肽 -1（GLP-1）受体激动剂是一类抗糖尿病药物，属于肠促胰岛素类似物。包括葡萄糖依赖性促胰岛素多肽（GIP）和 GLP-1 在内的肠促胰岛素是在进食时从肠内内分泌细胞释放的肠激素。GLP-1 激动剂通过刺激胰岛素分泌、抑制胰高血糖素分泌，以及抑制食物摄入和食欲来发挥作用。除了维持血糖稳定，GLP-1 激动剂还能减轻体重，改善血脂异常，并适度降低血压。它们减轻体重的效果有助于改善代谢综合征的多个危险因素，如 BMI、葡萄糖耐受不良、T2DM、非酒精性脂肪性肝病和脂肪性肝炎。减轻体重还可以改善高胰岛素血症和 IR。基于这些鼓舞人心的结果，过去 10 年里，学者们尝试和检测了许多不同的 GLP-1 激动剂在 PCOS 患者中的作用。首先，人们在 2008 年研究了艾塞那肽对 PCOS 患者的治疗效果。之后，在利拉鲁肽的各项研究中它表现出减重、减轻 HA 和改善月经的效果。

有多种不同的 GLP-1 受体激动剂可供选择。从历史上看，所有可用的 GLP-1 制剂都是注射剂，并通过皮下途径给药，因为口服途径的生物利用度较低。利拉鲁肽和利司那肽是每日单次注射剂，而度拉糖肽、司美格鲁肽和阿比鲁肽可以每天两次或每周一次给药。司美格鲁肽口服制剂已获得美国食品药品监督管理局（FDA）的批准。一种新型的 GLP-1 类似物他珀鲁肽的临床试验和研究已暂停，因为它引起了胃肠道相关的副作用和过敏反应。

2. 代谢效应和内分泌效应

证据表明，艾塞那肽和利拉鲁肽在单独使用或与二甲双胍联合使用时显著减轻了 PCOS 患者的体重。它们通过改善 BMI 和腰围来减轻体重。也有一些研究报告称，它们可以使雄激素水平下降，月经情况得到改善。GLP-1 激动剂治疗后，IR 指数［稳态模型评估（HOMA）］和睾酮水平也有所改善。几乎所有这些结果都与 GLP-1 激动剂导致的体重减轻有关。

然而，大多数评估 GLP-1 激动剂在 PCOS 中作用的研究被认为是证据力度不足的，因为样本量小，并且泛化性差，只纳入了超重和肥胖的 PCOS 患者。简言之，GLP-1 激动剂可能有助于改善 PCOS 患者的代谢结果，但它们在生育力方面的作用仍然是实验性的（表 17.1 和表 17.2）。

表 17.1　胰岛素增敏剂在多囊卵巢综合征中的内分泌效果

药物名称	月经情况	排卵率	高雄激素血症
二甲双胍	改善	改善	轻微改善
噻唑烷二酮类药物	改善	未改善或轻微改善	未改善或轻微改善
胰高血糖素样肽-1（GLP-1）受体激动剂（GLP-1 RA）	改善[a]	—	改善[a]
肌醇	—	改善[a]	—
α-硫辛酸	改善[a]	—	—

注：[a] 很少证据支持其效果。

表 17.2　胰岛素增敏剂在多囊卵巢综合征中的代谢效果

药物名称	葡萄糖耐受不良	体重	胰岛素敏感性
二甲双胍	改善	未改善或轻微降低	改善
噻唑烷二酮类药物	改善	未改善或轻微增加	改善
胰高血糖素样肽-1（GLP-1）受体激动剂（GLP-1 RA）	改善	体重减轻	改善[b]
肌醇	—	无影响	改善[a]
α-硫辛酸	—	—	改善[a]

注：[a] 很少证据支持其效果。
[b] 有限的证据支持其效果。

3. 副作用

GLP-1 受体激动剂最常见的副作用包括胃肠道症状（如恶心、呕吐、腹泻）、头痛、头晕和虚弱。恶心和呕吐通常是暂时的，在一两周内会消失。这些药物的其他常见不良反应包括注射部位反应、头痛和鼻咽炎。药物的费用和非肠道给药途径可能会影响治疗的依从性。

（四）其他药物

肌醇，特别是 myoinositol（MI）和 D-chiro-inositol（DCI），有利于胰岛素第二信使的形成，可能导致 IR 的减少。证据表明，DCI 有助于改善排卵率，但对 BMI、WHR 或血压没有影响。除了对血清 SHBG 水平、空腹血糖、空腹胰岛素和血脂（总胆固醇、甘油三酯）有一定效果，DCI 对其他激素参数没有任何影响。因此，国际上关于 PCOS 管理的指南建议谨慎使用肌醇，并将其视为 PCOS 患者的实验性疗法。

α-硫辛酸（alpha-lipoic acid，ALA）是一种生物抗氧化剂，学者们正在研究其作为胰岛素增敏剂的作用。基于氧化应激和 IR 的强烈关联，学者们曾在 T2DM 患者中对 ALA 进行过研究。数据显示，ALA 可能增强外周组织的胰岛素敏感性，并有助于改善糖尿病患者的血糖稳态。

ALA 的使用被认为是 PCOS 的独特治疗方法。对于其在体形偏瘦和超重女性中的效果都有所研究。在每日一次 400 mg 剂量给药后，ALA 可以改善甘油三酯、胰岛素敏感性、月经周期规律性和肝功能参数。多项研究报告了含有 ALA 的不同制剂，特别是 ALA 与 MI 联合的治疗效果。当将每天 3 g 的二甲双胍与 ALA、MI 和二甲双胍（每天 1.7 g）联合治疗进行比较时，在 BMI、HA 和 HOMA 指数方面可以观察到很好的反应。

四、不同胰岛素增敏剂的比较研究

关于在 PCOS 患者中使用不同胰岛素增敏剂的比较数据很少，然而，就内分泌结果而言，二甲双胍与 TZD 或肌醇相比，并未观察到显著差异。就代谢结果而言，当二甲双胍与 TZD 进行比较时，在具有代谢综合征高风险的人群中，二甲双胍对甘油三酯的降低有一定效果，但在 HOMA 指数和空腹胰岛素上则观察到相反的效果。二甲双胍与肌醇相比，两者对代谢结局的影响几乎没有差异。

五、结论

PCOS 的管理对医师来说仍是一项挑战，因为没有单一的治疗方案被证明有效，也无法解决 PCOS 的不同病理生理和表型差异。学者们已经研究和推出了多种胰岛素增敏剂，但它们仍远远未达到应用于 PCOS 临床治疗的程度。二甲双胍是唯一在 PCOS 患者治疗中看到希望的胰岛素增敏剂。然而，它被视为超说明书用药。其他可用的选择（TZD、肌醇、ALA 和 GLP-1 激动剂）大多是实验性的，并且数据显示在联合治疗、剂量和目标对象方面存在巨大的差异。尽管有一些研究展示出有希望的临床结果，但所有该类药物在针对 PCOS 患者的治疗中都被认为是实验性的。

参考文献

1. He L, Wondisford FE. Metformin action: concentrations matter. Cell Metab. 2015;21(2):159-162.
2. Romualdi D, Versace V, Lanzone A. What is new in the landscape of insulin-sensitizing agents for polycystic ovary syndrome treatment. Ther Adv Reprod Health. 2020;14. doi:10.1177/2633494120908709.
3. Tang T, Lord JM, Norman RJ, Yasmin E, Balen AH. Insulin-sensitising drugs (metformin, rosiglitazone, pioglitazone, D-chiro-inositol) for women with polycystic ovary syndrome, oligo amenorrhoea and subfertility. Cochrane Database Syst Rev. 2012;(5):CD003053.
4. Sam S, Ehrmann DA. Metformin therapy for the reproductive and metabolic consequences of polycystic ovary syndrome. Diabetologia. 2017;60(9):1656-1661.
5. Miller RA, Chu Q, Xie J, Foretz M, Viollet B, Birnbaum MJ. Biguanides suppress hepatic glucagon signalling by decreasing production of cyclic AMP. Nature. 2013;494(7436):256-260.
6. Nanjan M, Mohammed M, Kumar BP, Chandrasekar M. Thiazolidinediones as antidiabetic agents: a critical review. Bioorg Chem. 2018;77:548-567.
7. Lamos EM, Malek R, Davis SN. GLP-1 receptor agonists in the treatment of polycystic ovary syndrome. Expert Rev Clin Pharmacol. 2017;10(4):401-408.

阅读清单

1. He L, Wondisford FE. Metformin action: concentrations matter. Cell Metab. 2015;21(2):159-162.
2. Kim LH, Taylor AE, Barbieri RL. Insulin sensitizers and polycystic ovary syndrome: can a diabetes medication treat infertility? Fertil Steril. 2000;73(6):1097-1098.
3. Lamos EM, Malek R, Davis SN. GLP-1 receptor agonists in the treatment of polycystic ovary syndrome. Expert Rev Clin Pharmacol. 2017;10(4):401-408.
4. Nanjan MJ, Mohammed M, Kumar BP, Chandrasekar MJN. Thiazolidinediones as antidiabetic agents: a critical review. Bioorg Chem. 2018;77:548-567.
5. Pasquali R, Gambineri A. Insulin-sensitizing agents in polycystic ovary syndrome. Eur J Endocrinol. 2006;154(6):763-775.
6. Romualdi D, Versace V, Lanzone A. What is new in the landscape of insulin-sensitizing agents for polycystic ovary syndrome treatment. Ther Adv Reprod Health. 2020;14. doi:10.1177/2633494120908709.
7. Sam S, Ehrmann DA. Metformin therapy for the reproductive and metabolic consequences of polycystic ovary syndrome. Diabetologia. 2017;60(9):1656-1661.
8. Stracquadanio M, Ciotta L. Metabolic Aspects of PCOS. Heidelberg, NY: Springer; 2015.
9. Tang T, Lord JM, Norman RJ, Yasmin E, Balen AH. Insulin-sensitising drugs (metformin, rosiglitazone, pioglitazone, D-chiro-inositol) for women with polycystic ovary syndrome, oligo amenorrhoea and subfertility. Cochrane Database Syst Rev. 2012;(5):CD003053.
10. Xing C, Li C, He B. Insulin sensitizers for improving the endocrine and metabolic profile in overweight women with PCOS. J Clin Endocrinol Metab. 2020;105(9):2950-2963.
11. Zhao H, Xing C, Zhang J, He B. Comparative efficacy of oral insulin sensitizers metformin, thiazolidinediones, inositol, and berberine in improving endocrine and metabolic profiles in women with PCOS: a network meta-analysis. Reprod Health. 2021;18(1):171.

第十八章 降低多囊卵巢综合征患者的心血管疾病风险

一、引言

心血管疾病（CVD）是女性死亡最常见的原因。多囊卵巢综合征（PCOS）患者普遍存在 CVD 的典型风险因素，包括代谢综合征（MetS）。PCOS 与血脂异常、肥胖和糖尿病（DM）相关。此外，研究发现 PCOS 患者存在亚临床 CVD 标志物的增加，如冠状动脉钙化（coronary calcium，CAC）、C 反应蛋白（CRP）和内皮功能障碍。这主要基于观察性研究。目前尚缺乏大型前瞻性研究探讨 PCOS 与 CVD（包括急性冠脉综合征和缺血性脑卒中）之间的因果关系。

在 PCOS 患者中进行 CVD 风险评估可以提供有效的 CVD 预防窗口。PCOS 女性应该进行早期风险分层以实现预防效果。虽然目前已经确定了 CVD 风险增强因素和 PCOS 之间的关联，但不确定该关联是否会转化为临床和亚临床 CVD 的直接风险。本章将回顾 PCOS 患者中 CVD 风险因素及其管理。

二、多囊卵巢综合征中的心血管疾病风险因素

高血压、DM 和肥胖是 PCOS 患者发生 CVD 的主要风险因素。代谢和激素紊乱是 PCOS 的标志，在高血压、DM、血脂异常和其他 CVD 风险增强因素的发病机制中起着重要作用。

（一）高血压和多囊卵巢综合征

高血压是 CVD 重要的已知风险因素。虽然没有基于人口的大规模研究支持该关联，但小型观察性研究报告称，与匹配的对照组相比，年轻的 PCOS 女性普遍存在更高的高血压患病率。

PCOS 中的高血压可能与体重指数（BMI）和肥胖无关。Joham 等在大型队列中证明，育龄女性中，PCOS 女性发生高血压比非 PCOS 女性更常见。在亚组分析中，非 PCOS 患者中高血压与 BMI 有关，但在 PCOS 患者中无关，提示 PCOS 和高血压之间的关系独立于 BMI。

尽管 PCOS 患者发生高血压是多因素导致的，但醛固酮是高血压发展的关键因素。与健康女性相比，年轻的 PCOS 患者醛固酮水平更高。PCOS 患者的高雄激素血症（HA）可能会引起高血压。在一项实验研究中，虽然机制不详，但将雄激素给予卵巢切除的雌

鼠可以引起剂量依赖性的血压升高。当阻断肾素-血管紧张素系统（renin-angiotensin system，RAS）时，未观察到这种效应。

增加的雄激素已被认为与血管紧张素原的表达增加有关。研究表明PCOS和月经稀发者体内的肾素和肾素原水平较高。这解释了雄激素通过RAS途径在PCOS患者高血压病理生理中的可能作用。Chen等研究了150例年轻PCOS患者中雄激素和高血压之间的关系，并发现在校正BMI和血脂异常后，收缩压（SBP）和舒张压（DBP）都与游离雄激素指数（FAI）强相关。SBP最高四分位数的女性FAI水平也高于SBP较低（$P = 0.0006$）和SBP最低（$P = 0.019$）的四分位数组。

同样，血管病变的标志物内皮素-1是PCOS相关高血压的另一个可能介质。PCOS患者的内皮素-1水平高于对照组（$P < 0.02$）。高胰岛素血症也被认为是高血压的风险因素，原因是自主神经失衡、钠潴留和一氧化氮生成受损。

（二）肥胖、代谢综合征与多囊卵巢综合征

肥胖在PCOS患者中很常见。多达80%的PCOS患者肥胖或超重。与年龄匹配的健康人群相比，PCOS女性的腰臀比（WHR）较高。对来自34个研究的14 000多名研究对象进行的系统回顾和荟萃分析发现，PCOS患者中向心性肥胖的患病率较高［风险比（RR）：1.73］，这与年龄和地理分布无关。MetS和PCOS可能有共同的发病机制。向心性肥胖、血脂异常、胰岛素抵抗（IR）、高血压和空腹血糖升高等经典风险因素的重叠提示存在共同的通路。

Ehrmann等调查了394例PCOS患者，其中MetS的患病率为33.4%。不同种族/民族之间的患病率没有差异，其中50%的亚洲人、34%的高加索人、26%的非裔美国人和31%的西班牙裔有MetS的症状。与没有MetS的PCOS患者相比，该队列中存在MetS的PCOS患者与更高的SBP、DBP、BMI、WHR以及更宽的腰围相关联。

PCOS患者的肥胖可能是由于IR和升高的胰岛素水平。高胰岛素血症促进了卵巢中类固醇的合成，并抑制肝脏中雄激素结合球蛋白的产生。由此引发的游离雄激素水平升高导致内脏脂肪积累和体重增加。

MetS是一组心血管代谢风险因素的集合，包括腰围增加、甘油三酯升高、高密度脂蛋白胆固醇（HDL-C）降低、高血压和血糖升高。对来自15个研究的6000多名女性进行的荟萃分析显示，与非PCOS的女性相比，PCOS女性更容易患MetS（OR：2.8）。因此，IR和高胰岛素血症在MetS的发病机制和临床表现中起着核心作用。

（三）胰岛素抵抗、糖尿病和多囊卵巢综合征

超过1/3的PCOS患者检测结果提示存在糖耐量减低（IGT），有7%~10%的PCOS患者患有DM。无论年龄和BMI如何，PCOS患者患DM的风险增加。此外，与非DM人群相比，DM年轻女性患者中PCOS的患病率更高。

专家共识认为，PCOS是DM的一个风险因素，而DM是CVD的一个已知风险因素。

这是因为 PCOS 女性无论 BMI 如何，她们的 IR 都升高。荟萃分析显示，与对照组相比，PCOS 患者的胰岛素敏感性（IS）较低（平均效应：−27%，99%CI：±6%）。然而，在 BMI 较高的患者中，IS 进一步降低了 15%，而在性激素结合球蛋白（SHBG）较低的患者中会再降低 10%。

PCOS 中的 IR 和 DM 的发病机制在文献中有非常详尽的描述。胰岛素信号通路的缺陷和胰岛素受体及其底物的磷酸化障碍是 IR 和 DM 的主要原因。其他因素包括脂肪组织中葡萄糖转运体水平降低、肝脏中胰岛素清除能力下降、线粒体功能障碍，以及丝氨酸激酶的活化。

（四）血脂异常和多囊卵巢综合征

血脂异常，尤其是低密度脂蛋白（LDL）水平的升高与 CVD 密切相关。PCOS 女性常见的血脂异常包括甘油三酯（TG）和 LDL 水平的增加，以及高密度脂蛋白（HDL）水平的降低。一项对 30 余个研究进行的荟萃分析显示，与匹配年龄的非 PCOS 女性相比，PCOS 女性的 TG 水平高出 26 mg/dL，低密度脂蛋白胆固醇（LDL-C）水平高出 12.6 mg/dL，而高密度脂蛋白胆固醇（HDL-C）水平低于 6 mg/dL。PCOS 患者的血脂异常主要是受 IR、肥胖和 HA 的影响。

三、多囊卵巢综合征和心血管疾病

PCOS 包含多种代谢异常，这些异常是 CVD 的主要危险因素。然而，有关 PCOS 与临床 CVD 之间直接关联的数据却有限。PCOS 中 CVD 风险的增加是基于 PCOS 女性存在的动脉粥样硬化性心血管疾病（ASCVD）风险因素推断的。

（一）临床心血管疾病

一项来自丹麦的大规模人群研究（对 7 万多名女性进行了研究，并对其进行了 10 年以上的随访）显示，与匹配年龄的对照组相比，PCOS 患者发展为临床 CVD 的风险比（hazard ratio，HR）为 1.7。PCOS 患者诊断 CVD 的中位年龄为 35 岁。肥胖、DM 和不孕症都与 CVD 的发病率增加有关。

澳大利亚的一项针对 2.5 万名女性的大规模人群研究报告称，PCOS 组的缺血性心脏病和脑血管疾病发病率较匹配年龄的对照组高，校正后的 HR 分别为 2.8 和 2.5。另一项对 5 项研究进行的荟萃分析显示，经过 BMI 校正后，PCOS 组患 CVD 的风险是对照组的两倍。还有一项由 Luqian Zhao 等进行的荟萃分析显示，PCOS 女性患 CVD 的发病率更高（OR：1.30）。

另一项针对 8 项研究的荟萃分析显示，PCOS 患者脑血管意外的发病风险升高（OR：1.36）。然而，在校正 BMI 后，这种差异在统计上不具有显著性（OR：1.24，95%CI：0.98～1.59）。

（二）亚临床心血管疾病

多项研究对 PCOS 患者亚临床 CVD 的标志物进行了研究，包括冠状动脉钙化评分、内膜中层厚度、炎症标志物（如 CRP）和内皮素 -1（一种血管内皮功能障碍的标志物）。

Rose C. Cristian 等的研究报告称，与匹配的对照组相比，PCOS 女性冠状动脉钙化的患病率增加。另一项研究显示，在校正年龄和 BMI 后，PCOS 患者冠状动脉钙化评分较高。

一项荟萃分析显示，PCOS 女性的颈动脉内膜中层厚度（carotid intima-media thickness，CIMT）明显升高，较非 PCOS 组更容易患临床 CVD。PCOS 患者 CIMT 增加的原因可能与向心性肥胖，胰岛素、炎症标志物、TG 和 LDL-C 的水平升高，以及 HDL-C 水平降低有关。

针对 5000 多名女性进行的 45 项研究的荟萃分析报告称，PCOS 组的 CRP 和同型半胱氨酸水平显著升高。荟萃分析进一步显示，PCOS 女性的纤溶酶原激活物抑制物 -1、内皮素 -1 和血管内皮生长因子水平升高。多项研究已报道 PCOS 中存在内皮功能障碍，并进一步显示内皮功能障碍与炎症标志物（包括 CRP）水平升高同时存在，这提供了慢性炎症导致内皮功能障碍和动脉粥样硬化的间接证据。

四、多囊卵巢综合征患者的心血管疾病风险管理

PCOS 患者 CVD 风险的降低需要对经典的风险因素进行有效管理，并且医师及患者都需要对增加的 CVD 风险有基本的理解。在 PCOS 中实现对 CVD 风险的最佳识别和管理需要专注于早期代谢筛查和干预，给予营养和运动指导，并提供行为和心理支持的多学科团队合作。鉴于 PCOS 患者 CVD 风险因素的普遍存在，应采用个体化方法在每次就诊中对患者进行 CVD 风险分层。每次接诊都是识别高风险患者并向他们宣传健康生活方式的机会。专家们目前认为，在 PCOS 患者中降低 CVD 风险的关键潜在治疗靶点是胰岛素 - 糖代谢和控制 DM 发病风险，这是 CVD 的核心风险因素。

雄激素过多和多囊卵巢综合征协会（AE-PCOS）的共识声明建议根据患者的风险将患者分为"有风险"和"高风险"两种。"有风险"的类别是指肥胖、吸烟成瘾、高血压、血脂异常、任何亚临床血管疾病或 IGT 的证据，以及早发 CVD 阳性家族史的患者。此外，已确诊的 MetS 或 2 型糖尿病（T2DM），以及明显的肾血管疾病的 PCOS 患者属于高风险类别。

根据新近 CVD 的相关文献，可在以下策略上努力：

- 所有患者在每次就医时应进行 BMI 和腰围测量以评估腹型肥胖。
- 与美国心脏协会（American Heart Association，AHA）女性 CVD 预防指南一致，需在两年或更早的时间内（如果体重增加）进行完整的血脂检查。对于没有额外 CVD 风险因素的女性，目标 LDL 水平应小于 130 mg/dL，所有"高风险"患者的 LDL-C 水

平应降至 100 mg/dL 以下。

- 应对所有患者进行 IGT 筛查。每两年或更频繁地对高风险患者进行 2 小时 75 g 口服葡萄糖耐量试验。BMI 超过 30 kg/m² 或有晚期肾血管疾病的女性应重点筛查。IGT 检测结果阳性的患者应每年接受 T2DM 筛查。这些患者的 HbA1c 阈值应保持在 6.5%。
- 每次接诊应测量血压以便发现早发的高血压。目标血压为 120/80 mmHg 或更低。
- 应建议 PCOS 患者进行强化的生活方式干预。这将降低 IGT 转化为 T2DM 的风险。
- 开具复方口服避孕药（COC）治疗月经不规律的医师应注意，COC 可能会导致 CVD 风险增加。
- 使用二甲双胍会导致 IGT 减少且有利于血脂的纠正。理论上，这可以间接改善长期心血管结局。
- 需要强有力的社会心理支持来鼓励 PCOS 患者坚持生活方式干预和对抗抑郁。文献表明患有抑郁症和 T2DM 的患者对生活方式干预的依从性较弱。
- 对于高血压和血脂异常的患者，采用指南指定的药物治疗有利于达到目标水平。

五、降低多囊卵巢综合征患者心血管疾病风险的主要策略

（一）生活方式干预

生活方式干预是 PCOS 患者的一线治疗方法，包括减重、戒烟、每天达到推荐运动量和饮食调整。减重有望降低 CVD 风险。患者应力求每天减少摄入 500~1000 kcal 的热量，脂肪摄入不超过总热量的 30%，饱和脂肪摄入不超过总热量的 10%。至少进行 30 分钟中等强度的锻炼。超重患者应该首先力争减轻 5%~10% 的体重，长期目标是减轻 10%~20% 的体重，并使腰围小于 88 cm。

（二）药物治疗

治疗药物包括胰岛素增敏剂、降低胆固醇药物和降压药物。

六、结论

PCOS 患者中出现典型 CVD 风险因素的发生率更高，IR 在这些风险因素的发生机制中起到了重要作用。虽然向心性肥胖可能会加剧动脉粥样硬化，但无论 BMI 如何，PCOS 患者都存在较高的 CVD 风险。此外，与对照组相比，PCOS 患者亚临床 ASCVD 的患病率更高。然而，关于 PCOS 与临床 ASCVD（心肌梗死和脑卒中）之间直接关联的数据有限。需要进行基于人群的研究以建立 PCOS 与临床 CVD 之间的直接关联。生活方式干预，包括健康饮食、体育活动、减重和戒烟，可以降低 PCOS 患者的 CVD 风险。所有 PCOS 患者应定期进行 ASCVD 风险筛查，并保持健康的生活方式。

参考文献

1. Centre for Disease Control and Prevention. Women and Heart Disease. 2022. https://www.cdc.gov/heartdisease/women.
2. Zhu T, Cui J, Goodarzi MO. Polycystic ovary syndrome and risk of type 2 diabetes, coronary heart disease, and stroke. Diabetes. 2021;70(2):627-637.
3. Diamanti-Kandarakis E, Alexandraki K, Piperi C, et al. Inflammatory and endothelial markers in women with polycystic ovary syndrome. Eur J Clin Invest. 2006;36(10):691-697.
4. Osibogun O, Ogunmoroti O, Michos ED. Polycystic ovary syndrome and cardiometabolic risk: opportunities for cardiovascular disease prevention. Trends Cardiovasc Med. 2020;30(7):399-404.
5. Young L, Cho L. Unique cardiovascular risk factors in women. Heart. 2019;105(21):1656-1660.
6. Osibogun O, Ogunmoroti O, Michos ED. Polycystic ovary syndrome and cardiometabolic risk: opportunities for cardiovascular disease prevention. Trends Cardiovasc Med. 2020;30(7):399-404.
7. Marchesan LB, Spritzer PM. ACC/AHA 2017 definition of high blood pressure: implications for women with polycystic ovary syndrome. Fertil Steril. 2019;111(3):579-587.e1.
8. Joham AE, Boyle JA, Zoungas S, Teede HJ. Hypertension in reproductive-aged women with polycystic ovary syndrome and association with obesity. Am J Hypertens. 2015;28(7):847-851.
9. Cascella T, Palomba S, Tauchmanovà L, et al. Serum aldosterone concentration and cardiovascular risk in women with the polycystic ovarian syndrome. J Clin Endocrinol Metab. 2006;91(11):4395-4400.
10. Reckelhoff JF. Gender differences in the regulation of blood pressure. Hypertension. 2001;37(5):1199-1208.
11. Uncu G, Sözer MC, Develioğlu O, Cengiz C. The role of plasma renin activity in distinguishing patients with polycystic ovary syndrome (PCOS) from oligomenorrheic patients without PCOS. Gynecol Endocrinol. 2002;16(6):447-452.
12. Chen MJ, Yang WS, Yang JH, Chen CL, Ho HN, Yang YS. Relationship between androgen levels and blood pressure in young women with polycystic ovary syndrome. Hypertension. 2007;49(6):1442-1447.
13. Diamanti-Kandarakis E, Spina G, Kouli C, Migdalis I. Increased endothelin-1 levels in women with polycystic ovary syndrome and the beneficial effect of metformin therapy. J Clin Endocrinol Metab. 2001;86(10):4666-4673.
14. Sam S. Obesity and polycystic ovary syndrome. Obes Manag. 2007;3(2):69-73.
15. Lim SS, Davies MJ, Norman RJ, Moran LJ. Overweight, obesity and central obesity in women with polycystic ovary syndrome: a systematic review and meta-analysis. Hum Reprod Update. 2012;18(6):618-637.
16. Third Report of the National Cholesterol Education Program (NCEP) expert panel on detection, evaluation, and treatment of high blood cholesterol in adults (Adult Treatment Panel III) final report. Circulation. 2002;106(25):3143-3421.
17. Rachoń D, Teede H. Ovarian function and obesity-interrelationship, impact on women's reproductive lifespan and treatment options. Mol Cell Endocrinol. 2010;316(2):172-179.
18. Grundy SM, Cleeman JI, Daniels SR, et al. Diagnosis and management of the metabolic syndrome: an American Heart Association/National Heart, Lung, and Blood Institute Scientific Statement. Circulation. 2005;112(17):2735-2752.
19. Moran LJ, Misso ML, Wild RA, Norman RJ. Impaired glucose tolerance, type 2 diabetes and metabolic syndrome in polycystic ovary syndrome: a systematic review and meta-analysis. Hum Reprod Update. 2010;16(4):347-363.
20. Lim SS, Kakoly NS, Tan JWJ, et al. Metabolic syndrome in polycystic ovary syndrome: a systematic review, meta-analysis, and meta-regression. Obes Rev. 2019;20(2):339-352.
21. Salley KE, Wickham EP, Cheang KI, Essah PA, Karjane NW, Nestler JE. Glucose intolerance in polycystic ovary syndrome-a position statement of the Androgen Excess Society. J Clin Endocrinol Metab. 2007;92(12):4546-4556.

22. Kakoly NS, Earnest A, Teede HJ, Moran LJ, Joham AE. The impact of obesity on the incidence of type 2 diabetes among women with polycystic ovary syndrome. Diabetes Care. 2019;42(4):560-567.
23. Sirmans SM, Pate KA. Epidemiology, diagnosis, and management of polycystic ovary syndrome. Clin Epidemiol. 2013;6:1-13.
24. Cassar S, Misso ML, Hopkins WG, Shaw CS, Teede HJ, Stepto NK. Insulin resistance in polycystic ovary syndrome: a systematic review and meta-analysis of euglycaemic-hyperinsulinaemic clamp studies. Hum Reprod. 2016;31(11):2619-2631.
25. Anagnostis P, Tarlatzis BC, Kauff man RP. Polycystic ovarian syndrome (PCOS): long-term metabolic consequences. Metabolism. 2018;86:33-43.
26. Weitgasser R, Ratzinger M, Hemetsberger M, Siostrzonek P. [LDL-cholesterol and cardiovascular events: the lower the better?]. Wien Med Wochenschr. 2018;168(5-6):108-120.
27. Wild RA, Rizzo M, Clifton S, Carmina E. Lipid levels in polycystic ovary syndrome: systematic review and meta-analysis. Fertil Steril. 2011;95(3):1073-1079.e1-11.
28. Diamanti-Kandarakis E, Spina G, Kouli C, Migdalis I. Increased endothelin-1 levels in women with polycystic ovary syndrome and the beneficial effect of metformin therapy. J Clin Endocrinol Metab. 2001;86(10):4666-4673.
29. Wild RA. Polycystic ovary syndrome: a risk for coronary artery disease? Am J Obstet Gynecol. 2002;186(1):35-43.
30. Glintborg D, Rubin KH, Nybo M, Abrahamsen B, Andersen M. Cardiovascular disease in a nationwide population of Danish women with polycystic ovary syndrome. Cardiovasc Diabetol. 2018;17(1):37.
31. Corrigenda. J Clin Endocrinol Metab. 2015;100(6):2502.
32. de Groot PC, Dekkers OM, Romijn JA, Dieben SW, Helmerhorst FM. PCOS, coronary heart disease, stroke and the influence of obesity: a systematic review and meta-analysis. Hum Reprod Update. 2011;17(4):495-500.
33. Zhao L, Zhu Z, Lou H, et al. Polycystic ovary syndrome (PCOS) and the risk of coronary heart disease (CHD): a meta-analysis. Oncotarget. 2016;7(23):33715-33721.
34. Zhou Y, Wang X, Jiang Y, et al. Association between polycystic ovary syndrome and the risk of stroke and all-cause mortality: insights from a meta-analysis. Gynecol Endocrinol. 2017;33(12):904-910.
35. Christian RC, Dumesic DA, Behrenbeck T, Oberg AL, Sheedy PF II, Fitzpatrick LA. Prevalence and predictors of coronary artery calcification in women with polycystic ovary syndrome. J Clin Endocrinol Metab. 2003;88(6):2562-2568.
36. Talbott EO, Zborowski JV, Rager JR, Boudreaux MY, Edmundowicz DA, Guzick DS. Evidence for an association between metabolic cardiovascular syndrome and coronary and aortic calcification among women with polycystic ovary syndrome. J Clin Endocrinol Metab. 2004;89(11):5454-5461.
37. Meyer ML, Malek AM, Wild RA, Korytkowski MT, Talbott EO. Carotid artery intima-media thickness in polycystic ovary syndrome: a systematic review and meta-analysis. Hum Reprod Update. 2012;18(2):112-126.
38. Cascella T, Palomba S, De Sio I, et al. Visceral fat is associated with cardiovascular risk in women with polycystic ovary syndrome. Hum Reprod. 2008;23(1):153-159.
39. Saha S, Sarkar C, Biswas SC, Karim R. Correlation between serum lipid profile and carotid intima-media thickness in polycystic ovarian syndrome. Indian J Clin Biochem. 2008;23(3):262-266.
40. Toulis KA, Goulis DG, Mintziori G, et al. Meta-analysis of cardiovascular disease risk markers in women with polycystic ovary syndrome. Hum Reprod Update. 2011;17(6):741-760.
41. Diamanti-Kandarakis E, Alexandraki K, Piperi C, et al. Inflammatory and endothelial markers in women with polycystic ovary syndrome. Eur J Clin Invest. 2006;36(10):691-697.
42. Wild RA, Carmina E, Diamanti-Kandarakis E, et al. Assessment of cardiovascular risk and prevention of cardiovascular disease in women with the polycystic ovary syndrome: a consensus statement by the Androgen Excess and Polycystic Ovary Syndrome (AE-PCOS) Society. J Clin Endocrinol Metab. 2010;95(5):2038-2049.

43. Mosca L. Guidelines for prevention of cardiovascular disease in women: a summary of recommendations. Prev Cardiol. 2007;10(suppl 4):19-25.
44. Knowler WC, Barrett-Connor E, Fowler SE, et al. Reduction in the incidence of type 2 diabetes with lifestyle intervention or metformin. N Engl J Med. 2002;346(6):393-403.
45. Kaminski P, Szpotanska-Sikorska M, Wielgos M. Cardiovascular risk and the use of oral contraceptives. Neuro Endocrinol Lett. 2013;34(7):587-9. PMID: 24464000.
46. Roach RE, Helmerhorst FM, Lijfering WM, Stijnen T, Algra A, Dekkers OM. Combined oral contraceptives: the risk of myocardial infarction and ischemic stroke. Cochrane Database of Systematic Reviews. 2015(8).
47. Sumlin LL, Garcia TJ, Brown SA, et al. Depression and adherence to lifestyle changes in type 2 diabetes: a systematic review. Diabetes Educ. 2014;40(6):731-744.
48. McCartney CR, Marshall JC. CLINICAL PRACTICE. polycystic ovary syndrome. N Engl J Med. 2016;375(1):54-64.

第十九章 多囊卵巢综合征患者低生育力的管理

一、引言

多囊卵巢综合征（PCOS）是最常见的内分泌紊乱疾病，影响着约 20% 的育龄期女性。该综合征表现多样，包括临床或生化高雄激素血症（HA）、排卵功能障碍，以及超声检查提示多囊卵巢形态（PCOM）（表 19.1）。

表 19.1 多囊卵巢综合征的诊断标准

标准	描述
雄激素过多	临床[a] 和（或）生化高雄激素血症[b]
卵巢功能障碍	稀发排卵或无排卵和（或）多囊卵巢形态[c]
排除其他原因	其他病因导致的雄激素过多或排卵障碍[d]

改编自：Azziz R. Diagnostic criteria for polycystic ovary syndrome: A reappraisal. Fertil Steril. 2005；83(5): 1343–1346.

注：[a] 如多毛症。
[b] 高雄激素血症，如总睾酮水平或游离睾酮水平升高。
[c] 定义为中等大小的卵泡数量（直径为 2～9 mm 的卵泡＞8 个）和（或）卵巢体积增大（即＞10 cm³），伴有月经周期不规律（周期＞35 天或＜21 天）。
[d] 包括但不限于 21-羟化酶缺乏症、非经典肾上腺增生、甲状腺功能异常、高催乳素血症、分泌雄激素的肿瘤或药物引起的雄激素过多。

PCOS 是一个多因素疾病，涉及遗传、激素、神经内分泌和环境等不同因素。高胰岛素血症是 PCOS 的特征，它与胰岛素抵抗（IR）、雄激素和黄体生成素（LH）分泌增加相关，可对该综合征的激素、代谢和生殖效应起作用。PCOS 属于世界卫生组织（WHO）Ⅱ型排卵障碍，涵盖正常促性腺激素性腺功能减退。根据 2012 年美国国立卫生研究院（NIH）的标准，PCOS 的 A 型、B 型和 D 型存在排卵功能障碍（表 19.2）。

表 19.2 2012 年美国国立卫生研究院标准将多囊卵巢综合征分为 4 种表型

序号	表型	特征
1	A 型	高雄激素血症+排卵功能障碍+PCOM
2	B 型	高雄激素血症+排卵功能障碍
3	C 型	高雄激素血症+PCOM
4	D 型	排卵功能障碍+PCOM

注：PCOM，多囊卵巢形态。

这些女性通常表现为月经不规律（从月经稀发到闭经）和不孕症，但并非所有 PCOS 患者都难以怀孕，由于排卵障碍，75%～80% 的患者存在不孕症。

二、促性腺激素刺激卵巢的生理学原则

在出生时，每侧卵巢中有100万～200万个原始卵泡。这个数量逐渐减少，到青春期时只剩下3000个卵泡。在未知的刺激下，这些原始卵泡逐渐发展成为初级、次级和小窦状卵泡。初级发育（促性腺激素应答）需要70～80天，在这个阶段，直径为2～5 mm的小卵泡开始对低水平的促性腺激素有反应。一旦卵泡达到窦状卵泡阶段，其生长即转变为卵泡刺激素（FSH）依赖性模式，并具有了周期性募集的能力（促性腺激素依赖）。在青春期，下丘脑-垂体系统的成熟刺激FSH分泌，达到激发排卵周期的水平。从小窦状卵泡阶段发展成为排卵前卵泡需要两种促性腺激素的共同作用（即FSH和LH）。在卵泡期的前半段，FSH占主导地位，在这个阶段的后半段则由LH起主导作用。通常情况下，LH作用于卵泡膜细胞并激活LH受体以促进雄激素的产生，而FSH作用于卵巢颗粒细胞，将雄激素转化为雌激素（图19.1）。

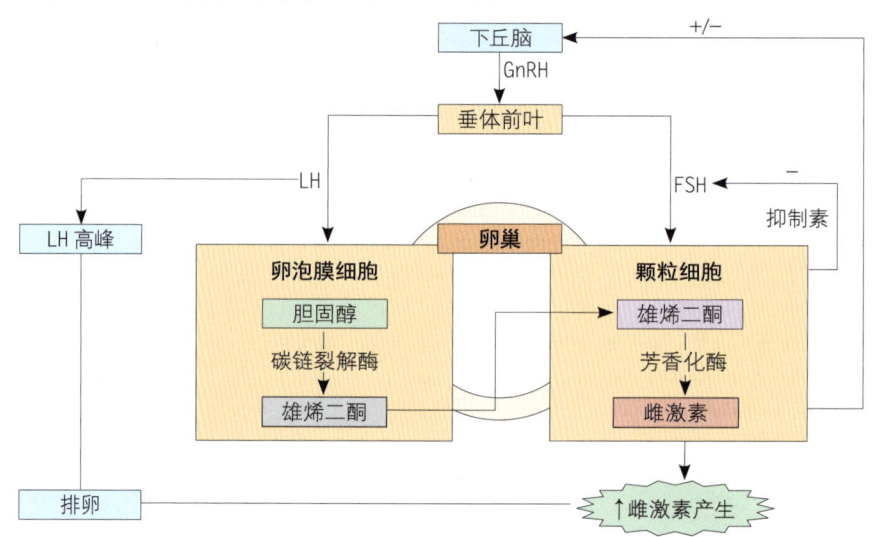

FSH，卵泡刺激素；GnRH，促性腺激素释放激素；LH，黄体生成素。
图19.1 下丘脑-垂体轴、"两种细胞-两种促性腺激素"概念和激素相互作用

（一）卵泡刺激素阈值/窗口期概念

在月经周期中，FSH水平在黄体后期逐渐上升，使得一组小窦状卵泡被募集（解除闭锁）并进一步生长（图19.2）。在卵泡期的早期到中期，血清FSH水平上升超过特定的水平（FSH阈值）并持续一段时间，这段时间被称为FSH窗口期。一旦出现一个直径为9～10 mm的主导卵泡，FSH水平就会下降到阈值以下（图19.2）。在FSH的作用下，主导卵泡的颗粒细胞获得LH受体，排卵前卵泡进一步发育，变得依赖LH（图19.3）。其余的卵泡由于FSH水平较低而发生闭锁。这种阈值/窗口期概念对于单卵泡的发育非常重要。如果FSH窗口期扩大并且FSH水平在阈值以上保持的时间更长，就会发生多卵泡发育，而在阈值以上的时间较短则会导致单卵泡排卵。

第十九章　多囊卵巢综合征患者低生育力的管理

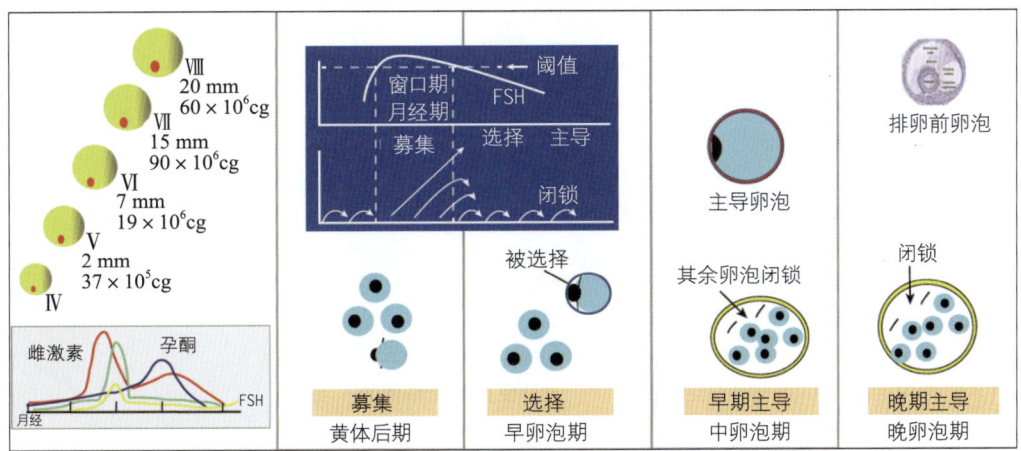

FSH，卵泡刺激素；LH，黄体生成素。
图19.2　促性腺激素依赖性卵泡生长和卵泡刺激素窗口期概念
来源：http://slideplayer.com/slide/575035/

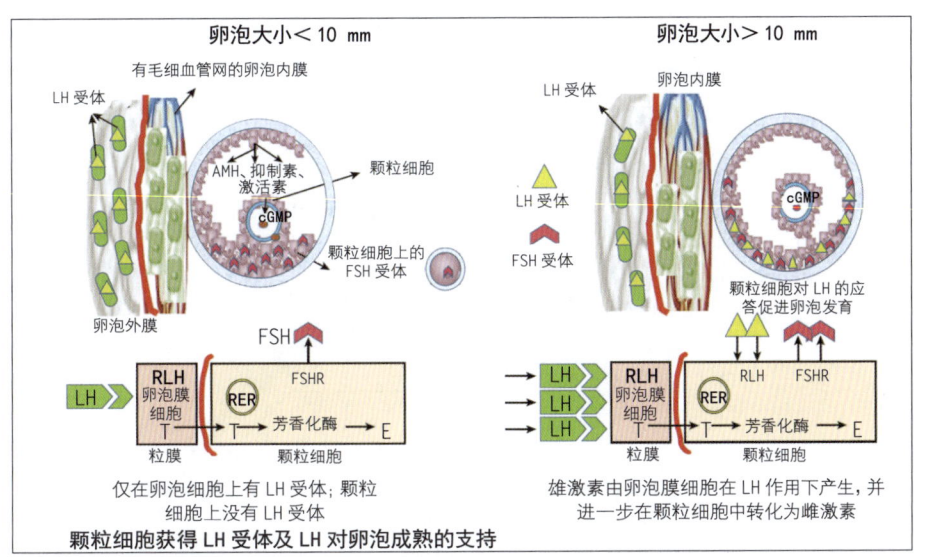

AMH，抗米勒管激素；cGMP，环磷酸鸟苷；E，雌激素；FSH，卵泡刺激素；LH，黄体生成素；RER，粗面内质网；RLH，黄体生成素受体；FSHR，卵泡刺激素受体；T，睾酮。
图19.3　黄体生成素受体的获取

改编自：https://clinicalgate.com/getting-ready-for-pregnancy/ and Slide player Regulation of Menstural Cycle: by CEM FICICIOGLU, M.D, Ph.D, AA, MBA

（二）黄体生成素在卵泡发育中的作用

最佳的卵泡发育也取决于LH的最低暴露水平。在晚卵泡期，上升的LH水平促进卵泡萎缩，维持优势卵泡生长，并诱导单卵泡排卵。LH阈值对卵泡发育至关重要，因为过高的水平（如在PCOS患者中所观察到的）会妨碍卵泡发育并导致过早黄体化，而低水平则会导致雄激素和雌激素合成不足、卵泡发育受损，以及子宫内膜增生不充分（图19.4）。

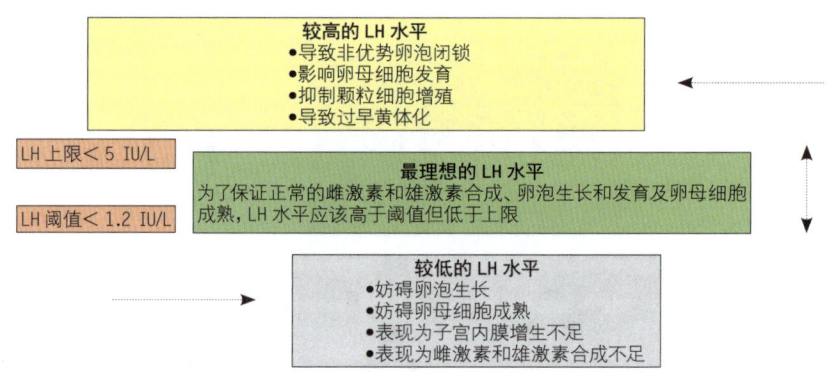

图 19.4 黄体生成素上限概念

（三）抗米勒管激素和卵泡发育

卵泡发育的另一个重要调节因子是抗米勒管激素（AMH），它属于生长因子受体β超家族。AMH 主要由直径不超过 4 mm 的窦前卵泡和小窦状卵泡的颗粒细胞产生。它作为"卵泡池的护卫"，使 FSH 受体和芳香化酶表达降低。此外，AMH 会阻止渐进性卵泡发育和早期静止卵泡进展为活跃卵泡。一旦卵泡直径＞ 8 mm，AMH 的影响就会减少，这些卵泡会变得对 FSH 的作用更加敏感（图 19.5）。这种转变促进了生长卵泡中雌激素分泌的不断增加，并导致优势卵泡被选择并排卵。

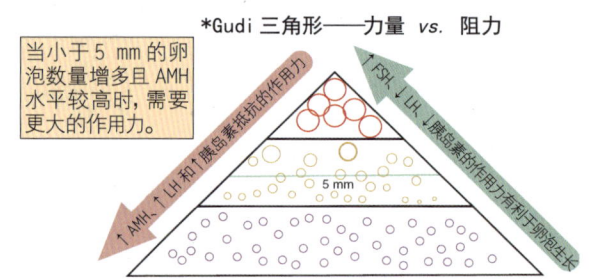

AMH，抗米勒管激素；FSH，卵泡刺激素；LH，黄体生成素。

图 19.5 克服阻力的力量

* 感谢 Anil Gudi 教授和 Fertility Plus http://www.fertilityplu.org.uk/

三、病理生理学：多囊卵巢综合征对生育力的影响

有关更多信息，请参阅第七章——"多囊卵巢综合征和低生育力：排卵调节障碍和生育力问题"。

PCOS 的病理生理学涉及下丘脑 – 垂体 – 卵巢（HPO）轴的紊乱、胰岛素分泌和雄激素水平的增加及卵巢功能的改变。PCOS 可以通过不同的方式影响生育力。这些患者的生育潜力降低归因于慢性无排卵和子宫内膜容受性的改变。在 PCOS 中，LH 和 FSH 失衡，雄激素和胰岛素水平升高。这三重激素变化，以及低维生素 D 水平增强了 AMH 的表达，并导致排卵功能障碍。高水平的 AMH 会抑制芳香化酶的表达，影响 FSH 的释

放，增加卵泡对 FSH 作用的抵抗。最终，卵泡的发育受到阻碍，它们的生长停滞在直径 4～8 mm。由于没有优势卵泡的发育，排卵和卵子受精也不会发生，最终导致不孕症。即使排卵发生，激素失衡也会影响子宫内膜并干扰受精卵的着床（表 19.3）。

表 19.3　多囊卵巢综合征中出现的问题

问题	描述
促性腺激素分泌异常	• 促性腺激素释放激素（GnRH）脉冲幅度增加 • LH 的过度分泌；在瘦型 PCOS 表型中尤为明显 • FSH 作用的内在缺陷 • 吻素水平升高
胰岛素抵抗	• 高胰岛素血症 • 高雄激素血症（包括子宫内暴露于高雄激素水平）
类固醇合成异常	• 卵巢的雄激素和雌激素产生增加 • 卵泡对 FSH 作用的抵抗增加，导致卵泡成熟和排卵障碍，并抑制芳香化酶的表达 • 大量小卵泡发育停滞（但能对外源性 FSH 做出反应）
子宫内膜容受性受影响	PCOS 女性的子宫内环境发生的变化有以下几方面： • 孕酮敏感性 • 黏附分子 • 细胞因子 • 炎症级联反应 • 氧化状态
微量营养素受影响（缺乏和代谢紊乱）	• 维生素 D 缺乏 • 通过甲基四氢叶酸还原酶基因的改变干扰叶酸代谢

改编自：Azziz R, Carmina E, Chen Z, et al. Polycystic ovary syndrome. Nature Rev Dis Primers. 2016: 11; 2(1): 1-8.

四、多囊卵巢综合征患者不孕症的检查

PCOS 通常表现为 LH 水平和空腹血清胰岛素水平升高，以及 LH∶FSH 反转。然而，PCOS 的确诊仍基于其他无排卵原因的排除，包括甲状腺疾病、21- 羟化酶缺乏症、高催乳素血症、库欣综合征和分泌雄激素的肿瘤。对于想要怀孕的 PCOS 患者，应考虑进行以下检测：

• 激素水平检测，包括血清睾酮、促甲状腺激素（TSH）、催乳素和月经第 3 天 FSH 水平，以了解月经稀发/无排卵情况。

• 超声检查，以评估 PCOM 和监测卵泡。

• 所有接受诱导排卵治疗的 PCOS 患者需进行精液分析检查。

• 35 岁以上的女性且临床病史提示输卵管或子宫病变时，在开始诱导排卵前应进行子宫输卵管造影联合精液分析。

• AMH 检测目前不推荐用于筛查 PCOS 和 PCOM，因为缺乏标准化且未建立统一诊断值。新证据支持 AMH 的检测有助于预测卵泡数量和治疗反应。AMH 水平大于 5 ng/mL 具有 97% 的特异性，且敏感性高于当前 PCOM 标准。AMH 可帮助指导体外受精（IVF）患者在卵巢刺激前选择恰当的方案，并最大限度地降低卵巢过度刺激综合征（ovarian hyperstimulation syndrome，OHSS）的风险。

五、多囊卵巢综合征患者无排卵性不孕的治疗原则

目前尚无药物可明确治愈 PCOS，但可以采用治疗策略改善其临床症状，改善代谢和生殖功能。在 PCOS 中，不孕的主要原因是无排卵，因此成功恢复排卵可以帮助大多数患者实现妊娠。在优化健康状况后，可通过纠正排卵功能障碍来诱导正常的排卵周期。这可以通过提高 FSH 水平来实现，FSH 是将卵泡生长从雄激素环境转变为雌激素环境的驱动力。在使用这种驱动力时应注意，因为有大量小卵泡发育停滞。这种驱动力应足够克服阻力以允许单卵泡排卵，但同时不应超过过度刺激的水平（图 19.5）。AMH 水平可以在一定程度上提供指导；如果其水平较高，则可能存在更大的阻力。此外，PCOS 中的慢性无排卵与高胰岛素血症和肥胖相关，这些代谢异常也应纳入考虑以有效改善排卵功能。因此，为恢复排卵功能，生育管理应基于 3 个原则：

- 通过生活方式干预（如饮食、锻炼和减重）和胰岛素增敏剂改善 IR。
- 通过口服抗雌激素药物［如来曲唑、枸橼酸氯米芬（clomiphene citrate，CC）］或非肠道途径的促性腺激素疗法增加 FSH 水平，或采用 IVF。
- 通过腹腔镜卵巢手术降低高 LH 水平。

PCOS 患者治疗不孕症前，应考虑以下先决条件（方框 19.1）。

方框 19.1　多囊卵巢综合征患者治疗不孕症的先决条件

- 在开始治疗前，应该对闭经或月经稀发的患者排除妊娠
- 在开始促排卵治疗之前，建议优化健康状况（如肥胖女性需减重）
- 应确保充足的维生素 D 和叶酸补充剂摄入
- 诱导排卵的目标是恢复单卵泡排卵
- 在 PCOS 中，需要考虑患者教育、咨询、生活方式建议和心理健康，同时结合药物治疗
- 在推荐药物治疗时，应考虑患者的个人特点、偏好和价值取向
- 在开处方之前，应考虑治疗的益处、不良反应和禁忌证
- 应避免多个卵泡的发育，因为会产生不良后果：OHSS 和多胎妊娠
- 来曲唑和二甲双胍用于诱导排卵属于超说明书用药，但它们在 PCOS 中的使用是基于证据的，并且在许多国家是允许的

六、治疗管理

PCOS 的生育管理涉及非药物、药物和手术干预的联合治疗（流程规则 19.1）。非药物疗法包括生活方式干预；药物治疗包括口服促排卵药，如枸橼酸氯米芬和来曲唑，以及外源性促性腺激素。它们还包括一线和二线疗法的结合及胰岛素增敏剂，如二甲双胍和肌醇。手术治疗涉及腹腔镜卵巢手术，包括卵巢打孔术和经阴道注水腹腔镜检查（transvaginal hydrolaparoscopy，THL）。对于常规诱导排卵方法无效的病例可考虑 IVF。体外成熟（vitro maturation，IVM）对患 PCOS 的年轻女性来说是一种有前景的替代传统 IVF 技术的方法。

第十九章 多囊卵巢综合征患者低生育力的管理

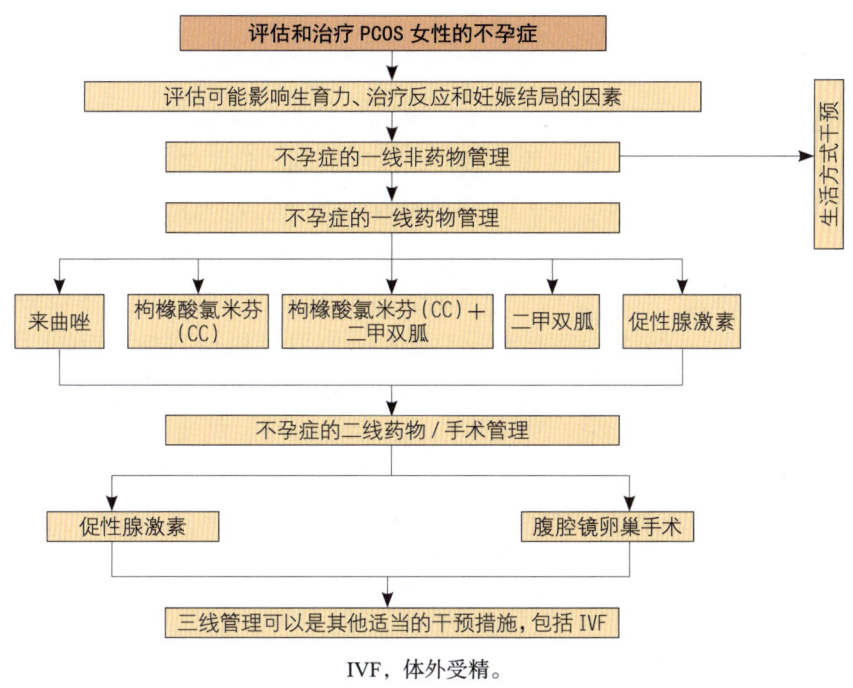

流程规则 19.1　多囊卵巢综合征患者不孕症的治疗管理

IVF，体外受精。

（一）改善胰岛素抵抗

1. 生活方式干预和减重

在 PCOS 患者中，月经不规律和无排卵与患者的体重指数（BMI）相关。被诊断为 PCOS 的患者中至少有一半是肥胖的（BMI > 30 kg/m^2）。由于超声扫描难以清晰显示卵巢，对肥胖的 PCOS 患者进行治疗和监测常具有挑战性。这增加了多卵泡发育和多胎妊娠的漏诊风险。

在开始任何生育治疗之前，生活方式干预被视为 BMI ≥ 25 kg/m^2 的 PCOS 患者的一线干预措施。对于病态肥胖的患者，理想情况下应将促排卵治疗推迟到 BMI < 35 kg/m^2。然而，对于卵巢储备正常的年轻女性，减少体重至 BMI < 30 kg/m^2 更为合适。生活方式建议有饮食改变、定期体育锻炼和减重策略，以及药物治疗和手术治疗。即使体重减轻 5%～10% 也有助于实现诱导排卵和改善所有生育治疗方式的效果。在使用药物减重前，应考虑药物在早孕期的安全性。

二甲双胍是一种胰岛素增敏药物，本身并不能用于减重治疗；然而，当与生活方式干预结合使用时，它可以改善体重。减肥药只能提供短期效果。对于病态肥胖的患者，如果通过常规方法无法减轻体重，则应考虑进行减重手术。PCOS 患者的减重术适应证与普通人群类似（BMI ≥ 40 kg/m^2）。对于那些具有糖尿病（DM）等合并症的患者，应考虑更低水平的 BMI（35 kg/m^2）。减重术后可以实现明显的体重减轻，并降低血清总睾酮和游离睾酮的水平。此外，多达 53% 和 96% 的女性多毛症和排卵功能障碍得到了改善。

2. 胰岛素增敏剂

（1）二甲双胍

二甲双胍可通过降低胰岛素水平、促进正常的促性腺激素释放激素（GnRH）和促性腺激素释放来改善生育率。由于作用缓慢，二甲双胍的临床效果可能只有在数周治疗后才会显现。在 PCOS 患者中，单用二甲双胍的效果不如枸橼酸氯米芬（CC）；然而，在无其他治疗选择时，它可以作为一线药物。与 CC 相比，二甲双胍的效果似乎是 BMI 依赖性的。二甲双胍在非肥胖女性中更有效，而在肥胖女性中，它会导致活产率下降。二甲双胍是 CC 耐药患者最常推荐的辅助疗法。二甲双胍和 CC 联合疗法可用作无排卵肥胖 PCOS 患者的一线药物治疗，因为它可以提高排卵率和妊娠率，而对活产率没有影响。目前没有足够的证据支持将二甲双胍作为来曲唑和腹腔镜卵巢打孔术（laparoscopic ovarian drilling，LOD）的附加疗法。二甲双胍应被考虑作为促性腺激素和 IVF 治疗的辅助疗法，因为它显著降低了 OHSS 的发生率。

二甲双胍的推荐剂量为每日 1500～2500 mg，持续 4～60 周。二甲双胍的长期使用是安全的；然而，在间隔期需要考虑是否继续治疗，因为使用该药可能会导致维生素 B_{12} 水平降低，如恶心、呕吐和其他胃肠不适等副作用。然而，通过逐渐增加剂量（每 1～2 周增加 500 mg）和使用缓释制剂可以改善二甲双胍的治疗依从性。乳酸酸中毒是二甲双胍的一种罕见并发症。二甲双胍通过肾脏排泄，在开始使用前应确认血清肌酐 < 1.4 mg/dL。

（2）肌醇

肌醇是一种新兴的胰岛素增敏剂，适用于 PCOS 患者。最常用的两种肌醇异构体是 myoinositol（MI）和 D-chiro inositol（DCI）。这些异构体作用于不同的通路：MI 可以发挥对卵巢和非卵巢的作用，而 DCI 具有非卵巢的胰岛素增敏效果。研究表明，当以符合血浆生理比例（MI：DCI = 40：1）的联合形式给药时，两者对 PCOS 的协同治疗效果更为显著。肌醇作为细胞内信使，调节着 TSH、FSH 等激素和胰岛素的活动。既往研究强调了肌醇在人类生殖中的作用。Pundir 等发现，肌醇治疗有助于提高排卵率和月经周期的频率。PCOS 患者的肌醇代谢可能有改变，因此给予肌醇可以帮助改善胰岛素敏感性（IS），改善代谢效应，并进一步改善胚胎质量和提高受精率。同样，在接受 IVF 治疗的 PCOS 患者中，肌醇的使用显示出积极的效果。目前没有证据表明它对妊娠、流产和活产率具有改善作用。建议每天使用 2～4 g 的 MI 和 1000～1200 mg 的 DCI。肌醇可以单独使用或与其他疗法联合使用，但使用肌醇被认为是实验性的。

3. 其他降低胰岛素的治疗方法

噻唑烷二酮类药物（TZD）（如吡格列酮和罗格列酮）被作为 PCOS 患者的二线治疗选择。TZD 治疗被认为对于肥胖或有高胰岛素血症的患者是有效的。

艾塞那肽是一种胰高血糖素样肽-1（GLP-1）受体激动剂，可以减轻胰岛素抵抗，并在 2 型糖尿病（T2DM）管理方面非常有效。它可以改善 IS 并有助于减轻体重。在肥胖的 PCOS 患者中，这种药物可以改善月经，减轻体重并降低雄激素水平。与二甲双胍相比，艾塞那肽可以更好地改善 IS 和提高怀孕率。联合使用二甲双胍和 GLP-1 受体激动剂在管理 PCOS 的代谢和生殖紊乱问题上比单一治疗更有效。需要进一步研究探讨 GLP-1 类似物在肥胖 PCOS 女性中的有效性。

（二）提高卵泡刺激素：黄体生成素水平

1. 一线治疗

（1）枸橼酸氯米芬

由于 CC 成本相对较低、易用性较好、副作用较少、监测要求较低，以及药物安全数据的可获得性，它已被用作 PCOS 女性诱导排卵的一线药物。

1）作用机制

CC 是一种选择性雌激素受体调节剂，能够在内分泌腺（下丘脑、垂体和卵巢）中竞争性结合内源性雌激素受体结合位点。CC 具有雌激素激动剂和拮抗剂两种属性；然而，CC 的临床效果主要是由其拮抗作用。CC 长时间地结合下丘脑雌激素受体，切断了内源性雌激素和雌二醇的负反馈环路。这会导致 GnRH 的分泌增加。上升的 GnRH 提高了血浆 LH 和 FSH 的水平，并促进卵泡成熟和最终排卵（图 19.6）。

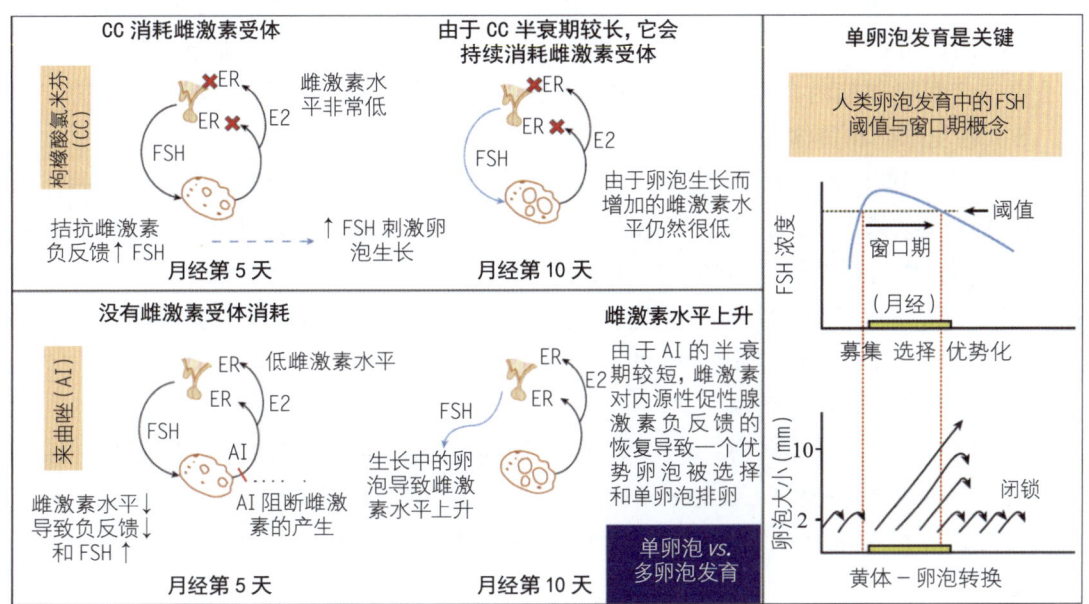

AI，芳香化酶抑制剂；E2，雌二醇；ER，雌激素受体；FSH，卵泡刺激素。

图 19.6 枸橼酸氯米芬与来曲唑在卵泡发育中的作用机制比较

来源：Yang A-M, Cui N, Sun Y-F and Hao G-M (2021) Letrozole for Female Infertility. Front. Endocrinol. 12: 676133.doi: 10.3389/fendo.2021.676133 and B.C.J.M Fauser, A.M van Heusden, Manipulation of human ovarian function: physiological concepts and clinical consequences. Endocr Rev, 18 (1997), p. 71-106.

2）患者的选择

对于具有正常 FSH 和雌二醇（E2）水平的无排卵型 PCOS 患者，可以开具 CC。表型 A、肥胖、高胰岛素血症、雄激素水平升高、高 LH 水平和年龄大等因素会影响 CC 治疗的效果。与之类似，AMH 水平升高的患者在 CC 治疗后排卵率和妊娠率低于 AMH 水平较低的患者。升高的 AMH 水平与发育阻滞的中间卵泡池的扩大相关，并对治疗有抵抗反应（图 19.5）。因此，使用血清 AMH 水平可以预测卵巢对 CC 的反应，以 3.4 ng/mL 作为截断值。

3）剂量

CC 的起始剂量为每天 50 mg，从自然周期或使用孕酮撤退性出血的第 2 天到第 5 天起连续服用 5 天。通常在最后一天服药后的 5～10 天内发生排卵。如果未能达到排卵，剂量逐渐增加至每天 150 mg。如果成功排卵，相同剂量可持续使用 3～6 个周期。更高剂量（200 mg）可以提高疗效，但不会带来额外的好处。如果每日 50 mg 引起过度反应，则应将剂量减至每日 25 mg。

4）检测

超声监测方面，第一周期建议至少在月经第 12～14 天（或最后一次剂量后 7 天）进行超声排卵监测，以便调整后续周期的剂量。这也有助于追踪卵泡，并提供有关子宫内膜厚度的信息。当存在一个直径为 18～25 mm 的主导卵泡，且子宫内膜厚度大于 7 mm 时，可认为反应是适当的。在使用 CC 期间可能出现功能性卵巢囊肿。它们通常会在一个月经周期内自行消失。若出现囊肿，治疗应暂停，直到囊肿消失。

5）触发排卵和黄体期支持

CC 治疗周期中不推荐使用人绒毛膜促性腺激素（hCG）作为排卵扳机药。它的使用不会改善生殖结果。然而，在个体化的基础上，也可以考虑在监测周期中使用 hCG。如果推荐使用，则可以在经阴道超声检查显示反应适当时给予 hCG（5000～10 000 IU）。在以 hCG 扳机的 CC 治疗期间，不需要进行黄体期支持；但如果经阴道超声检查显示子宫内膜厚度低于 6 mm，则可以考虑进行黄体期支持。

6）枸橼酸氯米芬的疗效

使用 CC 的排卵率为 75%～80%，每个周期的妊娠率可达 22%。排卵率和妊娠率之间约 40% 的差异主要与 CC 对子宫内膜和宫颈黏液的低雌激素作用有关。对 CC 有反应的女性，治疗应限制在 6 个周期内。妊娠率可达 50%～60%，但此后 CC 的疗效显著下降。

7）枸橼酸氯米芬的安全性

CC 促排卵治疗后的双胎和三胎妊娠率分别为 5%～7% 和 0.3%，OHSS 的风险极低（小于 1%），因此不需要进行定期的周期监测。CC 被认为是一种安全的药物，根据报道，其（遗传和结构性）先天畸形发生率为 3.9%，与自然妊娠相当。使用 CC 超过 12 个周期与患交界性卵巢恶性肿瘤和乳腺癌的风险有关，但并未被证实存在因果关系。

第十九章　多囊卵巢综合征患者低生育力的管理

CC 的副作用包括潮热、视觉障碍（如复视，此时应立即停药）、腹部胀气、情绪波动、乳房胀痛和恶心。应避免在存在卵巢囊肿、未控制的甲状腺功能异常和肝功能受损的患者中使用 CC。

8）枸橼酸氯米芬的耐药和失败

每天服用 150 mg 剂量的 CC 连续 3 个周期后仍无排卵，被认为是 CC 耐药；15%～40% 的 PCOS 患者对 CC 无反应。6 个有排卵周期后未能怀孕，被认为是 CC 失败。对于 CC 耐药和失败的病例，应评估其他代谢和不孕因素。为了提高反应率，应考虑使用替代疗法和二线治疗。

连续 10 天延长使用每天 150 mg 剂量的 CC 是一种安全有效的选择，但妊娠率会更低。在使用 CC 时与二甲双胍联合使用可以改善排卵和提高临床妊娠率，在采取更积极的治疗选择之前应考虑该治疗。有研究报道，可以对 CC 耐药、硫酸脱氢表雄酮（DHEAS）水平升高的患者使用 CC 与糖皮质激素联合治疗。对于有反应的患者，可以在月经周期的第 5～14 天使用泼尼松（每日 5 mg）或地塞米松（每日 0.5～2.0 mg）进行 3～6 个周期的联合治疗。这种联合治疗可以提高排卵率，但不推荐作为常规做法。

在 CC 耐药的病例中，已经开始使用 CC 与来曲唑联合治疗，并取得了良好的结果，排卵率和妊娠率提高，风险降低，成本更低。

（2）芳香化酶抑制剂

来曲唑和阿那曲唑是第三代芳香化酶抑制剂，用于 PCOS 患者的诱导排卵治疗。与阿那曲唑相比，来曲唑具有更高的妊娠率。

来曲唑在许多国家被视为治疗无排卵性不孕的超说明书用药。来自欧洲人类生殖与胚胎学协会和美国生殖医学协会 2018 年共识指南及 WHO 的新证据支持来曲唑作为诱导排卵的一线药物。在来曲唑不可用或不允许使用，或者治疗选择受到费用影响的情况下，可以使用 CC 作为一线治疗。此外，在 CC 耐药的病例中，在促排卵和妊娠率方面来曲唑比促性腺激素效果更好。

1）作用机制

来曲唑在卵泡、外周组织和大脑中对芳香化酶产生局部作用，阻止雄激素向雌激素的转化。由于其双重作用，来曲唑阻止雄烯二酮向雌酮的转化，以及睾酮向雌二醇的转化，从而阻止了系统性雌激素的生物合成。低水平的雌激素会对 HPO 轴产生负反馈，并促进 GnRH 的释放，刺激 FSH 的产生。升高的 FSH 水平促进了卵泡发育和成熟，随后进行排卵（图 19.6）。

2）剂量

来曲唑的剂量范围为每天 2.5～7.5 mg，具体剂量取决于治疗反应。在月经周期的第 3 天到第 7 天连续使用 5 天。有报道称，在第 3 天单次高剂量（20 mg）的使用也取得了良好的效果。通常建议使用来曲唑治疗 6 个排卵周期。支持黄体期使用来曲唑治疗的数据不足。

3）来曲唑和枸橼酸氯米芬的比较

PCOS 的女性使用来曲唑后，排卵和活产的可能性比 CC 更高，后者是以前的一线药物。与 CC 相比，使用来曲唑的活产率可增加 40%～60%。同样，与 CC 相比，来曲唑的排卵失败（来曲唑耐药）率更低。

如表 19.4 所示，CC 的半衰期为 5～7 天。其延长的半衰期导致雌激素受体的消耗，并破坏了 HPO 轴的长时间平衡。持续升高的 FSH 水平会导致多卵泡生长，并增加多胎妊娠的风险。与 CC 相比，来曲唑的半衰期仅为 2 天，并且不影响雌激素受体。由于其半衰期较短，中枢反馈机制保持完好。成长中的优势卵泡会使雌激素水平升高，并通过中枢负反馈抑制 FSH 的产生，导致小卵泡的闭锁。这种效应为来曲唑提供了独特的安全优势，并预防了 OHSS 和多胎妊娠。

表 19.4 氯米芬和来曲唑的比较

参数	氯米芬	来曲唑
作用机制	选择性雌激素受体调节剂	芳香化酶抑制剂
半衰期	长，5～7 天	短，45 小时
抗雌激素效应	子宫内膜薄，宫颈黏液改变	子宫内膜厚，良好的宫颈黏液
子宫血流	降低	增加
流产风险	可能高	发生率较低
卵巢过度刺激综合征风险	高	低
多胎妊娠	高	低
致畸性		相似

CC 会导致子宫内膜变薄并影响宫颈黏液，而来曲唑则不会引起雌激素受体拮抗作用。这解释了为什么来曲唑对子宫内膜和宫颈黏液没有抗雌激素作用。使用来曲唑或 CC 观察到的畸形患病率均低于 5%（自然怀孕预期畸形率为 5%～8%）。据报道，CC 和来曲唑的致畸性风险相似。

潮热在来曲唑使用中比 CC 更少见，但疲劳和头晕在来曲唑中更常见。与 CC 相比，来曲唑在促排卵方面对于患有 PCOS 的肥胖患者具有独特的益处。

来曲唑与促性腺激素方案联合使用可减少促性腺激素的需求，妊娠率也与单独使用促性腺激素相当。芳香化酶抑制剂在辅助生殖技术（assisted reproductive treatments，ART）中的作用有待证实。

（3）他莫昔芬

他莫昔芬是一种抗雌激素的抗癌药物，用于女性乳腺癌患者。对于未能或未对 CC 产生反应者，他莫昔芬被用作诱导排卵的替代选择。他莫昔芬具有与 CC 类似的作用，但对宫颈黏液和子宫内膜具有益处。然而，他莫昔芬的效果不如 CC，因此并不作为首选疗法。他莫昔芬的剂量为每日两次 20 mg，持续 5 天，可使 70%～80% 的患者排卵，妊娠率为 35%～40%。

2. 二线治疗

（1）促性腺激素

对于对一线促排卵药物无反应或有抗药性的患者，通常会将外源性促性腺激素作为二线治疗药物。然而，对于年龄较大的 PCOS 患者，FSH 可作为不孕症的一线治疗药物。促性腺激素治疗的目的是实现无排卵 PCOS 患者的单卵泡排卵，而对于具有正常排卵功能的女性，使用促性腺激素有助于实现多卵泡排卵。

1）治疗前提条件

应由经过专业培训且具备经验的专家来提供使用促性腺激素治疗的建议。在开始治疗之前，应排除其他不孕因素，如子宫腔异常（肌瘤、粘连）、输卵管阻塞、子宫内膜异位症和精液异常。同样，应进行评估以排除高催乳素和异常甲状腺素水平。

2）作用机制

促性腺激素（LH 和 FSH）是由垂体腺自然产生的，对卵泡生长和排卵起着至关重要的作用。在 PCOS 患者中，虽然 CC 和来曲唑相较于促性腺激素更易于使用且成本效益更高，因而被视为首选治疗方法，但使用促性腺激素可能会在不孕症治疗中产生更大的效果。

3）促性腺激素的选择

促性腺激素有尿源和重组两种形式。这两种制剂在诱导排卵方面同样有效，二者诱发排卵的疗效、OHSS 风险，以及多胎妊娠的风险也没有差异。从理论上讲，由于 PCOS 患者内源性 LH 水平较高，最好选择不含有 LH 的促性腺激素制剂。然而，在 PCOS 患者中，同时含有 FSH 和 LH 的制剂，以及单纯的 FSH 制剂都可成功诱导排卵。

4）PCOS 患者的促性腺激素治疗方案

PCOS 无排卵患者的小窦状卵泡数目增加。这些生长停滞的卵泡在内源性 FSH 功能异常的情况下无法被刺激排卵。然而，通过给予外源性 FSH，这些卵泡会出现过度反应，导致多卵发育。为了避免多囊卵巢的高度反应性，不推荐对 PCOS 患者采用传统的高剂量（150 IU）梯度方案，而是推荐低剂量治疗方案（图 19.7）。低剂量方案可采用递增、递减或序贯方式。

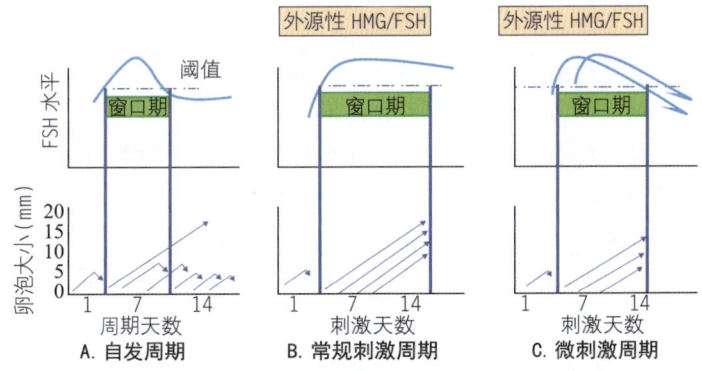

HMG，人绝经期促性腺激素；FSH，卵泡雌激素。
图 19.7 卵泡刺激素窗口期概念与促性腺激素刺激

来源：Macklon NS, Stouffer RL, Giudice LC, Fauser BC: The science behind 25 years of ovarian stimulation for in vitro fertilization. Endocr Rev 27[2]: 170–207, 2006.

①低剂量起始缓慢递增方案

低剂量起始缓慢递增方案被认为是PCOS患者诱导排卵的首选方法。通过低剂量递增给药，使FSH逐渐升高到略高于FSH阈值，有助于避免过度反应，以及降低与OHSS和多胎妊娠相关的风险。该方案从每天小剂量的FSH开始（通常为37.5～75.0 IU），通常保持该剂量持续14天。然后，每5～7天逐渐增加剂量，每次增加25.0～37.5 IU，直到在监测过程中观察到一个优势卵泡。该方案可达到最佳效果，单囊泡排卵率达到70%，每个周期妊娠率为20%（每位患者为40%），并将多胎妊娠和OHSS的风险分别降至5%和1%。然而，长时间的治疗是一个问题，因此有研究者尝试将周期持续时间从初始的14天减少到7天。结果显示成功率相似，但7天周期方案轻微提高了多胎妊娠率（图19.8）。

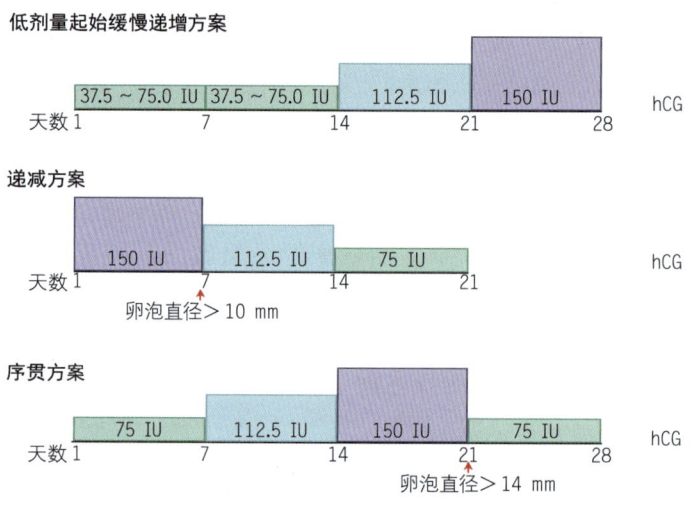

hCG，人绒毛膜促性腺激素。
图19.8 多囊卵巢综合征患者的促性腺激素方案
改编自：Amer S. Gonadotropin induction of ovulation. Obstet Gynaecol Reprod Med. 2007; 17 (7): 205-10.

②递减方案

该方案模拟了生理学上的FSH阈值/窗口期概念。治疗开始时使用高剂量的FSH（每天150 IU FSH），直到适当的卵巢反应（图19.8）。然后，通过两个步骤按37.5 IU逐渐减量。首先，当观察到一个直径为10 mm的卵泡时，开始减量，并且如果卵泡继续生长，每3天减少相同的剂量。剂量逐渐减少到每天75 IU，然后维持到hCG注射当日。这种方案在实现单卵泡发育方面与低剂量起始缓慢递增方案一样成功，但治疗时间更短。然而，由于频繁的剂量调整，通常需要进行密集的卵泡监测。

③序贯方案

该方案是递增和递减方案的组合，起始阶段采用递增方案。一旦出现优势卵泡，则转为递减方案。

5）治疗监测

建议促性腺激素治疗只做 6 个排卵周期。在治疗周期中，需要进行多次的超声监测，以确定卵泡在促性腺激素刺激下的生长和发育情况。单排卵周期是指只有 1 个直径为 16 mm 的卵泡，且没有其他直径＞12 mm 的卵泡。因此，需要考虑到所有卵泡的数量，并对直径＞10 mm 的卵泡进行记录。如果存在 3 个以上直径＞14 mm 的卵泡和血清雌二醇水平超过 15 000 pmol/L，则需考虑取消该周期。如果存在 2 个以上直径为 16 mm 或更大的卵泡，或者存在 1 个直径≥16 mm 的卵泡和另外 2 个直径为 14 mm 或更大的卵泡，则应禁止使用 hCG 以降低多胎妊娠和 OHSS 的风险。

建议在使用促性腺激素治疗期间进行黄体期支持，因为它可以提高临床妊娠率和活产率。促性腺激素的使用会影响下丘脑对 LH 的分泌，从而影响黄体对孕酮的释放，导致黄体期缩短。孕酮补充剂和 hCG 都可以使用。然而，由于 hCG 使用时可能会出现副作用（OHSS），因此建议使用孕酮补充剂。阴道给药的孕酮制剂优于口服制剂，因为其成本低且副作用较少。促性腺激素治疗时可考虑联合使用二甲双胍，因为它可以改善排卵、提高妊娠率和活产率，并有助于降低 OHSS 的风险。

促性腺激素治疗周期

- 月经来潮的第一天被视为月经周期的第 1 天。
- 在月经周期第 2 天或第 3 天进行经阴道超声基线检查，以排除潜在的卵巢囊肿。
- 如果超声检查正常，治疗从周期的第 2 天开始，使用相对较低剂量的促性腺激素（每天 37.5～75.0 IU）。
- 通常在每天晚上固定时间（下午 5:00—8:00）进行皮下注射（subcutaneous, SC）或肌内注射（intramuscularly, IM）。
- 超声和雌二醇水平检查（每 2～3 天 1 次）安排在上午（8:00—10:00）进行。
- 超声检查可以评估卵泡的发育情况，通常在治疗开始后的 4～5 天进行，之后根据治疗反应和所使用的方案间隔 1～3 天进行。
- 治疗的刺激阶段通常持续 7～14 天。
- 在周期第 8 天后的所有监测都是根据最大卵泡的大小安排的。
- 一旦有 1 个成熟的卵泡发育，通常平均直径为 16～18 mm，会给予 hCG 5000～10 000 IU IM 或 SC。
- 尽管没有关于最佳时机的具体指南，但当观察到至少 1 个、理想情况下不超过 2 个直径＞16 mm 的卵泡时，可以给予排卵扳机。
- 预计在 hCG 注射后的 24～48 小时内会发生排卵。因此，在此时间段内进行性交可以最大限度地增加受孕的可能性。
- 在促性腺激素治疗周期更建议做宫腔内人工授精，安排在扳机后 24～36 小时。
- 应考虑使用孕酮作为黄体支持。

6）患者咨询

在使用促性腺激素治疗之前，对患者进行咨询非常重要。应该讨论的内容包括治疗计划、成本和治疗反应，以及相关的高序多胎妊娠和 OHSS 的风险。在进行治疗之前，需要在严格的周期性标准上与患者达成共识。不同的人对促性腺激素发生反应的速度不同，即使是同一个人在每个周期中也不会以相同的方式对治疗做出反应。因此，需要调整促性腺激素剂量并进行密切监测，以实现成功的治疗反应。使用促性腺激素治疗，每个周期的妊娠率为 15%～20%，自然流产率为 20%～25%，略高于自然妊娠。然而，促性腺激素治疗并不会增加先天畸形的风险。

7）口服和非肠道给药联合诱导排卵治疗

在 CC 抵抗的 PCOS 患者中，可将 CC 和促性腺激素联合使用进行诱导排卵。新近的研究也支持联合使用来曲唑和促性腺激素。来曲唑加促性腺激素的效果比单独使用来曲唑更好，具有更高的排卵率、较低的取消率和更好的子宫内膜厚度，并且比 CC 加促性腺激素的风险更小（流程规则 19.2）。然而，这种治疗方案会增加多胎妊娠的风险。来曲唑、CC，以及促性腺激素联合治疗也已经被尝试使用，并且可能适用于对促性腺激素敏感的患者。

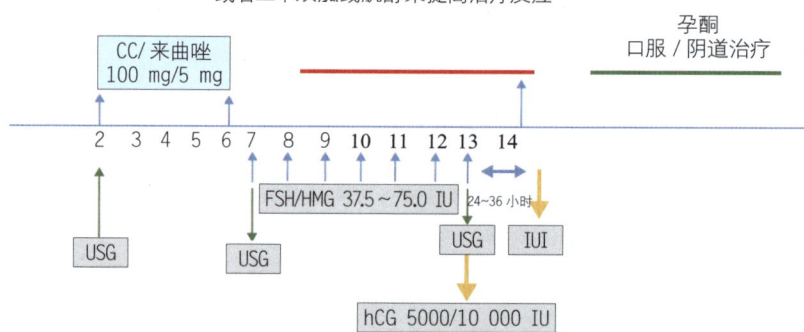

CC，枸橼酸氯米芬；FSH，卵泡刺激素；GTN，促性腺激素；IUI，宫腔内人工授精；USG，超声检查；HMG，人绝经期促性腺激素。

流程规则 19.2　口服和注射联合治疗流程

8）促性腺激素治疗的风险

尽管促性腺激素疗法在诱导排卵方面非常有效，但它与多胎妊娠和 OHSS 的风险显著相关。

①多胎妊娠

近年来，由于使用促性腺激素进行诱导排卵、控制性超促排卵和辅助生殖技术，多胎妊娠显著增加。多胎妊娠被认为是高风险的，与相关的孕产并发症有关，会影响围产期结局，增加新生儿的发病率和死亡率。

为了最大限度地减少多胎妊娠的风险，治疗应旨在诱导所有无排卵女性的单卵泡排卵。应对周期进行仔细监测，当有过多成熟卵泡时应考虑取消周期。

②卵巢过度刺激综合征

OHSS 是与促性腺激素治疗相关的一种潜在危及生命的并发症。大约有 1% 的患者在诱导排卵治疗后出现严重的 OHSS。它的特点是细胞内液体向细胞外转移，导致血管内容量减少、低血容量和血液浓缩。

OHSS 的确切机制尚不清楚；然而，hCG（无论是外源性还是内源性）被认为是主要的触发因素。可能是 hCG 激活卵巢释放了某些血管活性介质［如血管内皮生长因子（VEGF）］。这些因子在体内引发一系列事件，导致 OHSS 的病理生理后果。此外，在 PCOS 患者中，大量的中等大小卵泡都对外源性 FSH 敏感，一旦受到刺激就会导致雌激素水平升高。升高的血清雌二醇介导了 hCG 对血管系统的影响。除此之外，改善胰岛素水平增强了促性腺激素对颗粒细胞和卵泡膜细胞的作用。最后，多囊卵巢中 VEGF 的过表达增加了血管通透性。这导致胞内液体向胞外转移，导致血管内容量减少、低血容量和血液浓缩。

OHSS 有两种类型，早发型和晚发型，取决于 hCG 的来源。早发型 OHSS 是由外源性 hCG 引起的，症状在其给药后的 3～7 天内出现。晚发型 OHSS 是由早期妊娠的滋养层产生的内源性（胎盘）hCG 引起的，症状在 hCG 给药后的 12～17 天出现。OHSS 可以是轻度、中度或重度的，通常是自限性的，几天内会自行缓解。晚发型 OHSS 可能会加重并持续更长时间，因为妊娠仍在持续中。

瘦型 PCOS 患者接受高剂量促性腺激素治疗，并且曾经有过该综合征的病史，被认为是 OHSS 的高风险人群。大量中等大小的卵泡、高雌二醇水平（2500 pg/mL）和使用 hCG 进行黄体期支持都增加了发生 OHSS 的风险。

在促性腺激素刺激期间怀疑存在 OHSS 风险时，应考虑停用 hCG。另一种方法是停止进一步的促性腺激素刺激，并延迟 1～3 天，直到雌二醇水平稳定或下降后再给予 hCG。如有必要，黄体期支持应使用孕酮而不是 hCG。对于有过 OHSS 病史的患者，可以考虑低剂量刺激方案。

③卵巢恶性肿瘤

在未生育的女性中，使用促排卵药物可能与交界性浆液性卵巢肿瘤的发病率增加有关，但与浸润性癌无关。然而，并没有观察到促性腺激素治疗与卵巢癌之间的因果关系。一些大型研究也未证明存在这种风险。

（2）手术诱导排卵

1）腹腔镜卵巢打孔术（LOD）

对于 CC 抵抗的患者来说，LOD 是一种促性腺激素的替代疗法。这种手术已经取代了更具破坏性的卵巢楔形切除术。LOD 特别适用于未能对一线不孕治疗产生反应或需要腹腔镜盆腔评估，并因不能频繁监测而无法接受促性腺激素治疗的 PCOS 患者。年轻患者和 LH 水平持续升高的患者更有可能从 LOD 中受益，而肥胖、高雄激素水平或不孕时间较长的患者更有可能发生抵抗。与 CC 相比，LOD 在一线治疗中没有优势；然而，它在治疗 CC 耐药的 PCOS 方面显示出与促性腺激素类似的疗效。

①方法

LOD 在全身麻醉下进行，使用 1 根 10 mm 的传统内镜通过脐下切口，并配备 2 个额外的穿刺器。LOD 常用的方法包括单极或双极电凝和激光，效果相当。卵巢穿刺次数可以根据卵巢体积的大小而有所不同。较多的穿刺次数与卵巢组织的创伤程度增加和早期卵巢功能衰竭的风险增加有关。根据 Adam Balen 和 Armer 的技术，应该优先选择在 4 个部位进行打孔，避免损伤卵巢皮质，深度为 4 mm，持续 4 秒，功率为 40 W，以减少对卵巢的损伤。术后向腹腔注入等渗溶液可以预防卵巢受热损伤，并降低粘连的风险。单侧或双侧进行 LOD 的结果没有明显差异，但为了减少不良反应的发生率，一侧手术更受青睐。LOD 可以达到 86% 的排卵率和妊娠率。

②作用机制

LOD 直接破坏卵巢组织，包括卵泡和周围的基质，从而降低 AMH 水平和减少雄激素的产生。这有助于降低 LH 和睾酮的水平，并促进 FSH 的释放，从而支持卵泡生长和排卵。此外，它提高了 LH：FSH，降低了雄烯二酮和 DHEAS 水平，并增加了性激素结合球蛋白（SHBG）的水平（图 19.9）。LOD 手术的效果还包括卵巢接受热刺激后抑制素水平的降低和多种生长因子（胰岛素样生长因子 -1）的产生增加。这些改变增强了 FSH 的活性，促使卵泡发育。LOD 还减少了卵巢和基质体积，增加了 IS。这些变化也提高了其对外源 FSH 刺激的反应性。

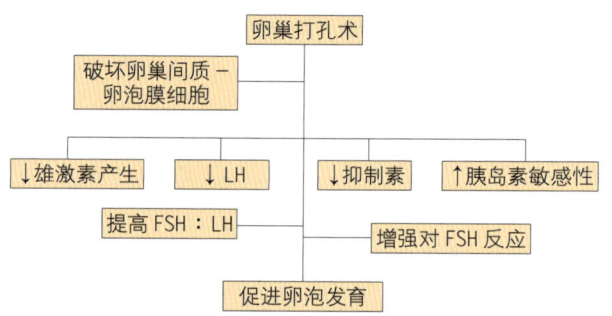

FSH，卵泡刺激素；LH，黄体生成素。
图 19.9 腹腔镜卵巢打孔术的作用机制

来源：Julie Collée, Marie Mawet, Linda Tebache, Michelle Nisolle & Géraldine Brichant (2021) Polycystic ovarian syndrome and infertility: overview and insights of the putative treatments, Gynecological Endocrinology,37: 10, 869-874, DOI: 10.1080/09513590.2021.1958310.

③副作用

LOD 可能与术后并发症有关，包括出血、感染和较小的术后粘连。由于 LOD 对卵巢功能的影响不是永久性的，所以随着时间的推移，月经不规律可能会再次出现。此外，存在一定理论上的卵巢储备减少风险，需要在患者咨询时予以考虑。在手术过程中应避免使用过度激进的方法，因为它可能会导致广泛的卵巢损伤并导致过早绝经。然而，通过更安全的方法和先进的技术，可以将这种风险最小化。

④优点

LOD 不需要超声监测，因为它能诱导单卵泡发育。与其他诱导排卵疗法相比，LOD 的多胎妊娠和 OHSS 的风险较低。通过 LOD，排卵率和妊娠率分别为 30%～80% 和 60%。选择的技术可能也会影响 LOD 的功效。Giampaolino 等报道了 THL 后 6 个月的排卵率和妊娠率分别为 82.9% 和 70%。

除了在妊娠率方面的功效外，LOD 还具有长期的好处。研究表明，手术后 PCOS 症状的改善可以持续 20 年。这种长期疗效是其他治疗选择所无法达到的（除非长时间进行生活方式干预）。在 2020 年的一项回顾性研究中，Debras 等表明，对于符合适应证的患者，LOD 有助于实现自然怀孕并具有长期效果。

⑤成功的预测因素

大约 30% 的 PCOS 患者对 LOD 无反应。当闭经和无排卵状态持续至术后 8 周时，治疗被视为失败。增强 LOD 效果的因素是高 LH 浓度（＞ 10 IU/L）、不孕症持续时间短（＜ 3 年）、年龄小于 35 岁和窦状卵泡数量少（＜ 50 个）。导致 LOD 反应差的相关因素见方框 19.2。

方框 19.2　导致腹腔镜卵巢打孔术反应差的相关因素

- 不孕症持续时间超过 3 年
- 基础 LH 水平＜ 10 IU/L
- 睾酮水平＞ 4.5 nmol/L
- 抗米勒管激素（AMH）基线水平高（＞ 7.7 ng/mL）
- 高体重指数（BMI ＞ 35 kg/m^2）
- 胰岛素抵抗

来源：Debras E, Fernandez H, Neveu M-E, Deffieux X, Capmas P. Ovarian drilling in polycystic ovarian syndrome. Long-term pregnancy rate. Euro J Obstet Gynaecol Reprod Biol. 2019.

在接受 LOD 治疗的患者中，大约有 50% 需要辅助治疗。如果未检测到排卵，可以在手术后 12～24 周使用口服促排卵药物，而在手术后 6 个月可以考虑使用促性腺激素治疗。

2）经阴道注水腹腔镜检查（THL）

THL 是一种可以在脊髓麻醉下进行的新兴手术。在 THL 中，通过腹腔内注入生理盐水。内镜的角度为 30°，可以更好地检查整个盆腔。它还可以通过输卵管镜检查同时评估输卵管和伞部。

该手术的安全性受到技术选择的影响。与腹腔镜相比，THL 的操作速度更快，降低了粘连的风险，并且术后疼痛较轻。这些好处可能是由于腹腔内注射生理盐水、时间较短、使用双极电凝，以及与 LOD 相比对卵巢的操作较少而导致出血较少。THL 也适用于肥胖患者。最后，与腹腔镜相比，THL 的学习曲线较短。

这种技术存在 0.5% 的直肠穿孔风险，通常可以使用抗生素保守治疗。在这种情况下，需要进行第二次腹腔镜检查以确认是否恢复，包括腹腔镜多针刺卵巢介入术和超声引导下经阴道卵巢打孔术等目前正在试验中的技术。

3）宫腔内人工授精（IUI）

IUI 适用于不明原因的不孕症、轻度子宫内膜异位症或轻度男性因素不孕。对于 PCOS 患者，如果口服、联合口服和非肠道治疗或单纯非肠道治疗的诱导排卵失败 2～3 个周期，并且存在男性因素不孕，可以考虑将 IUI 作为补充治疗选择。可在促排周期的 hCG 扳机后 24～36 小时进行 IUI。据报道，促性腺激素联合 IUI 的妊娠率为 11%～20%。

3. 三线治疗

IVF 被认为是 PCOS 患者无排卵性不孕的三线治疗。这种治疗方式并不直接建议作为一种选择，只有在二线治疗方案失败或存在其他相关不孕因素，包括男性因素、输卵管阻塞和子宫内膜异位症时才推荐使用。此外，对生育潜力有担忧的年轻 PCOS 女性，可以考虑卵子冷冻。

对于 PCOS 患者，IVF 面临多重挑战，包括反应差到反应过度之间的把控，获卵数和卵泡数比值的调节，受精率和囊胚形成率低，以及 OHSS 风险（5%～10%）和多胎妊娠风险（10%）增加。为了避免这些并发症，应考虑个体化的治疗方法。根据患者窦状卵泡数量、AMH 和 LH 水平来精细规划卵巢刺激方案。IVF 治疗涉及低剂量促性腺激素刺激结合 GnRH 激动剂和拮抗剂的使用。对于 PCOS 患者，GnRH 拮抗剂短方案优于 GnRH 激动剂长方案。对于拮抗剂治疗，GnRH 激动剂被认为是促进最终卵母细胞成熟的最佳扳机药，而不是 hCG。对于那些具有 OHSS 高风险的人，建议选择冷冻胚胎。同样，促排卵期间使用二甲双胍（1500～2550 mg）作为辅助治疗，有助于提高妊娠率并降低 OHSS 风险。

体外成熟（IVM）是一种新兴的 ART，可以帮助年轻的 PCOS 女性避免与 IVF 相关的 OHSS 风险。这种治疗方式被认为是经济有效的，因为它只涉及短期的促性腺激素刺激，并且不需要使用注射药物扳机。此外，相比传统的 IVF，当卵泡处于 10～11 mm 大小时就会取出卵子，这种早期干预有助于减少促性腺激素的刺激。取出的未成熟卵子（减数分裂和成熟度为第二次减数分裂中期）的进一步成熟过程发生在体外。在最终成熟阶段，给予 hCG 扳机，并在 36 小时后进行取卵，然后进行卵胞质内精子注射程序。然而，该程序的妊娠率较低（流程规则 19.3）。

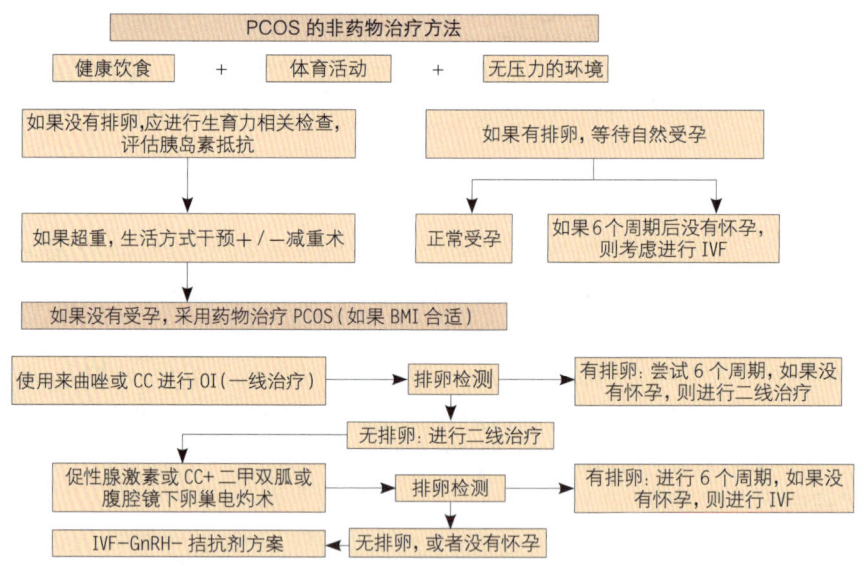

BMI，体重指数；CC，枸橼酸氯米芬；GnRH，促性腺激素释放激素；IVF，体外受精；OI，诱导排卵；PCOS，多囊卵巢综合征。

流程规则 19.3 多囊卵巢综合征女性的生育治疗

改编自：Adapted and simplified for book chapter from: Balen AH., et al. The management of anovulatory infertility in women with polycystic ovarian syndrome; ana analysis of evidence to support the development of global WHO guidance. Hum Reprod Update 2016.

七、结论

对于患有 PCOS 的肥胖患者，生活方式干预是一线干预措施，并且对于正常 BMI 的女性来说，这也是一种预防策略。诱导排卵的首选药物是来曲唑。在没有来曲唑可用，或者不允许使用来曲唑，或者成本影响治疗选择的情况下，可以将 CC 作为一线治疗方法。与单独使用 CC 或者单独使用二甲双胍相比，二甲双胍与 CC 联合使用在肥胖女性中更有效。肌醇在 IVF 治疗中显示出了理想的结果，但其使用被认为是实验性的。促性腺激素是用于 CC 耐药的 PCOS 患者诱导排卵的二线治疗方法。在年龄较大的 PCOS 女性中，它们比 CC 更有效，并且在具备监测设施和对患者进行多胎妊娠和 OHSS 相关风险咨询的情况下，可以作为一线治疗方法。对于 LH 浓度高、不孕时间短、怀孕年龄较小的非肥胖 PCOS 患者，LOS 作为二线治疗方法是有效的。在其他改善排卵治疗方法无效的情况下，可以考虑进行 IVF（流程规则 19.4 和方框 19.3）。

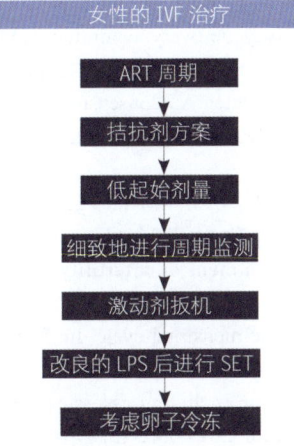

ART，辅助生殖技术；LPS，黄体期支持；SET，选择性胚胎移植。
流程规则 19.4　多囊卵巢综合征女性的体外受精（IVF）治疗

方框 19.3　总结：多囊卵巢综合征无排卵性不孕的管理

- 建议生活方式干预作为一线治疗方法
- 如果 BMI ≥ 35 kg/m² 且生活方式疗法无效，可以考虑进行减重术
- 来曲唑是首选药物：CC 和来曲唑都可以作为无排卵的一线药物治疗
- 二甲双胍和肌醇都可以改善卵泡环境，从而提高受精率，但对活产率无影响
- CC＋二甲双胍可用于 CC 抵抗病例
- 低剂量促性腺激素治疗和 LOD 可作为二线管理方法
- 对生活方式干预和 OI 无反应的患者，或者存在其他不孕因素的患者，可以采用 GnRH 拮抗剂方案进行 IVF。IVM 是一种作为三线治疗的新兴技术
- 如果使用 GnRH 激动剂方案，辅助使用二甲双胍可能会降低 OHSS 的风险

注：BMI，体重指数；GnRH，促性腺激素释放激素；IVF，体外受精；IVM，体外成熟；LOD，腹腔镜卵巢打孔术；OHSS，卵巢过度刺激综合征；OI，诱导排卵。

参考文献

1. Azziz R, Carmina E, Dewailly D, et al. Positions statement: criteria for defining polycystic ovary syndrome as a predominantly hyperandrogenic syndrome: an Androgen Excess Society guideline. J Clin Endocrinol Metab. 2006;91(11):4237-4245.
2. Bozdag G, Mumusoglu S, Zengin D, et al. The prevalence and phenotypic features of polycystic ovary syndrome: a systematic review and meta-analysis. Hum Reprod. 2016;31(12):2841-2855.
3. Escobar-Morreale HF. Polycystic ovary syndrome: definition, aetiology, diagnosis, and treatment. Nat Rev Endocrinol. 2018;14(5):270.
4. Azziz R. Diagnostic criteria for polycystic ovary syndrome: a reappraisal. Fertil Steril. 2005;83(5):1343-1346. doi:10.1016/j.fertnstert.2005.01.085.
5. Minocha N. Polycystic ovarian disease or polycystic ovarian syndrome: how to identify and manage—a review. Arch Pharm Pract. 2020;11(2):102-106.
6. Dennett CC, Simon J. The role of polycystic ovary syndrome in reproductive and metabolic health: overview and approaches for treatment. Diabetes Spectr. 2015;28(2):116-120. Available at: https://doi.org/10.2337/diaspect.28.2.116.
7. Witchel SF, Oberfield SE, Peña AS. Polycystic ovary syndrome: pathophysiology, presentation, and treatment with emphasis on adolescent girls. J Endocr Soc. 2019;3(8):1545-1573.
8. Fauser B, Tarlatzis B, Rebar R, Legro R, Balen A. Consensus on women's health aspects of polycystic ovary syndrome (PCOS): the Amsterdam ESHRE. Paper presented at: ASRM-sponsored 3rd PCOS Consensus Workshop Group. Fertil Steril. 2011;97:28.
9. Lizneva D, Gavrilova-Jordan L, Walker W, Azziz R. Androgen excess: investigations and management. Best Pract Res Clin Obstet Gynaecol. 2016;30:1-21. Available at: https://doi.org/10.1016/j.bpobgyn.2016.05.003.
10. Melo AS, Ferriani RA, Navarro PA. Treatment of infertility in women with polycystic ovary syndrome: approach to clinical practice. Clinics. 2015;70(11):765-769.
11. Taylor HS, Pal L, Seli E. Regulation of the menstrual cycle. In: Speroff's Clinical Gynecologic Endocrinology and Infertility. Philadelphia: Lippincott Williams & Wilkins; 2019:137-173.
12. Lew R. Natural history of ovarian function including assessment of ovarian reserve and premature ovarian failure. Best Pract Res Clin Obstet Gynaecol. 2019;55:2-13.
13. Pellatt L, Rice S, Mason HD. Anti-Müllerian hormone and polycystic ovary syndrome: a mountain too high? Reproduction. 2010;139:825-833.
14. Pellatt L, Rice S, Dilaver N, et al. Anti-Müllerian hormone reduces follicle sensitivity to follicle-stimulating hormone human granulosa cells. Fertil Steril. 2011;96:1246-1251.
15. Mascarenhas M, Balen AH. Treatment update for anovulation and subfertility in polycystic ovary syndrome. Curr Opin Endocr Metab Res. 2020;12:53-58.
16. Conway G, Dewailly D, Diamanti-Kandarakis E, et al. The polycystic ovary syndrome: a position statement from the European Society of Endocrinology. Eur J Endocrinol. 2014;171(4):P1-P29.
17. Bhide P, Homburg R. Anti-Müllerian hormone, and polycystic ovary syndrome. Best Prac Res Clin Obstet Gynaecol. 2016;37:38-45.
18. Seifer D, Tal R. Anti-Mullerian Hormone: Biology, Role in Ovarian Function and Clinical Significance. Obstetrics and Gynecology Advances. Nova Science Publishers, Inc.; 2016.
19. Wang F, Niu W, Kong H, Guo YH, Sun Y. The role of AMH and its receptor SNP in the pathogenesis of PCOS. Mol Cell Endocrinol. 2017;439:363-368.
20. Porter DT, Moore AM, Cobern JA, et al. Prenatal testosterone exposure alters GABAergic synaptic inputs to GnRH and KNDy neurons in a sheep model of polycystic ovarian syndrome. Endocrinology. 2019;160:2529-2542.
21. de Assis Rodrigues NP, Laganà AS, Zaia V, et al. The role of Kisspeptin levels in polycystic ovary syndrome: a

systematic review and meta-analysis. Arch Gynecol Obstet. 2019;300:1423-1434.
22. Homburg R. Androgen circle of polycystic ovary syndrome. Hum Reprod. 2009;24:1548-1555.
23. Ferreira SR, Motta AB. Uterine function: from normal to polycystic ovarian syndrome alterations. Curr Med Chem. 2018;25:1792-1804.
24. National Institute for Health and Care Excellence. Fertility: Assessment and Treatment for People with Fertility Problems. CG156. London: NICE; 2013. Available at: http://www.nice.org.uk/CG156.9.
25. Teede HJ, Misso ML, Costello MF, et al. Recommendations from the international evidence-based guideline for the assessment and management of polycystic ovary syndrome. Hum Reprod. 2018;33(9):1602-1618.
26. Balen AH. Polycystic ovary syndrome (PCOS). Obstet Gynaecol. 2017;19(2):119-129.
27. Dewailly D, Lujan ME, Carmina E, et al. Definition and significance of polycystic ovarian morphology: a task force report from the Androgen Excess and Polycystic Ovary Syndrome Society. Hum Reprod Update. 2014;20(3):334-352.
28. Escobar-Morreale HF. Polycystic ovary syndrome: definition, aetiology, diagnosis, and treatment. Nat Rev Endocrinol. 2018;14(5):270.
29. Christiansen SC, Eilertsen TB, Vanky E, Carlsen SM. Does AMH reflect follicle number similarly in women with and without PCOS? PLoS One. 2016;11(1):e0146739.
30. Grisendi V, La Marca A. Individualization of controlled ovarian stimulation in vitro fertilization using ovarian reserve markers. Minerva Ginecol. 2017;69(3):250-258.
31. Costello MF, Misso ML, Wong J, et al. The treatment of infertility in polycystic ovary syndrome: a brief update. Aust N Z J Obstet Gynaecol. 2012;52:400-403.
32. Walls ML, Hunter T, Ryan JP, Keelan JA, Nathan E, Hart RJ. In vitro maturation as an alternative to standard in vitro fertilization for patients diagnosed with polycystic ovaries: a comparative analysis of fresh, frozen and cumulative cycle outcomes. Hum Reprod. 2015;30:88-96.
33. Balen AH, Anderson R. Impact of obesity on female reproductive health. British Fertility Society, Police and Practice Guidelines. Hum Fertil. 2007;10:195-206.
34. Naderpoor N, Shorakae S, de Courten B, Misso ML, Moran LJ, Teede HJ. Metformin and lifestyle modification in PCOS: systematic review and meta- analysis. Hum Reprod Update. 2015;21:560-574.
35. Azziz R, Carmina E, Dewailly D, et al. The Androgen Excess and PCOS Society criteria for the polycystic ovary syndrome: the complete task force report. Fertil Steril. 2009;91(2):456-488.
36. Ali SS, Rehman R. Polycystic ovary syndrome and subfertility. In: Subfertility. Amsterdam: Elsevier Inc.; 2021:115-134.
37. Pasquali R. Contemporary approaches to the management of polycystic ovary syndrome. Ther Adv Endocrinol Metab. 2018;9:123-134.
38. Goodman NF, Cobin RH, Futterweit W, Glueck JS, Legro RS, Carmina E. American Association of Clinical Endocrinologists, American College of Endocrinology, and Androgen Excess and PCOS Society disease state clinical review: guide to the best practices in the evaluation and treatment of polycystic ovary syndrome-part 1. Endocr Pract. 2015;21(11):1291-1300.
39. Nestler JE. Metformin in the treatment of infertility in PCOS: an alternative perspective. Fertil Steril. 2008;90:14-16.
40. Morley LC, Tang T, Yasmin E, Norman RJ, Balen AH. Insulin-sensitising drugs (metformin, rosiglitazone, pioglitazone, D-chiro-inositol) for women with polycystic ovary syndrome, oligo amenorrhoea and subfertility [Internet]. Cochrane Database Syst Rev. 2017. Available at: https://www.cochranelibrary.com/cdsr/doi/10.1002/14651858.CD003053.pub6/full.
41. Tso LO, Costello MF, Albuquerque LET, Andriolo RB, Macedo CR. Metformin treatment before and during IVF or ICSI in women with polycystic ovary syndrome. Cochrane Database Syst Rev. 2014;2014:CD006105.
42. Collée J, Mawet M, Tebache L, Nisolle M, Brichant G. Polycystic ovarian syndrome and infertility: overview

and insights of the putative treatments. Gynecol Endocrinol. 2021;37(10):869-874. doi:10.1080/09513590.2021.1958310.

43. Facchinetti F, Bizzarri M, Benvenga S, et al. Results from the international consensus conference on myo-inositol and D-chiro-inositol in obstetrics and gynecology: the link between metabolic syndrome and PCOS. Eur J Obstet Gynecol Reprod Biol. 2015;195:72-76.

44. Baillargeon JP, Iuorno MJ, Jakubowicz DJ, Apridonidze T, He N, Nestler JE. Metformin therapy increases insulin-stimulated release of D-chiro-inositol-containing inositolphosphoglycan mediator in women with polycystic ovary syndrome. J Clin Endocrinol Metab. 2004;89(1):242-249.

45. Pundir J, Psaroudakis D, Savnur P, et al. Inositol treatment of anovulation in women with polycystic ovary syndrome: a meta-analysis of randomised trials. BJOG. 2018;125(3):299-308.

46. Atay V, Cam C, Muhcu M, Cam M, Karateke A. Comparison of letrozole and clomiphene citrate in women with polycystic ovaries undergoing ovarian stimulation. J Int Med Res. 2006;34(1):73-76.

47. Stout DL, Fugate SE. Thiazolidinediones for treatment of polycystic ovary syndrome. Pharmacotherapy. 2005;25:244-252.

48. Sanchez-Garrido MA, Tena-Sempere M. Metabolic dysfunction in polycystic ovary syndrome: pathogenic role of androgen excess and potential therapeutic strategies. Mol Metab. 2020;35:100937.

49. Practice Committee of the American Society for Reproductive Medicine. Use of clomiphene citrate in infertile women: a committee opinion. Fertil Steril. 2013;100:341-348.

50. Clark JH, Markaverich BM. The agonistic and antagonistic effects of short acting estrogens: a review. Pharmacol Ther. 1983;21(3):429-453.

51. Use of clomiphene citrate in infertile women: a committee opinion. Fertil Steril. 2013;100:341-348.

52. Ege S, Bademkıran MH, Peker N, Tahaoğlu AE, Çaça FNH, Özçelik SM. A comparison between a combination of letrozole and clomiphene citrate versus gonadotropins for ovulation induction in infertile patients with clomiphene citrateresistant polycystic ovary syndrome—a retrospective study. Ginekol Pol. 2020;91(4):185-188.

53. Shokeir T, El-Kannishy G. Rosiglitazone as treatment for clomiphene citrate-resistant polycystic ovary syndrome: factors associated with clinical response. J Womens Health (Larchmt). 2008;17(9):1445-1452.

54. Mahran A, Abdelmeged A, El-Adawy AR, Eissa MK, Shaw RW, Amer SA. The predictive value of circulating anti-Müllerian hormone in women with polycystic ovarian syndrome receiving clomiphene citrate: a prospective observational study. J Clin Endocrinol Metab. 2013;98(10):4170-4175.

55. Thomas S, Sudharshini S. Polycystic ovarian syndrome: treatment options for infertility. Curr Med Issues. 2016;14(4):87.

56. George K, Kamath MS, Nair R, Tharyan P. Ovulation triggers in anovulatory women undergoing ovulation induction. Cochrane Database Syst Rev. 2014;31(1):CD006900. Available at: https://www.cochranelibrary.com/cdsr/doi/10.1002/14651858.CD006900.pub3/abstract.

57. Hill MJ, Whitcomb BW, Lewis TD, et al. Progesterone luteal support after ovulation induction and intrauterine insemination: a systematic review and meta-analysis. Fertil Steril. 2013;100(5):1373-1380.

58. Thessaloniki ESHRE/ASRM-Sponsored PCOS Consensus Workshop Group. Consensus on infertility treatment related to polycystic ovary syndrome. Hum Reprod. 2008;23:462-477.

59. Dickey RP, Taylor SN, Lu PY, et al. Effect of diagnosis. Age, sperm quality and number of preovulatory follicles on the outcome of multiple cycles of clomiphene citrate-intrauterine insemination. Fertil Steril. 2002;78:1088-1095.

60. Sharma S, Ghosh S, Singh S, et al. Congenital malformations among babies born following letrozole or clomiphene for infertility treatment. PLoS One. 2014;9(10):e108219.

61. Mbi Feh MK, Wadhwa R. Clomiphene. In: StatPearls [Internet]. Treasure Island, FL: StatPearls Publishing; 2021.

62. Abu Hashim H, Foda O, Ghayaty E. Combined metformin-clomiphene in clomiphene-resistant polycystic ovary syndrome: a systematic review and meta-analysis of randomized controlled trials. Acta Obstet Gynecol Scand.

2015;94:921-930.
63. Omara MA, El Khouly NI, Salama HT, Solyman AE. Extended use of clomiphene citrate in induction of ovulation in polycystic ovary syndrome with clomiphene citrate resistance. Egypt J Hosp Med. 2021;82(3):567-573.
64. Mejia RB, Summers KM, Kresowik JD, Van Voorhis BJ. A randomized controlled trial of combination letrozole and clomiphene citrate or letrozole alone for ovulation induction in women with polycystic ovary syndrome. Fert Steril. 2019;111(3):571-578.
65. Balen AH, Morley LC, Misso M, et al. The management of anovulatory infertility in women with polycystic ovary syndrome: an analysis of the evidence to support the development of global WHO guidance). Hum Reprod Update. 2016;22(6):687-708. doi:10.1093/humupd/dmw025.
66. Dawood AS, Abdelghaffar SD, Borg HM. Letrozole versus gonadotropins for ovulation induction in clomiphene citrate resistance: a randomized controlled study. Ann Gynecol Obstet. 2021;5(1):127-132.
67. Holzer H, Casper RR, Tulandi T. A new era in ovulation Induction. Fertil Steril. 2006;85(2):277-284.
68. Mitwally MF, Casper RF. Single-dose administration of an aromatase inhibitor for ovarian stimulation. Fertil Steril. 2005;83:229-231.
69. Legro RS, Brzyski RG, Diamond MP, et al. Letrozole versus clomiphene for infertility in the polycystic ovary syndrome. N Engl J Med. 2014;371:119-129.
70. Franik S, Kremer JA, Nelen WL, Farquhar C. Aromatase inhibitors for subfertile women with polycystic ovary syndrome. Cochrane Database Syst Rev. 2014;(2):CD010287.
71. Badawy A, Gibreal A. Clomiphene citrate versus tamoxifen for ovulation induction in women with PCOS: a prospective randomized trial. Eur J Obstet Gynecol Reprod Biol. 2011;159:151-154.
72. Steiner AZ, Terplan M, Paulson RJ. Comparison of tamoxifen and clomiphene citrate for ovulation induction: a meta-analysis. Hum Reprod. 2005;20:1511-1515.
73. Royal Collegue of Obstetricians and Gynaecologists. Long-Term Consequences of Polycystic Ovary Syndrome: Green-Top Guideline no. 33. 2014. Available at: https://www.rcog.org.uk/globalassets/documents/guidelines/gtg_33.pdf.
74. Homburg R, Hendriks ML, Konig TE, et al. Clomifene citrate or low-dose FSH for the first-line treatment of infertile women with anovulation associated with polycystic ovary syndrome: a prospective randomized multinational study. Hum Reprod. 2012;27:468-473.
75. Weiss NS, Kostova E, Nahuis M, et al. Gonadotrophins for ovulation induction in women with polycystic ovary syndrome. Cochrane Database Syst Rev. 2019;(1):CD010290. doi:10.1002/14651858.CD010290.pub3.
76. Melo AS, Ferriani RA, Navarro PA. Treatment of infertility in women with polycystic ovary syndrome: approach to clinical practice. Clinics. 2015;70:765-769.
77. Dafopoulos K, Tarlatzis BC. Hormonal treatments in the infertile women. In: Petraglia F, Fauser B, eds. Female Reproductive Dysfunction. Endocrinology. Springer, Cham; 2020:247-261.
78. Della Corte L, Foreste V, Barra F, et al. Current and experimental drug therapy for the treatment of polycystic ovarian syndrome. Expert Opin Investig Drugs. 2020;29(8):819-830. Available at: https://doi.org/10.1080/13543784.2020.1781815.
79. Sood A, Mathur R. Ovarian hyperstimulation syndrome. Obstet Gynaecol Reprod Med. 2020;30(8):251-255. Available at: https://doi.org/10.1016/j.ogrm.2020.05.004.
80. Du DF, Li MF, Li XL. Ovarian hyperstimulation syndrome: a clinical retrospective study on 565 inpatients. Gynecol Endocrinol. 2020;36(4):313-317.
81. El-Sayed Abd El-Maksoud A, Zakaria El-Sheikha K, El-Sayed Ibrahim A. Comparison between letrozole alone versus letrozole-gonadotrophins combination in versus clomiphene citrate–gonadotrophins combination in ovarian induction for PCOS patient undergoing intrauterine insemination. Al Azhar Med J. 2021;50(1):253-264.
82. Xi W, Liu S, Mao H, Yang Y, Xue X, Lu X. Use of letrozole and clomiphene citrate combined with gonadotropins in clomiphene-resistant infertile women with polycystic ovary syndrome: a prospective study. Drug Des Devel Ther. 2015;9:6001-6008.
83. Amer SA, Li TC, Metwally M, Emarh M, Ledger WL. Randomized controlled trial comparing laparoscopic

ovarian diathermy with clomiphene citrate as a first-line method of ovulation induction in women with polycystic ovary syndrome. Hum Reprod. 2009;24(1):219-225.
84. Abu Hashim H, Foda O, Ghayaty E, Elawa A. Laparoscopic ovarian diathermy after clomiphene failure in polycystic ovary syndrome: is it worthwhile? A randomized controlled trial. Arch Gynecol Obstet. 2011;284(5):1303-1309.
85. Farquhar C, Brown J, Marjoribanks J. Laparoscopic drilling by diathermy or laser for ovulation induction in anovulatory polycystic ovary syndrome. Cochrane Database Syst Rev. 2012;(6):CD001122.
86. Roy KK, Baruah J, Moda N, Kumar S. Evaluation of unilateral versus bilateral ovarian drilling in clomiphene citrate resistant cases of polycystic ovarian syndrome. Arch Gynecol Obstet. 2009;280(4):573-578.
87. Lebbi I, Ben Temime R, Fadhlaoui A, Feki A. Ovarian drilling in PCOS: is it really useful? Front Surg. 2015;2:30.
88. Gjonnaess H. Polycystic ovarian syndrome treated by ovarian electrocautery through the laparoscope. Fertil Steril. 1984;41(1):20-25.
89. Ott J, Mayerhofer K, Nouri K, Walch K, Seemann R, Kurz C. Perioperative androstenedione kinetics in women undergoing laparoscopic ovarian drilling: a prospective study. Endocrine. 2014;47(3):936-942.
90. Felemban A, Tan SL, Tulandi T. Laparoscopic treatment of polycystic ovaries with insulated needle cautery: a reappraisal. Fertil Steril. 2000;73:266-269.
91. Saleh AM, Khalil HS. Review of nonsurgical and surgical treatment and the role of insulin-sensitizing agents in the management of infertile women with polycystic ovary syndrome. Acta Obstet Gynecol Scand. 2004;83:614-621.
92. Debras E, Fernandez H, Neveu ME, Deffieux X, Capmas P. Ovarian drilling in polycystic ovary syndrome: long term pregnancy rate. Eur J Obstet Gynecol Reprod Biol X. 2019;4:100093.
93. Bordewijk EM, Ng KY, Rakic L, et al. Laparoscopic ovarian drilling for ovulation induction in women with anovulatory polycystic ovary syndrome. Cochrane Database Syst Rev. 2020;2:CD001122.
94. Seow KM, Juan CC, Hwang JL, Ho LT. Laparoscopic surgery in polycystic ovary syndrome: reproductive and metabolic effects. Semin Reprod Med. 2008;26(1):101-110.
95. Practice Committee of American Society for Reproductive Medicine. Diagnostic evaluation of the infertile female: a committee opinion. Fertil Steril. 2012;98(2):302-307. doi:10.1016/j.fertnstert.2012.05.032.
96. Giampaolino P, Morra I, Tommaselli GA, Di Carlo C, Nappi C, Bifulco G. Post-operative ovarian adhesion formation after ovarian drilling: a randomized study comparing conventional laparoscopy and transvaginal hydrolaparoscopy. Arch Gynecol Obstet. 2016;294(4):791-796.
97. Giampaolino P, De Rosa N, Della Corte L, et al. Operative transvaginal hydrolaparoscopy improve ovulation rate after clomiphene failure in polycystic ovary syndrome. Gynecol Endocrinol. 2018;34(1):32-35.
98. Ezedinma NA, Phelps JY. Transvaginal hydrolaparoscopy. JSLS. 2012;16(3):461-465.
99. Nguyen TT, Doan HT, Quan LH, Lam NM. Effect of letrozole for ovulation induction combined with intrauterine insemination on women with polycystic ovary syndrome. Gynecol Endocrinol. 2020;36(10):860-863.
100. Giudice LC. Endometrium in PCOS: implantation and predisposition to endocrine CA. Best Pract Res Clin Endocrinol Metab. 2006;20:235-244.
101. Walls ML, Hart RJ. In vitro maturation. Best Pract Res Clin Obstet Gynaecol. 2018;53:60-72.
102. Thakre N, Homburg R. A review of IVF in PCOS patients at risk of ovarian hyperstimulation syndrome. Expert Rev Endocrinol Metab. 2019;14(5):315-319.
103. Walls ML, Hunter T, Ryan JP, Keelan JA, Nathan E, Hart RJ. In vitro maturation as an alternative to standard in vitro fertilization for patients diagnosed with polycystic ovaries: a comparative analysis of fresh, frozen and cumulative cycle outcomes. Hum Reprod. 2015;30:88-96.

第二十章 多囊卵巢综合征患者妊娠相关风险的管理

多囊卵巢综合征（PCOS）是育龄期妇女最常见的内分泌紊乱疾病之一，影响着 5%～20% 的女性。它与高雄激素血症（HA）、排卵功能障碍，以及超声下单侧或双侧多囊卵巢形态（PCOM）有关。PCOS 的发病机制是多因素的。患者具有潜在的遗传易感性，并且因为雄激素过多、高胰岛素血症和升高的黄体生成素水平而导致过度肥胖和激素失调。

在妊娠期间，生理性胰岛素抵抗（IR）导致妊娠后半期产生代偿性高胰岛素血症。这种生理性 IR 是为了限制母体葡萄糖的利用，从而增加向发育中胎儿的葡萄糖供应。这一过程得益于妊娠激素，包括雌二醇（E2）、孕酮（P2）、催乳素、皮质醇、人绒毛膜促性腺激素、胎盘生长激素和人胎盘催乳素。其中妊娠期 IR 主要由后两种激素引起。

HA 和 IR 是 PCOS 患者的特征性表现，这些特征不仅限于肥胖女性，瘦型 PCOS 患者也可能存在 IR。因为存在过多的脂肪组织，肥胖进一步加重了 PCOS 患者的 IR。随着女性进入妊娠期，这种基线 IR 进一步加重，从而增加了妊娠并发症的风险。PCOS 患者在妊娠期间更容易发生自发流产、妊娠期糖尿病（GDM）、妊娠高血压综合征（pregnancy induced hypertension syndrome，PIH）、早产（preterm birth，PTB）和小于胎龄儿（small-for-gestational-age，SGA）。尽管 GDM、PIH、子痫前期和剖宫产（cesarean section，CS）的发生率因研究而异，但即使对体重指数（BMI）进行校正后，这些风险仍然显著增加。因此，PCOS 会对女性的身体和心理健康产生深远的影响，对生殖结果也会产生重要的影响。妊娠相关代谢和生殖问题的管理是 PCOS 管理的基石。

一、多囊卵巢综合征女性妊娠期病理生理变化的可能潜在机制

（一）多囊卵巢综合征表型

IR 是 PCOS 的标志，与肥胖无关；然而，肥胖会进一步加重 IR。因此，风险会因不同表型而异，并与 BMI 呈线性相关。一些研究报告称，HA、IR 和（或）高胰岛素血症的组合可能会通过改变正常的胎盘植入而导致 PCOS 患者在妊娠期间发生并发症的风险增加，如流产、宫内发育受限、GDM、PIH、子痫前期、PTB 和妊娠期出血。文献已证实，即使采取不同诊断标准，无论何种表型的 PCOS 患者都需要进行筛查和管理以预防不良妊娠结局。

（二）胰岛素抵抗的影响

IR 和高胰岛素血症是 HA 的典型特征，它们出现在超过一半的 PCOS 患者中。在妊娠期间，PIH 和既往已存在的 IR 的结合，增加了发展至 GDM 的风险。尽管一些研究未能显示出这种关联，但其他研究则明确提示这种关系的存在。IR 导致血管收缩，在 PIH 的发展中起作用。它还提高了促凝和促纤维化作用，并引起了钠摄入后血压反应的增强。这种综合效应导致了子痫前期的发展。与之类似，继发于 IR 的血管功能障碍与 PTB 和胎儿生长障碍，如大于胎龄儿（large-for-gestational-age，LGA）和 SGA 的风险增加有关。

（三）肥胖和孕期体重增加的影响

约 61% 的 PCOS 患者超重或肥胖。孕前 BMI 和不良妊娠结局直接相关。如果孕前 BMI > 25 kg/m^2，则 PCOS 是 GDM 的最重要的预测因素。

（四）炎症的影响

HA 可以在 PCOS 患者的组织中制造一种慢性低度炎症环境。这导致炎症标志物的增加，如白细胞计数、C 反应蛋白、炎症细胞因子［如白细胞介素 -6（IL-6）和 IL-8］、细胞黏附分子［如可溶性内皮白细胞黏附分子 -1（sE-selectin）、可溶性细胞间黏附分子 -1（sICAM-1）和可溶性血管细胞黏附分子 -1（sVCAM-1）］。具体机制及其与 PCOS 的不良妊娠结局的关联尚不清楚。

（五）不孕症和多胎的影响

绝大多数 PCOS 患者能够自然受孕，但超过 3/4 的 PCOS 患者需要凭借辅助受孕或对不孕症进行治疗。其中很多女性需要辅助生殖技术（ART），比例在 17%～40%。文献综述表明，在低生育力的女性中，即使是自然受孕，也存在更高的不良妊娠结局风险，如 PTB、低出生体重（low birth weight，LBW）、先天畸形、GDM 和 PIH。ART 与不良妊娠结局的高发率有关，包括 PTB、LBW、SGA 胎儿、围产儿死亡和先天畸形。因此，与低生育力相关的 PCOS 不良妊娠结局的风险进一步增加，可能是由于生育治疗和多胎等因素的影响。

二、多囊卵巢综合征相关的妊娠风险

（一）早期流产

PCOS 患者由于排卵障碍面临着生育问题。随着 ART 的进展，PCOS 的受孕率显著提高。关于 PCOS 患者是否更容易发生早期流产（第一孕期流产）的证据并不一致。早期流产的潜在原因包括子宫内膜环境的改变，以及继发于高胰岛素血症和 HA 的胚胎植入率降低。与非 PCOS 的女性相比，患有 PCOS 的女性妊娠流产的风险增加了 2.9 倍。然而，BMI 和 ART 是主要的混杂因素，因为两者都是流产的独立风险因素。肥胖加剧的高胰岛素血症可能与纤溶酶原激活物抑制物-1的水平增加有关，后者是纤溶作用的强力抑制物，也是导致流产的可能因素。此外，许多前瞻性及回顾性队列研究已经显示出PCOS有明显增加的流产风险。

（二）妊娠期糖尿病

GDM常见于PCOS患者的妊娠。不同的荟萃分析显示PCOS患者具有明显较高的GDM风险。一项研究发现，40%～50%的妊娠被诊断为GDM。当将PCOS和非PCOS女性进行年龄和BMI匹配时，研究发现PCOS女性在BMI为正常到超重范围内的GDM风险更高，但在BMI＞30 kg/m^{2}的女性中，二者GDM的风险相似。

（三）妊娠高血压综合征

患有PCOS的妊娠女性患高血压疾病的风险增加可高达4倍，包括妊娠高血压和子痫前期。根据现有数据，妊娠PCOS患者中妊娠高血压和子痫前期的患病率分别为10%～30%和8%～15%。另外，在PCOS患者中使用ART而导致的多胎妊娠率较高，这也是一个潜在的混杂因素。高胰岛素血症引起的血管功能障碍可能是PCOS患者发生PIH的一个主要原因。

（四）早产

PCOS和PTB之间并不直接相关。各种研究报告了PCOS患者早产率较高的情况。在PCOS患者中使用诱导排卵药物可能导致多胎妊娠，而多胎妊娠本身与PTB和SGA直接相关。Boomsma等对PCOS女性的不良结局进行的荟萃分析清楚地显示了其早产风险显著增加，然而在这个荟萃分析中，PCOS患者与正常人群相比，多胎妊娠的发生率没有差异。这个荟萃分析纳入的研究结果具有明显的统计学异质性。此外，这些研究中没有将早产按原因分层。因此，其他混杂因素，如胎盘功能不全、高血压或糖尿病等医源性分娩指征也可能导致早产。另一项荟萃分析未发现PCOS对PTB的影响。Naver等证实了伴有HA的PCOS患者早产的风险增加。这一发现与Qin等的荟萃分析结果不一致，后者指出并不存在这种关联。

（五）小于胎龄儿

关于PCOS女性与SGA的证据也不一致。虽然Boomsma等报道PCOS与SGA没有显著关联，但几年后进行的另一项荟萃分析显示，PCOS患者患SGA的风险增加了近2倍。其他研究报告了PCOS与LGA的关联，这可能受到母体高胰岛素血症和妊娠期糖尿病的影响。相较于非肥胖对照组，这种关联在肥胖PCOS患者中更为明显。这可能是由于HA、IR和高胰岛素血症之间的复杂相互作用。

关于PCOS妊娠中CS风险的数据不一致。一些研究显示PCOS患者的CS率显著升高，而另外一些研究则提示与非PCOS的妊娠相比，CS率相似。荟萃分析显示PCOS母亲的新生儿入住新生儿重症监护室的风险增加。可能的解释是PTB增加，以及随后出现的呼吸窘迫综合征等并发症。同样，围产儿死亡率也因多胎率和早产率增加而增加。

三、多囊卵巢综合征患者妊娠并发症的管理

PCOS 是育龄女性中最常见的内分泌疾病之一，具有重要意义。PCOS 患者应该接受孕前咨询，了解 PCOS 的代谢、心理和生殖后果，并听取关于生活方式、肥胖和年龄对生育力影响的建议。应强调 PCOS 对生殖结局的影响。应向这些女性提供有关计划妊娠和妊娠前健康优化的重要建议。在孕前访视和首次产前访视中，应探讨 GDM 的风险并提供筛查。根据美国糖尿病协会的建议，PCOS 也被列为妊娠人群进行第一次产前访视时 2 型糖尿病（T2DM）筛查的一个风险因素。良好的血糖控制可能会提高 PCOS 妊娠的成功率。应建议补充叶酸，尽可能戒烟。

（一）生活方式干预

生活方式管理在 PCOS 患者中起着至关重要的作用，是首选的治疗策略。包括饮食、运动和行为管理在内的多学科干预，旨在达到适当的 BMI。对于 PCOS 女性来说，孕前减重（体重的 5%～10%）与改善妊娠结局相关联，尤其是在减重后立即开始妊娠效果更好。所有肥胖的孕妇都应该接受有关饮食和（或）体育活动对妊娠期体重增加的有益影响的指导。美国医学研究所提出了不同 BMI 水平的孕期体重增加目标。应鼓励妇女摄入适量的蔬菜、水果、谷物食品、蛋白质食品、乳制品及替代食物，并限制含有饱和脂肪的食物、精制碳水化合物及添加盐和糖的食物摄入量，同时减少酒精的摄入。应避免摄入含汞量高的鱼类。虽然这些建议并不特定针对 PCOS 患者，但在孕前适度减重，保持适度的体育活动和摄入健康食物以达到基于孕前 BMI 的增重目标，可以改善这些高风险病例的生殖结局。

（二）二甲双胍

二甲双胍在糖尿病（DM）管理中已经使用了几十年，即使在妊娠期间也可以使用，因为它是一种公认的便宜且安全的口服降血糖药物，它可以穿过胎盘。然而，关于其在 PCOS 中效果的数据有限。一项系统评价显示，与安慰剂相比，孕前使用二甲双胍对流产没有保护作用。然而，一些研究表明，在妊娠期间使用二甲双胍可以预防 GDM 和子痫前期。一项荟萃分析未能证实这一发现。同样，一些研究显示，使用二甲双胍可以预防早产。使用二甲双胍还与较低的孕期体重增加相关。关于这种保护性关系的证据仍然有限。虽然该药物无致畸作用，但对后代的长期影响尚不清楚，因此不建议在没有 GDM 的 PCOS 女性中使用二甲双胍。

（三）肌醇

肌醇是一种天然存在于动植物细胞中的环多醇，具有类似胰岛素的特性，可改善

IR 和 DM 中的代谢异常。关于其有效性的数据显示，肌醇对流产率没有益处，但在父母患有 T2DM 的患者中，GDM 的发生率较低。肌醇在 PCOS 妊娠中的作用仍不清楚。

四、结论

总之，应向孕妇宣传 PCOS 的 IR 和高雄激素状态与不良妊娠结局风险增加的相关性。优化孕前健康，密切监测孕期母婴健康状况，并及时提供预防和治疗干预措施，以确保 PCOS 女性获得良好的分娩结局。

参考文献

1. Boomsma CM, Eijkemans MJ, Hughes EG, Visser GH, Fauser BC, Macklon NS. A meta-analysis of pregnancy outcomes in women with polycystic ovary syndrome. Hum Reprod Update. 2006;12:673-683.
2. March WA, Moore VM, Willson KJ, Phillips DI, Norman RJ, Davies MJ. The prevalence of polycystic ovary syndrome in a community sample assessed under contrasting diagnostic criteria. Hum Reprod. 2010;25:544-551.
3. Fauser BC, Tarlatzis BC, Rebar RW, et al. Consensus on women's health aspects of polycystic ovary syndrome (PCOS): the Amsterdam ESHRFJASRM-Sponsored 3rd PCOS Consensus Workshop Group. Fertil Steril. 2012;97:28-38.
4. Azziz R, Carmina E, Chen Z, et al. Polycystic ovary syndrome. Nat Rev Dis Primers. 2016;2:16057.
5. Homburg R. Polycystic ovary syndrome. Best Pract Res Clin Obstet Gynaecol. 2008;22(2):261-274.
6. Kamalanathan S, Sahoo JP, Sathyapalan T. Pregnancy in polycystic ovary syndrome. Indian J Endocrinol Metab. 2013;17(1):37-43.
7. Kjerulff LE, Sanchez Ramos L, Duffy D. Pregnancy outcomes in women with polycystic ovary syndrome: a meta analysis. Am J Obstet Gynecol. 2011;204:558.e16.
8. Al-Biate MA. Effect of metformin on early pregnancy loss in women with polycystic ovary syndrome. Taiwan J Obstet Gynecol. 2015;54:266-269.
9. Sir-Petermann T, Hitchsfeld C, Maliqueo M, et al. Birth weight in offspring of mothers with polycystic ovarian syndrome. Hum Reprod. 2005;20:2122-2126.
10. Mumm H, Jensen DM, Sorensen JA, et al. Hyperandrogenism and phenotypes of polycystic ovary syndrome are not associated with differences in obstetric outcomes. Acta Obstet Gynecol Scand. 2015;94:204-211.
11. Lovvik TS, Wikstrom AK, Neovius M, Stephansson O, Roos N, Vanky E. Pregnancy and perinatal outcomes in women with polycystic ovary syndrome and twin births: a population-based cohort study. BJOG. 2015;122:1295-1302.
12. Palomba S, Falbo A, Chiossi G, et al. Low-grade chronic inflammation in pregnant women with polycystic ovary syndrome: a prospective controlled clinical study. J Clin Endocrinol Metab. 2014;99:2942-2951.
13. Wolf M, Sandler L, Hsu K, Vossen-Smirnakis K, Ecker JL, Thadhani R. First-trimester C-reactive protein and subsequent gestational diabetes. Diabetes Care. 2003;26:819-824.
14. Kollmann M, Klaritsch P, Martins WP, et al. Maternal and neonatal outcomes in pregnant women with PCOS: comparison of different diagnostic definitions. Hum Reprod. 2015;30:2396-2403.
15. Teede H, Deeks A, Moran L. Polycystic ovary syndrome: a complex condition with psychological, reproductive and metabolic manifestations that impacts on health across the lifespan. BMC Med. 2010;8:41.
16. Bjercke S, Dale PO, Tanbo T, Storeng R, Ertzeid G, Abyholm T. Impact of insulin resistance on pregnancy complications and outcome in women with polycystic ovary syndrome. Gynecol Obstet Invest. 2002;54:94-98.
17. Nouh AA, Shalaby SM. The predictive value of uterine blood flow in detecting the risk of adverse pregnancy

outcome in patients with polycystic ovary syndrome. Middle East Fertil Soc J. 2011;16:284-290.
18. Aktun HL, Yorgunlar B, Acet M, Aygun BK, Karaca N. The effects of polycystic ovary syndrome on gestational diabetes mellitus. Gynecol Endocrinol. 2016;32:139-142.
19. Zhou M-S, Schulman IH, Zeng Q. Link between the renin-angiotensin system and insulin resistance: implications for cardiovascular disease. Vasc Med. 2012;17:330-341.
20. Bennett SN, Tita A, Owen J, Biggio JR, Harper LM. Assessing White's classification of pregestational diabetes in a contemporary diabetic population. Obstet Gynecol. 2015;125:1217.
21. Lim SS, Davies MJ, Norman RJ, Moran LJ. Overweight, obesity and central obesity in women with polycystic ovary syndrome: a systematic review and meta-analysis. Hum Reprod Update. 2012;18:618-637.
22. Yu HF, Chen HS, Rao DP, Gong J. Association between polycystic ovary syndrome and the risk of pregnancy complications: a PRISMA-compliant systematic review and meta-analysis. Medicine. 2016;95:e4863.
23. Turhan NO, Seckin NC, Aybar F, Inegol I. Assessment of glucose tolerance and pregnancy outcome of polycystic ovary patients. Int J Gynaecol Obstet. 2003;81:163-168.
24. Diamanti-Kandarakis E, Paterakis T, Alexandraki K, et al. Indices of low-grade chronic inflammation in polycystic ovary syndrome and the beneficial effect of metformin. Hum Reprod. 2006;21:1426-1431.
25. Hudecova M, Holte J, Olovsson M, Sundström Poromaa I. Long-term follow-up of patients with polycystic ovary syndrome: reproductive outcome and ovarian reserve. Hum Reprod. 2009;24:1176-1183.
26. Joham AE, Teede HJ, Ranasinha S, Zoungas S, Boyle J. Prevalence of infertility and use of fertility treatment in women with polycystic ovary syndrome: data from a large community-based cohort study. J Womens Health. 2015;24:299-307.
27. Zhu JL, Obel C, Bech BH, Olsen J, Basso O. Infertility, infertility treatment and fetal growth restriction. Obstet Gynecol. 2007;110:1326.
28. Zhu JL, Basso O, Obel C, Bille C, Olsen J. Infertility, infertility treatment, and congenital malformations: Danish national birth cohort. BMJ. 2006;333:679.
29. Qin JB, Wang H, Sheng X, Xie Q, Gao S. Assisted reproductive technology and risk of adverse obstetric outcomes in dichorionic twin pregnancies: a systematic review and meta-analysis. Fertil Steril. 2016;105:1180-1192.
30. Homburg R. Pregnancy complications in PCOS. Best Pract Res Clin Endocrinol Metab. 2006;20:281-292.
31. Wang JX, Davies MJ, Norman RJ. Polycystic ovarian syndrome and the risk of spontaneous abortion following assisted reproductive technology treatment. Hum Reprod. 2001;16:2606-2609.
32. Elkholi DG, Nagy HM. The effects of adipocytokines on the endocrino-metabolic features and obstetric outcome in pregnant obese women with polycystic ovary syndrome. Middle East Fertil Soc J. 2014;19:293-302.
33. Li HW, Lee VC, Lau EY, Yeung WS, Ho PC, Ng EH. Cumulative live-birth rate in women with polycystic ovary syndrome or isolated polycystic ovaries undergoing in-vitro fertilisation treatment. J Assist Reprod Genet. 2014;31:205-211.
34. Qin JZ, Pang LH, Li MJ, Fan XJ, Huang RD, Chen HY. Obstetric complications in women with polycystic ovary syndrome: a systematic review and meta-analysis. Reprod Biol Endocrinol. 2013;11:56.
35. Veltman Verhulst SM, van Haeften TW, Eijkemans MJ, de Valk HW, Fauser BC, Goverde AJ. Sex hormonebinding globulin concentrations before conception as a predictor for gestational diabetes in women with polycystic ovary syndrome. Hum Reprod. 2010;25:31233128.
36. de Vries MJ, Dekker GA, Schoemaker J. Higher risk of preeclampsia in the polycystic ovary syndrome: a case control study. Eur J Obstet Gynecol Reprod Biol. 1998;91-95.
37. Naver KV, Grinsted J, Larsen SO, et al. Increased risk of preterm delivery and pre-eclampsia in women with polycystic ovary syndrome and hyperandrogenaemia. BJOG. 2014;121:575-581.
38. Roos N, Kieler H, Sahlin L, Ekman-Ordeberg G, Falconer H, Stephansson O. Risk of adverse pregnancy outcomes in women with polycystic ovary syndrome: population-based cohort study. Br Med J. 2011;343:d6309.

39. Mikola M, Hiilesmaa V, Halttunen M, Suhonen L, Tiitinen A. Obstetric outcome in women with polycystic ovarian syndrome. Hum Reprod. 2001;16:226-229.
40. Fridstrom M, Nisell H, Sjoblom P, Hillensjo T. Are women with polycystic ovary syndrome at an increased risk of pregnancyinduced hypertension and/or preeclampsia? Hypertens Pregnancy. 1999;18:73-80.
41. American Diabetes Association. Standards of medical care in diabetes—2011. Diabetes Care. 2011;34:S11-S61.
42. Moran LJ, Hutchison SK, Norman RJ, Teede HJ. Lifestyle changes in women with polycystic ovary syndrome. Cochrane Database Syst Rev. 2011;7:CD007506.
43. Legro RS, Dodson WC, Kunselman AR, et al. Benefit of delayed fertility therapy with preconception weight loss over immediate therapy in obese women with PCOS. J Clin Endocrinol Metab. 2016;101:2658-2666.
44. Agha M, Agha RA, Sandell J. Interventions to reduce and prevent obesity in pre-conceptual and pregnant women: a systematic review and meta-analysis. PLoS One. 2014;9:e95132.
45. NICE. Weight Management Before, During and After Pregnancy (ed. N. I. o. C. Excellence). London, UK: NICE; 2010.
46. Kominiarek Michelle A, Priya Rajan. Nutrition Recommendations in Pregnancy and lactation. The Medical Clinics of North America. 2016;100(6):1199-1215. doi:10.1016/j.mcna.2016.06.004. In this issue.
47. Vanky E, Zahlsen K, Spigset O, Carlsen SM. Placental passage of metformin in women with polycystic ovary syndrome. Fertil Steril. 2005;83:1575-1578.
48. Palomba S, Falbo A, Orio Jr F, Zullo F. Effect of preconceptional metformin on abortion risk in polycystic ovary syndrome: a systematic review and meta-analysis of randomized controlled trials. Fertil Steril. 2009;92:1646-1658.
49. Khattab S, Mohsen IA, Aboul Foutouh I, et al. Can metformin reduce the incidence of gestational diabetes mellitus in pregnant women with polycystic ovary syndrome? Prospective cohort study. Gynecol Endocrinol. 2011;27:789-793.
50. Vanky E, Stridsklev S, Heimstad R, et al. Metformin versus placebo from first trimester to delivery in polycystic ovary syndrome: a randomized, controlled multicenter study. J Clin Endocrinol Metab. 2010;95:E448-E455.
51. Croze ML, Soulage CO. Potential role and therapeutic interests of myo-inositol in metabolic diseases. Biochimie. 2013;95:1811-1827.
52. Pundir J, Psaroudakis D, Savnur P, et al. Inositol treatment of anovulation in women with polycystic ovary syndrome: a meta-analysis of randomised trials. BJOG. 2018;125:509-510.
53. D'Anna R, Scilipoti A, Giordano D, et al. myo-Inositol supplementation and onset of gestational diabetes mellitus in pregnant women with a family history of type 2 diabetes: a prospective, randomized, placebo-controlled study. Diabetes Care. 2013;36:854-857.

第二十一章 生活方式干预的重要性

一、引言

生活方式干预对多囊卵巢综合征（PCOS）管理的重要性是不言而喻的，它被认为是 PCOS 管理的第一步。现有证据显示，生活方式干预如改变饮食、限制热量、运动训练和行为改变，无论是单用其中一种方法还是几种方法联合应用，均可改善 PCOS。然而，关于最佳的饮食和运动策略，以及明确的目标和终点仍然缺乏统一的准则。患者和医务工作者对生活方式干预措施方面知识的缺乏，可能会影响治疗效果。

本章旨在回顾有关生活方式干预对 PCOS 患者生化、代谢、心血管和生殖健康影响的现有证据。

二、病理生理学/机制

胰岛素抵抗（IR）和高雄激素血症（HA）是 PCOS 的标志。内在性 IR 是超重、肥胖，以及低体重 PCOS 患者多种临床表现的促成因素。高胰岛素血症以多种方式导致雄激素的产生。胰岛素水平升高会降低性激素结合球蛋白（SHBG）在肝脏的分泌，导致游离循环雄激素水平升高。肥胖，特别是腹型肥胖会加重这种情况，导致雄激素分泌增加；而雄激素分泌增加会反过来导致腹部脂肪组织增加，形成了恶性循环。有 HA 的 PCOS 患者，可表现为月经不规律、排卵障碍、痤疮和多毛症。胰岛素抵抗、高胰岛素血症、超重/肥胖也会增加心血管疾病的风险，如代谢综合征（MetS）、糖代谢受损和血脂异常。

通过生活方式干预，如饮食改变、运动和行为疗法来减重，会使 PCOS 患者受益。减重 5%～10% 可显著改善临床症状。减重可提高胰岛素敏感性，并降低与 PCOS 相关的代谢风险，如 MetS、血脂异常、糖代谢受损和心血管疾病风险。生活方式干预除了对 PCOS 患者的生活质量和社会心理健康有显著影响外，也增加了自然妊娠的机会（图 21.1）。

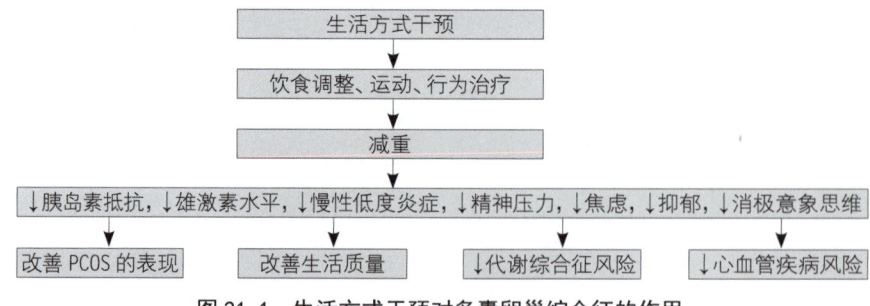

图 21.1 生活方式干预对多囊卵巢综合征的作用

三、饮食调整

同普通人一样，改变饮食也是 PCOS 患者减重的主要方法。关于 PCOS 患者理想饮食的具体搭配，没有统一的指导方针。多个随机对照试验（RCT）比较了不同饮食方案，如高蛋白质饮食与高碳水化合物饮食比较，以及高蛋白质饮食与正常蛋白质饮食比较，没有显示哪种饮食方案更有优越性。总体上，证据支持通过限制热量减重的饮食方案。为实现减重，建议肥胖或超重的女性将总热量摄入量减少 30% 左右或 500～750 kcal/d。重点是将健康饮食习惯作为一种生活方式，而不是短期行为。饮食方案应根据患者的营养需求、基线体重和能量消耗水平进行个性化定制。在制订个人营养计划时，应考虑患者的偏好、选择、文化多样性，以及患者能力的可行性。在制订营养计划时，避免不必要的营养缺失至关重要。

低糖饮食对 PCOS 有积极影响。这种影响可能是通过减缓葡萄糖吸收，降低胰岛素水平来实现的。富含纤维的饮食也可能通过减重对 PCOS 产生积极影响，因为摄入富含纤维的饮食会较早产生饱腹感，从而减少食物摄入量。一个有趣的发现是，膳食纤维摄入量与 PCOS 特征，如 IR、空腹胰岛素水平、餐后血糖水平、甘油三酯和睾酮水平呈负相关，与高密度脂蛋白（HDL）水平呈正相关。这一发现来自小样本研究，因此需要进一步研究以提出明确的建议。

低碳水化合物饮食，即热量低于 45% 的饮食，使体重指数（BMI）、IR 和循环胰岛素水平、总胆固醇和低密度脂蛋白（LDL）胆固醇都有显著改善。此外，研究表明，低碳水化合物/低脂肪饮食（定义为含有低于 45% 的碳水化合物和少于 35% 的脂肪），使 PCOS 患者的卵泡刺激素（FSH）和 SHBG 水平显著增加，血清睾酮水平降低。如果食用低碳水化合物饮食超过 4 周，效果会进一步增强。这种饮食的有益作用是由胰岛素水平降低和胰岛素敏感性提高引起的，然后通过对卵巢和肾上腺的影响来降低雄激素水平。高胰岛素血症对卵巢的直接影响和黄体生成素（LH）：FSH 的增加，是抑制卵泡发育和排卵的关键因素。胰岛素水平降低和 FSH 水平增加可改善月经周期和多毛症，提高排卵率、生育力。

四、运动

大量数据显示，运动对 PCOS 的代谢、性激素和社会心理具有有益影响。临床中提出的建议主要来自综述和荟萃分析；然而，没有关于运动干预的最佳类型、持续时间和强度的统一指南。

已有文献报告了许多使 PCOS 患者受益的不同运动模型。一项荟萃分析对关于各种有氧运动项目的研究进行了分析，从 12 周到 6 个月不等，每周至少 3 天，每次持续 30～60 分钟的中等强度到高强度运动，结果都显示对空腹胰岛素水平和胰岛素敏感性有所改善。

另一项荟萃分析将运动和饮食组与单独运动组对比，得出的结论是，运动与饮食组和单独运动组均可以改善 PCOS 女性的 SHBG、FSH、雄烯二酮、睾酮水平和 Ferriman-Gallwey 多毛症评分。Hakimi 报告，即使不节食，定期锻炼也会降低肥胖或超重 PCOS 女性的胰岛素和雄激素水平，并恢复排卵。一项关于运动干预研究的荟萃分析显示，运动是改善 IR 和排卵的独立因素。有氧运动通过不同病理生理途径改善 IR，如减少脂肪因子、氧化应激和炎症反应，以及通过不同的细胞和分子途径改善胰岛素的信号转导，直接提高胰岛素敏感性。虽然数据有限，但有文献显示运动可以改善血清甘油三酯、总胆固醇、HDL、LDL 的水平。

最近，国际循证指南提出了一些针对特定年龄的运动建议，以防止 PCOS 患者的体重增加。根据这些指南，对于 18～64 岁的女性，建议每周至少进行 75 分钟的剧烈运动，或每周 150 分钟的中等强度体育活动，或两者的组合，包括每周至少非连续两天进行肌肉强化运动。对于青少年，建议每周至少 3 次进行每天至少 60 分钟的中等强度到高强度的体育活动，包括肌肉和骨骼强化活动。该指南建议，体育活动应至少进行 10 分钟或约 1000 步，目标是在大多数日子里每天至少花费 30 分钟进行体育锻炼。为了减重，建议每周至少 150 分钟的剧烈活动或每周 250 分钟的中等强度活动，或两者相结合，以及每周至少非连续两天进行增强大肌群肌肉力量的活动。

在制订结构化运动计划时，应考虑文化、个人和家庭偏好。解决 PCOS 患者的心理问题很重要。与对照组相比，PCOS 患者更有可能自卑、焦虑和抑郁。体育活动已被证明可以改善情绪健康，减少焦虑和抑郁，并改善普通人群的情绪。生活方式干预，包括饮食和运动，也显示出对 PCOS 患者的抑郁和自尊有所改善，但需要进一步研究以阐明运动对 PCOS 患者心理社会健康和生活质量的独立影响。

五、行为策略

PCOS 患者经常需要与心理问题做斗争，如焦虑、抑郁、饮食障碍和消极体象。心理问题往往成为有效管理 PCOS 的障碍。动机和情感障碍，如缺乏即时的鼓励和抑郁，会降低患者对生活方式干预的依从性。

此外，据报道，这些心理问题与下丘脑－垂体－肾上腺轴失调有关，可导致慢性炎症、皮质醇轻度增加，以及 IR、HA、PCOS 整体症状的加重（图 21.2）。

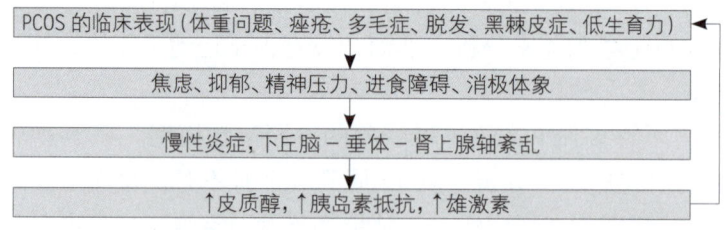

图 21.2　多囊卵巢综合征的临床表现与心理问题之间的恶性循环

这些因素对整体疾病谱系影响巨大，所以医疗保健人员识别和解决这些因素非常重要。

研究表明，增加与医疗保健人员的接触频率、提高社会支持和积极性、设定现实的目标和定期自我监测等策略可以提高患者对生活方式干预的坚持。认知行为干预应包括增加患者的支持、参与、依从性，维持长期健康生活方式。

六、维生素 D

PCOS 患者常伴有维生素 D 缺乏。有研究表明，维生素 D 低水平与 IR、多毛症、HA、排卵和月经不规律、低妊娠率、超重/肥胖，以及远期心血管疾病风险升高均有关。一些证据表明，补充维生素 D 可以改善 PCOS 患者的月经失调和 IR。有研究证明，补充维生素 D 可改善空腹胰岛素、甘油三酯、SHBG、总睾酮和游离雄激素指数（FAI），但数据有限。在提出对所有 PCOS 患者常规给予维生素 D 治疗的建议之前，仍需要进一步的研究支持。

七、环境内分泌干扰物

接触环境内分泌干扰物（environmental endocrine disruptors，EED）对 PCOS 的整体疾病谱产生重大影响。据报道，EED 会在多个层面上干扰性激素的调节，如增加雌激素水平、促进 HA、增加体重、促进高胰岛素血症和糖代谢受损。吸烟、打鼾、室内装饰和使用塑料餐具等 EED，与月经不规律相关。除了上述情况，接触双酚 A 也会影响生育力。然而，EED 的确切影响仍有待研究。但根据现有文献，可以得出结论：除了生活方式干预外，PCOS 患者还应减少对 EED 的暴露。

八、总结

生活方式干预仍然是 PCOS 的一线治疗。现有文献证明，饮食调整、运动和减重有益于改善 IR、月经不规律、排卵和 HA，以及降低心血管风险。但针对 PCOS 患者提供明确的、既现实又可持续的标准化结构化的生活方式干预模型，仍需要进一步研究。

参考文献

1. Moran LJ, Tassone EC, Boyle J, et al. Evidence summaries and recommendations from the international evidence-based guideline for the assessment and management of polycystic ovary syndrome: lifestyle management. Obes Rev. 2020;21(10):e13046. doi:10.1111/obr.13046.
2. Goodman NF, Cobin RH, Futterweit W, Glueck JS, Legro RS, Carmina E. American Association of Clinical Endocrinologists, American College of Endocrinology, and Androgen Excess and PCOS Society Disease State Clinical Review: guide to the best practices in the evaluation and treatment of polycystic ovary syndrome – part 2. Endocr Pract. 2015;21(12):1415-1426. doi:10.4158/Ep15748.Dscpt2.
3. Legro RS, Arslanian SA, Ehrmann DA, et al. Diagnosis and treatment of polycystic ovary syndrome: an

Endocrine Society clinical practice guideline. J Clin Endocrinol Metab. 2013;98(12):4565-4592. doi:10.1210/jc.2013-2350.
4. Hoeger KM, Dokras A, Piltonen T. Update on PCOS: consequences, challenges, and guiding treatment. J Clin Endocrinol Metab. 2021;106(3):e1071-e1083. doi:10.1210/clinem/dgaa839.
5. Ibáñez L, Oberfield SE, Witchel S, et al. An international consortium update: pathophysiology, diagnosis, and treatment of polycystic ovarian syndrome in adolescence. Horm Res Paediatr. 2017;88(6):371-395. doi:10.1159/000479371.
6. Teede H, Misso M, Costello M, et al. On behalf of the International PCOS Network. International Evidence Based Guideline for the Assessment and Management of Polycystic Ovary Syndrome. Melbourne, Australia: Monash University; 2018.
7. Gibson-Helm M, Tassone EC, Teede HJ, Dokras A, Garad R. The needs of women and healthcare providers regarding polycystic ovary syndrome information, resources, and education: a systematic search and narrative review. Semin Reprod Med. 2018;36(1):35-41. doi:10.1055/s-0038-1668086.
8. Gibson-Helm M, Teede H, Dunaif A, Dokras A. Delayed diagnosis and a lack of information associated with dissatisfaction in women with polycystic ovary syndrome. J Clin Endocrinol Metab. 2017;102(2):604-612. doi:10.1210/jc.2016-2963.
9. Stepto NK, Cassar S, Joham AE, et al. Women with polycystic ovary syndrome have intrinsic insulin resistance on euglycaemic-hyperinsulaemic clamp. Hum Reprod. 2013;28(3):777-784. doi:10.1093/humrep/des463.
10. Alzanati N. Polycystic Ovarian Syndrome and Adipose Tissue: Contribution of Peripheral Androgen Synthesis to Hyperandrogenism in Polycystic Ovarian Syndrome. University of Nottingham; 2017. https://eprints.nottingham.ac.uk/39390/.
11. Teede HJ, Misso ML, Costello MF, et al. Recommendations from the international evidence-based guideline for the assessment and management of polycystic ovary syndrome. Hum Reprod. 2018;33(9):1602-1618. doi:10.1093/humrep/dey256.
12. Costello MF, Misso ML, Balen A, et al. Evidence summaries and recommendations from the international evidence-based guideline for the assessment and management of polycystic ovary syndrome: assessment and treatment of infertility. Hum Reprod Open. 2019;2019(1):hoy021. doi:10.1093/hropen/hoy021.
13. Eslamian G, Baghestani AR, Eghtesad S, Hekmatdoost A. Dietary carbohydrate composition is associated with polycystic ovary syndrome: a case-control study. J Hum Nutr Diet. 2017;30(1):90-97. doi:10.1111/jhn.12388.
14. Cutler D. The Impact of Lifestyle on the Reproductive, Metabolic, and Psychological Well-Being of Women with Polycystic Ovary Syndrome (PCOS). University of British Columbia; 2019. https://dx.doi.org/10.14288/1.0378929.
15. Aly JM, Decherney AH. Lifestyle modifications in PCOS. Clin Obstet Gynecol. 2021;64(1):83-89. doi:10.1097/grf.0000000000000594.
16. Zhang X, Zheng Y, Guo Y, Lai Z. The effect of low carbohydrate diet on polycystic ovary syndrome: a meta-analysis of randomized controlled trials. Int J Endocrinol. 2019;2019:4386401. doi:10.1155/2019/4386401.
17. de Luis DA, Izaola O, Aller R, de la Fuente B, Bachiller R, Romero E. Effects of a high-protein/low carbohydrate versus a standard hypocaloric diet on adipocytokine levels and insulin resistance in obese patients along 9 months. J Diabetes Complications. 2015;29(7):950-954. doi:10.1016/j.jdiacomp.2015.06.002.
18. Jonard S, Dewailly D. The follicular excess in polycystic ovaries, due to intra-ovarian hyperandrogenism, may be the main culprit for the follicular arrest. Hum Reprod Update. 2004;10(2):107-117. doi:10.1093/humupd/dmh010.
19. Crosignani PG, Colombo M, Vegetti W, Somigliana E, Gessati A, Ragni G. Overweight and obese anovulatory patients with polycystic ovaries: parallel improvements in anthropometric indices, ovarian physiology and fertility rate induced by diet. Hum Reprod. 2003;18(9):1928-1932. doi:10.1093/humrep/deg367.
20. Thomson RL, Buckley JD, Brinkworth GD. Exercise for the treatment and management of overweight women

with polycystic ovary syndrome: a review of the literature. Obes Rev. 2011;12(5):e202-e210. doi:10.1111/j.1467-789X.2010.00758.x.
21. Marzouk TM, Sayed Ahmed WA. Effect of dietary weight loss on menstrual regularity in obese young adult women with polycystic ovary syndrome. J Pediatr Adolesc Gynecol. 2015;28(6):457-461. doi:10.1016/j.jpag.2015.01.002.
22. Shele G, Genkil J, Speelman D. A systematic review of the effects of exercise on hormones in women with polycystic ovary syndrome. J Funct Morphol Kinesiol. 2020;5(2):35. doi:10.3390/jfmk5020035.
23. Haqq L, McFarlane J, Dieberg G, Smart N. Effect of lifestyle intervention on the reproductive endocrine profile in women with polycystic ovarian syndrome: a systematic review and meta-analysis. Endocr Connect. 2014;3(1):36-46. doi:10.1530/ec-14-0010.
24. Hakimi O, Cameron LC. Effect of exercise on ovulation: a systematic review. Sports Med. 2017;47(8):1555-1567. doi:10.1007/s40279-016-0669-8.
25. Harrison CL, Lombard CB, Moran LJ, Teede HJ. Exercise therapy in polycystic ovary syndrome: a systematic review. Hum Reprod Update. 2011;17(2):171-183. doi:10.1093/humupd/dmq045.
26. Yaribeygi H, Atkin SL, Simental-Mendía LE, Sahebkar A. Molecular mechanisms by which aerobic exercise induces insulin sensitivity. J Cell Physiol. 2019;234(8):12385-12392. doi:10.1002/jcp.28066.
27. Kite C, Lahart IM, Afzal I, et al. Exercise, or exercise and diet for the management of polycystic ovary syndrome: a systematic review and meta-analysis. Syst Rev. 2019;8(1):1-28.
28. Brown AJ, Setji TL, Sanders LL, et al. Effects of exercise on lipoprotein particles in women with polycystic ovary syndrome. Med Sci Sports Exerc. 2009;41(3):497-504. doi:10.1249/MSS.0b013e31818c6c0c.
29. Sayyah-Melli M, Alizadeh M, Pourafkary N, et al. Psychosocial factors associated with polycystic ovary syndrome: a case control study. J Caring Sci. 2015;4(3):225-231. doi:10.15171/jcs.2015.023.
30. Guszkowska M. [Effects of exercise on anxiety, depression and mood]. Psychiatr Pol. 2004;38(4):611-620.
31. Jiskoot G, Dietz de Loos A, Beerthuizen A, Timman R, Busschbach J, Laven J. Long-term effects of a three-component lifestyle intervention on emotional well-being in women with polycystic ovary syndrome (PCOS): a secondary analysis of a randomized controlled trial. PLoS One. 2020;15(6):e0233876. doi:10.1371/journal.pone.0233876.
32. Alur-Gupta S, Chemerinski A, Liu C, et al. Body-image distress is increased in women with polycystic ovary syndrome and mediates depression and anxiety. Fertil Steril. 2019;112(5):930-938.e1. doi:10.1016/j.fertnstert.2019.06.018.
33. Cooney LG, Lee I, Sammel MD, Dokras A. High prevalence of moderate and severe depressive and anxiety symptoms in polycystic ovary syndrome: a systematic review and meta-analysis. Hum Reprod. 2017;32(5):1075-1091. doi:10.1093/humrep/dex044.
34. Lim S, Smith CA, Costello MF, MacMillan F, Moran L, Ee C. Barriers and facilitators to weight management in overweight and obese women living in Australia with PCOS: a qualitative study. BMC Endocr Disord. 2019;19(1):106. doi:10.1186/s12902-019-0434-8.
35. Rudnicka E, Suchta K, Grymowicz M, et al. Chronic low grade inflammation in pathogenesis of PCOS. Int J Mol Sci. 2021;22(7):3789. doi:10.3390/ijms22073789.
36. Wang F, Zhang ZH, Xiao KZ, Wang ZC. Roles of hypothalamic-pituitary-adrenal axis and hypothalamus-pituitary-ovary axis in the abnormal endocrine functions in patients with polycystic ovary syndrome. Zhongguo Yi Xue Ke Xue Yuan Xue Bao. 2017;39(5):699-704. doi:10.3881/j.issn.1000-503X.2017.05.017.
37. Greaves CJ, Sheppard KE, Abraham C, et al. Systematic review of reviews of intervention components associated with increased effectiveness in dietary and physical activity interventions. BMC Public Health. 2011;11:119. doi:10.1186/1471-2458-11-119.
38. Brennan L, Teede H, Skouteris H, Linardon J, Hill B, Moran L. Lifestyle and behavioral management of polycystic ovary syndrome. J Womens Health (Larchmt). 2017;26(8):836-848. doi:10.1089/jwh.2016.5792.

39. He C, Lin Z, Robb SW, Ezeamama AE. Serum vitamin D levels and polycystic ovary syndrome: a systematic review and meta-analysis. Nutrients. 2015;7(6):4555-4577. doi:10.3390/nu7064555.
40. Thomson RL, Spedding S, Buckley JD. Vitamin D in the aetiology and management of polycystic ovary syndrome. Clin Endocrinol (Oxf). 2012;77(3):343-350. doi:10.1111/j.1365-2265.2012.04434.x.
41. Miao CY, Fang XJ, Chen Y, Zhang Q. Effect of vitamin D supplementation on polycystic ovary syndrome: a meta-analysis. Exp Ther Med. 2020;19(4):2641-2649. doi:10.3892/etm.2020.8525.
42. Menichini D, Facchinetti F. Effects of vitamin D supplementation in women with polycystic ovary syndrome: a review. Gynecol Endocrinol. 2020;36(1):1-5. doi:10.1080/09513590.2019.1625881.
43. Zhao JF, Li BX, Zhang Q. Vitamin D improves levels of hormonal, oxidative stress and inflammatory parameters in polycystic ovary syndrome: a meta-analysis study. Ann Palliat Med. 2021;10(1):169-183. doi:10.21037/apm-20-2201.
44. Gore AC, Chappell VA, Fenton SE, et al. EDC-2: The endocrine society's second scientific statement on endocrine-disrupting chemicals. Endocr Rev. 2015;36(6):E1-E150. doi:10.1210/er.2015-1010.
45. Wang Y, Zhu Q, Dang X, He Y, Li X, Sun Y. Local effect of bisphenol A on the estradiol synthesis of ovarian granulosa cells from PCOS. Gynecol Endocrinol. 2017;33(1):21-25. doi:10.1080/09513590.2016.1184641.
46. Kandaraki E, Chatzigeorgiou A, Livadas S, et al. Endocrine disruptors and polycystic ovary syndrome (PCOS): elevated serum levels of bisphenol A in women with PCOS. J Clin Endocrinol Metab. 2011;96(3):E480-E484. doi:10.1210/jc.2010-1658.
47. Zhang B, Zhou W, Shi Y, Zhang J, Cui L, Chen ZJ. Lifestyle and environmental contributions to ovulatory dysfunction in women of polycystic ovary syndrome. BMC Endocr Disord. 2020;20(1):19.
48. Pivonello C, Muscogiuri G, Nardone A, et al. Bisphenol A: an emerging threat to female fertility. Reprod Biol Endocrinol. 2020;18(1):22. doi:10.1186/s12958-019-0558-8.

第二十二章 补充和替代治疗在多囊卵巢综合征中的作用

一、引言

多囊卵巢综合征（PCOS）是一种内分泌紊乱疾病，它可引起月经异常、体重增加、多毛症和肥胖等症状，通常伴有胰岛素抵抗（IR）和代谢紊乱。PCOS 的发展及其并发症是内分泌、遗传和环境因素相互作用的结果。现如今，由于城市化、不健康的生活方式、不平衡的饮食习惯，以及突发的心理和社会经济压力，全球范围内 PCOS 发病率上升了 5%～10%。在巴基斯坦，PCOS 发病率为 15.7%～37.0%，影响了约 10% 的育龄女性。大多数患者受教育程度不高，对 PCOS 的临床表现不了解；因此，及时追踪该疾病仍很困难，这导致并发症难以控制。

二、病因学

PCOS 的病因尚不清楚，但与多毛症和月经失调相关。PCOS 的临床表现包括多毛症、月经不规律、肥胖、痤疮和交感神经活动的改变。其诊断可通过鹿特丹诊断标准进行确认。PCOS 的诊断标准包括排卵功能障碍和高雄激素血症（HA），或伴有雄激素分泌肿瘤、肾上腺羟化酶缺乏和高催乳素血症。PCOS 的诊断依靠体格检查、血液检查和超声检查。

PCOS 涉及的主要功能障碍具有多方面病因，还包括涉及卵巢外因素导致的卵巢行为改变。PCOS 最突出的临床特征是由于稀发排卵/无排卵引起的月经周期紊乱；HA 和卵巢的形态变化可能导致多囊卵巢的发生发展。多囊卵巢可以存在于先前没有症状或体征的患者中，然而，具有多囊卵巢的女性容易在体重增加时导致这组疾病的发病。作为一种多因素疾病，PCOS 的不同症状与不同的遗传变异相关。黄体生成素（LH）浓度在 PCOS 患者中增加了 95%，LH 升高导致女性患者怀孕的概率降低和流产的可能性增加；高水平的 LH 分泌导致雄激素（如睾酮）水平增加，而卵泡刺激素（FSH）水平降低，这些均可能导致卵母细胞发育不良，从而导致不孕症（因为无法排卵）。理论上，PCOS 患者的 HA 会导致多毛症和痤疮，但这些症状的确切存在和患病率仍然存在争议。尽管一些研究与临床证据存在冲突，血生化指标提示 HA 与 PCOS 的关系更密切。血清睾酮浓度大于 4.8 nmol/L 是存在 PCOS 的证据，但前提是已经排除了库欣综合征、先天性肾上腺皮质增生症和卵巢及肾上腺分泌雄激素的肿瘤。因此，可以通过平衡透析、硫酸铵沉淀和性激素结合球蛋白（SHBG）方法测量的游离雄激素指数（FAI）来评估 HA。

（一）高雄激素血症

PCOS 患者的 HA 导致类固醇激素合成失调。类固醇激素合成的初始步骤是胆固醇转化为孕烯醇酮，再经历 17α- 羟基化后转化为脱氢表雄酮（DHEA），进而形成睾酮。卵泡膜细胞和肾上腺皮质的束状带通过 LH 和促肾上腺皮质激素（ACTH）的调控负责产生 50% 的睾酮，卵巢内的睾酮有助于正常的卵泡生长和雌二醇合成。LH 作用于卵巢膜细胞使其分泌雄激素，而 FSH 作用于颗粒细胞，使雄激素被芳香化酶转化为雌激素。PCOS 的异常调节是因卵泡成熟不良和雌激素形成异常，导致卵泡闭锁，从而影响生殖能力。另一项研究给予 PCOS 患者外源性促性腺激素释放激素（GnRH）时机体可产生雄烯二酮、睾酮和雌二醇，进一步证明了其异常。因此，卵巢内雄激素合成失调，卵巢对促性腺激素变得过度敏感，导致雌激素浓度增加。

（二）高胰岛素血症

高胰岛素血症是 PCOS 的另一特征，几乎所有 PCOS 患者中均见报道存在更高程度的 IR；特别是在南亚人群中，IR 更为严重。由于高体重指数（BMI）和肥胖抑制肝脏产生胰岛素样生长因子 -1（IGF-1）和胰岛素样生长因子结合蛋白 -1（IGFBP-1），导致 IGF-1 和 IGF-2 的生物可用性增加，进而导致排卵功能障碍和 HA 的恶化，卵泡成熟受损，并通过增加 LH 对卵泡膜细胞的作用来增加类固醇激素合成。

三、治疗方法

根据病因及其临床特征，PCOS 可采用不同的治疗方法，包括体重管理、定期锻炼、改善 IR、降低雄激素水平、调节月经周期和促排卵，如图 22.1 所示。

（一）传统治疗方法

二甲双胍、人骨髓间充质干细胞和血管紧张素转化酶抑制剂都可以用于 PCOS 的治疗。PCOS 涉及一系列炎症标志物［如 C 反应蛋白（CRP）、白细胞介素 -1（IL-1）和白细胞介素 -6（IL-6）］的持续表达，代表着慢性炎症状态。选

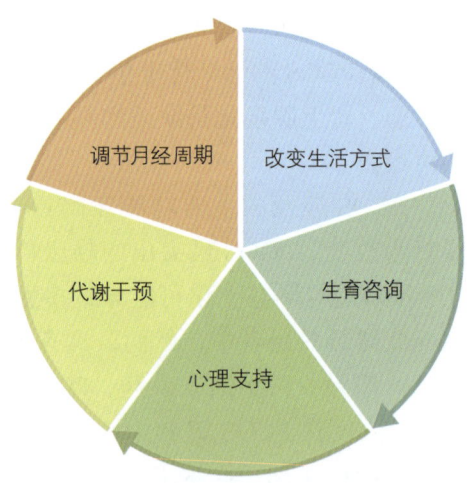

图 22.1　多囊卵巢综合征的管理流程

择性孕酮受体调节剂被发现对慢性炎症性疾病有益，但临床试验仍在进一步研究中。赖诺普利已在来曲唑诱导的啮齿类 PCOS 模型中进行了实验，研究发现它能够抑制纤溶酶原激活物抑制物 -1，从而逆转来曲唑的作用，其应用仍在进一步研究中。二甲双胍的不良反应包括虚弱、腹泻、胃肠胀气、无力和肌肉痛，它还会引起胃肠不适和低血糖，少

见乳酸酸中毒。赖诺普利会导致心力衰竭、低血压和咳嗽，长期使用还会导致肌酐水平升高和高钾血症。这些药物的副作用限制了它们在长期治疗中的作用。副作用较少的补充和替代治疗（complementary and alternative medicine，CAM）在 PCOS 的治疗中可以发挥有益作用。

（二）补充疗法

尽管对 PCOS 有传统治疗方法，但经常出现患者依从性不佳、药物不良反应和成功率较低的情况。因此，有必要找到对 PCOS 有效且患者适应的替代治疗方法。CAM 独立于西医，但在全球医疗系统中被广泛使用。大量文献已强调了 CAM 对抗 PCOS 的疗效和患者接受程度。根据各地的本土习俗和资源，CAM 在不同地区有所不同。例如，在中国，中草药、针灸和气功已被用于有效治疗 PCOS；在巴基斯坦，北部地区的草药、坚果和本土功能性食品，以及冥想疗法是治疗各种慢性疾病（包括 PCOS）的流行方式，如图 22.2 所示。

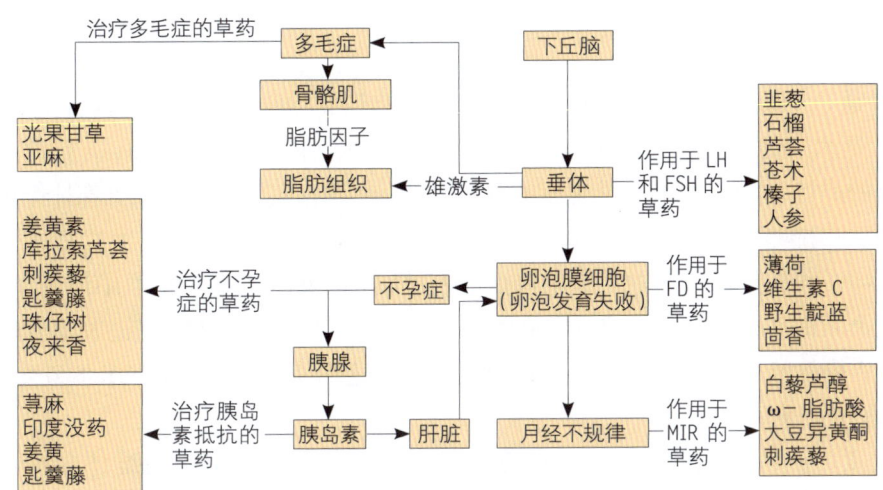

FD，卵泡发育；FSH，卵泡刺激素；LH，黄体生成素；MIR，月经不规律。

图 22.2　不同治疗方式治疗多囊卵巢综合征的机制

四、补充和替代治疗

CAM 在全球医疗系统中被广泛应用。许多研究表明，包括针灸、中草药、太极、瑜伽和气功在内的 CAM 的使用也可以有效地治疗 PCOS，并且副作用较少。基于此，本综述的目的是提供更准确的证据，证明 CAM 对 PCOS 的治疗有效，并分析其潜在机制。

传统疗法在治疗 PCOS 方面是有效的，但长期使用可能会导致副作用。患有 PCOS 的患者可以使用替代疗法来管理其不孕问题。因此，目前的科学研究重点是基于证据的临床前评估结果，以总结草药在 PCOS 中的重要性。

（一）植物和维生素成分在多囊卵巢综合征治疗中的作用

1. 白藜芦醇

白藜芦醇是一种天然多酚（植物成分），存在于坚果、浆果和葡萄中，具有抗氧化、心脏保护和抗炎作用，它也可以治疗与PCOS相关的不孕、卵巢储备减少和肥胖；但由于其抗蜕膜化作用，应避免在妊娠期和黄体期使用。它还通过抑制细胞内维A酸结合蛋白2（CRABP2-RAR）的表达来对抗编码IGF-1和催乳素的蜕膜基因表达过程。临床研究表明，使用白藜芦醇后，患者流产率增加、怀孕率降低。据报道，补充白藜芦醇未能增加胰岛素敏感性。

2. 黄酮和类似物

柚皮素来源于不同的植物物种及柚子，是一种常见的黄酮。文献表明，它具有抗炎和细胞保护作用，在PCOS中发挥治疗作用。柚皮素可降低患者的雌二醇和睾酮水平，增加活性氧自由基清除酶的浓度，并对PCOS患者的体重增加产生有益影响。芦丁是另一种黄酮类化合物，也被用于治疗PCOS。

3. 维生素C

维生素C，即抗坏血酸，对身体细胞的生长起到有效的作用，并且具有抗氧化性质。维生素C是水溶性的，会随尿液排出，需要持续通过膳食摄入。Olaniyan等调查了拥有多囊卵巢的雌性Wistar大鼠中维生素C相关的代谢变化，发现其水平随着月经周期的变化而波动。在排卵前，维生素C水平下降，而在排卵后体温升高时维生素C水平也相应升高。抗坏血酸在月经周期中的作用包括促进排卵（在排卵前期的摄取中体现），并刺激孕酮和催产素的产生，与卵泡和黄体的生长相关联。维生素C能够促进胶原合成，有助于在排卵后修复卵巢组织。维生素C缺乏会影响上述功能，并导致PCOS的发生。

4. 维生素E

维生素E是脂溶性的维生素，储存在肝脏中并以微量释放，易维持在正常生理水平。它是一种抗氧化剂，因此能够中和自由基并促进细胞更新。由于其抗氧化和抗凝血性质，它可以改善特发性不孕患者的子宫内膜厚度。虽然辅酶Q10和维生素E的治疗降低了PCOS患者的SHBG水平并降低了血浆睾酮水平，但也已证明短期给予维生素E可以诱导PCOS患者排卵。使用维生素E还有助于减少氧化应激和人绝经期促性腺激素（HMG）的促排剂量。

5. 维生素D

维生素D是一种甾体类物质，具有类孕激素样作用。它能够促进骨骼矿化和维持钙平衡。维生素D需要经过两个羟化步骤才能变为活性形式；首先生成钙化醇［25-羟基胆钙化醇或25（OH）D］这一前体物质，然后生成激素活化维生素D［1,25-二羟基胆钙化醇或1,25（OH）2D］。在炎症、PCOS、生育力降低、IR和血脂异常患者中都可以观察到维生素D缺乏。一些研究观察了PCOS患者和月经失调患者接受促性腺激素时联用钙－维生素D与二甲双胍，在PCOS患者和维生素D缺乏的患者中，维生素D

和钙补充剂能够促进二甲双胍的作用，但对 IGF-1 系统和促性腺激素的作用没有显著影响。也有研究指出，维生素 D 补充对 BMI、DHEAS、甘油三酯或 HDL 胆固醇水平没有积极影响。维生素 D 补充剂可以减少 PCOS 患者的雄激素和减轻 IR。一些研究观察到维生素 D 补充剂能够使口服葡萄糖耐量试验后 1 小时内血浆中葡萄糖水平降低、子宫内膜厚度增加，进而增加维生素 D 水平正常的女性受孕的可能性。维生素 D 通过降低晚期糖基化终末产物的作用来降低 PCOS 患者的雄激素和卵泡的合成。

6. 脂肪酸

ω-3 是一种多不饱和脂肪酸，来源于鲱鱼、三文鱼、金枪鱼、蓝鱼和鲭鱼等富含油脂的鱼类。在多不饱和脂肪酸中，二十二碳六烯酸（docosahexaenoic acid，DHA）和二十碳五烯酸（eicosatetraenoic acid，EPA）是具有生物活性的。它们具有抗氧化、增强胰岛素敏感性、抗肥胖和抗炎的特性，被认为通过增加抗炎脂连蛋白分泌并减少如 IL-6 和肿瘤坏死因子-α（TNF-α）等炎性细胞因子的产生，增强胰岛素的敏感性。而肥胖和 IR 可以导致 40 岁以后出现高血压、糖尿病（DM）和血脂异常。

在 Sadeghi 等的研究中，他们发现在 PCOS 患者中，补充 ω-3 脂肪酸并不能改善 IR。在非 PCOS 患者中，它增加了高密度脂蛋白（HDL）、低密度脂蛋白（LDL）、甘油三酯含量，并增加了腰围，使月经周期更加规律。此外，Yang 等的研究显示，IR 与补充 ω-3 脂肪酸有关，因为 ω-3 可导致 LDL、总胆固醇和甘油三酯增加，但它又通过降低促炎细胞因子和增加抗炎脂连蛋白的产生来提高胰岛素敏感性。在 PCOS 患者中，由于抗炎脂连蛋白水平增加和 C 反应蛋白水平降低，炎症状态反而会减轻。

ω-3 脂肪酸的日摄入量仅为身体需求的 0.5%～2.0%，而 EPA：DHA 的最低需求量为每天 500 mg，对于甘油三酯水平发生变化的人群为每天 2000～4000 mg。ω-3 脂肪酸的副作用包括肠积气、肠道不适、头痛、恶心和腹泻，正在服用抗凝血和抗血小板药物治疗的患者禁忌使用，怀孕期间慎用，因为它会干扰药物并引起副作用。由于 EPA 干扰胎儿阶段所需的花生四烯酸的作用，怀孕期间应避免使用 EPA。考虑到 ω-3 脂肪酸的高热量，应谨慎使用其治疗肥胖患者，以避免对 PCOS 患者的心脏代谢产生有害影响。

（二）药用植物在多囊卵巢综合征治疗中的作用

1. 野生靛蓝（紫花毛茛）

紫花毛茛被用作治疗女性生殖系统疾病和炎症性疾病，它的提取物被用于增强来曲唑诱导 PCOS 大鼠排卵的有效性。这种治疗被用来使类固醇激素和发情周期的激素水平恢复正常，但垂体分泌的 FSH 和 LH 没有受到影响，所以紫花毛茛的作用仅限于卵巢。为了检查大鼠生育力，通过交配实验确认怀孕情况。

2. 茴芹籽（茴香）

茴香是伊朗的传统药物。它含有茴香油、甲基香草醇、茴香醛和丁香酚，用于治疗癫痫和癫痫发作，也可以作为退烧药、抗真菌剂、抗细菌剂，对消化系统有帮助。当使用 200 mg/kg 和 400 mg/kg 的茴香油提取物时，可以减轻大鼠卵巢组织中 PCOS 的症状。

3. 夜来香（棚架藤）

棚架藤含有三萜类化合物、类固醇化合物、皂苷、生物碱和强心苷，它被用作抗糖 DM 药物、护肝药和抗生育药。在通过睾酮丙酸酯诱导 PCOS 的大鼠中，与单独使用二甲双胍治疗相比，二甲双胍和棚架藤的联合作用被发现更有效。通过测量孕酮、雌二醇、睾酮、FSH 和 LH 的血浆水平，可以证实肥胖对 PCOS 大鼠的影响。结果显示，治疗 PCOS 中的冠心病和肥胖可以预防大鼠的动脉粥样硬化。因此，棚架藤是降低血清胆固醇水平和治疗 PCOS 的有效药用植物。

4. 芦荟（库拉索芦荟）

传统上芦荟被用来控制高血压，治疗 DM 及一些消化和皮肤问题，包括皮肤癌和烧伤。一些研究者使用芦荟来治疗大鼠的 PCOS。首先，他们使用来曲唑诱导大鼠的 PCOS，之后使用芦荟来控制症状，持续 2 个月之后，大鼠怀孕并在妊娠后期被处死以检查调节蛋白和激素状态。一系列分析显示，芦荟直接参与调节一些主要受体的作用，包括 LH 受体、芳香化酶受体和雄激素受体。这证明对于有 PCOS 症状的人来说，芦荟是一种良好的孕前使用药物。

5. 苍术（白术）

白术（*Atractylodes macrocephala* Koidz，AMK）是一种用于治疗 PCOS 的草药，被用于评估治疗 PCOS 大鼠 HA 模型的活性，HA 状态是通过睾酮丙酸酯诱导的。

研究使用了 5 组动物，通过睾酮丙酸酯诱导 PCOS。使用酶联免疫吸附法测量总睾酮（total testosterone，TT）、SHBG、雄烯二酮、FSH、LH 和抗米勒管激素。聚合酶链反应和生物化学方法测量了 FSH 和水通道蛋白 -9 的表达。AMK 的提取物通过改善动情周期和降低 TT 和雄烯二酮的血浆水平来缓解 PCOS，它还减少了大鼠卵巢中 FSH 受体的表达，并增加了水通道蛋白 -9 的表达。

6. 印度没药（乳香）

Kavitha 等在一项实验中研究了乳香的作用，该实验涉及 4 组大鼠，使用 DHEA 诱导 PCOS。另外给予这些动物二甲双胍和乳香后评估了其血清葡萄糖和类固醇的水平，结果表明，乳香通过减少卵巢滤泡的形态异常，在减轻 DHEA 诱导的 PCOS 症状方面发挥了很好的作用。

7. 三角榕

实验将大鼠分为 6 组，使用来曲唑诱导 PCOS。在实验大鼠中研究了黄肉桂（*Ficus deltoidea*）对生殖器官的影响，并使用不同浓度的枸橼酸氯米芬作为标准进行处理；在治疗周期结束时收集了其卵巢和子宫，并评估了它们的重量。组织病理学显示，经过该物质处理的组织显示出较少的囊性卵泡，它减少了卵巢湿重，增加了子宫湿重。另一项研究表明，这些植物药对抗 PCOS 有良好的效果。

8. 甘草（光果甘草）

甘草以其抗菌和降血糖作用而闻名。甘草中提取的甘草素和异黄酮是两种天然化合物，表现出雌激素活性，它们在减肥方面非常有效，并且当与螺内酯一起用于治疗多毛症时，可以保护由螺内酯引起的有效血容量不足，并增强其抗雄激素作用。

9. 薄荷（欧薄荷）

薄荷（唇形科）以其抗菌、抗肿瘤、抗炎和抗过敏性质而闻名，由于其抗雄激素作用，它还可以降低血液中的游离睾酮水平。因此，它已被用作 PCOS 的替代疗法。

10. 人参属（人参）

人参在草药医学中被用作滋补剂，并以其抗衰老性质而闻名。研究发现，人参可以调节 PCOS 患者的黄体生成素水平，从而通过调节内分泌功能来改善排卵障碍。

11. 蒺藜（刺蒺藜）

实验证明，蒺藜是治疗 PCOS 患者使其获得优良生育力的草药。研究发现，蒺藜可以通过改善类固醇激素水平来促进卵泡生长、排卵和调节月经周期。因此，它被认为是一种有效的卵巢刺激剂。

12. 武靴叶（匙羹藤）

匙羹藤（萝藦科）以其降糖和降脂的特性而闻名。实验证明，匙羹藤具有治疗 IR 的效果，以及降低血清甘油三酯水平的特性，它在 DM 的治疗中非常有益。

13. 枫香树（珠仔树）

珠仔树属于山矾科。在来曲唑诱导的 PCOS 大鼠模型中，发现枫香树能够改善睾酮、雌激素和孕酮水平。因此，它在治疗 PCOS 中具有抗雄激素作用，有助于改善生育力。此外，它还能够使卵巢组织恢复正常，从而改善 PCOS 中的卵巢功能。

14. 贞洁树（黄荆）

贞洁树属于马鞭草科，以其抗菌、抗炎和止痛效果而闻名。在妇科疾病的治疗中，发挥抗雄激素和抗雌激素的作用。在使用来曲唑诱导的 PCOS 大鼠的实验中发现贞洁树具有多种益处，能够改善 FSH、LH、血清性激素水平，以及治疗高血糖、高脂血症和月经周期不规律。

15. Licogliflozin

PCOS 中的高胰岛素血症导致雄激素增加。Licogliflozin 是一种钠 - 葡萄糖协同转运蛋白 1 和 2 抑制剂，可改善 2 型糖尿病（T2DM）和高胰岛素血症中的 IR。一项关于其疗效的研究表明，它显著降低了高胰岛素血症和雄激素水平。

16. 刺槐

长期以来，印度人一直使用刺槐（*Caesalpinia bonduc*）来退烧和消炎。现在它也被发现可以纠正 PCOS 中月经周期的失调。

17. 人类抑制素

人类抑制素是一种线粒体来源的肽。一项研究表明，当给 PCOS 的大鼠补充人类抑制素时，可以降低空腹血糖和胰岛素水平，从而缓解 IR。该作用机制通过多囊卵巢患者卵泡液中人类抑制素浓度降低得以印证。此外，它还能刺激运动信号通路，有助于减轻体重，从而改善 PCOS 症状。

（三）功能性食物在多囊卵巢综合征治疗中的作用

1. 大豆异黄酮（大豆）

大豆（*Glycine max*）含有异黄酮，被用作更年期女性的内分泌替代治疗。Rajan 等研究了使用来曲唑诱导的 PCOS 大鼠的身体、内分泌和代谢参数，通过组织病理学，研究了大鼠的特征性卵巢变化。大豆异黄酮在临床和生化参数及治疗 PCOS 方面表现出有益的效果。

2. 姜黄（姜黄素）

姜黄素是姜黄根茎的重要成分，它被用作食品添加剂，并具有抗炎、降脂、降血糖和抗氧化性能。一项实验对使用来曲唑诱导 PCOS 的 5 组大鼠进行了姜黄素的性能评估，通过评估空腹血糖、糖化血红蛋白和血脂谱的实验室结果，比较了姜黄素和枸橼酸氯米芬的治疗效果。过氧化氢酶和超氧化物歧化酶活性的测定结果确定了姜黄素的抗氧化性能。实验结果显示，姜黄素直接参与降低空腹血糖和糖化血红蛋白水平。姜黄素对治疗来曲唑诱导的 PCOS 是有益的。

3. 洋葱（韭葱）

韭葱在亚洲除了作为食物之外，还被当作传统药物而广泛应用。研究发现，韭葱提取物疗法能够通过使 LH 和 FSH 水平正常化来治疗排卵障碍，它还能够使卵泡生长和卵巢囊肿正常化。

4. 亚麻籽（亚麻）

亚麻籽是从食物木质素中提取的。研究发现，亚麻籽是治疗多毛症、雄激素过多的有效药物，它能够使 PCOS 中的雄激素水平正常化，还能改善高脂血症。此外，它还能促进卵泡生长，减少卵巢体积，并调节月经周期。

5. 石榴

石榴属于石榴科。这种水果富含叶酸、硫胺素、维生素 C、有机酸，以及饱和与不饱和脂肪酸。在实验性诱导 PCOS 的动物（大鼠）研究中发现，石榴能够使激素失衡恢复正常，并减少与 PCOS 相关的并发症。

6. 肉桂皮（肉桂）

肉桂属于樟科，可以增强胰岛素的促葡萄糖摄取作用，并促进糖原的合成。在对患有 PCOS 的患者进行的研究中发现，肉桂表现出显著的降血糖作用。它含有原花青素和酚类化合物，可以通过增强胰岛素信号通路来增加胰岛素的敏感性。在另一个实验中，肉桂被发现可以使月经周期规律，并改善 PCOS 的代谢功能障碍。

（四）坚果食物在多囊卵巢综合征治疗中的作用

1. 榛子

Demirel 评估了榛子油在来曲唑诱导的 PCOS 中的治疗效果，评估参数包括血清 FSH、LH、雌二醇、睾酮、孕酮、脂质、瘦素和葡萄糖，以及榛子油的抗氧化活性和植物甾醇含量。结果显示，治疗组中 HDL 浓度较高，而葡萄糖和瘦素浓度较低。该油含有生育酚、谷固醇、角鲨烯、蓖麻固醇和豆固醇，对 PCOS 确实有效。

2. 核桃

有实验分别研究了杏仁和核桃作为单不饱和脂肪酸和多不饱和脂肪酸（polyunsaturated fatty acids，PUFA）的来源，并比较了它们在 PCOS 患者中的效果。结果表明，食用核桃显著增加了脂肪酸和 α-硫辛酸的浓度；然而，EPA 和 DHA 的血清浓度保持不变。食用核桃的 PCOS 患者组显示了升高的 SHGB 和脂连蛋白血清浓度，而 LDL 胆固醇和载脂蛋白 H 水平的浓度得到了降低。

3. 杏仁

在 PCOS 患者中，血清氨基酸、SHBG 和脂连蛋白浓度增加，而 FAI 值降低，这表明脂连蛋白水平的增加对胰岛素敏感性没有影响。血清促炎细胞因子（IL-6 和 IL-1）和 CRP 的浓度没有显著变化。研究得出结论，核桃作为 PUFA 的来源可能显著改善 PCOS 患者的激素和脂质谱，并降低心血管疾病的风险。如图 22.2 所示，摄入坚果对 PCOS 患者的血浆脂质和雄激素水平可产生有益影响。

参考文献

1. Sneha S. Effect of high levels of testosterone on cardiovascular risk in polycystic ovary syndrome (PCOS). Int J Res Rev. 2020;7(7):285-289.
2. Hachey LM, Kroger-Jarvis M, Pavlik-Maus T, Leach R. Clinical implications of polycystic ovary syndrome in adolescents. Nurs Womens Health. 2020;24(2):115-126.
3. Haq N, Khan Z, Riaz S, et al. Prevalence and knowledge of polycystic ovary syndrome (PCOS) among female science students of different public universities of Quetta, Pakistan. Imp J Interdiscip Res. 2017;35(6):385-392.
4. Anjum N, Zohra S, Arif A, et al. Prevalence of metabolic syndrome in Pakistani women with polycystic ovarian syndrome. Pak J Biochem Mol Biol. 2013;46(3):97-100.
5. Hamza DH, Hassan SA. Polycystic ovary syndrome and some hormonal and physiological changes: a review. Eur Asian J BioSci. 2020;14(2):5149-5156.
6. Ibáñez L, Oberfield SE, Witchel S, et al. An international consortium update: pathophysiology, diagnosis, and treatment of polycystic ovarian syndrome in adolescence. Horm Res Paediatr. 2017;88:371-395.
7. Azziz R, Kintziger K, Li R, et al. Recommendations for epidemiologic and phenotypic research in polycystic ovary syndrome: an androgen excess and PCOS society resource. Hum Reprod. 2019;34(11):2254-2265.
8. Rosenfield RL, Ehrmann DA. The pathogenesis of polycystic ovary syndrome (PCOS): the hypothesis of PCOS as functional ovarian hyperandrogenism revisited. Endocr Rev. 2016;37(5):467-520.
9. Shukla P, Mukherjee S. Mitochondrial dysfunction: an emerging link in the pathophysiology of polycystic ovary syndrome. Mitochondrion. 2020;52:24-39.
10. Hart R, Hickey M, Franks S. Definitions, prevalence and symptoms of polycystic ovaries and polycystic ovary

syndrome. Best Pract Res Clin Obstet Gynaecol. 2004;18(5):671-683.

11. Asghari R, Shokri V, Rezaei H, et al. Alteration of TGFB1, GDF9, and BMPR2 gene expression in preantral follicles of an estradiol valerate-induced polycystic ovary mouse model can lead to anovulation, polycystic morphology, obesity, and absence of hyperandrogenism. Korean J Fertil Steril. 2021;48(3):245-254.

12. Soumya V. Polycystic ovary disease (PCOD)-an insight into rodent models, diagnosis and treatments. J Clin Med Img. 2021;5(11):1-13.

13. Kabil Kucur S, Kurek Eken M, Sanli I, et al. Predictive value of serum and follicular fluid chemerin concentrations during assisted reproductive cycles in women with polycystic ovary syndrome. Gynecol Endocrinol. 2021;37(9):814-818.

14. Amin S, Nabi M, Andrabi SM, et al. Androgen receptor coregulator long non coding RNA CTBP1-AS is associated with polycystic ovary syndrome in Kashmiri women. Endocrine. 2022;75(2):614-622.

15. Escobar-Morreale HF. Polycystic ovary syndrome: definition, aetiology, diagnosis and treatment. Nat Rev Endocrinol. 2018;14(5):270-284.

16. Laven JS, Imani B, Eijkemans MJ, Fauser BC. New approaches to PCOS and other forms of anovulation. Obstet Gynecol Surv. 2002;57:755-767.

17. Ferk P, Perme MP, Teran N, Gersak K. Androgen receptor gene (CAG) n polymorphism in patients with polycystic ovary syndrome. Fertili Steril. 2008;90(3):860-863.

18. Keevil BG, Adaway J. Assessment of free testosterone concentration. J Steroid Biochem Mol Biol. 2019;190:207-211.

19. Rosenfield RL. Ovarian and adrenal function in polycystic ovary syndrome. Endocrinol Metab Clin North Am. 1999;28(2):265-293.

20. Zeng X, Xie YJ, Liu YT, Long SL, Mo ZC. Polycystic ovarian syndrome: correlation between hyperandrogenism, insulin resistance and obesity. Clinica Chimica Acta. 2022;502:214-221.

21. Hsueh AJ, Adashi EY, Jones PB, Welsh Jr TH. Hormonal regulation of the differentiation of cultured ovarian granulosa cells. Endocr Rev. 1984;5(1):76-127.

22. White DW, Leigh A, Wilson C, et al. Gonadotrophin and gonadal steroid response to a single dose of a long-acting agonist of gonadotrophin-releasing hormone in ovulatory and anovulatory women with polycystic ovary syndrome. Clin Endocrinol. 1995;42:475-481.

23. Ezeh U, Ida Chen YD, Azziz R. Racial and ethnic differences in the metabolic response of polycystic ovary syndrome. Clin Endocrinol. 2020;93(2):163-172.

24. Di Bari F, Catalano A, Bellone F, Martino G, Benvenga S. Vitamin D, bone metabolism, and fracture risk in polycystic ovary syndrome. Metabolites. 2021;11(2):116.

25. Speelman DL. Nonpharmacologic management of symptoms in females with polycystic ovary syndrome: a narrative review. Int J Osteopath Med. 2019;119(1):25-39.

26. Paris VR, Walters KA. Humanin: a potential treatment for PCOS? Endocrinology. 2021;162(8);bqab085.

27. Regidor PA, Mueller A, Sailer M, Gonzalez Santos F, Rizo JM, Moreno Egea F. Chronic inflammation in PCOS: the potential benefits of specialized pro-resolving lipid mediators (SPMs) in the improvement of the resolutive response. Int J Mol Sci. 2021;22(1):384.

28. Chugh RM, Park HS, El Andaloussi A, et al. Mesenchymal stem cell therapy ameliorates metabolic dysfunction and restores fertility in a PCOS mouse model through interleukin-10. Stem Cell Res Ther. 2021;12(1):388.

29. Coskun B, Ercan CM, Togrul C, et al. Effects of lisinopril treatment on the pathophysiology of PCOS and plasminogen activator inhibitor-1 concentrations in rats. Reprod Biomed Online. 2021;42(1):16-25.

30. Naz S, Anjum N, Gul I A Community based cross sectional study on prevalence of polycystic ovarian syndrome (PCOS) and health related quality of life in Pakistani females. Research square. 2020:1-8.

31. Gale N. The sociology of traditional, complementary and alternative medicine. Sociol Compass. 2014;8(6):805-822.

32. Pan SY, Gao SH, Zhou SF, Tang MK, Yu ZL, Ko KM. New perspectives on complementary and alternative

medicine: an overview and alternative therapy. Altern Ther Health Med. 2012;18(4):20-36.
33. Ben-Nun L. Treatment of infertility.
34. Hamza DH, Hassan SA. Polycystic ovary syndrome and some hormonal and physiological changes: a review. Eur Asian J BioSci. 2020;14(2):5149-5156.
35. Ibáñez L, Oberfield SE, Witchel S, et al. An international consortium update: pathophysiology, diagnosis, and treatment of polycystic ovarian syndrome in adolescence. Horm Res Paediatr. 2017;88:371-395.
36. Park YL, Canaway R. Integrating traditional and complementary medicine with national healthcare systems for universal health coverage in Asia and the Western Pacific. Health Syst Reform. 2019;5(1):24-31.
37. Jia LY, Feng JX, Li JL, et al. The complementary and alternative medicine for polycystic ovary syndrome: a review of clinical application and mechanism. Evid Based Complement Alternat Med. 2021;2021:5555315.
38. Devaki R. Preclinical Evaluation of Siddha Poly-Herbal Formulation Ashuwathi Chooranam for its Naturally Curing PCOS. Doctoral Dissertation. Chennai: Government Siddha Medical College; 2017.
39. Farkhondeh T, Folgado SL, Pourbagher-Shahri AM, Ashrafizadeh M, Samarghandian S. The therapeutic effect of resveratrol: Focusing on the Nrf2 signaling pathway. Biomed Pharmacother. 2020;127:110234.
40. Zhang T, Zhou Y, LI L, et al. SIRT1, 2, 3 protect mouse oocytes from postovulatory aging. Aging (Albany NY). 2016;8(4):685.
41. Cabello E, Garrido P, Morán J, et al. Effects of resveratrol on ovarian response to controlled ovarian hyperstimulation in ob/ob mice. Fertil Steril. 2015;103(2):570-579.
42. Ortega I, Duleba AJ. Ovarian actions of resveratrol. Ann N Y Acad Sci. 2015;1348(1):86-96.
43. Iervolino M, Lepore E, Forte G, Laganà AS, Buzzaccarini G, Unfer V. Natural molecules in the management of polycystic ovary syndrome (PCOS): an analytical review. Nutrients. 2021;13(5):1677.
44. Benrick A, Maliqueo M, Miao S, et al. Resveratrol is not as effective as physical exercise for improving reproductive and metabolic functions in rats with dihydrotestosterone-induced polycystic ovary syndrome. Evid Based Complement Alternat Med. 2013;2013:964070.
45. Hong Y, Yin Y, Tan Y, Hong K, Zhou H. The flavanone, naringenin, modifies antioxidant and steroidogenic enzyme activity in a rat model of letrozole-induced polycystic ovary syndrome. Med Sci Monit. 2019;25:395.
46. Mihanfar A, Nouri M, Roshangar L, Khadem-Ansari MH. Polyphenols: natural compounds with promising potential in treating polycystic ovary syndrome. Reprod Biol. 2021;21(2):100500.
47. Wawrzkiewicz-Jałowiecka A, Kowalczyk K, Trybek P, et al. In search of new therapeutics—molecular aspects of the PCOS pathophysiology: genetics, hormones, metabolism and beyond. Int J Mol Sci. 2020;21(19):7054.
48. Hong Y, Yin Y, Tan Y, Hong K, Zhou H. The flavanone, naringenin, modifies antioxidant and steroidogenic enzyme activity in a rat model of letrozole-induced polycystic ovary syndrome. Med Sci Monit. 2019;25:395.
49. Jahan S, Munir F, Razak S, et al. Ameliorative effects of rutin against metabolic, biochemical and hormonal disturbances in polycystic ovary syndrome in rats. J Ovarian Res. 2016;9(1):1-9.
50. Pehlivan FE. Vitamin C: an antioxidant agent. Vitamin C. 2017;2:23-35.
51. Olaniyan OT, Femi A, Iliya G, et al. Vitamin C suppresses ovarian pathophysiology in experimental polycystic ovarian syndrome. Pathophysiology. 2019;26(3-4):331-341.
52. Bendich A, Machlin LJ, Scandurra O, Burton GW, Wayner DD. The antioxidant role of vitamin C. Adv Free Radic Biol Med. 1986;2(2):419-444.
53. Chandrasekhar U. Unit-7 Fat-Soluble Vitamins: Vitamin A, D, E, and K. New Delhi: Indira Gandhi National Open University; 2021.
54. Ebhohimen IE, Okanlanwon TS, Osagie AO, Izevbigie ON. Vitamin E in Human Health and Oxidative Stress Related Diseases. Diseases and Health Aspects. IntechOpen. 2021.
55. Cicek N, Eryilmaz OG, Sarikaya E, Gulerman C, Genc Y. Vitamin E effect on controlled ovarian stimulation of unexplained infertile women. J Assist Reprod Genet. 2012;29(4):325-328.
56. Izadi A, Ebrahimi S, Shirazi S, et al. Hormonal and metabolic effects of coenzyme Q10 and/or vitamin E in patients with polycystic ovary syndrome. J Clin Endocrinol Metab. 2019;104(2):319-327.

57. Monastra G, De Grazia S, De Luca L, Vittorio S, Unfer V. Vitamin D: a steroid hormone with progesterone-like activity. Eur Rev Med Pharmacol Sci. 2018;22(8):2502-2512.
58. Goltzman D, Miao D, Panda DK, Hendy GN. Effects of calcium and of the Vitamin D system on skeletal and calcium homeostasis: lessons from genetic models. J Steroid Biochem Mol Biol. 2004;89:485-489.
59. Holick MF. Vitamin D deficiency. N Engl J Med. 2007;357(3):266-281.
60. Iervolino M, Lepore E, Forte G, Laganà AS, Buzzaccarini G, Unfer V. Natural molecules in the management of polycystic ovary syndrome (PCOS): an analytical review. Nutrients. 2021;13(5):1677.
61. Kadoura S, Alhalabi M, Nattouf AH. Effect of calcium and vitamin D supplements as an adjuvant therapy to metformin on menstrual cycle abnormalities, hormonal profile, and IGF-1 system in polycystic ovary syndrome patients: a randomized, placebo-controlled clinical trial. Adv Pharmacol Sci. 2019;2019:9680390.
62. Iervolino M, Lepore E, Forte G, Laganà AS, Buzzaccarini G, Unfer V. Natural molecules in the management of polycystic ovary syndrome (PCOS): an analytical review. Nutrients. 2021;13(5):1677.
63. Lerchbaum E, Rabe T. Vitamin D and female fertility. Curr Opin Obstet Gynecol. 2014;26(3):145-150.
64. Merhi Z, Buyuk E, Cipolla MJ. Advanced glycation end products alter steroidogenic gene expression by granulosa cells: an effect partially reversible by vitamin D. Mol Hum Reprod. 2018;24(6):318-326.
65. Oliver L, Dietrich T, Marañón I, Villarán MC, Barrio RJ. Producing omega-3 polyunsaturated fatty acids: a review of sustainable sources and future trends for the EPA and DHA market. Resources. 2020;9(12):148.
66. Watanabe Y, Tatsuno I. Omega-3 polyunsaturated fatty acids focusing on eicosapentaenoic acid and docosahexaenoic acid in the prevention of cardiovascular diseases: a review of the state-of-the-art. Expert Rev Clin Pharmacol. 2021;14(1):79-93.
67. Monk JM, Turk HF, Liddle DM, et al. n-3 polyunsaturated fatty acids and mechanisms to mitigate inflammatory paracrine signaling in obesity-associated breast cancer. Nutrients. 2014;6(11):4760-4793.
68. Bellver J, Rodríguez-Tabernero L, Robles A, et al. Polycystic ovary syndrome throughout a woman's life. J Assist Reprod Genet. 2018;35(1):25-39.
69. Sadeghi A, Djafarian K, Mohammadi H, Shab-Bidar S. Effect of omega-3 fatty acids supplementation on insulin resistance in women with polycystic ovary syndrome: meta-analysis of randomized controlled trials. Diabetes Metab Syndr. 2017;11(2):157-162.
70. Yang K, Zeng L, Bao T, Ge J. Effectiveness of omega-3 fatty acid for polycystic ovary syndrome: a systematic review and meta-analysis. Reprod Biol Endocrinol. 2018;16(1):1-13.
71. Tosatti JA, Alves MT, Cândido AL, Reis FM, Araújo VE, Gomes KB. Influence of n-3 fatty acid supplementation on inflammatory and oxidative stress markers in patients with polycystic ovary syndrome: a systematic review and meta-analysis. Br J Nutr. 2021;125(6):657-668.
72. Tu Wei-Chun. Effects of Dietary Alpha Linolenic Acid on Biosynthesis of N-3 Long Chain Polyunsaturated Fatty Acids in Animals (Doctoral Dissertation). 2011.
73. Sheehan MT. Polycystic ovarian syndrome: diagnosis and management. Clin Med Res. 2004;2(1):13-27.
74. Thakor AP, Patel AJ. Normalizing of estrous cycle in polycystic ovary syndrome (PCOS) induced rats with Tephrosia purpurea (Linn.) Pers. J Appli Nat Sci. 2014;6(1):197-201.
75. Mahood RAH. Effects of Pimpinella anisum oil extract on some biochemical parameters in mice experimentally induced for human polycystic ovary syndrome. J Biotec Res Cent. 2012;6:67-73.
76. Bhuvaneshwari S, Poornima R, Averal HI. Comparative study of Pergularia daemia and Citrullus colocynthis in polycystic ovarian syndrome induced albino wistar rats. Int J Multidisc Res Dev. 2015;2(9):207-212.
77. Radha MH, Laxmipriya NP. The role of Aloe Barbadensis Mill. As a possible pre-conceptive herb for the management of polycystic ovarian syndrome: a rodent model study. Austin J Reprod Med Infertil. 2016;3(2):1040.
78. Zhou J, Qu F, Barry JA, et al. An atractylodes macrocephala koidz extract alleviates hyperandrogenism of polycystic ovarian syndrome. Int J Clin Exp Med. 2016;9(2):2758-2767.

79. Kavitha A, Babu AN, Kumar MS, Kiran SV. Evaluation of effects of Commiphora wightii in dehydroepiandrosterone (DHEA) induced polycystic ovary syndrome (PCOS) in rats. Pharma Tutor. 2016;4(1):47-55.
80. Suhaimi NA, Nooraain H, Nurdiana S. Effects of Ficus deltoidea Ethanolic leaves extract on female reproductive organs among Letrozole-induced polycystic ovarian syndrome rats. J Sci Res Dev. 2016;3(4):8-14.
81. Yang H, Kim HJ, Pyun BJ, Lee HW. Licorice ethanol extract improves symptoms of polycystic ovary syndrome in Letrozole-induced female rats. Integr Med Res. 2018;7(3):264-270.
82. Amoura M, Lotfy ZH, Neveen E, Khloud, A. Potential effects of Mentha piperita (peppermint) on Letrozole-induced polycystic ovarian syndrome in female albino rat. Int J. 2015;3(10):211-226.
83. Choi JH, Jang M, Kim EJ, et al. Korean Red Ginseng alleviates dehydroepiandrosterone-induced polycystic ovarian syndrome in rats via its antiinflammatory and antioxidant activities. J Ginseng Res. 2020;44(6):790-798.
84. Saiyed A, Jahan N, Makbul SAA, Ansari M, Bano H, Habib SH. Effect of combination of Withania somnifera Dunal and Tribulus terrestris Linn on letrozole induced polycystic ovarian syndrome in rats. Integr Med Res. 2016;5(4):293-300.
85. Sudhakar P, Suganeswari M, Pushkalai PS, Haripriya S. Regulation of estrous cycle using combination of Gymnema sylvestre and Pergularia daemia in estradiol valerate induced PCOS rats. Asian J Res Pharm Sci. 2018;8(1):4-8.
86. Jadhav M, Menon S, Shailajan S. Anti-androgenic effect of Symplocos racemosa Roxb. Against letrozole induced polycystic ovary using rat model. J Coast life Med. 2013;1(4):309-314.
87. Kakadia N, Patel P, Deshpande S, Shah G. Effect of Vitex negundo L. seeds in letrozole induced polycystic ovarian syndrome. J Tradit Complement Med. 2019;9(4):336-345.
88. Tysoe O. Licogliflozin effective in PCOS treatment. Nat Rev Endocrinol. 2021;17(10):577.
89. Kandasamy V, Balasundaram U. Caesalpinia bonduc (L.) Roxb. As a promising source of pharmacological compounds to treat poly cystic ovary syndrome (PCOS): a review. J Ethnopharmacol. 2021;279:114375.
90. Paris VR, Walters KA. Humanin: a potential treatment for PCOS? Endocrinology. 2021;162(8);bqab085.
91. Rajan RK, Balaji B. Soy isoflavones exert beneficial effects on letrozole-induced rat polycystic ovary syndrome (PCOS) model through anti-androgenic mechanism. Pharm Biol. 2017;55(1):242-251.
92. Reddy PS, Begum N, Mutha S, Bakshi V. Beneficial effect of Curcumin in Letrozole induced polycystic ovary syndrome. Asian Pac J Reprod. 2016;5(2):116-122.
93. Lee YH, Yang H, Lee SR, Kwon SW, Hong EJ, Lee HW. Welsh onion root (Allium fistulosum) restores ovarian functions from letrozole induced-polycystic ovary syndrome. Nutrients. 2018;10(10):1430.
94. Jelodar G, Masoomi S, Rahmanifar F. Hydroalcoholic extract of flaxseed improves polycystic ovary syndrome in a rat model. Iran J Basic Med Sci. 2018;21(6):645.
95. Hossein KJ, Leila KJ, koukhdan Ebrahim T, Nazanin SJ, Farzad P, Elham R. The effect of pomegranate juice extract on hormonal changes of female Wistar rats caused by polycystic ovarian syndrome. Biomed Pharmacol J. 2015;8(2):971-977.
96. Wang JG, Anderson RA, Graham GM III, et al. The effect of cinnamon extract on insulin resistance parameters in polycystic ovary syndrome: a pilot study. Fertil Steril. 2007;88(1):240-243.
97. Demirel MA, Ilhan M, Suntar I, Keles H, Akkol EK. Activity of Corylus avellana seed oil in letrozole-induced polycystic ovary syndrome model in rats. Rev Bras Farmacognosia. 2016;26:83-88.
98. Kalgaonkar S, Almario RU, Gurusinghe D, et al. Differential effects of walnuts vs almonds on improving metabolic and endocrine parameters in PCOS. Eur J Clin Nutr. 2011;65(3):386-393.

第二十三章 基于循证的临床实践推荐（未来的研究与实践方向）

一、引言

多囊卵巢综合征（PCOS）是女性常见疾病，其疾病表型在女性一生的不同阶段有所不同。为了更好地识别疾病表型，PCOS 的诊断标准发生了变化。PCOS 表型受遗传、激素、生活方式等复杂因素相互影响，但尚缺乏这方面的文献支持，尤其缺乏中低收入国家（low-and middle-income country，LMIC）的文献报道。这些国家累计有 65 亿人口，存在一些共同特点。在其中一些国家，每年有许多青春期女性步入生育活跃阶段，人口生育率高但卫生健康系统薄弱。PCOS 与非传染性疾病（noncommunicable disease，NCD）之间的关系众所周知。全世界每年约有 4100 万人死于 NCD，其中 85% 发生在 LMIC；在 LMIC 每年有 1500 万人在 30～69 岁过早死亡。同样具有挑战性的是，心血管疾病、糖尿病（DM）、呼吸系统疾病、癌症和精神障碍在 NCD 中占比高。

PCOS 评估和管理的国际循证指南包括一篇对已有文献和已发布指南的深入综述。该综述明确提出 PCOS 的诸多影响因素，但这些影响因素在青少年和 PCOS 患者中缺乏循证证据。循证证据的缺乏体现出未来对该领域相关理论和调查研究的需求，特别是关于社会因素、遗传因素、不同社会背景下的生活方式，以及不同地域不同种族和民族背景对 PCOS 的影响（有迹象表明 PCOS 在特定人群中患病率更高）。加强对 PCOS 的整体认知，有助于建立对疾病筛查、早期干预和改善远期预后的切实有效手段。本节内容的主旨是提出一些关键的研究问题，为本领域的未来科研提供引领性参考。PCOS 领域在不断发展，因此这些问题并不是未来探索的全部问题。应鼓励研究人员和公共卫生人员发现关键问题并推动其开展调查研究。

二、关于多囊卵巢综合征诊断标准的探讨与建立的问题

- PCOS 诊断过程中评价高雄激素血症（HA）的最有效方法是什么？对于有 PCOS 临床表现的女性，不同生命阶段关于雄激素异常的诊断标准分别是什么？
- 超声检查在 PCOS 诊断中起什么作用？提高超声检查分辨率是否会影响 PCOS 的诊断标准？
- 如何利用抗米勒管激素（AMH）提高 PCOS 的诊断率？（引申问题：在中低收入国家中实施该检测是否可行？）

三、关于改善多囊卵巢综合征治疗和干预措施的问题

- PCOS 患者妊娠后可能有哪些不良预后？有哪些干预措施？
- 在 PCOS 患者中，控制体重、代谢、妊娠、生育力、生活质量（QoL）、情绪健康的生活方式干预有效吗？（引申问题：对于青春期和成年女性，哪些行为改变可以促进健康的生活方式？）
- 如何利用社交媒体和电子健康平台，提高 PCOS 及合并症高风险人群对生活方式调整的关注度？（引申问题：作为心血管疾病高风险人群，PCOS 患者可以接受何种程度的宣教干预？应在哪个生命阶段进行干预？）
- 复方口服避孕药的孕激素成分中，哪种孕激素可以有效调整青春期和成年 PCOS 患者的性激素水平并控制临床症状？（引申问题：在不同年龄、不同文化背景的人群中，复方口服避孕药的接受度如何？）
- 除了常规措施，还有哪些干预措施能够管理成年和青少年 PCOS 患者的肥胖问题？（引申问题：二甲双胍单药或与其他药物联合应用对青少年和成年 PCOS 患者调整性激素水平、缓解临床症状和控制体重是否有效？减肥药对 PCOS 患者的性激素水平和临床症状有改善作用吗？肌醇单药或与其他治疗联合应用对控制青春期和成年 PCOS 患者的性激素水平、临床症状和体重有效吗？减肥药在改善 PCOS 患者生育力中的作用是什么？）
- 哪些干预措施能有效解决 PCOS 患者的不孕问题？（引申问题：不同诱导排卵方案分别有哪些远期风险？能否为 LMIC 的 PCOS 不孕女性制定一个低风险、低剂量的标准化促性腺激素方案？减重术能否改善 PCOS 患者的生育力和妊娠结局？超声引导下经阴道卵巢穿刺术对促排耐药的 PCOS 不孕患者是否有意义？）

四、关于识别多囊卵巢综合征患者身心共病的问题

- 哪些危险因素可以用于预测 PCOS 患者未来发生心血管疾病的风险？（引申问题：青少年和成年 PCOS 患者可能合并哪些躯体或心理健康疾病？）
- PCOS 患者诊断 2 型糖尿病特异性最高的检测方法是什么？
- PCOS 患者绝经后如何监测并筛查子宫内膜癌？（引申问题：不同年龄段 PCOS 女性患癌症的风险是多少？如何将危险因素筛查纳入 PCOS 患者的日常妇科临床实践，实现癌症早筛查、早治疗？尽早干预对减少绝经前和绝经后 PCOS 女性癌症发生风险的效果如何？）
- 综合管理方案如何保护青春期和成年 PCOS 患者避免合并精神心理疾病？（引申问题：青少年和成年女性诊断 PCOS 后，焦虑和抑郁程度如何？）

五、关于影响多囊卵巢综合征预后的环境因素和社会因素问题

- PCOS 人群分布的种族差异和地理环境差异是什么？能否整合各个国家数据，比

较不同种群间的 PCOS 差异或相似之处？

- PCOS 患者绝经后应该如何监测子宫内膜癌？
- 如何筛查和预防 PCOS 对青少年和成年患者 QoL 的早期负面影响？（引申问题：PCOS 对青少年和成年患者的 QoL 产生哪些影响？改善 QoL 是否有助于改善 PCOS 的预后？）
- 青少年和成年 PCOS 患者的性心理异常状态如何？（引申问题：PCOS 如何影响 LMIC 青少年和成年 PCOS 患者的社会交往？哪些方法可以有效减少青春期和成年 PCOS 女性性心理异常的发生？）
- 诊断 PCOS 后，可以利用哪些方法筛查患者的消极体象（通常由多个躯体问题引起）？
- 诊断 PCOS 后，可以使用哪些方法筛查患者可能存在的进食障碍并评估其严重程度？

六、关于加强卫生系统能力建设、满足多囊卵巢综合征患者或易感人群服务需求和组织准备的问题

- 在世界不同地区有哪些不同的医疗照护模式？这些模式在患者满意度、生育力和高雄激素治疗方面的成功之处是什么？不同文化和语言背景下如何提供适当照护？
- 需要对社区工作者及非专业人员进行哪些培训，以帮助这些心血管疾病和 PCOS 的高风险人群？（引申问题：如何将这些内容融入他们的日常培训，并利用技术手段强化认识？）
- 卫生健康政策如何能加强资源匮乏地区 PCOS 人群的识别、治疗和长期随访支持？
- 将 PCOS 的综合照护方案整合到医疗机构和社区机构中有什么意义？（引申问题：系统性的 PCOS 管理在资源匮乏或农村地区面临哪些挑战？）

七、结束语

研究表明，PCOS 存在遗传和生活方式相关问题。家族性发病很常见，这反映出遗传因素对 PCOS 的影响。全基因组关联研究已经发现一些 PCOS 基因位点，未来需要进一步研究致病突变及其对 PCOS 病理生理机制的影响。

以往对大脑与神经内分泌变化的动物模型研究提示，下丘脑-垂体轴及其功能参与成年 PCOS 患者临床表型的发病机制，未来需要对 PCOS 女性开展研究以验证这些机制。

是否有人觉察到青春期男女两性在肥胖及随之发生的躯体、精神和心理问题上存在相似之处？既然已经在女性中发现（即 PCOS），那么在男性中会有相关问题吗？

第二十三章　基于循证的临床实践推荐（未来的研究与实践方向）

参考文献

1. March WA, Moore VM, Willson KJ, Phillips DI, Norman RJ, Davies MJ. The prevalence of polycystic ovary syndrome in a community sample assessed under contrasting diagnostic criteria. Hum Reprod. 2010;25(2):544-551.
2. Rotterdam ESHRE/ASRM-Sponsored PCOS Consensus Workshop Group. Revised 2003 consensus on diagnostic criteria and long-term health risks related to polycystic ovary syndrome. Fertil Steril. 2004;81(1):19-25.
3. Bozdag G, Mumusoglu S, Zengin D, Karabulut E, Yildiz BO. The prevalence and phenotypic features of polycystic ovary syndrome: a systematic review and meta-analysis. Hum Reprod. 2016;31(12):2841-2855.
4. Sexton C, Snyder HM, Chandrasekaran L, Worley S, Carrillo MC. Expanding representation of low and middle income countries in global dementia research: commentary from the Alzheimer's Association. Front Neurol. 2021;12:633777.
5. Mills A. Health care systems in low-and middle-income countries. N Engl J Med. 2014;370(6):552-557.
6. Tosatti JA, Sóter MO, Ferreira CN, et al. The hallmark of pro-and anti-inflammatory cytokine ratios in women with polycystic ovary syndrome. Cytokine. 2020;134:155187.
7. Cooney LG, Dokras A. Beyond fertility: polycystic ovary syndrome and long-term health. Fertil Steril. 2018;110(5):794-809.
8. Teede H, Misso M, Costello MF, et al. International Evidence-Based Guideline for the Assessment and Management of Polycystic Ovary Syndrome 2018. National Health and Medical Research Council (NHMRC), Monash University; 2018:1-198.
9. Rosenfield RL, Ehrmann DA. The pathogenesis of polycystic ovary syndrome (PCOS): the hypothesis of PCOS as functional ovarian hyperandrogenism revisited. Endocr Rev. 2016;37(5):467-520.
10. Rackow BW, Brink HV, Hammers L, Flannery CA, Lujan ME, Burgert TS. Ovarian morphology by transabdominal ultrasound correlates with reproductive and metabolic disturbance in adolescents with PCOS. J Adolesc Health. 2018;62(3):288-293.
11. Teede HJ, Misso ML, Boyle JA, et al. Translation and implementation of the Australian-led PCOS guideline: clinical summary and translation resources from the international evidence-based guideline for the assessment and management of polycystic ovary syndrome. Med J Aust. 2018;209:S3-S8.
12. Teede H, Misso M, Tassone EC, et al. Anti-müllerian hormone in PCOS: a review informing international guidelines. Trends Endocrinol Metab. 2019;30(7):467-478.
13. Artini PG, Obino MER, Sergiampietri C, et al. PCOS and pregnancy: a review of available therapies to improve the outcome of pregnancy in women with polycystic ovary syndrome. Expert Rev Endocrinol Metab. 2018;13(2):87-98.
14. Lim S, Wright B, Savaglio M, Goodwin D, Pirotta S, Moran L. An analysis on the implementation of the evidence-based PCOS lifestyle guideline: recommendations from women with PCOS. Paper presented at the Semin Reprod Med. 2021;39(3-4):153-160.
15. Abroms LC. Public health in the era of social media. Am J Public Health Assoc. 2019;109:S130-S131.
16. Stellefson M, Paige SR, Chaney BH, Chaney JD. Evolving role of social media in health promotion: updated responsibilities for health education specialists. Int J Environ Res Public Health. 2020;17(4):1153.
17. Fraison E, Kostova E, Moran LJ, et al. Metformin versus the combined oral contraceptive pill for hirsutism, acne, and menstrual pattern in polycystic ovary syndrome. Cochrane Database Syst Rev. 2020;8(8):CD005552.
18. Pundir J, Psaroudakis D, Savnur P, et al. Inositol treatment of anovulation in women with polycystic ovary syndrome: a meta-analysis of randomised trials. BJOG. 2018;125(3):299-308.
19. Cena H, Chiovato L, Nappi RE. Obesity, polycystic ovary syndrome, and infertility: a new avenue for glp-1 receptor agonists. J Clin Endocrinol Metab. 2020;105(8):e2695-e2709.
20. Zhang J, Tang L, Kong L, et al. Ultrasound-guided transvaginal ovarian needle drilling for clomiphene-resistant

polycystic ovarian syndrome in subfertile women. Cochrane Database Syst Rev. 2019;7(7):CD008583.
21. Glueck CJ, Goldenberg N. Characteristics of obesity in polycystic ovary syndrome: etiology, treatment, and genetics. Metabolism. 2019;92:108-120.
22. Saboor Aftab S, Kumar S, Barber T. The role of obesity and type 2 diabetes mellitus in the development of male obesity-associated secondary hypogonadism. Clin Endocrinol. 2013;78(3):330-337.
23. Hiam D, Moreno-Asso A, Teede HJ, et al. The genetics of polycystic ovary syndrome: an overview of candidate gene systematic reviews and genome-wide association studies. J Clin Med. 2019;8(10):1606.
24. Coutinho EA, Kauffman AS. The role of the brain in the pathogenesis and physiology of polycystic ovary syndrome (PCOS). Med Sci. 2019;7(8):84.

第四篇

多囊卵巢综合征的全球治疗方式

第二十四章 南亚多囊卵巢综合征的现状分析

多囊卵巢综合征（PCOS）是育龄期女性最常见的内分泌疾病，根据使用的诊断标准不同，其发病率为4%～25%。PCOS的特征包括月经稀发、闭经/无排卵、痤疮、多毛症等高雄激素血症（HA）表现，以及超声可见的卵巢改变。2003年鹿特丹标准是临床和研究中最常用的标准。据估计，PCOS人群的肥胖率为50%，高于人群中的平均肥胖率。代谢方面，PCOS主要表现为胰岛素抵抗（IR），这可能影响未来其他疾病的发病率。

"南亚人群"是对印度、巴基斯坦、斯里兰卡、孟加拉国和尼泊尔等国族裔的统称。这些国家人口稠密，并且与世界许多地区一样，也存在PCOS患者。南亚裔占全球人口的20%。事实上，在2000年，美国居民中有160万人是南亚人（0.7%）。同样，在2011年，加拿大居民中有100万人口是南亚人，澳大利亚也有100万人口是南亚族裔（占总人口的1.3%）。在英国，5.7%的居民认为自己是南亚裔或英国籍亚裔人，这使得南亚族裔在2001年成为英国最大的少数族裔群体，占全国人口的4%。考虑到全球PCOS患病人数众多，有必要进一步了解PCOS的患病情况及疾病对患者的影响，并根据患者的需求展开治疗。

PCOS在不同地区的表现存在种族差异（图24.1）。然而，关于PCOS的许多认识都源于以欧洲女性为主的研究。英国一项基于社区的研究发现，高加索女性的多囊卵巢（PCO）患病率（22%）低于和她们情况相似的南亚女性（52%）。斯里兰卡的一项以社区为基础的研究发现 PCOS 的患病率为 6.3%。此外，南亚族裔中 IR 和 2 型糖尿病（T2DM）患病率较高，这可能会增加 PCOS 患者未来患其他疾病的风险（表 24.1）。

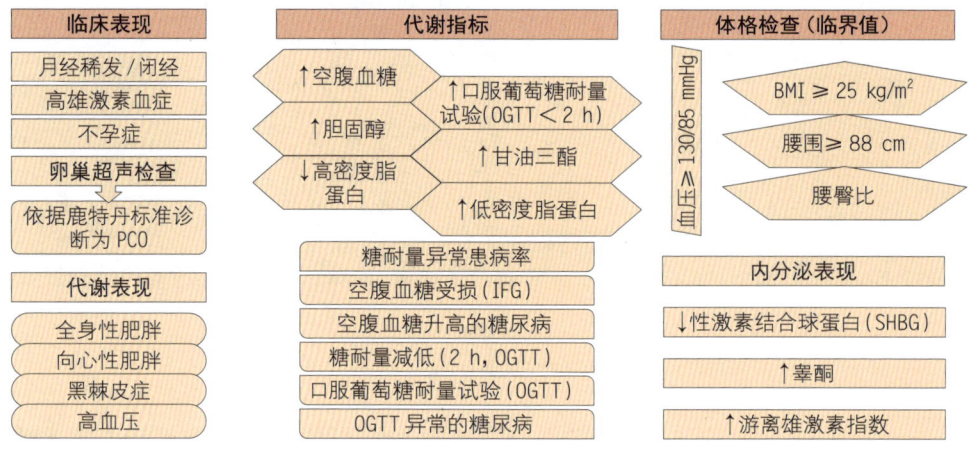

图 24.1　南亚女性多囊卵巢综合征的异质性表现（临床表现、体格检查及代谢方面损害）

表 24.1　全球育龄期女性多囊卵巢综合征患病率比较

作者	研究人群	患病率
Kumarapeli 等	南亚女性	6.3%（鹿特丹标准）
Ding 等	中国女性	5.6%（鹿特丹标准）
Chen 等	中国南方女性	2.2%[美国国立卫生研究院（NIH）标准]
Moran 等	墨西哥城女性	6.0%（NIH 标准）
Goodarzi 等	墨西哥裔美国女性	13%
Knochenhauer 等	美国东南部高加索女性	4.7%（NIH 标准）
Knochenhauer 等	美国东南部黑种人女性	3.4%（NIH 标准）
Vaduneme KO	非洲尼日利亚女性	5%~10%（鹿特丹标准）
Gabrielli L G	巴西女性	8.5%（鹿特丹标准）
Sarah C Hillman 和 Jeremy Dale A	英国女性	2.27%（鹿特丹标准）
Richard Scott Lucidi, Medscape	美国女性	4%~12%

来源：Wolf WM, Wattick RA, Kinkade ON, Olfert MD. Geographical prevalence of polycystic ovary syndrome as determined by region and race/ethnicity. *Int J Environ Res Public Health*. 2018; 15[11]: 2589.

一、多囊卵巢综合征的遗传学研究

毫无疑问，PCOS 的发病存在遗传因素，然而其相关基因还有待确定。此外，其遗传模式仍存在争议，证据也不足。

既往有许多在 PCOS 患者兄弟姐妹中开展的研究，旨在建立 PCOS 的遗传联系。

Kaushal 等研究者发现，南亚族裔 PCOS 患者兄弟患糖尿病（DM）、内皮细胞功能障碍和早发性男性型秃发的风险增加。

Siddamalla 等研究了抑癌基因 *PTEN* 在南印度女性中的单核苷酸多态性（SNP），探索其与 PCOS 发病的相关性。*PTEN* 基因是细胞增殖、迁移和凋亡的重要调控因子，其 rs1903858A/G、rs185262832G/A、rs10490920T/C 位点及基因多态性与 PCOS 相关，这意味着这些基因是南印度女性患 PCOS 的遗传风险因素。

此外，Tumu 等发现白细胞介素 -6（IL-6）基因启动子多态性在南亚 PCOS 患者中显著升高，并进一步在斯里兰卡人群的研究中发现了线粒体 DNA 拷贝数和位移环的改变。

有趣的是，*FTO* 基因（与脂肪量、肥胖相关）广泛存在于包括脂肪组织、脑和肌肉在内的多个器官中，可参与体重的调节。该基因位于 16 号染色体，已有多个 SNP 位点研究。研究最广泛的 rs9939609 位点是 *FTO* 的第一个内含子，由 2 个等位基因（A 和 T）组成。A 等位基因与肥胖和 T2DM 的风险增加有关。

Branavan 等研究了 *FTO*（rs9939609）的多态性，发现其与斯里兰卡年轻 PCOS 女性的代谢紊乱和高睾酮水平相关。*FTO* 基因变异位点 rs9939609 与代谢性疾病的体征和 HA，以及吻素和睾酮在内的激素标记物升高有关，这些都是 PCOS 的特征性表现。

Guruvajah 等发现，在南印度女性中，另一个遗传性因素是血管内皮生长因子（VEGF）+ 405G/C 多态性。

卵泡抑制素（follistatin，FST）是一种在卵巢等多种组织中表达的单链糖蛋白，其主要功能是拮抗激活素的活性，导致血清卵泡刺激素（FSH）降低、卵泡发育障碍及卵巢雄激素合成增加等 PCOS 特征性表现。由于 *FST* 基因的功能及其表现出的强连锁反应，研究者认为 *FST* 基因是 PCOS 潜在致病基因 / 易感基因。已有少量研究试图确定该基因的序列变异及其与 PCOS 的相关性，但目前尚没有明确的结论。一项包括 150 个家系的大规模研究探索了 37 个候选基因与 PCOS 的连锁证据或关联证据，其中连锁证据最强的是 *FST* 基因区域。然而，Dasgupta 等关于南亚人群的研究中未发现 *FST* 基因附近的外显子变异，该研究推论，*FST* 基因表达因研究对象种族而异。

二、多囊卵巢综合征女性的代谢疾病及其他疾病

代谢综合征（MetS）是代谢紊乱性疾病的统称，包括各种导致动脉粥样硬化和内皮功能障碍的疾病，如高脂血症、高血压和 DM/DM 前期。

据报道，英国南亚裔人群（BMI > 25 kg/m² 的患者）MetS 的患病率是高加索裔人群的 4.6 倍。然而，在患有 PCOS 的肥胖南亚裔女性中，这一比例甚至更高。

PCOS 的临床表现存在种族差异。Apridonidze 等对 30～39 岁的女性进行研究，发现对于 BMI 相似的女性，PCOS 患者的 MetS 患病率几乎是正常人的 2 倍（43% *vs.* 24%）。PCOS 患者的 MetS 患病率在其他研究中结果类似（33%～46%）。尽管部分研究结果

尚存在争议，但 PCOS 患者的 MetS 患病率及其特征（空腹血糖、空腹甘油三酯、腰围、高密度脂蛋白、高血压等方面）确实存在种族差异。

Kudesia 等对 52 名南亚裔和 52 名高加索女性不孕症患者进行了横断面分析，两组患者的 BMI 相似，且总体上都没有达到肥胖标准。尽管如此，南亚裔组女性患代谢性疾病（IR、DM、血脂异常）和子宫内膜疾病（子宫内膜增生及息肉）的比例较高。整体而言，南亚裔人群年龄较小，PCOS 发病率较高，代谢异常和子宫内膜异常发生率较高。

这一研究发现在 Chahal 等的多种族横断面研究中得到进一步证实，在研究对象的 BMI 和年龄相匹配情况下，东亚和南亚女性（25～30 岁和＞30 岁年龄组）与高加索女性相比，前者 2 小时胰岛素水平更高。

在一项关于斯里兰卡育龄期女性不同 PCOS 的表现研究中，Wijeyaratne 等对比了同时患有 PCOS 和 MetS 的女性与仅患有 PCOS 的女性，发现两组患者具有相似的睾酮浓度。然而，同时患有 PCOS 和 MetS 的患者其 BMI、BP、空腹血糖、胰岛素和甘油三酯更高，高密度脂蛋白和性激素结合球蛋白更低。该研究还发现，肥胖在月经稀发的 PCOS 患者中更常见。与对照组相比，黑棘皮症（AN）这一 IR 的强烈标志，在同时患有 PCOS 和 MetS 的患者中更常见。事实上，研究者对 PCOS 患者进行了多变量逻辑回归分析，发现年龄 ≥ 35 岁、BMI ≥ 25 kg/m^2 和 AN 等可作为 MetS 的预测因子。此外，研究者还通过病例对照分析发现了其他 MetS 预测因素，包括高腰围、高舒张压、空腹血脂紊乱、高空腹胰岛素水平和高睾酮水平。

Sundararaman 等调查了南印度 PCOS 患者，将血糖∶胰岛素和颈动脉内中膜厚度作为血管病变的标志物。研究的主要假设是南亚人自幼年起就有 IR 和 MetS 的倾向。该研究发现，南印度 PCOS 患者的 IR 更严重，颈动脉内中膜厚度更厚，因此她们的动脉粥样硬化风险也更高。

在南亚人群中，PCOS 与非酒精性脂肪性肝病（NAFLD）正相关，特别是在高 BMI 和 HA 患者中。研究进一步证实 IR 和 HA 是预测南亚 PCOS 患者发生 NAFLD 的独立危险因素，这也为在特定人群中开展筛查提供了依据，以提高早期发现率并指导治疗。

还有一个重要的发现是，南亚 PCOS 女性缺乏维生素 D。Azhar 等发现，该人群中维生素 D 缺乏的患病率高达 85%。另有研究发现，南亚 PCOS 患者的 MetS 的发病率与低维生素 D 水平有关。

Romitti 等对 PCOS 与自身免疫性甲状腺疾病（AITD）的关系进行了系统综述和荟萃分析，发现高达 40% 的 PCOS 患者同时被诊断为 AITD。与其他种族相比，亚洲 PCOS 患者患 AITD 的风险更高。

由于南亚女性患心脏代谢性疾病的风险较高，筛查及后续治疗将使该人群获益。

三、多囊卵巢综合征患者的生育力和妊娠

由于 PCOS 的重要特点之一是稀发排卵/无排卵，所以低生育力是 PCOS 公认的

不良后果。无排卵性不孕的患者在生殖医院中占很大比例，而 PCOS 则是无排卵性不孕最常见的病因。由此可推断，接受辅助生殖技术（ART）的人群中，有相当比例的人患 PCOS。

这一情形同样出现在南亚裔女性中。与高加索女性相比，南亚裔女性体外受精活产率较低。此外，南亚裔女性更早因生育问题就诊，并有更严重的多毛症、不孕症和痤疮问题。事实上，与其他种族相比，南亚裔 PCOS 女性生育力问题往往更早地表现出来，ART 结局更差（研究报告显示，南亚裔女性的 ART 成功率比同等条件下的高加索女性低 2.5 倍）。

此外，南亚裔 PCOS 患者的妊娠风险很高，其在妊娠期发生宫颈机能不全和妊娠期糖尿病（GDM）的风险也会增加。尽管 Feigenbaum 等的回顾性队列研究样本量较小，但这一研究发现，2.9% 的 PCOS 患者存在宫颈机能不全，其中南亚裔和黑种人女性的比例偏高。

Wijeyaratne 等发现该女性群体的产后风险仍然较高。一项对 274 名斯里兰卡 PCOS 患者的病例对照研究发现，怀孕期间患有 GDM 的女性，其产后 3 年患 MetS 的风险显著增加。Kousta 等研究了既往诊断过 GDM 同时伴有 PCO 和月经周期不规律情况的女性，进一步证实了 PCOS 和 GDM 之间的关系。

在英国，女性在被转诊到产前咨询门诊或进行糖耐量试验前，会先根据其现存风险和家族史进行分层，而南亚血统和患 PCOS 并不作为分层依据。或许是时候重新审视分层依据，并相应改变女性围妊娠期管理方式，以改善其妊娠结局，降低远期发病率。

四、多囊卵巢综合征患者的身体特征及其对生活的影响

健康相关生活质量、情绪和性健康是评估患者整体情况的重要参数。不幸的是，PCOS 相关症状会在上述方面影响患者生活，且该影响难以客观测量。有证据表明，PCOS 患者比其他慢性病（如哮喘、关节炎或心脏病）患者会遭受更多的情绪困扰。与 PCOS 相关的多毛症、肥胖和痤疮等症状，以及月经不规律和不孕症，会引起更严重的心理困扰，而且精确测量这些影响有一定难度。

南亚 PCOS 患者与高加索患者，在身体特征方面似乎有细微差异。她们可能有更高的 Ferriman-Gallwey 评分，更严重的 AN 和痤疮症状。

有趣的是，与高加索女性相比，南亚裔女性对肥胖的困扰较小，但对多毛症的困扰要大。对肥胖的不同态度或许能通过文化差异来解释。由于衣着习惯不同，南亚人对外貌和向心性肥胖的观念可能与西方世界不同。然而，Jones 等的研究表明，生活在英国的南亚裔女性对自己的体重也产生了类似的苦恼，这表明生活在西方社会改变了南亚裔女性的文化信仰。

然而，不在意向心性肥胖会使南亚女性对减肥策略和体育锻炼的依从性较差。肥胖是 MetS 病情发展的已知因素，也与远期患病率的升高相关。因此，这应该是对该群

体患者进行教育和改变观念的关键。

PCOS 的遗传学研究是一个复杂的课题，在候选基因方面仍存在很大空白。越来越多证据表明，不同种族将显示出不同的基因表达，在南亚人群中也是如此。然而，基因表达差异不仅仅局限于遗传学。南亚裔女性似乎有最严重的 PCOS 表现，以至于面临更高的远期发病率和死亡率。亟待在英国乃至世界范围内的指南中反映这一情况并付诸行动，以降低该群体患者的发病和死亡风险。

参考文献

1. Hart R, Hickey M, Franks S. Definitions, prevalence and symptoms of polycystic ovaries and polycystic ovary syndrome. Best Pract Res Clin Obstet Gynaecol. 2004;18:671-683. Available at: https://doi.org/10.1016/j.bpobgyn.2004.05.001.

2. Jones GL, Palep-Singh M, Ledger WL, et al. Do South Asian women with PCOS have poorer health-related quality of life than Caucasian women with PCOS? A comparative cross-sectional study. Health Qual Life Outcomes. 2010;8:149. Available at: https://doi.org/10.1186/1477-7525-8-149.

3. Homburg R. Choices in the treatment of anovulatory PCOS. In: Balen A, Franks S, Homburg R, Kehoe S, eds. Current Management of Polycystic Ovary Syndrome. Cambridge, UK: Cambridge University Press; 2010:143-152.

4. Fauser BCJM, Tarlatzis B, Rebar R, et al. Revised 2003 consensus on diagnostic criteria and long-term health risks related to polycystic ovary syndrome. Hum Reprod. 2004;19:41-47. Available at: https://doi.org/10.1093/humrep/deh098.

5. Gambineri A, Pelusi C, Vicennati V, Pagotto U, Pasquali R. Obesity and the polycystic ovary syndrome. Int J Obes. 2002;26:883-896. Available at: https://doi.org/10.1038/sj.ijo.0801994.

6. Reeves TJ, Bennett CE, Sweeney J, et al. We the People: Asians in the United States. Census 2000 Special Reports. U.S. Census Bureau; 2004. Available at: https://www.scirp.org/(S(351jmbntvnsjt1aadkposzje))/journal/paperinformation.aspx?paperid=16896.

7. Tran K, Kaddatz J, Allard P. South Asians in Canada: Unity Through Diversity. n.d. Available at: https://www150.statcan.gc.ca/n1/en/catalogue/11-008-X20050028455.

8. Deleted in review.

9. Office for National Statistics. Coronavirus (COVID-19). n.d. Available at: https://www.ons.gov.uk/. Accessed December 4, 2021.

10. Office for National Statistics. Ethnic Group, National Identity and Religion. n.d. Available at: https://www.ons.gov.uk/methodology/classificationsandstandards/measuresequality/ethnicgroupnationalidentityandreligion. Accessed December 4, 2021.

11. Rodin DA, Bano G, Bland JM, Taylor K, Nussey SS. Polycystic ovaries and associated metabolic abnormalities in Indian subcontinent Asian women. Clin Endocrinol (Oxf). 1998;49:91-99. Available at: https://doi.org/10.1046/j.1365-2265.1998.00492.x.

12. Wijeyaratne CN, Balen AH, Barth JH, Belchetz PE. Clinical manifestations and insulin resistance (IR) in polycystic ovary syndrome (PCOS) among South Asians and Caucasians: is there a difference? Clin Endocrinol (Oxf). 2002;57:343-350. Available at: https://doi.org/10.1046/j.1365-2265.2002.01603.x.

13. Wild S, Roglic G, Green A, Sicree R, King H. Global prevalence of diabetes: estimates for the year 2000 and projections for 2030. Diabetes Care. 2004;27:1047-1053. Available at: https://doi.org/10.2337/diacare.27.5.1047.

14. Kaushal R, Parchure N, Bano G, Kaski JC, Nussey SS. Insulin resistance and endothelial dysfunction in the brothers of Indian subcontinent Asian women with polycystic ovaries. Clin Endocrinol (Oxf). 2004;60:322-328. Available at: https://doi.org/10.1111/j.1365-2265.2004.01981.x.

15. Siddamalla S, Govatati S, Venu VK, et al. Association of genetic variations in phosphatase and tensin homolog (PTEN) gene with polycystic ovary syndrome in South Indian women: a case control study. Arch Gynecol Obstet. 2020;302:1033-1040. Available at: https://doi.org/10.1007/s00404-020-05658-4.
16. Tumu VR, Govatati S, Guruvaiah P, Deenadayal M, Shivaji S, Bhanoori M. An interleukin-6 gene promoter polymorphism is associated with polycystic ovary syndrome in South Indian women. J Assist Reprod Genet. 2013;30:1541-1546. Available at: https://doi.org/10.1007/s10815-013-0111-1.
17. Reddy TV, Govatati S, Deenadayal M, Sisinthy S, Bhanoori M. Impact of mitochondrial DNA copy number and displacement loop alterations on polycystic ovary syndrome risk in south Indian women. Mitochondrion. 2019;44:35-40. Available at: https://doi.org/10.1016/j.mito.2017.12.010.
18. Branavan U, Wijesundera S, Chandrasekaran V, Arambepola C, Wijeyaratne C. In depth analysis of the association of FTO SNP (rs9939609) with the expression of classical phenotype of PCOS: A Sri Lankan study. BMC Med Genet. 2020;21:30. Available at: https://doi.org/10.1186/s12881-020-0961-1.
19. Guruvaiah P, Govatati S, Reddy TV, et al. The VEGF -405 G>C 5' untranslated region polymorphism and risk of PCOS: a study in the South Indian Women. J Assist Reprod Genet. 2014;31:1383-1389. Available at: https://doi.org/10.1007/s10815-014-0310-4.
20. Guo Q, Kumar TR, Woodruff T, Hadsell LA, DeMayo FJ, Matzuk MM. Overexpression of mouse follistatin causes reproductive defects in transgenic mice. Mol Endocrinol. 1998;12:96-106. Available at: https://doi.org/10.1210/mend.12.1.0053.
21. Mather JP, Moore A, Li RH. Activins, inhibins, and follistatins: further thoughts on a growing family of regulators. Exp Biol Med. 1997;215:209-222. Available at: https://doi.org/10.3181/00379727-215-44130.
22. Urbanek M. The genetics of the polycystic ovary syndrome. Nat Clin Pract Endocrinol Metab. 2007;3:103-111. Available at: https://doi.org/10.1038/ncpendmet0400.
23. Dasgupta S, Pisapati SVS, Kudugunti N, Godi S, Kathragadda A, Reddy MM. Does follistatin gene have any direct role in the manifestation of polycystic ovary syndrome in Indian women. J Postgrad Med. 2012;58:190-193. Available at: https://doi.org/10.4103/0022-3859.101386.
24. Deleted in review.
25. Apridonidze T, Essah PA, Iuorno MJ, Nester JE. Prevalence and characteristics of the metabolic syndrome in women with polycystic ovary syndrome. J Clin Endocrinol Metab. 2005;90(4):1929-1935. Available at: https://doi.org/10.1210/jc.2004-1045.
26. Chahal N, Quinn M, Jaswa EA, Kao CN, Cedars MI, Huddleston HG. Comparison of metabolic syndrome elements in White and Asian women with polycystic ovary syndrome: results of a regional, American cross-sectional study. F S Rep. 2020;1:305-313. Available at: https://doi.org/10.1016/j.xfre.2020.09.008.
27. Kudesia R, Illions EH, Lieman HJ. Elevated prevalence of polycystic ovary syndrome and cardiometabolic disease in South Asian infertility patients. J Immigr Minor Heal. 2017;19:1338-1342. Available at: https://doi.org/10.1007/s10903-016-0454-7.
28. Sundararaman PG, Manomani R, Sridhar GR, Sridhar V, Sundaravalli A, Umachander M. Risk of atherosclerosis in women with polycystic ovary syndrome: a study from South India. Metab Syndr Relat Disord. 2003;1:271-275. Available at: https://doi.org/10.1089/1540419031361435.
29. Shengir M, Krishnamurthy S, Ghali P, et al. Prevalence and predictors of nonalcoholic fatty liver disease in South Asian women with polycystic ovary syndrome. World J Gastroenterol. 2020;26:7046-7060. Available at: https://doi.org/10.3748/wjg.v26.i44.7046.
30. Harsha Varma S, Tirupati S, Pradeep TVS, Sarathi V, Kumar D. Insulin resistance and hyperandrogenemia independently predict nonalcoholic fatty liver disease in women with polycystic ovary syndrome. Diabetes Metab Syndr Clin Res Rev. 2019;13:1065-1069. Available at: https://doi.org/10.1016/j.dsx.2018.12.020.
31. Azhar A, Abid F, Rehman R. Polycystic ovary syndrome, subfertility and vitamin D deficiency. J Coll Physicians Surg Pak. 2020;30:545-546. Available at: https://doi.org/10.29271/jcpsp.2020.05.545.

32. Tuz F, Aalpona Z. Association of vitamin D status with metabolic syndrome and its components in polycystic ovary syndrome. Mymensingh Med J. 2019;28(3):547-552.
33. Romitti M, Fabris VC, Ziegelmann PK, Maia AL, Spritzer PM. Association between PCOS and autoimmune thyroid disease: a systematic review and meta-analysis. Endocr Connect. 2018;7:1158-1167. Available at: https://doi.org/10.1530/EC-18-0309.
34. Mehta J, Kamdar V, Dumesic D. Phenotypic expression of polycystic ovary syndrome in South Asian women. Obstet Gynecol Surv. 2013;68:228-234. Available at: https://doi.org/10.1097/OGX.0b013e318280a30f.
35. Palep-Singh M, Picton HM, Yates ZR, Barth J, Balen AH. Polycystic ovary syndrome and the single nucleotide polymorphisms of methylenetetrahydrofolate reductase: a pilot observational study. Hum Fertil. 2007;10:33-41. Available at: https://doi.org/10.1080/14647270600950157.
36. Feigenbaum SL, Crites Y, Hararah MK, Yamamoto MP, Yang J, Lo JC. Prevalence of cervical insufficiency in polycystic ovarian syndrome. Hum Reprod. 2012;27:2837-2842. Available at: https://doi.org/10.1093/humrep/des193.
37. Wijeyaratne CN, Waduge R, Arandara D, et al. Metabolic and polycystic ovary syndromes in indigenous South Asian women with previous gestational diabetes mellitus. BJOG. 2006;113:1182-1187. Available at: https://doi.org/10.1111/j.1471-0528.2006.01046.x.
38. Kousta E, Cela E, Lawrence N, et al. The prevalence of polycystic ovaries in women with a history of gestational diabetes. Clin Endocrinol (Oxf). 2000;53:501-507. Available at: https://doi.org/10.1046/j.1365-2265.2000.01123.x.
39. National Institute for Health and Care Excellence (NICE). Diabetes in pregnancy: management from preconception to the postnatal period. n.d. Available at: https://www.nice.org.uk/guidance/ng3.
40. Afifi L, Saeed L, Pasch LA, et al. Association of ethnicity, Fitzpatrick skin type, and hirsutism: a retrospective cross-sectional study of women with polycystic ovarian syndrome. Int J Womens Dermatol. 2017;3:37-43. Available at: https://doi.org/10.1016/j.ijwd.2017.01.006.
41. Kumarapeli VL, De A Seneviratne R, Wijeyaratne CN. Health-related quality of life and psychological distress in polycystic ovary syndrome: a hidden facet in South Asian women. BJOG. 2011;118:319-328. Available at: https://doi.org/10.1111/j.1471-0528.2010.02799.x.

第二十五章 中亚和东亚多囊卵巢综合征的现状分析

一、引言

亚洲面积最大，约占地球陆地总面积的 1/3，截至 2021 年亚洲人口约为 46.8 亿人。亚洲有 5 个主要地区：中亚、东亚、南亚、东南亚和西亚，而北亚目前定义为包括西伯利亚和东北部地区。这 5 个主要地区的国家有着不同的人口、民族、文化、疾病流行情况和模式。

PCOS 影响着全球近 6%～10% 的育龄期女性，患者可能同时出现生殖和代谢功能障碍，如肥胖、糖耐量减低、痤疮、多毛症和无排卵。目前公认的 PCOS 病因是遗传因素，但其表型不容忽视。在全球不同种族中，东亚女性 PCOS 的发病率低于白种人女性，且不同种族患者对治疗方案的反应也不尽相同。

PCOS 发病率的计算是基于特定人群的诊断标准。在不同的研究中，相似人群选择不同的诊断标准，得到的发病率可能受到影响，从而波动于 1.6%～18.0%。因此，相当一部分患者可能因为诊断不明而未能得到有效诊治。

二、发病率、诊断和治疗的影响因素

环境中的社会与自然条件变化是影响特定人群的健康、疾病和损伤模式的关键因素。种族、医疗保健系统、常用保健药物的种类、人群的求医行为（health-seeking behavior，HSB）、饮食文化及习惯、医疗服务的便利性和可负担性、生活模式及疾病本身的发病率等因素，均直接或间接地影响 PCOS 的发病率、诊断和治疗。

（一）种族

全基因组关联研究是为了评估 PCOS 发病相关风险因素之间的关联性，相似的风险因素可能出现在具有相同主诉的两组不同人群中。一般来说，多毛症在东亚人群中不太常见，诊断界值也低于白种人。月经周期不规律则是东亚人群常见的症状，而白种人不太常见。胰岛素抵抗（IR）的比例升高是各种族的共同特征，虽然东亚女性的 BMI 较低且代谢异常较少，但糖尿病（DM）的发病率依旧提示了代谢并发症的存在。

与白种人女性相比（发病率为 11%～20%），某些特定东亚人群（如韩国、中国和泰国女性）的 PCOS 发病率较低（约 5%）。由于不同种族人群对于治疗的反应不同，在制订治疗计划的时候需要考虑到种族的差别。

（二）多囊卵巢综合征患者的生活行为方式和饮食习惯

生活方式主要体现在饮食和运动上，不良的生活方式会导致体脂含量增加并诱发IR。这些因素导致体内氧化环境的产生，是PCOS发病的重要机制。每个社会均有自己特定的饮食偏好，如有些种族偏好吃鱼，而其他种族则有进食米饭或高脂食品的传统，同样，有些社会中人们更喜欢消费饮料和快餐。由高纤维抗炎成分、低精细碳水化合物和反式脂肪组成的饮食结构会减少机体氧化应激，并对PCOS患者的激素水平产生影响。PCOS患者常被诊断为心脏病、糖耐量减低和MetS，相当一部分患者表现为肥胖，这可能是遗传因素造成，也可能是生活方式和环境因素造成。特定社会环境中的氧化应激水平可能反映了这部分人群对于特定饮食因素的文化消费，且可能与某些疾病（如肥胖和心血管疾病）有显著关联。

三、中亚地区

中亚是亚洲最被忽视的地区。该地区有5个国家：哈萨克斯坦、吉尔吉斯斯坦、塔吉克斯坦、土库曼斯坦、乌兹别克斯坦。

（一）医疗保健系统

中亚各国自独立以来一直面对不利的政治和经济条件，各国均实施了一些政策来提高医疗标准和质量。迄今为止，该地区有关女性健康的文献很少，人口详情见表25.1。

表25.1 中亚地区国家医疗保健概况

国家	CPR[%(年)]	EmOC设备	ANC[%(年)]	SBA[%(年)]	CS（%）	IMR（截至2020年）（%）	MMR[%(年)]
哈萨克斯坦	53（2018）	245	99（2015）	100（2018）	11.5	9	9（2015）
吉尔吉斯斯坦	39（2018）	71	100（2018）	100（2018）	58.36	16	30（2016）
塔吉克斯坦	29（2017）	88	92（2017）	95（2017）	2.8	28	7（2016）
土库曼斯坦	50（2019）	59	100（2019）	100（2016）	4	36	3（2015）
乌兹别克斯坦	65（2006）	2775	99（2015）	100（2018）	6.3	13	18（2016）

来源：Rehman, R., Alam, F. and Khan, R., 2022. World Bank Open Data | Data . [online] Data.worldbank.org. Available at: < https://data.worldbank.org/ > [Accessed 7 October 2022].

注：ANC，产前保健；CPR，避孕普及率；CS，剖宫产；EmOC，产科急诊；IMR，婴儿死亡率（每1000例活产）；MMR，孕产妇死亡率（每10万例活产）；SBA，熟练助产率。

（二）求医行为

自1990年以来，每个国家均开展了卫生部门改革，但由于预算有限、卫生系统员工缺乏培训和服务资源短缺等，改革仍在进行之中。在一项针对不同国家进行的评估中，死亡率和发病率上升的原因是自行用药和治疗费用高。关于该地区健康模式及其影响因素的已发表研究少之又少（关键词：医疗保健服务）。

（三）多囊卵巢综合征发病率与女性健康问题

近几十年来，女性健康（包括孕产妇和新生儿健康指标）受到了关注，除PCOS，还有其他女性健康相关研究发表。根据16篇相关的研究文章，中亚地区PCOS发病率为14.24%。2016年全球疾病负担研究显示，哈萨克斯坦发病率为42%。

（四）生活方式

中亚地区"游牧民族"的生活习惯可以从他们的环境条件、当地经济情况及与饮食相关的仪式和宗教观念中看出。他们饲养牲畜，饮食以牛奶、奶制品和肉类为主。除水果和蔬菜之外，干果的摄入量也很多。

（五）文化对于求医行为的影响

关于中亚地区各人群亚组的就医行为的数据很少。由于各种政治、地理和经济等不稳定因素的影响，超过一半的人选择自行用药治疗，并认为可以靠自己缓解健康问题。加上治疗费用超出人们的负担能力，医疗设施要么关闭、要么太远，或无法提供优质的服务。

（六）心理影响

"使人人享有优质医疗服务"是该地区政策制定者面临的一项挑战，不仅仅从人权发展的角度来看很重要，从人类发展的角度来看也同样重要。中亚各国的发展前景依赖于人力、社会和智力资本。

四、东亚地区

东亚地区覆盖面积约为 11 839 074 km^2，人口超过 16.41 亿。东亚地区包括中国、日本、蒙古国、朝鲜、韩国（表25.2）。

（一）中国

1. 多囊卵巢综合征发病率、诊断和治疗的影响因素

在中国，直接或间接影响PCOS发病率、诊断和治疗的因素包括种族、医疗保健系统、医疗保健服务类型和健康观念。

（1）种族

中国是个多民族统一的国家，其中汉族人口最多。基于证据的研究结果显示，种族会影响PCOS的临床特征。

（2）医疗保健系统

中国有人口居住在山区，这些地区医疗资源相对有限。2009年的改革弥补了西部地区医疗保健系统的不足，改善了孕产妇和新生儿保健的多项指标。

表 25.2　东亚地区国家和地区医疗保健概况

国家和地区		大概死亡率（%）（截至2020年）	IMR（%）（截至2020年）	新生儿 MR（%）（截至2020年）	≤5 MR（%）（截至2020年）	ANC [%（年）]	SBA [%（年）]	MMR [%（年）]
中国	中国大陆	7	6	4	7	100（2018）	100（2016）	27（2013）
	中国香港	7	NA	NA	NA	NA	100（2005）	NA
	中国澳门	4	NA	NA	NA	NA	100（2004）	NA
	中国台湾	7.89	3.42	NA	4.33	NA	NA	NA
日本		11	2	0.84	3	100[a]	100（2018）	4（2014）
蒙古国		6	13	8.14	15	99（2018）	99（2018）	49（2016）
朝鲜		9	12	2	17	100（2017）	100（2017）	8（2016）
韩国		6	3	NA	3	98.1[a]	100（2015）	11（2016）

来源：Rehman, R., Alam, F. and Khan, R., 2022. *World Bank Open Data / Data*. [online] Data.worldbank.org. Available at: < https://data.worldbank.org/ > [Accessed 7 October 2022].

注：IMR，婴儿死亡率（每1000例活产）；新生儿 MR，新生儿死亡率；≤5 MR，5 岁以下儿童死亡率；ANC，产前保健；SBA，熟练助产率；MMR，孕产妇死亡率（每 10 万例活产）；NA，不详。

[a] 译者注：原著中未标注年份。

（3）医疗保健服务类型

中国有中医、西医两种医疗保健服务，人们可以选择自己喜欢的医疗保健服务类型（图 25.1）。

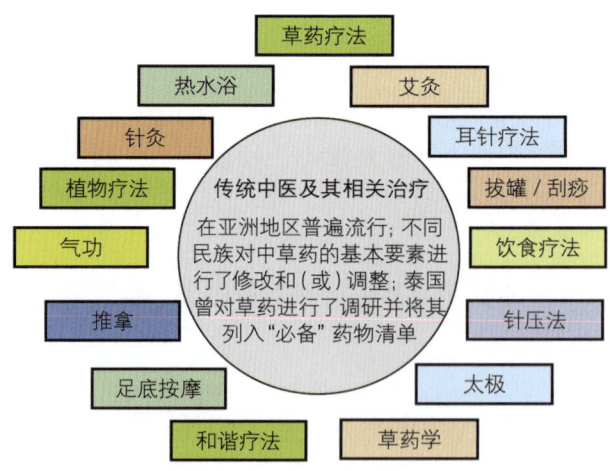

图 25.1　传统／经典中医及其相关治疗在亚洲地区普遍流行，也用于治疗多囊卵巢综合征

- 西部地区医疗保健系统为近 95% 的人口提供服务。"健康中国 2020"战略旨在将患有慢性病的老年人群纳入其中，但服务的使用情况主要取决于人群的求医习惯。

- 传统中医药诊疗体系强调生活方式调整，常采用草药与针灸等疗法，主张优先替代部分化学药物及侵入性手术。中医师通过开具中药处方调和人体阴阳气血平衡。中药学与中医辨证论治共同构成传统中医的核心框架。
- 中医治疗手段涵盖针灸、推拿（含穴位按摩）、气功及食疗。推拿师运用手法刺激经络穴位，调节机体功能。

2. 多囊卵巢综合征的发病率

循证研究结果显示，同一地区中不同种族和出身的人 PCOS 发病率和表现可能有所不同。根据鹿特丹标准，中国女性 PCOS 的发病率为 5.6%，而西方人群中这一比例为 15.0%。泰国女性为 5.7%，斯里兰卡女性为 6.3%，伊朗女性为 14.3%。因此，根据鹿特丹标准，中国女性的 PCOS 发病率在各大洲中最低。

3. 多囊卵巢综合征的特征

（1）**多毛症**

在对不同群体进行比较时发现，亚洲女性多毛症发生率低于白种人。

（2）**表型**

一项大型研究显示，中国汉族女性中 PCOS 发病率为 5.6%。年轻女性更有可能患 PCOS 并伴有月经不规律、高雄激素血症（HA）、超声下多囊卵巢样表现和不孕症。肥胖女性患 MetS 和 IR 的风险也随年龄增长而增加。根据 1990 年美国国立卫生研究院（NIH）标准，中国南方女性 PCOS 的发病率为 2.2%。

（3）**总发病率**

中国 PCOS 的总发病率为 0.45%～35.14%，综合发病率为 10.01%。地区分析显示，西部地区发病率为 13.35%，东部地区为 7.82%，中部地区为 24.00%，东北地区为 8.68%。不孕症的发病率为 13.69%。

（4）**族群比较**

斯里兰卡 PCOS 发病率为 6.3%（nhp.gov.in），与白种人女性相比，东亚华裔女性 PCOS 糖耐量低和 IR 的发病率较低。

（5）**发病率随年龄增长而下降的趋势**

在一项以社区为基础的横断面调查中，使用了 3 条标准进行 PCOS 的诊断，发现发病率随年龄增长而呈下降趋势，这表明 PCOS 是一种暂时性状态，会随年龄增长而减轻。

（6）**多囊卵巢综合征合并妊娠期糖尿病、肥胖和血脂异常病史**

根据修订后的超声标准，PCOS 发病率在既往妊娠期糖尿病（GDM）患者中更高。这些患者同样存在肥胖和 DM 伴空腹血糖及血脂升高的发病风险。

（7）**多囊卵巢综合征与糖尿病风险**

PCOS 女性与非 PCOS 女性相比，提前 10 年发生心脏病和 DM 的风险上升。

（8）**多囊卵巢综合征与肥胖**

对中国肥胖女性临床和代谢特征进行的分析表明，其血脂更高且与 IR 呈正相关。

（9）多囊卵巢综合征与高雄激素血症

中国 HA 女性的不良妊娠结局（早产和妊娠期高血压）风险是普通女性的两倍。

（10）多囊卵巢综合征与妊娠期糖尿病、高血压、早产之间的关系

对中国 32 个省的自然妊娠且单胎妊娠的孕产妇进行的调查发现，PCOS 女性发生妊娠期 DM、高血压和早产的风险增加。

注

【中国台湾地区】

（1）医疗保健系统

中国与韩国、新加坡近期的医疗改革显著提升了医疗卫生指标，为东亚其他 4 个国家提供了宝贵经验。改革措施包括：福利整合方案、保险费率调整、精细化成本控制、临床合理用药规范及医疗服务提供方的成本节约激励机制等。

（2）医疗保健服务类型

该地区并行发展西医与传统中医学，传统中医理论体系与中国大陆同源，治疗常结合中草药制剂与针灸等辅助疗法。

（3）健康理念及其对医疗保健的影响

该地区医疗系统覆盖约 99% 人口，可提供较高质量的医疗服务。然而，部分人受特定观念影响——将疾病视为"过失的惩罚"，隐瞒病情，导致求医行为受到干扰。

（4）女性多囊卵巢综合征的发病率与特征

目前尚缺乏该地区 PCOS 发病率数据。现有研究均是在不同地域、医院、族群及年龄段开展的。

①该地区数据库显示，年轻的 PCOS 女性（15～29 岁）患抑郁症的风险更高。

②超声提示多囊卵巢形态是该地区女性 PCOS 最常见表现。

③仅 28%～35% 的女性 PCOS 患者伴多毛症。

④超重女性痤疮发生率低于体重正常女性；肥胖女性 BMI 与血清总睾酮呈显著相关性。

⑤肥胖 PCOS 女性的黄体生成素与卵泡刺激素（比值显著低于非肥胖者；BMI 升高与黄体生成素水平下降呈相关性。

【中国香港地区】

（1）医疗保健系统

该地区医疗体系获加拿大皇家内科及外科医师学院（RCPSC）认证，提供公立与私立并行服务：公立医疗以低廉费用覆盖基础诊疗。

（2）传统中医药的应用

2002 年该地区就医需求调查显示，居民对中医药服务需求显著。政府通过制定相关条例将中医药纳入公共医疗体系，并制定系统化发展政策。

（3）多囊卵巢综合征特征

①按鹿特丹标准，该地区 PCOS 女性最常见表现为：无排卵性高雄激素血症（排除其他内分泌病因）、超声多囊卵巢形态（PCOM）、LH 升高、肥胖及胰岛素抵抗（IR）。

②该地区华裔 PCOS 患者代谢综合征患病率显著增高，校正年龄与 BMI 后代谢异常风险仍增加 5 倍。

③该地区 PCOS 女性糖尿病发病更早，患 2 型糖尿病风险为非 PCOS 者的 4 倍。

【中国澳门地区】

（1）医疗保健系统

该地区涵盖公立、私立等医院，卫生中心提供免费基础医疗及中医药服务。

（2）女性健康研究现状

该地区女性健康相关的文献尚缺乏。

（二）日本

2021 年日本人口为 125 932 148 人，面积为 364 555 km²。日本人口普查时将多民族背景的人群均视为日本人。日本的 HDI 名列前茅。

1. 医疗保健系统

日本人的预期寿命比其他任何国家都长，这可能是由于日本的医疗保健注重预防服务。日本人的饮食习惯、饮食结构及获得优质医疗服务的机会，都是日本人长寿的原因。在日本的医疗保健系统中，每个人均可以直接就诊于专科医师。日本是亚洲医疗保健体系达到发达国家水平的国家之一。

2. 民间疗法

一些民间疗法包括热桑拿浴和草药制剂成品，这些无须处方即可在药店购买。中医医师和熟练的针灸按摩师也可以提供传统治疗服务。

3. 文化影响

传统中医药学也是日本文化的一部分。中医医师在日本接受一定的培训后可以在日本进行执业。

4. 健康理念及其对护理教育者的影响

对临床和教学护士的调研显示，部分护士会向患者传递无科学证据证实的健康信息。

5. 种族

HA 不是日本 PCOS 女性的主要表现特征，因此也不作为日本诊断标准中的一条，取而代之的是 LH 的评估。

6. 饮食文化

根据联合国人居署的数据，日本女性的预期寿命最长，可达87岁。在日本文化中，人们不会过度饮食，一般仅进食至70%～80%的饱腹感。此外，他们的饮食简单，以米饭或面食为主，配以汤和鱼。日本人还非常注意锻炼身体，并饮用大量的水和茶。在发达国家中，日本人的肥胖率最低（3%）。

7. 女性多囊卵巢综合征的发病率和相关特征

（1）发病率

日本女性PCOS的发病率为3%～5%。

（2）多囊卵巢综合征与肥胖和多毛症

虽然日本PCOS患者的肥胖和多毛症发病率较低，但雄激素过多和IR的发病率却与美国和意大利相当。

（3）PCOM与1型糖尿病

患有1型DM的女性超声提示PCO特征的比例、硫酸脱氢表雄酮的水平和月经不规律的比例更高。

（4）肝酶和体重指数是多囊卵巢综合征的风险因素

PCOS患者的BMI和肝酶水平明显较高。

（5）多囊卵巢综合征和流产

在早孕期连续两次流产的日本女性中，尚无证据证实PCOS与流产之间有任何相关性。

（6）二甲双胍治疗多囊卵巢综合征与不孕症

对于枸橼酸氯米芬（CC）抵抗的日本不孕症女性，在3个周期的CC治疗中联合低剂量二甲双胍，可以提高排卵率。

（三）朝鲜

朝鲜人口估计为25 917 513人，主要为朝鲜族。医疗保健指标见表25.2。

1. 医疗保健系统

覆盖全民的普惠型医疗体系在饥荒期间崩溃，而未经认证的治疗方法和私立诊所遍地开花。草药和传统疗法成为那些因经济困难而无法获得正规医疗服务的个人常用方法。

2. 女性健康问题

朝鲜女性健康状态并不清楚。政府声称女性享有与男性平等的权利。

3. 族群构成

以本地朝鲜族为主，另有少数汉族等中国其他民族公民及日本侨民。

4. 饮食

饮食以米饭或面条为主，配以泡菜（每餐都有的蔬菜）、烤肉（如果有肉时）及烧酒（或汤）。近年来朝鲜啤酒也成为朝鲜文化的一部分。朝鲜人参茶作为一种抗氧化剂风靡全球。

5. 女性多囊卵巢综合征的相关特征

PCOS 患者葡萄糖耐受不良的发病率是普通女性的 28 倍，同样，偏瘦的 PCOS 患者葡萄糖耐受不良的发病率是匹配年龄后无 PCOS 朝鲜女性的 9.8 倍。

（四）韩国

韩国人口为 51 323 965 人，面积为 38 502 km²。韩国是多民族的国家，移民来自中国、北美国家、越南、俄罗斯、菲律宾和乌兹别克斯坦。

1. 医疗保健系统

韩国的医疗保健被评为世界第二高效的医疗保健系统，在全国范围内提供免费医疗服务，其中治疗性服务多于预防性服务，城镇医疗资源更多。随着老龄人口的增加，慢性退行性疾病造成的医疗负担相应加重。

2. 族群构成

除韩国本地人之外，还有一小部分中国人居住在该国。

3. 饮食文化

韩国饮食（又称 K 饮食）主要以米饭配以大量蔬菜、豆类和鱼。生菜、青椒、胡萝卜和黄瓜等生食蔬菜也非常普遍。

4. 女性多囊卵巢综合征的患病率和特征

（1）女性多囊卵巢综合征亚群的发病率

与白种人女性相比，韩国 PCOS 女性的 BMI 和血清性激素结合球蛋白（SHBG）水平较低。HA 也不是主要特征，这可能提示韩国女性与其他国家女性相比，发生代谢紊乱的风险较低。

（2）年轻人中多囊卵巢综合征的发病率

在学生中 PCOS 的发病率为 4.9%，肥胖和多毛症表现不常见。

（3）多囊卵巢综合征和促性腺激素分泌异常

在 PCOS 患者中，促性腺激素分泌异常与 BMI 呈负相关。

（4）多囊卵巢综合征女性的饮食与抑郁症的关系

韩国女性动物蛋白的摄入与精神健康症状有关。

（5）多囊卵巢综合征女性的血脂异常

脂连蛋白基因多态性与 PCOS 血脂异常有关。

五、结论

中亚自 1991 年独立以来，一直在实施新的卫生改革措施以降低孕产妇和新生儿发病率与死亡率等基本指标。随着该地区卫生系统的加强，学术和研究机构将获得更多机会解释流行疾病（如 PCOS）的发病模式。

东亚地区的研究发现，种族、生活方式、文化和宗教信仰，以及社区求医行为是该地区健康状态关键的决定性因素。PCOS 的识别、早期诊断和适当的治疗可以防止不孕症等并发症发生，这些并发症会导致医疗预算大幅上升。随着不同类型医疗模式的普及，治疗的依从性往往受到影响。因此，如何充分认识这一问题并就此进行健康教育和个体化咨询，依旧是一片值得研究的领域。

参考文献

1. Saharan T, Pfeffer K, Baud I. Urban livelihoods in slums of Chennai: developing a relational understanding. Eur J Dev Res. 2018;30(2):276-296.
2. Laven JS, Imani B, Eijkemans MJ, Fauser BC. New approaches to PCOS and other forms of anovulatory infertility. Obstet Gynecol Surv. 2002;57(11):755-767.
3. Huang Z, Yong EL. Ethnic differences: is there an Asian phenotype for polycystic ovarian syndrome? Best Pract Res Clin Obstet Gynaecol. 2016;37:46-55.
4. Amato MC, Galluzzo A, Finocchiaro S, Criscimanna A, Giordano CJ. The evaluation of metabolic parameters and insulin sensitivity for a more robust diagnosis of the polycystic ovary syndrome. Clin Endocrinol. 2008;69(1):52-60.
5. Kim JJ, Choi YM. Phenotype and genotype of polycystic ovary syndrome in Asia: ethnic differences. J Obstet Gynaecol Res. 2019;45(12):2330-2337.
6. Liepa GU, Sengupta A, Karsies D. Polycystic ovary syndrome (PCOS) and other androgen excess–related conditions: can changes in dietary intake make a difference? Nutr Clin Pract. 2008;23(1):63-71.
7. UNFPA. A Review of Progress in Maternal Health in Eastern Europe and Central Asia (unfpa.org). UNFPA; 2019.
8. McKee M, Healy J, Falkingham J. Health Care in Central Asia. London UK: Open University Press; 2002.
9. Wu Q, Gao J, Bai D, Yang Z, Liao Q. The prevalence of polycystic ovarian syndrome in Chinese women: a meta-analysis. Ann Palliat Med. 2021;10(1):74-87.
10. Omaleki V, Reed E. The role of gender in health outcomes among women in Central Asia: a narrative review of the literature. Paper presented at the Women's Studies International Forum; 2019.
11. Malik K. Human Development Report 2014: Sustaining Human Progress: Reducing Vulnerabilities and Building Resilience. New York: United Nations Development Programme; 2014.
12. Communiqué on Major Figures of the 2000 Population Census (No. 1). National Bureau of Statistics of China. 2002-04-23. Archived from the original on 2021-05-16. Retrieved 2021-05-16.
13. Capell J, Veenstra G, Dean EJ. Cultural competence in healthcare: critical analysis of the construct, its assessment and implications. J Theory Constr Test. 2007;11(1):30-37.
14. Cao R, Stone T, Petrini M, & Turale S. Nurses' perceptions of health beliefs and impact on teaching and practice: a Q-sort study. Int Nurs Rev. 2018;65(1):131-144.
15. Gupta VB. Impact of culture on healthcare seeking behavior of Asian Indians. J Cult Divers. 2010;17(1):13-19.
16. Ministry of Ecology and Environment of the People's Republic of China. Regular Press Conference (September) September 29, 2018. Paper presented at the 2018 Press Conference Records of Ministry of Ecology and Environment, the People's Republic of China. Springer; 2021.
17. Fang P, Han S, Zhao L, Fang Z, Zhang Y, Zou X. What limits the utilization of health services among the rural population in the Dabie Mountains-evidence from Hubei province, China? BMC Health Serv Res. 2014;14(1):1-7.
18. Yang Y, Wang S, Chen L, et al. Socioeconomic status, social capital, health risk behaviors, and health-related quality of life among Chinese older adults. Health Qual Life Outcomes. 2020;18(1):291.
19. Hong YA, Zhou Z. A profile of eHealth behaviors in China: results from a national survey show a low of usage and significant digital divide. Front Public Health. 2018;6:274.

20. Chang AY, Oshiro J, Ayers C, Auchus RJ. Influence of race/ethnicity on cardiovascular risk factors in polycystic ovary syndrome, the Dallas Heart Study. Clin Endocrinol. 2016;85(1):92-99.
21. Li R, Zhang Q, Yang D, et al. Prevalence of polycystic ovary syndrome in women in China: a large community-based study. Hum Reprod. 2013;28(9):2562-2569.
22. Fauser BC, Tarlatzis BC, Rebar RW, et al. Consensus on women's health aspects of polycystic ovary syndrome (PCOS): the Amsterdam ESHRE/ASRM-Sponsored 3rd PCOS Consensus Workshop Group. Fertil Steril. 2012;97(1):28-38.e25.
23. Vutyavanich T, Khaniyao V, Wongtra-ngan S, Sreshthaputra O, Sreshthaputra R, Piromlertamorn W. Clinical, endocrine and ultrasonographic features of polycystic ovary syndrome in Thai women. J Obstet Gynaecol Res. 2007;33(5):677-680.
24. Kumarapeli V, Seneviratne Rde A, Wijeyaratne CN, Yapa RM, Dodampahala SH. A simple screening approach for assessing community prevalence and phenotype of polycystic ovary syndrome in a semi-urban population in Sri Lanka. Am J Epidemiol. 2008;168(3):321-328.
25. Tehrani FR, Simbar M, Tohidi M, Hosseinpanah F, Azizi F. The prevalence of polycystic ovary syndrome in a community sample of Iranian population: Iranian PCOS prevalence study. Reprod Biol Endocrinol. 2011;9(1):1-7.
26. Ding T, Hardiman PJ, Petersen I, Wang FF, Qu F, Baio GJ. The prevalence of polycystic ovary syndrome in reproductive-aged women of different ethnicity: a systematic review and meta-analysis. Oncotarget. 2017;8(56):96351-96358.
27. Chen X, Yang D, Mo Y, et al. Prevalence of polycystic ovary syndrome in unselected women from southern China. Eur J Obstet Gynecol Reprod Biol. 2008;139(1):59-64.
28. Wei HJ, Young R, Kuo IL, Liaw CM, Chiang HS, Yeh CY. Prevalence of insulin resistance and determination of risk factors for glucose intolerance in polycystic ovary syndrome: a cross-sectional study of Chinese infertility patients. Fertil Steril. 2009;91(5):1864-1868.
29. Zhuang J, Liu Y, Xu L, et al. Prevalence of the polycystic ovary syndrome in female residents of Chengdu, China. Gynecol Obstet Invest. 2014;77(4):217-223.
30. Chan CC, Ng EH, Tang OS, Lee CP, Ho PC. The prevalence of polycystic ovaries in Chinese women with a history of gestational diabetes mellitus. Gynecol Endocrinol. 2006;22(9):516-520.
31. Ng NYH, Jiang G, Cheung LP, et al. Progression of glucose intolerance and cardiometabolic risk factors over a decade in Chinese women with polycystic ovary syndrome: a case-control study. PLoS Med. 2019;16(10):e1002953.
32. Shi Y, Guo M, Yan J, et al. Analysis of clinical characteristics in large-scale Chinese women with polycystic ovary syndrome. Neuro Endocrinol Lett. 2007;28(6):807-810.
33. Naver KV, Grinsted J, Larsen S, et al. Increased risk of preterm delivery and pre-eclampsia in women with polycystic ovary syndrome and hyperandrogenaemia. BJOG. 2014;121(5):575-581.
34. Li Y, Ruan X, Wang H, et al. Comparing the risk of adverse pregnancy outcomes of Chinese patients with polycystic ovary syndrome with and without antiandrogenic pretreatment. Fertil Steril. 2018;109(4):720-727.
35. Wagstaff A. Health systems in East Asia: what can developing countries learn from Japan and the Asian Tigers? Health Econ. 2007;16(5):441-456.
36. Chiu SL, Gee MJ, Muo CH, Chu CL, Lan SJ, Chen CL. The sociocultural effects on orthopedic surgeries in Taiwan. PLoS One. 2018;13(3):e0195183.
37. Harnod T, Chen W, Wang JH, Lin SZ, Ding DC. Association between depression risk and polycystic ovarian syndrome in young women: a retrospective nationwide population-based cohort study (1998-2013). Hum Reprod. 2019;34(9):1830-1837.
38. Hsu MI, Liou TH, Chou SY, Chang CY, Hsu CS. Diagnostic criteria for polycystic ovary syndrome in Taiwanese Chinese women: comparison between Rotterdam 2003 and NIH 1990. Fertil Steril. 2007;88(3):727-729.

39. Yang JH, Weng SL, Lee CY, Chou SY, Hsu CS, Hsu MI. A comparative study of cutaneous manifestations of hyperandrogenism in obese and non-obese Taiwanese women. Arch Gynecol Obstet. 2010;282(3):327-333.
40. Hsu MI. Clinical characteristics in Taiwanese women with polycystic ovary syndrome. Clin Exp Reprod Med. 2015;42(3):86-93.
41. Cheung L, Ma R, Lam P, et al. Cardiovascular risks and metabolic syndrome in Hong Kong Chinese women with polycystic ovary syndrome. Hum Reprod. 2008;23(6):1431-1438.
42. Stone TE, Kang SJ, Cha C, Turale S, Murakami K, Shimizu A. Health beliefs and their sources in Korean and Japanese nurses: a Q-methodology pilot study. Nurse Educ Today. 2016;36:214-220.
43. Sugimoto O. The Committee for Reproductive and Endocrine in Japan Society of Obstetrics and Gynecology. Annual report (1991-1992) for the determination of diagnostic criteria for polycystic ovary syndrome. Acta Obstet Gynaecol Jpn. 1993;45:1359-1367.
44. United Nations. Department of Economic, Social Affairs, Population Division. World Population Ageing. 2015;2015:1-164.
45. Baba T, Endo T, Ikeda K, et al. Distinctive features of female-to-male transsexualism and prevalence of gender identity disorder in Japan. J Sex Med. 2011;8(6):1686-1693.
46. Zhao Y, Qiao J. Ethnic differences in the phenotypic expression of polycystic ovary syndrome. Steroids. 2013;78(8):755-760.
47. Miyoshi A, Nagai S, Takeda M, et al. Ovarian morphology and prevalence of polycystic ovary syndrome in Japanese women with type 1 diabetes mellitus. J Diabetes Investig. 2013;4(3):326-329.
48. Sugiura-Ogasawara M, Sato T, Suzumori N, Kitaori T, Kumagai K, Ozaki YJ. The polycystic ovary syndrome does not predict further miscarriage in Japanese couples experiencing recurrent miscarriages. Am J Reprod Immunol. 2009;61(1):62-67.
49. Kurabayashi T, Suzuki M, Kashima K, et al. Effects of low-dose metformin in Japanese women with clomiphene-resistant polycystic ovary syndrome. Reprod Med Biol. 2004;3(1):19-26.
50. Lee H, Oh JY, Sung YA, Chung H, Cho WY. The prevalence and risk factors for glucose intolerance in young Korean women with polycystic ovary syndrome. Endocrine. 2009;36(2):326-332.
51. Kim SH, Kim MS, Lee MS, et al. Korean diet: characteristics and historical background. J Ethnic Foods. 2016;3(1):26-31.
52. Chae SJ, Kim JJ, Choi YM, et al. Clinical and characteristics of polycystic ovary syndrome in Korean women. Hum Reprod. 2008;23(8):1924-1931.
53. Byun EK, Kim HJ, Oh JY, Hong YS, Sung YA. The prevalence of polycystic ovary syndrome in college students from Seoul. J Korean Endocr Soc. 2005;20(2):120-126.
54. Shim AR, Im Hwang Y, Lim KJ, et al. Inappropriate gonadotropin secretion in polycystic ovary syndrome: the relationship with clinical, hormonal and metabolic characteristics. Korean J Obstet Gynecol. 2011;54(11):659-665.
55. Kim SH, Kim HS, Park SH, Hwang JY, Chung HW, Chang NS. Dietary intake, dietary habits, and depression in Korean women with polycystic ovary syndrome. J Nutr Health. 2012;45(3):229-239.
56. Lee H, Byun EK, Park HR, et al. Adiponectin and ghrelin polymorphism in Korean women with polycystic ovary syndrome. J Korean Endocr Soc. 2006;21(5):394-401.

第二十六章 东南亚多囊卵巢综合征的现状分析

一、文莱

文莱，又称文莱达鲁萨兰国，国土面积为 5765 km²，是一个有着丰富石油和天然气储备的高收入国家。根据人类发展指数（HDI），文莱在东南亚国家中排名第二（表 26.1）。

表 26.1 东南亚国家的主要健康指标

国家	人口（百万）[G]	总死亡率（%）[β]	IMR[β]	新生儿MR（%）[β]	≤5MR（%）[β]	SBA（%）[β]	MMR（%）[β]
文莱	0.449	4.7	10	6	12	100	31
印度尼西亚	275.5	7	20	12	23	95	282
柬埔寨	16.77	6	22	13	26	89	184
菲律宾	115.6	6	21	13	26	84	206
老挝	7.5	6	35	22	44	64	217
马来西亚	33.9	5	7	5	9	100	23
缅甸	54.2	8	35	22	45	60	244
新加坡	6.0	5	2	1	2	100	4
泰国	71.7	8	7	5	9	99	24
越南	98.2	6	17	9	21	94	42
东帝汶	1.3	6	37	19	42	57	129

注：[β] https://data.worldbank.org/ 2020
[G] South-Eastern Asia Population 2022 (Demographics, Maps, Graphs) (worldpopulationreview.com)
IMR，婴儿死亡率（每 1000 例活产）；MMR，孕产妇死亡率（每 10 万例活产）；MR，死亡率；SBA，熟练助产率。

（一）卫生保健系统

文莱拥有完善的公共医疗保健系统，国民可免费使用。政府、私立医院和社区健康中心提供初级医疗保健服务。农村地区也有特色医疗。公民还可以出国就医（https://www.everyculture.com/Bo-Co/Brunei-Darussalam.html）。

（二）求医行为

图 26.1 展示了与医疗服务使用率相关的指标。不过，男性使用医疗保健服务的情况较少，因为这被认为是缺乏男子气概的一种表现。

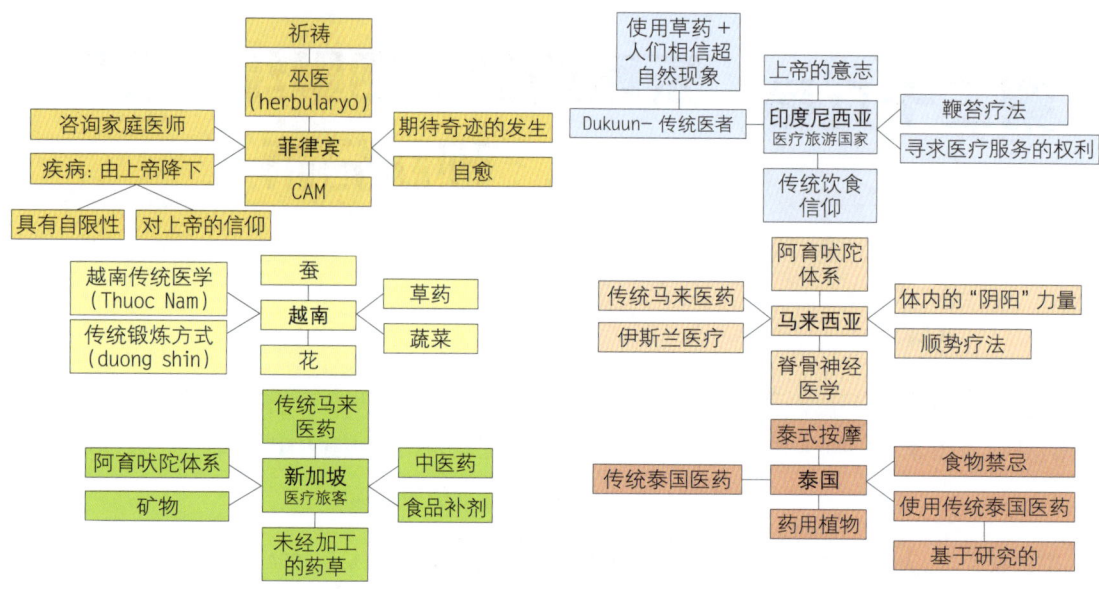

CAM，补充和替代治疗。

图 26.1　东南亚的文化信仰和民族健康行为影响了求医行为和治疗

（三）女性健康问题

女性可以在"Brunei Hive"这个旨在改善妇女健康和福祉的门户网站上分享她们的健康经历，同时该网站还提供有关妇女健康的"初级保健临床指南"。针对文莱女性最常见的三大癌症（乳腺癌、肠癌、宫颈癌），医院提供有补贴的"女性健康筛查服务"常规套餐。由于PCOS可能会导致癌症，文莱曾经开展过每年一次的PCOS筛查，并且在2020年重启了这一筛查。

二、柬埔寨

柬埔寨的国土面积为 181 035 km^2，人口数为 16 718 965 人，其中人口最多的民族是高棉族，约占总人口的90%。除此之外，柬埔寨还有越南人和华人。

（一）卫生保健系统

卫生部通过从基层到医院的一系列层级来监督医疗服务。保健中心提供预防和基本治疗服务，服务经费由政府提供，并可得到捐助者的资助。目前正在启动卫生改革，以降低疾病死亡率，延长预期寿命，解决营养不良问题，预防流行性传染病和新出现的非传染性疾病。

（二）孕产妇健康

柬埔寨在捐款资助下开展了降低孕产妇发病率和死亡率的改革。柬埔寨的PCOS发病率统计数据很难得到。

三、东帝汶

东帝汶是一个较低收入的国家,国土面积为 14 874 km^2,人口数为 1 267 974 人。东帝汶有多个民族,国民同时具有美拉尼西亚人和马来西亚人血统。

(一)卫生保健系统

东帝汶独立过程中的暴力冲击摧毁了公立和私立医院。大多数印度尼西亚籍的医务人员和专家也在 1999 年离开了东帝汶。2003 年,古巴和东帝汶达成了一项协议,让上百名东帝汶医学生在奖学金资助下前往古巴学习。古巴还派遣了医师在过渡时期管理东帝汶的医疗机构。世界卫生组织(WHO)、联合国人口基金、UNICEF,以及许多国际组织都正在致力于发展东帝汶基础医疗设施及培训人力资源。

与独立有关的暴力行为摧毁和破坏了公共和私营部门的保健中心和医院。大多数卫生工作者和医疗专业人员都是印度尼西亚国民,他们也于 1999 年离开了东帝汶。2003 年,古巴和东帝汶达成一项协议,东帝汶的数百名医科学生以奖学金的形式在古巴学习医学。古巴还安排古巴医师到东帝汶,在过渡时期管理卫生设施。WHO、联合国人口基金、UNICEF 和许多国际组织正在为东帝汶卫生系统基础设施的发展及人力资源培训提供服务。

(二)女性健康问题

表 26.1 列出的与女性健康相关的指标中,因为东帝汶连基础医疗需求都无法满足,所以在相关表格中没有找到与 PCOS 有关的信息。

四、印度尼西亚

印度尼西亚的国土面积为 1 904 569 km^2。根据 2020 年的人口普查结果,印度尼西亚总人口为 2.702 亿人,人口主要集中在爪哇岛。

(一)卫生保健系统

印度尼西亚的社区健康系统分为 3 级。健康系统的基本单位是卫生所(公共医疗中心),由受过培训的护士提供基本医疗服务,如疫苗接种、产前保健和伤口护理等。截至 2019 年,印度尼西亚设备齐全的公立和私立医院的数量近 2813 家,它们提供多种医疗服务,包括诊断和管理 PCOS。

(二)多囊卵巢综合征的患病率

PCOS 是一种育龄期女性的内分泌疾病,是印度尼西亚女性患不孕症的原因之一。印度尼西亚的医院能够诊治 PCOS。印度尼西亚的 PCOS 患病率为 5%～10%。

(三)多囊卵巢综合征和影响其发病的因素

由于其风险因素尚未得到认识,印度尼西亚 PCOS 得到的关注不多。一项研究发现,与 PCOS 发病最相关的因素是月经不规律。

(四)多囊卵巢综合征和不孕症的管理

采用二甲双胍和枸橼酸氯米芬联合疗法治疗 PCOS 患者,可降低 PCOS 女性的稳态模型评估 – 胰岛素抵抗指数(HOMA-IR)和雌二醇水平及卵泡直径,从而改善病情。

五、老挝

老挝的国土面积为 236 800 km^2。根据联合国最新数据进行预测,目前老挝的人口数为 7 404 929 人,其中 80% 的人口都居住在农村地区。

(一)卫生保健系统

老挝在 1975 年结束了内战,实现了政治稳定,但医疗系统依然资源不足,分布也不均衡,缺乏受过训练的医务人员、基础设施/设备和药物。老挝在疫苗接种、培训医务人员、加强妇幼保健方面都需要依靠国际援助(https://www.pacificbridgemedical.com/publication/healthcare-in-laos/)。目前,老挝 5 岁以下儿童死亡率仍然是东南亚国家中最高的(https://www.unicef.org/eap/what-we-do/health)。

(二)女性健康问题

表 26.1 展示了孕产妇和儿童健康指标。目前暂没有找到在老挝开展的关于 PCOS 的循证研究。

六、马来西亚

马来西亚的国土面积为 329 847 km^2,2020 年的人口规模为 32 365 999 人,是一个多民族国家。2019 年马来西亚的 HDI 非常高,达到了高收入国家的水平。

(一)医疗保健系统

大体上来说,马来西亚有着有效且广泛的双层医疗系统:公共全民医疗保健系统与私人医疗保健系统并行。尽管公共医疗保健服务是免费的,但在寻求专家看诊时,可能会出现等候时间过长的问题。

(二)求医行为(研究)

一项研究结果表明,马来西亚人的公立医院就医诉求最强烈,而马来西亚华人则更多在私立医院就医。同时,教育程度也影响求医行为。教育水平较低的人群倾向于在政府的医疗机构就医,而教育水平较高的人群倾向于在私立诊所就医。马来西亚的自我医疗率较高。

(三)女性健康问题

顶级医院可为不同年龄段的女性提供全面的健康检查服务。此外,还有专门的女性诊所为其提供各种健康服务。城市医院同样开展 PCOS 的筛查和管理服务。远程问诊也是可行的，由医师和资深医疗保健提供者管理。

（四）多囊卵巢综合征的患病率

马来西亚的 PCOS 患病率为 12.6%。

（五）多囊卵巢综合征和饮食补剂

一篇文章的研究结果推荐 PCOS 患者补充维生素 D 来减轻与 PCOS 相关的慢性炎症。研究同样发现，健康的肠道菌群有利于改善 PCOS 症状，提示使用益生元和益生菌可能是 PCOS 治疗的一部分。

（六）多囊卵巢综合征和马来西亚大学职工患者的特殊表型

据报道，马来西亚职工 PCOS 患病率为 12.6%，她们表现为高雄激素血症和多囊卵巢，其中 1 例患者确诊为不排卵。诊断结果与 BMI 和腰围增加、多毛症和闭经特征相关。该研究展示了这些女性中 PCOS 的主要表型。

（七）多囊卵巢综合征中代谢综合征的患病率

PCOS 患者代谢综合征（MetS）的患病率为 43.4%，这些患者更容易衰老，并且更有可能有糖尿病（DM）家族史。

（八）多囊卵巢综合征和代谢综合征患病率及高甘油三酯 – 腰围表型

PCOS 患者中高甘油三酯 – 腰围表型的患病率为 19.7%。根据国际糖尿病联盟的标准，97.5% 有高甘油三酯 – 腰围表型的患者都患有 MetS。

（九）多囊卵巢综合征和性功能障碍

62% 的 PCOS 患者存在与性唤起或润滑相关的性功能障碍。在合并抑郁、焦虑和压力症状的患者中性功能障碍更明显。

（十）多囊卵巢综合征及其治疗综述

该综述揭示了生活方式干预和二甲双胍治疗可能会提高胰岛素敏感性，并提高预防策略的效果。

七、缅甸

缅甸的国土面积为 676 578 km^2，2021 年人口数为 54 903 837 人。缅甸在 2011 年 3 月过渡为民选政府。这个国家有 135 个政府承认的民族。

缅甸的医疗系统是全世界最糟糕的医疗系统之一，亟须改善。这个国家正面临医务人员的短缺和卫生拨款的不足。缅甸的医疗系统受国际援助（https://borgenproject.org/healthcare-in-myanmar/）。表 26.1 展示了该国孕产妇和新生儿健康指标。

八、菲律宾

菲律宾的国土面积为 300 000 km^2，2020 年的人口数为 109 581 078 人。菲律宾的文化是东西方结合的。根据世界卫生组织的数据，约 90% 的菲律宾男性都行过割礼，菲律宾是全世界割礼率最高的国家。

（一）医疗保健系统

菲律宾的医疗保健机构包括私立、公立和乡镇健康中心。公立医疗机构的卫生专业人员只占医务人员的 30%，不能满足所有的医疗需求。因此，菲律宾的医疗保健负担由昂贵的私人医疗机构承担。菲律宾的孕产妇和婴儿健康指标都很差，参见表 26.1。

（二）多囊卵巢综合征的患病率

关于菲律宾当地 PCOS 的患病率的数据很少。一项针对确诊子宫内膜癌的菲律宾女性的研究表明，这些患者中 PCOS 的发病率较高（https://seud.org/wp-content/uploads/2017/07/2-2548.pdf）。

（三）多囊卵巢综合征和多毛症

在菲律宾 PCOS 患者中观察到生化 HA 和改良 Ferriman-Gallwey（mFG）评分系统的相关性。多毛症女性的 mFG 评分 ≥ 7 分。研究还发现游离睾酮与多毛症有显著关系。

九、新加坡

新加坡的国土面积为 719.2 km^2，2021 年的人口数为 5 925 000 人。新加坡的 HDI 排名靠前，拥有三所医学院和三类医院。

（一）医疗保健系统

新加坡以其堪称典范的医疗保健标准而闻名，有着亚洲最优秀的医疗系统之一。医疗保健由新加坡卫生部监管。新加坡有综合医院、社区医院和专科医院或机构，提供最全面的 PCOS 诊断和治疗服务。所有公民都可以获得公立或私立医疗机构的服务。远程咨询也是可行的。还设有可以提供咨询服务的女性论坛。有注册医师提供传统中医药、针灸、顺势疗法、自然疗法、整骨和补充医疗等服务。

（二）多囊卵巢综合征的患病率

事实上，多达 10% 的新加坡女性可能患有 PCOS（https://www.womensweekly.com.sg/gallery/beauty-and-health/living-with-pcos-symptoms-polycystic-ovarian-syndrome/）。在新加坡，PCOS 主要由妇科医师管理和随访，因为 PCOS 与一些疾病风险相关，如 DM 和心脏病。

（三）体重指数对多囊卵巢综合征表型特征的影响

新加坡 PCOS 患者的 BMI 较高，毛发较旺盛，mFG 评分平均差较高。这解释了

BMI 和 PCOS 对游离睾酮指数的影响。

（四）多囊卵巢综合征和改善生活方式的实践

一项研究根据最新的国家和全球循证指南分析了，在新加坡改变生活方式对治疗 PCOS 的重要性。

十、泰国

泰国也被称为"泰王国"，国土面积为 513 120 km²，2021 年的人口数为 69 799 978 人。这个国家因多样的地理环境、吸引游客的景观和热情的人民而有着"千笑之国"的称号。泰国人信仰佛教。

（一）医疗保健系统

泰国有"悠久且成功的卫生发展历史"。长期出现的非传染性疾病，以及疟疾和结核等传染病都是公共健康问题。在公共卫生部的监督下，公立医院网络为城市地区的所有人提供全民医疗保健服务，但一些农村地区则远远落后。大多数泰国医师是多语种专家，全科医师还非常少。医院都配备有诊断和治疗 PCOS 的设备。

（二）其他类型的医疗保健和公共卫生研究

泰国医疗保健的公共卫生视角是在评估公共卫生措施的研究网络中得到反映的。

（三）传统医学

泰国人可能会选择泰国传统医学（Thai traditional medicine，TTM）治疗，经研究，这种疗法已成功应用于泰国许多现代医院。这门学科被称为泰国传统医学应用（ATTM）。

（四）药用植物

由泰国公共卫生部和其他组织合作开展的"药用植物和初级卫生保健项目"，把药用植物列入了泰国国家基本药物清单。

（五）社区中的求医行为

研究观察到，自我医疗被认为是获得性轻微不适的根本原因。在评估对待流感这类疾病的求医行为时，医务人员展示了积极的卫生保健行为。

（六）多囊卵巢综合征的患病率

在一项研究中，泰国青少年的 PCOS 患病率为 5.29%。尽管中度痤疮是最重要的 PCOS 相关危险因素，但轻度痤疮、月经稀发/闭经也与 PCOS 有很大相关性。

另一项针对泰国患者的 PCOS 研究评估了临床 HA 和生化 HA 的关系。HA 的主要表现是月经稀发/闭经和痤疮（56.6%）。2/5 的患者有高浓度的血清游离睾酮（free testosterone，FT）。多毛症和 FT、多毛症和血清总睾酮（total testosterone，TT）水平、痤疮和 TT 之间有显著的统计学相关性。其他指标之间则没有显著关联。

十一、越南

越南的国土面积为 331 210 km², 2020 年的人口数为 97 141 003 人。越南文化是东南亚最古老的文化之一,深受中国文化的影响。迷信是越南文化和习俗中的一部分。

(一)医疗保健系统

越南的医疗保健是东西方医学的结合体。公立医院和私立医院都位于大城市,设备齐全,可提供优质服务,交通便利。公共卫生系统资金并不充足。私立医院收费较高,但可提供优质服务。这些医院都可以进行 PCOS 的诊断和管理。越南的医疗保健系统目前面向的是全民。如今,大多数越南民众需要自费支付医疗服务费用。越南也有传统中医药学,与中国传统医学非常相似。

(二)多囊卵巢综合征的患病率

1. 多囊卵巢综合征表型

越南的 PCOS 患者有着典型的瘦体形、面部以外部位多毛症、多囊卵巢、无排卵,以及典型的 PCOS 血浆激素标记物和低 MetS 风险。相较于 PCOS 患者的典型表型,越南患者的非典型 PCOS 表型明显更多。

2. 多囊卵巢综合征:意识和依从性

印度、中国、越南这些国家已经开始加强宣传活动来提高大众对 PCOS 的认识,重点是以证据为基础的 PCOS 管理建议,以及临床护理和筛查模式,并采取指导性干预措施。

3. 多囊卵巢综合征和不孕症管理

有一项研究在越南 PCOS 患者中采用低剂量、逐步加量的重组卵泡刺激素方案促排卵。该研究观察到,25 IU/d 的起始剂量对不排卵、低或正常 BMI 的越南 PCOS 患者来说是安全的。事实证明,这种方案的临床妊娠率和持续妊娠率都很高。

十二、结论

根据 WHO 2000 年发布的报告,东南亚的女性健康问题需要得到关注。援助组织根据这份报告来帮助那些性别不平等和女性生殖健康需要额外援助的国家。一篇 2018 年发布的文章显示,目前东南亚女性的处境仍处于较低水平。深入分析 PCOS 等问题,并对其进行及时、适当的管理,可以减轻卫生预算的负担。

参考文献

1. Idris DR, Hassan NS, Sofian N. Masculinity, ill health, health help-seeking behavior and health maintenance of diabetic male patients: preliminary findings from brunei darussalam. Belitung Nurs J. 2019;5(3):123-129.
2. Annear PL, Grundy J, Ir P, et al. World Health Organization. The Kingdom of Cambodia Health System Review.

Health Syst Transit. 2015;5(2). https://apps.who.int/iris/handle/10665/208213.
3. Dzykryanka SM, Yulistani Y, Santoso BJ. Analysis of homa-IR, follicle size, and estradiol after combination therapy of metformin and clomiphene citrate in polycystic ovary syndrome's patient. Folia Medica Indonesiana. 2015;51(3):162-167.
4. Okta PP. Faktor-Faktor Yang Mempengaruhi Kejadian Sindrom Ovarium Polikistik di RSUP Dr. M. Djamil Padang Tahun 2015-2019. Diploma Thesis: Univeritas Andalas; 2020.
5. Amal N, Paramesarvathy R, Tee G, Gurpreet K, Karuthan C. Prevalence of chronic illness and health seeking behaviour in Malaysian population: results from the Third National Health Morbidity Survey (NHMS III) 2006. Med J Malaysia. 2011;66(1):36-41.
6. Dawood OT, Hassali MA, Saleem F, Ibrahim IR, Abdulameer AH, Jasim HH. Assessment of health seeking behaviour and self-medication among general public in the state of Penang, Malaysia. Pharm Pract (Granada). 2017;15(3):991.
7. Dashti S, Abdul Hamid H, Mohamad Saini S, et al. Prevalence of polycystic ovary syndrome among Malaysian female university staff. J Midwifery Womens Health. 2019;7(1):1560-1568.
8. Mohammed SB, Nayak B. Polycystic ovarian syndrome trend in a nutshell. Int J Womens Health Reprod Sci. 2017;5(3):153-157.
9. Ishak A, Kadir AA, Hussain NHN, Ismail SB. Prevalence and characteristics of metabolic syndrome among polycystic ovarian syndrome patients in Malaysia. Int J Collab Res Intern Med Public Health. 2012;4(8):1577-1588.
10. Bee Jr YT, Haresh KK, Rajibans S. Prevalence of metabolic syndrome among Malaysians using the International Diabetes Federation, National Education Program and modified World Health Organization definitions. Malays J Nutr. 2008;14(1):65-77.
11. Dashti S, Latiff LA, Hamid HA, et al. Sexual dysfunction in patients with polycystic ovary syndrome in Malaysia. Asian Pac J Cancer Prev. 2016;17(8):3747-3751.
12. Dashti S, Latiff LA, Zulkefli NAB, et al. A review on the assessment of the efficacy of common treatments in polycystic ovarian syndrome on prevention of diabetes mellitus. J Family Reprod Health. 2017;11(2):56-66.
13. Ilagan MKCC, Paz-Pacheco E, Totesora DZ, Clemente-Chua LR, Jalique JRK. The modified Ferriman-Gallwey score and hirsutism among Filipino women. Endocrinol Metab (Seoul). 2019;34(4):374-381.
14. Neubronner SA, Indran IR, Chan YH, Thu AWP, Yong EL. Effect of body mass index (BMI) on phenotypic features of polycystic ovary syndrome (PCOS) in Singapore women: a prospective cross-sectional study. BMC Womens Health. 2021;21(1):1-12.
15. Ko H, Teede H, Moran L. Analysis of the barriers and enablers to implementing lifestyle management practices for women with PCOS in Singapore. BMC Res Notes. 2016;9(1):1-11.
16. Wibulpolprasert S, Fleck F. Thailand's health ambitions pay off. Bull World Health Organ. 2014;92(7):472-473.
17. Fakkham S, Sirithanawutichi T, Jarupoonpol V, Homjumpa P, Bunalesnirunltr M. The integration of the applied Thai traditional medicine into hospitals of the current health delivery system: the development of an administrative/management model. J Med Assoc Thai. 2012;95(2):257.
18. Andrade C, Gomes NG, Duangsrisai S, Andrade PB, Pereira DM, Valentao P. Medicinal plants utilized in Thai Traditional Medicine for diabetes treatment: ethnobotanical surveys, scientific evidence and phytochemicals. J Ethnopharmacol. 2020;263:113177.
19. Chotchoungchatchai S, Saralamp P, Jenjittikul T, Pornsiripongse S, Prathanturarug S. Medicinal plants used with Thai Traditional Medicine in modern healthcare services: a case study in Kabchoeng Hospital, Surin Province, Thailand. J Ethnopharmacol. 2012;141(1):193-205.
20. Sangngern L, Kanchanakhan N, Somrongthong RJ. Health status and health seeking behaviours among the elderly in the Donmuang slum community, Bangkok, Thailand. J Health Res. 2014;28(3):205-210.

21. Chaipung B, Chapman RS. Health seeking behaviors in influenza-like illness among healthcare providers in angthong province, Thailand. J Health Res. 2014;28(2):127-134.
22. Kaewnin J, Vallibhakara O, Arj-Ong Vallibhakara S, et al. Prevalence of polycystic ovary syndrome in Thai University adolescents. Gynecol Endocrinol. 2018;34(6):476-480.
23. Leerasiri P, Wongwananuruk T, Indhavivadhana S, Techatraisak K, Rattanachaiyanont M, Angsuwathana S. Correlation of clinical and biochemical hyperandrogenism in Thai women with polycystic ovary syndrome. J Obstet Gynaecol Res. 2016;42(6):678-683.
24. Cao NT, Le MT, Nguyen VQH, et al. Defining polycystic ovary syndrome phenotype in Vietnamese women. J Obstet Gynaecol Res. 2019;45(11):2209-2219.
25. Garad RM, Teede H Polycystic ovary syndrome: improving policies, awareness, and clinical care. Curr Opin Endocr Metab Res. 2020;12:112-118.
26. Lan VTN, Norman RJ, Nhu GH, Tuan PH, Tuong HM. Ovulation induction using low-dose step-up rFSH in Vietnamese women with polycystic ovary syndrome. Reprod Biomed Online. 2009;18(4):516-521.
27. Kumar S. WHO draws attention to women's health in south-east Asia. Lancet. 2000;356(9233):922.
28. Feng C, Lai Y, Li R, et al. Reproductive health in Southeast Asian women: current situation and the influence factors. Midwifery. 2018;2(1):32-41.

第二十七章 西亚多囊卵巢综合征的现状分析

西亚人口分布在 3 个地区。首先，新月沃地地区包括 9 个国家：伊朗、伊拉克、土耳其、叙利亚、黎巴嫩、以色列、巴勒斯坦、塞浦路斯和约旦。其次，西亚北部包括格鲁吉亚、亚美尼亚和阿塞拜疆。最后，阿拉伯半岛包括也门、阿曼苏丹国、阿拉伯联合酋长国、巴林、卡塔尔、科威特和沙特阿拉伯。各国的卫生健康状况见表 27.1。

表 27.1 西亚地区的国家人口数和健康概况

国家	人口（百万）[c]	粗死亡率[e]（‰）	IMR[e]（‰）	Neo MR[e]（‰）	≤5 MR[e]（‰）	SBA[e]（％）	MMR[e] [‰（年）]
亚美尼亚	2.96	10	10	6	11	100	7（2017）
阿塞拜疆	10.3	8	17	10	19	99	12（2017）
巴林	1.5	2	6	3	7	100	9（2014）
塞浦路斯	1.2	7	2	2	3	98	0（2016）
埃及	111	6	17	10	20	92	15（2015）
格鲁吉亚	3.7	13	8	5	9	99	14（2018）
伊拉克	44.5	5	21	14	25	96	60（2013）
伊朗	88.5	5	11	8	13	99	7（2015）
以色列	9	5	3	2	4	99	2（2017）
科威特	4.2	3	8	5	9	100	2（2012）
黎巴嫩	5.4	5	6	4	7	98	46（2018）
阿曼苏丹国	4.5	2	10	5	11	99	23（2018）
巴勒斯坦	5.2	NA	NA	NA	NA	NA	NA
卡塔尔	2.69	1	5	4	6	100	0（2016）
沙特阿拉伯	36.4	4	6	4	7	99	25（1998）
土耳其	85.3	5	8	5	10	98	16（2018）
阿拉伯联合酋长国	9.4	2	6	4	7	100	2（2009）
也门	33.7	6	46	28	60	45	137（2013）

注：[c] 来源：World Population Review (2022). https://worldpopulationreview.com/。
[e] 来源：World Bank Open Data (2022). https://data.worldbank.org/。
粗死亡率，每 1000 例活产；IMR，婴儿死亡率（每 1000 例活产）；Neo MR，新生儿死亡率（每 1000 例活产）；≤5 MR，5 岁以下儿童死亡率（每 1000 例活产）；SBA，熟练助产率；MMR，孕产妇死亡率（每 10 万例活产）(数据为全国估算结果，括号内为估算年份)。

一、位于西亚北部的国家

（一）亚美尼亚

亚美尼亚人口为 2 969 323 人，国土面积为 28 470 km²。当代亚美尼亚是一个发展中国家，98% 的人口为亚美尼亚族。亚美尼亚在科学、技术和教育领域不断发展。

1. 卫生服务提供系统

世界银行正向亚美尼亚提供咨询和财政支持，以改善其卫生服务提供系统。卫生指标见表 27.1。截至 2018 年，亚美尼亚共有 102 家医院分布在主要城市，此外还有遍布全国的医疗中心。农村地区卫生资源有限。亚美尼亚有 5 所西式医科大学和 1 所传统医科大学。新的卫生政策建议医师和护士接受教育。

2. 女性健康问题

新的卫生政策提出了研究倡议，以评估孕产妇和新生儿健康指标方面的差距。亚美尼亚有一些针对常见女性健康主题的学术文章，但目前尚缺乏关于 PCOS 的文章。尽管如此，城市地区的大医院还是可以对 PCOS 进行诊断和治疗。

（二）阿塞拜疆

阿塞拜疆人口为 10 244 502 人，国土面积为 82 658 km²。

1. 卫生服务提供系统

医疗保健是国家的责任。阿塞拜疆通过公共和私人医疗设施提供服务。国际组织［如美国国际开发署（United States Agency for International Development，USAID）、联合国儿童基金会（United Nations International Children's Emergency Fund，UNICEF）、世界卫生组织（WHO）、世界银行］正在为改善健康指标提供支持。然而，阿塞拜疆的医疗保健系统仍需要关注。卫生指标见表 27.1。

2. 女性健康问题

目前阿塞拜疆有基于捐赠的、有关孕产妇和新生儿健康指标的研究项目，但目前还没有发表关于女性健康（尤其是 PCOS）的学术文章。

（三）格鲁吉亚

格鲁吉亚人口为 3 977 281 人，国土面积为 69 490 km²。它与欧洲接壤，是许多欧洲组织的成员国之一。它拥有一所排名很高的医学院，该医学院附属的研究机构在其期刊上发表过学术文章。

1. 卫生服务提供系统

政府通过一项综合计划提供医疗服务，以改善所有公民的就医条件。自 2015 年 5 月以来，格鲁吉亚已采取重大措施加强孕产妇和新生儿医疗保健系统，并改善健康指标。当地医师在格鲁吉亚医学院接受学术和临床教育。

2. 女性健康问题

格鲁吉亚目前有各种研究项目关注孕产妇和新生儿健康指标。但目前还没有发表关于女性健康（尤其是PCOS）的学术文章。

二、位于西亚新月沃地的国家

（一）伊拉克

伊拉克人口为 41 423 242 人，国土面积为 434 320 km^2。大多数人（总人口的 3/4）是伊拉克族人。该国人预期寿命为 74.9 岁。伊拉克人主要由阿拉伯人组成，库尔德人和土库曼人的数量较少。

1. 医疗保健提供系统

伊拉克的医疗保健是由中央负责的，向全国人口提供免费医疗保健。由于海湾危机，以及政府对医疗系统重视不足，伊拉克正在WHO的财政和技术支持下，努力重建医疗系统。

2. 女性健康问题

在伊拉克，有关女性健康问题（除基本的孕产妇指标外）已得到应有的重视，并已开展研究以了解许多疾病的模式，从而提供适当的诊断服务和管理。

3. 多囊卵巢综合征的患病率和特征

在伊拉克一家教学医院的不孕症门诊开展的一项病例对照研究显示，因PCOS而导致不孕症的发生率约为12%。

（二）伊朗

该国人口为 85 286 927 人，国土面积为 1 628 550 km^2。居民主要是伊朗人，少数是来自阿富汗和伊拉克的难民。伊朗通过学校系统培养医学生。

1. 医疗保健提供系统

伊朗建立了一套完善的医疗服务系统，可深入基层民众。医师在该国的公立和私立医院接受医学教育和培训。在农村地区，初级服务由负责孕产妇护理的助产士（熟练助产）提供。在大城市，医院符合国际质量标准，拥有训练有素的医务人员，并配备了识别、诊断PCOS患者的全套设备。

2. 医疗系统的公共卫生倡议和研究文化

伊朗有持续的医学教育计划，本科生和研究生承担研究任务，并在当地和国际医学期刊上发表文章。PCOS是这项研究的议程之一，迄今为止，伊朗共发表了176篇关于PCOS疾病模式和管理的文章。伊朗是参与全球PCOS研究的6个西亚国家之一，共发表了17篇文章（图27.1）。

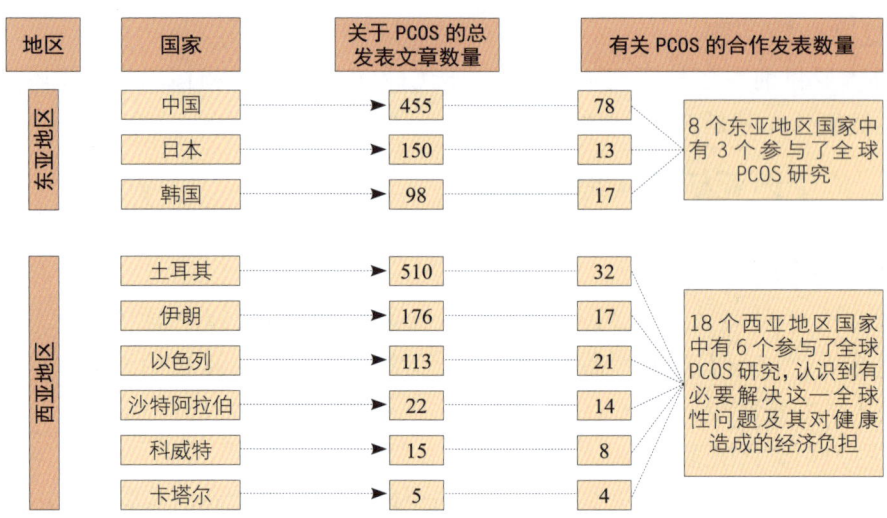

总发表数量反映了每个国家的公共卫生倡议。

图 27.1 亚洲国家在 PCOS 全球研究中的合作

来源：Brüggmann D, Berges L, Klingelhöfer D, et al. Polycystic ovary syndrome: analysis of the global research architecture using density equalizing mapping. Reprod Biomed Online. 2017; 34[6]: 627-638.

3. 多囊卵巢综合征的患病率和特征

（1）患病率

根据美国国立卫生研究院（NIH）的标准，该国估计的 PCOS 发病率为 7%；根据鹿特丹标准，发病率为 15.2%；根据雄激素过多协会（androgen excess society，AES）的标准，发病率为 7.92%。

在另一部分人群中，PCOS 的发病率为 7.1%～14.6%。受影响人群的主要特征依次为多毛症、不孕症和月经不规律。

（2）表现特征

特发性多毛症的发生率为 10.9%；稀发排卵/无排卵的发生率为 8.3%；多囊卵巢形态的发生率为 8.0%。根据不同的诊断标准，社区中 PCOS 的患病率为 7.1%（NIH 标准）、11.7%（AES 标准）和 14.6%（鹿特丹标准）。

（3）生化和激素紊乱与多囊卵巢综合征

PCOS 的相关症状，如多毛症、不孕症和月经问题等，都会影响生活质量。

（4）多囊卵巢综合征与健康相关生活质量

对健康相关生活质量（HRQoL）的深入了解表明，PCOS 对身体、性生活和心理方面的生活质量均有负面影响。

（5）多囊卵巢综合征和生活质量

影响患者生活的症状按严重程度排列分别是多毛症、高 BMI、月经失调和不孕。

（6）改良多囊卵巢综合征 HRQoL 问卷的质量

对于该问卷而言，其判别效度和收敛效度均显示其校准之间存在建设性关系。

（7）多囊卵巢综合征 HRQoL 问卷的质量

对于内部一致性和组内相关系数来说，该问卷定量和定性的有效性及可靠性都取得了令人满意的结果。

（8）多囊卵巢综合征问卷 -50（PCOSQ-50）

一项新的 50 项问卷（PCOSQ-50）被认为是评估与健康相关生活质量的一个有效和可靠的工具。这个新工具的设计旨在补充以前的 HRQoL 问卷中遗漏的方面。

（9）多囊卵巢综合征和维生素 D

维生素 D 水平被发现影响 PCOS 的氧化状态。在伊朗，补充维生素 D 能改善 PCOS 患者的免疫状态。研究人员在相同地域内也观察到了低生育力与维生素 D 水平之间的类似关联性。

（三）巴勒斯坦

巴勒斯坦的人口为 5 253 580 人，国土面积为 6020 km²。巴勒斯坦的主要族群是阿拉伯人。该国的识字率为 96.9%。

1. 医疗保健系统

根据世界卫生组织的报告，截至 2016 年，巴勒斯坦的全民医保覆盖率很高，并承诺通过捐助资金实现全民医保。持续的冲突导致巴勒斯坦对卫生服务需求和基础设施重建的要求增加，从而导致了购买基本药物和防止流行病方面的财政危机。专业劳动力和合格的卫生人员也在迁移。大学附属教学医院目前更侧重于救治紧急情况下的人员。

2. 女性健康问题

巴勒斯坦的女性健康计划是由不同领域捐助资金支持的工作组来负责的。这些工作组的目标是改善孕产妇保健和新生儿护理。

（四）塞浦路斯

塞浦路斯是一个拥有 1 217 746 人口和国土面积为 9240 km² 的岛屿。塞浦路斯最大的族群是希腊裔塞浦路斯人。其他居民主要包括土耳其人和一些俄罗斯人。

1. 医疗保健系统

塞浦路斯的公共医疗由卫生部提供补贴，与私人医疗相比非常便宜。农村地区有 42 个初级保健中心。农村和城市地区均设有医院，配有专业医疗人员。人们也经常向传统行医者求诊。

2. 女性健康问题

在塞浦路斯，健康相关数据通常局限于孕产妇保健、分娩和传染病等范畴。关于女性健康状况和相关合并症的数据不足，但该国对不孕症的诊断和管理护理水平很高。由于医疗费用相对较低，多家不孕症中心吸引着外籍人士前来就诊。

（五）土耳其

土耳其人口为 85 235 532 人，国土面积为 769 630 km²。人口由 75% 的土耳其人和

18% 的库尔德人构成。该国的识字率为 95.6%。

1. 医疗保健系统

2003 年,土耳其引入了一种名为"Genel Sağlık Sigortası"的全民医保制度,旨在通过循证医学研究来加强卫生系统并提高服务质量。公立和私立医院医师通过各自的机构提供服务。

2. 公共卫生倡议和研究文化

土耳其是一个注重研究的国家。该国在公共卫生倡议领域进行投资,以提高卫生系统的质量标准。土耳其共发表了 510 篇研究文章,旨在了解 PCOS 的发病模式和治疗方法。土耳其是参与全球 PCOS 研究计划的 6 个西亚地区国家之一,共发表了 32 篇文章。

3. 多囊卵巢综合征的患病率和特征

(1)表型

合并多毛症、无排卵的土耳其女性常具有 PCOS 的 3 种临床表型,其临床或生化特征相似。

(2)与肥胖相关的表型

具有第 1 表型(卵巢疾病 + HA + 多囊卵巢)特征的 PCOS 女性中,有 47.1% 合并黄体生成素(LH):卵泡刺激素(FSH)紊乱。BMI 的增加与血脂异常、空腹胰岛素异常和 IR(通过稳态模型评估 – 胰岛素抵抗指数)有关,表明肥胖在 PCOS 患者的代谢紊乱中起主要作用。

(3)不同标准的患病率

土耳其女性的患病率为 6.1%(NIH 标准)、19.9%(鹿特丹标准)和 15.3%(AES 标准),具体取决于所使用的标准。

(4)代谢综合征的风险

无论诊断标准如何,土耳其 PCOS 患者发生代谢异常的风险都是正常人水平的 2 倍。

(5)土耳其的患病率

土耳其的 PCOS 患病率估计为 11.4%。

(6)多囊卵巢综合征和子宫畸形

在土耳其东南部,寻求不孕症治疗的 PCOS 患者中 8% 合并子宫畸形。

(六)黎巴嫩

黎巴嫩是一个中等收入国家,人口为 6 761 926 人,国土面积为 10 230 km^2。黎巴嫩包括 150 万叙利亚人,47 万巴勒斯坦人和 5700 名伊拉克人。该国居民预期寿命约为 77.8 岁。

1. 医疗保健系统

黎巴嫩的医疗保健系统由初级医疗保健(primary healthcare,PHC)基础设施组成。尽管多个非政府组织正在支持卫生和社会福利,但其国内接二连三的危机和政治不稳定还是影响了卫生政策的实施。此外,双边机构正在提供资金和技术援助,以加强 PHC 系统。

2. 女性健康问题

目前，女性健康数据仅限于孕产妇和婴儿护理。

（七）叙利亚

叙利亚的人口为 18 439 007 人，包括伊拉克和巴勒斯坦难民。约 60% 的人口需要人道主义援助。叙利亚的国土面积为 183 630 km²。

1. 健康状况

自危机暴发以来，叙利亚的卫生基础设施已经崩溃。曾经用于初级和预防保健的公立医院和保健中心现在被用于急救和急诊。卡塔尔发展基金（Qatar fund for development，QFFD）和卡塔尔慈善机构提供的资金支持在叙利亚建立了 4 个初级医疗保健中心。

2. 女性健康问题

目前，女性健康不是优先考虑的问题。

（八）以色列

以色列的人口为 8 824 544 人，国土面积为 21 640 km²。以色列在人类发展指数（HDI）上排名很高。其人口主要由犹太裔公民构成。

1. 医疗保健系统

以色列向全体居民提供保险，尽管他们必须通过保险计划支付部分费用。这些战略具有创新性，并不断改进以建立质量标准。该系统在 2020 年被评为世界"第三高效"系统，它提供预防和治疗护理服务，并开展科研活动。

2. 女性健康问题

以色列在女性健康领域做了大量工作。有关 PCOS 的研究已发表了近 103 篇科学论文。其中，有 21 篇研究论文是"PCOS 全球战略"的合作成果。

（九）约旦

约旦的人口为 10 292 771 人，包括来自伊拉克、叙利亚、土耳其和伊朗的难民，国土面积为 88 780 km²。

1. 健康状况

约旦在医疗保健和卫生规划方面的远见卓识使得约旦的医疗保健系统可与许多发达国家相媲美。公立医疗和私立医疗都已建立完善。约旦共有 106 家医院，配备有诊断和手术设施。自 2001 年以来，约旦一直被认为是无疟疾国家。

2. 女性健康和多囊卵巢综合征

除了关注孕产妇和新生儿健康指标之外，约旦还致力于提高女性健康质量，并开展了相关研究等，以了解 PCOS 的模式和影响。

叙利亚和约旦的 PCOS 患者会接受教育以改善生活方式，如行为治疗、呼吸疗法，以及配合推荐饮食的锻炼，以减少应激。

三、位于阿拉伯半岛的国家

（一）沙特阿拉伯王国

沙特阿拉伯王国（KSA）人口为 35 476 659 人，国土面积为 2 149 690 km^2。该国在 HDI 排行中名列前茅。医学院附属于研究机构，卫生信息通过医学期刊传播。

1. 医疗保健系统

KSA 的医疗保健由私营部门提供支持，并由该部门提供高质量的医疗服务。医院配备有最先进的诊断设备和治疗设施。该国有一个用于记录所有健康数据的数据库，该数据库会定期进行维护并将其用于科学研究。医院护理符合国际质量标准。

2. 女性健康问题

癌症、肥胖和维生素 D 缺乏症在 KSA 女性中极为常见。女性肥胖是一个公共卫生问题，因为它是许多代谢问题和 PCOS 的危险因素。所有医院都配备了诊断和治疗设施，以应对 PCOS 等问题。从公共卫生的角度来看，改变生活方式和减轻体重尤为重要。《沙特医学年鉴》在著名的医学期刊上发表有关 PCOS 的模式、风险、识别和管理的文章。

3. 公共卫生倡议、研究机构和出版物

KSA 有 220 家医院，附属于 5 所医学院。该国通过一个有效的转诊系统，将所有医院与初级保健服务联系起来。评估 PCOS 模式和管理的循证医学研究通过 KSA 医学期刊和其他国际期刊进行传播。KSA 有关 PCOS 的研究共发表了 22 篇论文，其中 14 篇是合作发表的（图 27.1）。

4. 多囊卵巢综合征的患病率和特征

（1）**多囊卵巢综合征的患病率**

在麦地那，PCOS 的自我报告率为 32.5%。

（2）**多囊卵巢综合征的特征**

53.7% 的 KSA 未婚年轻女性患有 PCOM，伴有月经不规律和皮肤病表现。

（3）**多囊卵巢综合征和肥胖**

超重和肥胖女性自我报告的 PCOS 患病率较普通人群高出 16%，表明肥胖与 PCOS 之间呈正相关。

（4）**多囊卵巢综合征的风险因素**

肥胖被确认是与 PCOS 相关的危险因素。

（5）**多囊卵巢综合征和多毛症**

总体而言，82% 的 KSA 女性患有 PCOS，并伴有多毛症。

（6）**多囊卵巢综合征和不孕症管理**

在 BMI > 25 kg/m^2 的患者中，枸橼酸氯米芬和二甲双胍的联合使用在调节月经周期和改善生育力方面取得了满意疗效。

（7）多囊卵巢综合征与 BMI 和 LH ∶ FSH 的关系

在 PCOS 与 BMI 和循环激素水平［LH ∶ FSH、催乳素或促甲状腺激素（TSH）］之间尚未发现有明显相关性。

（8）多囊卵巢综合征和心身症状

受过大学教育的年轻女性（26～35岁）患压力症的概率最高，她们会出现月经周期紊乱、多毛症、痤疮和不孕症。抑郁和焦虑也会出现，但程度较轻。

（9）多囊卵巢综合征和糖代谢

KSA 女性糖代谢异常的患病率较高。

（10）多囊卵巢综合征的认知

KSA 女性对 PCOS 的认知水平较高。信息的主要来源是互联网。医学毕业生的认知水平较高。对症状的认知程度高于对并发症的认知。

（11）多囊卵巢综合征和生殖激素水平

研究发现，无论年龄和体重如何，KSA 女性的 LH ∶ FSH 水平和血清总睾酮水平都较高。此外，血清 FSH、性激素结合球蛋白（SHBG）和孕酮则低于对照组。

（二）阿拉伯联合酋长国

阿拉伯联合酋长国（UAE）由 7 个酋长国组成：阿布扎比、阿治曼、迪拜、富查伊拉、哈伊马角、沙迦和乌姆盖万。

UAE 的人口为 10 017 129 人，国土面积为 83 600 km^2。人口主要集中在阿布扎比、迪拜和沙迦。UAE 的大部分人口都是外籍人士，且年龄较小。

1. 医疗保健系统

居民的医疗保健费用由政府出资。每个酋长国都有自己的医疗保健系统，由卫生部负责管理，并由一个独立的卫生管理局负责监督。女性享有平等的医疗服务，医疗服务由女性提供。医院符合国际质量标准。

2. 关于多囊卵巢综合征日益增多的健康问题

用一位资深妇科医师的话说，PCOS 在 UAE 的发病率越来越高，但却没有采取任何措施来提高人们的预防意识。在 UAE，PCOS 的发病率相当高，这是因为该地区的生活方式舒适、过度放纵且缺乏运动。沙迦一家生殖医院的海湾阿拉伯裔女性研究显示，该地的 PCOS 的发病率为 39.38%，其中近 80.90% 的患者有 IR，而在全世界范围内这一比例仅为 50%～70%。

3. 多囊卵巢综合征的患病率和特征

（1）多囊卵巢综合征与血脂异常

在 UAE，糖尿病和 IR 与 PCOS 有关，但与血脂异常无关。血脂状况表明可能存在亚临床动脉粥样硬化。

（2）患病率

年龄在 18～24 岁的医学生中，PCOS 的发病率为 27.6%。肥胖是近一半 PCOS 患者的危险因素。月经不规律和多毛症是常见的症状。

（3）面向多囊卵巢综合征的结构化健康教育计划

一项旨在提高认识和传授健康教育的计划结果表明，通过事前和事后测试评估，人们对 PCOS 的认识和管理能力有了显著提高。

（4）多囊卵巢综合征的风险因素

研究发现，家族中有 PCOS 病史、常吃快餐和肥胖的女性患 PCOS 的风险更大。

（5）沙迦的多囊卵巢综合征患病率及其相关患病因素

PCOS 的患病率为 20%，其中 22% 的患者有 PCOS 家族史。

（6）多囊卵巢综合征的综合患病率

使用 NIH 标准，UAE 中 PCOS 的综合患病率为 8.9%，而海湾阿拉伯国家的患病率则为 18.8%。

（7）生殖健康和多囊卵巢综合征的认知

通过探究 PCOS 患者中对病情理解方面的差距，制定结构化的健康教育和宣传活动，从而促进健康的生活方式，预防不孕症和相关问题的发生。

（三）巴林

巴林人口为 1 760 392 人，国土面积为 760 km²。该国人口主要为巴林籍公民。亚洲人、阿拉伯人和其他移民约占总人口的 52.6%。

1. 医疗保健系统

巴林政府为所有本国公民提供免费医疗服务，并为非本国公民提供医疗补贴。巴林医疗设施达世界一流水平，医护人员专业素质高，公民均可便捷获取医疗服务。此外，该国医疗卫生类高校也日益注重科研发展。

2. 多囊卵巢综合征的患病率和特征

（1）确定合适的内分泌标志物

胰岛素和 LH：FSH 最好通过游离雄激素指数（FAI）来确定，而性激素结合容量可用于估计 IR、异常的促性腺激素分泌和雄激素过多。

（2）巴林阿拉伯女性中的 *DENND1A* 基因变异

未发现 *DENND1A* 基因变异与 PCOS 之间有关联，在亚洲人和巴林阿拉伯女性中也未观察到这种关联。

（3）卵巢打孔术和妊娠结局

尽管 PCOS 孕妇会更易出现糖代谢异常和高血压，但在其新生儿预后或早产方面并没有发现明显的差异。

（4）作为生物标志物的 C 反应蛋白：白蛋白

发现 PCOS 患者的 C 反应蛋白：白蛋白水平会升高，可将其用作生物标志物。

(四)阿曼苏丹国

阿曼苏丹国人口为 5 255 727 人,国土面积为 309 500 km²。人口主要由来自不同种族和民族的外籍人士组成。政府希望能提高阿曼苏丹国人民的生活水平。

1. 卫生保健系统

卫生部负责人民的医疗保健工作。医院设备齐全,提供各种服务。卫生教育是政府的优先事项,大学附属医学院提供研究生和文凭课程,以及短期继续教育和进修课程。

2. 多囊卵巢综合征的患病率和特征

(1)患病率

在阿曼苏丹国 25~34 岁的女性中,PCOS 的患病率为 7%。

(2)多囊卵巢综合征和情绪障碍

患有 PCOS 的女性出现情绪障碍的风险更高,但其压力、焦虑和抑郁水平没有出现统计学差异的改变。

(3)多囊卵巢综合征和氧化应激风险

氧化应激在 PCOS 发病机制中的作用已得到证实,并可用于识别高危人群。

(4)布赖米地区的患病率和特征

在阿曼苏丹国,PCOS 的发病率为 7%,常见症状包括月经不规律、不孕、异常子宫出血和多毛症。

(五)卡塔尔

卡塔尔的人口为 2 944 736 人,国土面积为 11 610 km²。从族群构成来看,居民主要为阿拉伯人(半岛原住民),亦有部分阿曼侨民。卡塔尔是一个富裕的国家,其为加强社会建设投入了大量资源。

1. 卫生服务系统

公共卫生部负责卡塔尔人民的医疗保健。卡塔尔的医疗质量标准位列世界前五。医院设备齐全,提供各种服务。继续教育和科学研究也得到了重视。

2. 公共卫生倡议和出版物

以证据为基础的研究已在许多期刊上发表。卡塔尔共发表了 5 篇关于 PCOS 的出版物,其中 4 篇是涉及 PCOS 全球策略的合作出版物(图 27.1)。

3. 多囊卵巢综合征的患病率和特征

(1)多囊卵巢综合征的代谢特征

研究发现,月经不规律的卡塔尔女性(18~40 岁)患 PCOS 的概率为 12.1%。这些女性的 FAI 值是正常值的 4.5 倍,且代谢水平较高。

(2)代谢比较:卡塔尔女性与英国女性

英国队列中女性的 BMI、腰围和臀围测量值、收缩压和舒张压及甘油三酯较高,而卡塔尔女性的睾酮、高密度脂蛋白(HDL)和 C 反应蛋白较高。

（3）多囊卵巢综合征和糖尿病风险

卡塔尔 PCOS 患者更容易患 DM，但较不易患心血管疾病。

（六）科威特

科威特人口为 4 352 157 人，国土面积为 17 820 km^2。科威特人占总人口的 28%～32%，其余为外籍人士。

1. 医疗保健系统

科威特为科威特国民提供由国家资助的医疗保健系统。非科威特国民可以通过支付费用获得保险。科威特政府的愿景是提高国家医疗质量和标准。

2. 公共卫生倡议和出版物

科威特的公共卫生倡议聚焦于发表有关女性健康问题（如 PCOS）的科研成果。卡塔尔分享了 15 篇关于 PCOS 的出版物，其中 8 篇是与全球研究者合作发表的（图 27.1）。

3. 多囊卵巢综合征的发病率和特征

（1）发病率

在科威特，患有 PCOS 的女性比例为 37%。这些患者超重但不肥胖。

（2）不孕症和多囊卵巢综合征

PCOS 是科威特不孕症的主要原因之一。

（3）腹腔镜卵巢打孔术和抗米勒管激素水平

抗米勒管激素水平和卵巢打孔术前后的多普勒血流指数改变程度与是否患有 PCOS 有显著关系。

（4）多囊卵巢综合征与肥胖

在不孕症的 PCOS 女性中，肥胖会影响不孕症治疗计划，从而降低临床妊娠率。

参考文献

1. World population review, 2022. https://worldpopulationreview.com/.
2. Mousa BA. The Prevalence of PCOS in Infertile Women According to Clinical Features and its Associated Hormonal Changes in Al-Hilla City, Iraq. Indian J Public Health Res Dev. 2019;10(10).
3. Brüggmann D, Berges L, Klingelhöfer D, et al. Polycystic ovary syndrome: analysis of the global research architecture using density equalizing mapping. Reprod Biomed Online. 2017;34(6):627-638.
4. Mehrabian F, Khani B, Kelishadi R, Ghanbari E. The prevalence of polycystic ovary syndrome in Iranian women based on different diagnostic criteria. Endokrynol Pol. 2011;62(3):238-242.
5. Behboodi Moghadam Z, Fereidooni B, Saffari M, Montazeri A. Polycystic ovary syndrome and its impact on Iranian women's quality of life: a population-based study. BMC Womens Health. 2018;18(1):1-8.
6. Tehrani FR, Simbar M, Tohidi M, Hosseinpanah F, Azizi F. The prevalence of polycystic ovary syndrome in a community sample of Iranian population: Iranian PCOS prevalence study. Reprod Biol Endocrinol. 2011;9(1):1-7.
7. Taghavi SA, Bazarganipour F, Hugh-Jones S, Hosseini N. Health-related quality of life in Iranian women with polycystic ovary syndrome: a qualitative study. BMC Womens Health. 2015;15(1):1-8.
8. Khomami MB, Tehrani FR, Hashemi S, Farahmand M, Azizi F. Of PCOS symptoms, hirsutism has the most significant impact on the quality of life of Iranian women. PLoS One. 2015;10(4):e0123608.

9. Bazarganipour F, Ziaei S, Montazeri A, Foroozanfard F. Iranian version of modified polycystic ovary syndrome health-related quality of life questionnaire: discriminant and convergent validity. Iran J Reprod Med. 2013;11(9):753.
10. Bazarganipour F, Ziaei S, Montazeri A, Faghihzadeh S, Frozanfard F. Psychometric properties of the Iranian version of modified polycystic ovary syndrome health-related quality-of-life questionnaire. Hum Reprod. 2012;27(9):2729-2736.
11. Nasiri-Amiri F, Tehrani FR, Simbar M, Montazeri A, Mohammadpour RA. Health-related quality of life questionnaire for polycystic ovary syndrome (PCOSQ-50): development and psychometric properties. Qual Life Res. 2016;25(7):1791-1801.
12. Masjedi F, Keshtgar S, Agah F, Karbalaei N. Association between sex steroids and oxidative status with vitamin D levels in follicular fluid of non-obese PCOS and healthy women. J Reprod Infertil. 2019;20(3):132.
13. Azhar A, Abid F, Rehman R. Polycystic ovary syndrome, subfertility and vitamin D deficiency. J Coll Physicians Surg Pak. 2020;30(5):545-546.
14. Hassa H, Tanir H, Yildiz Z. Comparison of clinical and laboratory characteristics of cases with polycystic ovarian syndrome based on Rotterdam's criteria and women whose only clinical signs are oligo/anovulation or hirsutism. Arch Gynecol Obstet. 2006;274(4):227-232.
15. Ates S, Sevket O, Sudolmus S, et al. Different phenotypes of polycystic ovary syndrome in Turkish women: clinical and endocrine characteristics. Gynecol Endocrinol. 2013;29(10):931-935.
16. Yildiz BO, Bozdag G, Yapici Z, Esinler I, Yarali H. Prevalence, phenotype and cardiometabolic risk of polycystic ovary syndrome under different diagnostic criteria. Hum Reprod. 2012;27(10):3067-3073.
17. Miazgowski T, Martopullo I, Widecka J, Miazgowski B, Brodowska A. National and regional trends in the prevalence of polycystic ovary syndrome since 1990 within Europe: the modeled estimates from the Global Burden of Disease Study 2016. Arch Med Sci. 2021;17(2):343.
18. Ege S, Peker N, Bademkıran MH. The prevalence of uterine anomalies in infertile patients with polycystic ovary syndrome: a retrospective study in a tertiary center in Southeastern Turkey. Turk J Obstet Gynecol. 2019;16(4):224.
19. Lai L, Flower A, Moore M, Prescott P, Lewith G. Polycystic ovary syndrome: a randomised feasibility and pilot study using Chinese Herbal medicine to explore Impact on Dysfunction (ORCHID)—study protocol. Eur J Integr Med. 2014;6(3):392-399.
20. Guraya SS. Prevalence and ultrasound features of polycystic ovaries in young unmarried Saudi females. J Microsc Ultrastruct. 2013;1(1-2):30-34.
21. Aldossary K, Alotaibi A, Alkhaldi K, Alharbi R. Prevalence of polycystic ovary syndrome, and relationship with obesity/overweight: cross-sectional study in Saudi Arabia. J Adv Pharm Educ Res. 2020;10(1):187.
22. Al-Ruhaily AD, Malabu UH, Sulimani RA. Hirsutism in Saudi females of reproductive age: a hospital-based study. Ann Saudi Med. 2008;28(1):28-32.
23. Ayaz A, Alwan Y, Farooq MU. Metformin—clomiphene citrate vs. clomiphene citrate alone: polycystic ovarian syndrome. J Hum Reprod Sci. 2013;6(1):15.
24. Saadia Z. Follicle stimulating hormone (LH: FSH) ratio in polycystic ovary syndrome (PCOS)-obese vs. non-obese women. Med Arch. 2020;74(4):289.
25. Asdaq SMB, Yasmin F. Risk of psychological burden in polycystic ovary syndrome: a case control study in Riyadh, Saudi Arabia. J Affect Disord. 2020;274:205-209.
26. Abdel-Rahman MY, Abdellah AH, Ahmad SR, Ismail SA, Frasure H, Hurd WW. Prevalence of abnormal glucose metabolism in a cohort of Arab women with polycystic ovary syndrome. Int J Gynecol Obstet. 2011;114(3):288-289.
27. Alessa A, Aleid D, Almutairi S, et al. Awareness of polycystic ovarian syndrome among Saudi females. Int J Med Sci Public Health. 2017;6(6):1013-1020.
28. Fakhoury H, Tamim H, Ferwana M, Siddiqui IA, Adham M, Tamimi W. Age and BMI adjusted comparison of reproductive hormones in PCOS. J Family Med Prim Care. 2012;1(2):132.

28a. Asma Alizain (2015). Polycystic Ovarian Syndrome on 'staggering' rise in UAE. Home/Health, Khaleej Times. Published 25th May, 2014. Available at: https://www.khaleejtimes.com/health/polycystic-ovarian-syndrome-on-staggering-rise-in-uae
29. Al Mulla A, El Sokkary A, Ekladiou S, Khamis AH. Prevalence of dyslipidemia among women with polycystic ovary syndrome based on body mass index. W J Gynecol Women's Health. 2020;4(1). doi:WJGWH.MS.ID.000580.
30. Saidunnisa B, Atiqulla S, Ayman G. Prevalence of polycystic ovarian syndrome among students of RAK Medical and Health Sciences University United Arab Emirates. IJMPS. 2016;109:118.
31. Shariff A, Begum GS, Ayman G, Mohammad B, Housam R, Khaled N. An interventional study on effectiveness of structured education programme in improving the knowledge of polycystic ovarian syndrome among female students of Ras Al Khaimah Medical & Health Sciences University, UAE. IJSR. 2016;5(1):1659-1663.
32. Attlee A, Nusralla A, Eqbal R, Said H, Hashim M, Obaid RS. Polycystic ovary syndrome in university students: occurrence and associated factors. Int J Fertil Steril. 2014;8(3):261.
33. Mousa M, Al-Jefout M, Alsafar H, et al. Prevalence of common gynecological conditions in the Middle East: systematic review and meta-analysis. Front Reprod Health. 2021;3:7.
34. Pramodh S. Exploration of lifestyle choices, reproductive health knowledge, and polycystic ovary syndrome (PCOS) awareness among female Emirati University students. Int J Womens Health. 2020;12:927.
35. Golbahar J, Al-Ayadhi M, Das NM, Gumaa K. Sensitive and specific markers for insulin resistance, hyperandrogenemia, and inappropriate gonadotrophin secretion in women with polycystic ovary syndrome: a case-control study from Bahrain. Int J Womens Health. 2012;4:201.
36. Gammoh E, Arekat MR, Saldhana FL, Madan S, Ebrahim BH, Almawi WY. DENND1A gene variants in Bahraini Arab women with polycystic ovary syndrome. Gene. 2015;560(1):30-33.
37. Al-Ojaimi EH. Pregnancy outcomes after laparoscopic ovarian drilling in women with polycystic ovarian syndrome. Saudi Med J. 2006;27(4):519.
38. Kalyan S, Goshtesabi A, Sarray S, Joannou A, Almawi WY. Assessing C reactive protein/albumin ratio as a new biomarker for polycystic ovary syndrome: a case–control study of women from Bahraini medical clinics. BMJ Open. 2018;8(10):e021860.
39. Al Khaduri M, Al Farsi Y, Al Najjar TAA, Gowri V. Hospital-based prevalence of polycystic ovarian syndrome among Omani women. Middle East Fertil Soc J. 2014;19(2):135-138.
40. Sulaiman MA, Al-Farsi YM, Al-Khaduri MM, Saleh J, Waly MI. Polycystic ovarian syndrome is linked to increased oxidative stress in Omani women. Int J Womens Health. 2018;10:763.
41. Varghese U, Varughese S. Prevalence of polycystic ovarian syndrome in the Buraimi region of Oman. Brunei Int Med J. 2012;8(5):248-252.
42. Dargham SR, Ahmed L, Kilpatrick ES, Atkin SL. The prevalence and metabolic characteristics of polycystic ovary syndrome in the Qatari population. PLoS One. 2017;12(7):e0181467.
43. Butler AE, Abouseif A, Dargham SR, Sathyapalan T, Atkin SL. Metabolic comparison of polycystic ovarian syndrome and control women in Middle Eastern and UK Caucasian populations. Sci Rep. 2020;10(1):1-5.
44. Dargham SR, El Shewehy A, Dakroury Y, Kilpatrick ES, Atkin SL. Prediabetes and diabetes in a cohort of Qatari women screened for polycystic ovary syndrome. Sci Rep. 2018;8(1):1-6.
45. Ching H, Burke V, Stuckey B. Quality of life and psychological morbidity in women with polycystic ovary syndrome: body mass index, age and the provision of patient information are significant modifiers. Clin Endocrinol. 2007;66(3):373-379.
46. Elmashad AI. Impact of laparoscopic ovarian drilling on anti-Müllerian hormone levels and ovarian stromal blood flow using three-dimensional power Doppler in women with anovulatory polycystic ovary syndrome. Fertil Steril. 2011;95(7):2342-2346.
47. Al-Azemi M, Omu FE, Omu AE. The effect of obesity on the outcome of infertility management in women with polycystic ovary syndrome. Arch Gynecol Obstet. 2004;270(4):205-210.

第二十八章 欧洲多囊卵巢综合征的现状分析

一、引言

多囊卵巢综合征（PCOS）在生育年龄女性中的患病率为 5%～10%。长期无排卵是 PCOS 的标志性特征，这最终将导致月经问题和较高的不孕症率。同时 PCOS 还可表现为面部多毛症和痤疮。

PCOS 患者普遍会出现内分泌异常，包括血清胰岛素、血糖水平、胰岛素抵抗（IR）稳态模型评估的异常，以及体重指数（BMI）和收缩压（SBP）与舒张压（DBP）的升高。然而，值得注意的是，不同种族和背景的患者在这些症状上可能会表现出显著的差异。此外，PCOS 的分布还受地理位置、民族和人种等因素的影响，变异很大。研究表明，基因型的累积效应并不是导致 PCOS 患者在数量或临床表现上存在差异的唯一因素。环境因素同样被认为在这些方面发挥着重要作用。越来越多的研究证据支持环境因素对患者临床表现的差异、生活方式干预对疾病的影响、疾病在不同背景人群中的显著差异，以及提升高危人群健康意识的重要性等方面的作用，这将为代谢和生育力低下提供更高质量的治疗方法。

二、多囊卵巢综合征的现状

欧洲不同地区的 PCOS 发病率各不相同，这高度提示了环境/遗传因素与 PCOS 密切相关。

2016 年的一项研究表明，捷克共和国的 PCOS 病例最多，而瑞典的病例最少。此外，该研究还发现，年龄对于 PCOS 的分布起着重要作用，在某些特别年龄组 PCOS 患者人数较多。总体来说，整个欧洲三大区域的数据都显示出随着年龄的增长，发病率逐渐上升的趋势，其中 35～39 岁和 40～44 岁的女性发病率最高；从 20 岁开始，东欧和中欧的 PCOS 发病率变化趋势几乎保持不变。事实上，在最年轻的年龄组（15～19 岁）中，只有极少数女性会出现这种疾病。在这个年龄组中，1990—2016 年，东欧的 PCOS 病例数增加了 0.73%［95% 的不确定性区间（UI）：-0.18～1.83］，中欧增加了 1.87%（95%UI：0.42～3.68），而西欧则减少了 1.30%（95%UI：4.65～2.64）（表 28.1）。

表 28.1　2016 年欧洲国家和地区 15～49 岁女性多囊卵巢综合征的患病数和趋势

国家和地区	患病例数 /100 000	下限	上限	总患病率（%）	下限	上限
阿尔巴尼亚	373.94	280.2	498.4	0.38	0.29	0.51
安多拉	119.88	90.26	158.8	0.12	0.09	0.16
奥地利	211.74	167.5	266.2	0.22	0.17	0.27
白俄罗斯	430.98	325.2	561.7	0.44	0.33	0.58
比利时	131.70	95.97	172.5	0.13	0.10	0.18
波黑	420.45	315.8	553.1	0.43	0.32	0.56
保加利亚	435.76	329.3	571.4	0.44	0.37	0.58
克罗地亚	415.90	312.2	546.1	0.43	0.32	0.56
捷克	460.60	346.2	602.1	0.47	0.35	0.62
丹麦	117.43	88.24	157.5	0.12	0.09	0.16
爱沙尼亚	432.44	326.2	567.4	0.44	0.34	0.56
芬兰	121.62	91.37	162.2	0.12	0.09	0.17
法国	120.68	90.61	160.1	0.12	0.09	0.16
德国	114.96	87.70	147.7	0.12	0.84	0.15
希腊	136.07	100.1	177.9	0.14	0.10	0.18
匈牙利	428.72	322.5	561.4	0.44	0.30	0.57
冰岛	120.65	90.51	161.6	0.12	0.09	0.16
爱尔兰	127.61	98.13	168.0	0.13	0.10	0.17
意大利	138.11	106.8	178.9	0.14	0.11	0.18
哈萨克斯坦	417.23	311.2	546.9	0.42	0.31	0.53
拉脱维亚	427.92	321.8	563.2	0.41	0.31	0.54
立陶宛	406.38	304.8	535.4	0.41	0.31	0.54
卢森堡	123.65	92.91	163.8	0.12	0.09	0.17
北马其顿	411.45	309.4	543.2	0.42	0.32	0.56
马耳他	123.51	92.99	164.1	0.13	0.09	0.17
摩尔多瓦	435.78	325.8	578.6	0.44	0.33	0.59
黑山	410.91	309.2	542.4	0.42	0.32	0.56
荷兰	117.50	88.29	156.3	0.12	0.09	0.16
挪威	106.55	80.62	137.9	0.11	0.08	0.14
波兰	447.22	336.3	588.9	0.46	0.34	0.60
葡萄牙	126.00	94.98	165.7	0.13	0.10	0.17
罗马尼亚	409.06	307.1	534.8	0.42	0.31	0 55
俄罗斯	443.14	333.9	583.2	0.45	0.34	0.59
塞尔维亚	409.00	308.5	536.5	0.42	0.32	0.55
斯洛伐克	437.15	328.6	573.7	0.45	0.34	0.59
斯洛文尼亚	402.66	302.6	528.0	0.41	0.31	0.54
西班牙	132.35	97.34	178.6	0.13	0.10	0.18
瑞典	34.10	24.59	45.77	0.04	0.03	0.05
瑞士	121.31	91.03	160.7	0.12	0.09	0.16
土耳其	258.52	195.3	333.2	0.26	0.20	0.34
乌克兰	428.91	321.5	565.3	0.44	0.33	0.57
英国	117.40	87.36	155.3	0.12	0.09	0.16
所有国家	276.35	207.8	363.2	0.28	0.23	0.37
西欧	123.42	93.04	162.3	0.13	0.13	0.17
中欧	408.68	307.4	536.7	0.42	0.32	0.55
东欧	427.79	321.3	562.8	0.43	0.33	0.56

来源：Miazgowski, et al. (2021). National and regional trends in the prevalence of polycystic ovary syndrome since 1990 within Europe: the modeled estimates from the Global Burden of Disease Study 2016. Arch Med Sci, 17 (2): 343-351.

三、多囊卵巢综合征患者的文化信仰和生活方式

有数据证实了环境因素和遗传因素与 PCOS 之间存在相关性。社会经济地位低下被认为是引起 PCOS 的关键环境因素之一；这种背景下的人们缺乏足够的知识，这会导致适应健康生活方式的能力较低，表现为体重增加、激素水平紊乱和 PCOS 易感性增加。

较低的社会经济地位可能意味着这些人获得医疗保健设施的机会较少，并且对 PCOS 的认识和知识也较少，从而增加了社区在 PCOS 方面的负担。由于管理 PCOS 需要多学科合作，因此管理这类患者始终是一个挑战。研究表明，从一开始，来自低社会经济背景的母亲所生的婴儿就因营养不良和孕期饮食不正确而导致宫内发育迟缓，这已被确定是日后患有 PCOS 的关键因素。

1990—2016 年，西欧、东欧和中欧国家的 PCOS 患病率几乎没有变化，但具体到某一地区时，则存在显著差异；这种差异可归因于卫生设施分配不均，这是由于该疾病需要多学科诊治，而许多国家无法精确计算其将造成的经济负担，因此分配给该疾病的资源较少。

由于临床表现各异（如涉及不同的身体系统），患者往往会去看不同的专科医师，如妇科医师、全科医师或内分泌科医师。在所有这些患者中，每个专业都有机会为管理提供建议。对于 PCOS 患者的管理，一个关键因素就是为他们提供相关知识和健康意识，因为如果进行简单的生活方式干预，大多数问题都可以解决。这就是全球范围内患者普遍认为他们所获得的疾病管理信息不足的原因，另一个重要因素是沟通的障碍。在欧洲，有不同背景和（或）来自不同地区的人们（移民），其中许多人并不理解他们所居住的那个特定国家的母语/官方语言，尤其是对于那些新移民来说。因此，如果某种特定语言是唯一可以供临床医师与患者沟通的工具，那么这将最终影响患者所获得的信息。由于 PCOS 的普遍存在及其对心理社会的影响，提高低经济水平人群对该疾病的认知至关重要。因为不同经济水平的人对于 PCOS 的理解和认知程度存在很大差异。来自较高经济水平的人群可能更容易获得信息和支持，而较低经济水平的人群可能面临更多的障碍和挑战。教育可以帮助患者家庭了解患者所面临的问题，以及这些问题对心理健康的严重影响。对于 PCOS 患者，不仅要解决其身体上的问题，如潜在的激素变化（如体重增加和不孕症），还要将心理健康视为同等重要的事项。通过安排教育课程可以提高人们的认识，这些课程应该关注患者的个人情况，并考虑他们的理解程度，以覆盖来自不同背景的患者。许多 PCOS 患者由于缺乏相关知识而未能得到正确诊断。营养师在帮助 PCOS 患者方面可以发挥重要作用，因为正确的饮食选择可以帮助他们减轻体重并尽可能减少 IR 的影响。

研究表明，患者和医疗专业人员面临的障碍、推动因素和满意度之间存在联系，并揭示了信息和社会情感支持的好处。PCOS 患者需要个体化的支持，因为这是一种长

期疾病。诊断信息不足可能导致患者在治疗中感到沮丧。

一项研究询问了 PCOS 患者关于他们的 PCOS 诊治经历，特别是从专业医务工作者那里得到的反馈，他们所面临的障碍是不能及时诊断出 PCOS，还有在不同种族和文化背景下患者对病情的接受度不同。这些反馈表明，女性通常会向医疗服务提供者提出她们的问题，但她们的症状要么被忽视，要么即使被诊断出来，提供的信息也少于所需。患者提出与医疗工作者的沟通效率不高。在很多情况下，教育不是个性化的，也没有号召家庭参与，这导致患者感到沮丧。护理工作中存在许多不足，患者不得不在线查找资料，但他们在网上找到的大部分信息都是商业化的。上述所有因素都会导致 PCOS 患者生活质量较差。有学者建议应为患者提供合适的课程和个性化教育，并向患者提供充分的信息，让他们有机会选择如何管理自己的病情。通常患者精神健康往往被忽视，医务人员只关注了患者体征方面的治疗（如痤疮、体重和不孕症）。因此，有必要采取更全面的管理方法。由于 PCOS 是一种慢性疾病，所以对患者进行教育将有助于他们管理自己的症状，并使他们为自己做出正确选择而变得更有信心。建议使用患者信息手册、电子和纸质媒体，以及 PCOS 讨论组等形式来提高患者对疾病的认识。这些都需要政府和慈善机构的支持。

据报道，有时仅针对患者个人的宣教并不足以解决这个问题。以家庭为整体进行健康宣教，并在讨论过程中让他们参与其中，最终让家庭成员了解患者的需求，这一点至关重要。数据显示，欧洲 PCOS 的患病率较高，部分原因是家庭对 PCOS 的诊断接受度较低、教育不足、文化程度较低（如不愿看男性医师），以及不认为体重增加是 PCOS 的原因。

四、心理影响

有人建议，应当对 PCOS 患者进行抑郁和焦虑的筛查，因为患者普遍存在这些症状，并且通常会被忽视。一旦诊断出抑郁症和焦虑症，应该进行相应的处理。同时，也要避免过度诊断。

有研究报道了一些 PCOS 患者存在基于认知、身体形象及抑郁的心理健康问题。性功能障碍在 PCOS 中的患病率为 13.3%～62.5%。研究已表明 PCOS 与心理性功能障碍之间的关系，以及 PCOS 如何导致自尊心低下、消极体象、女性认同感减弱和性满意度降低。

指南制定小组进行的一项系统性综述，确定了 18 项使用经过验证的性功能问卷和视觉模拟量表的相关研究。在性功能子量表方面发现了微小但显著的差异，与没有 PCOS 的女性相比，PCOS 患者的性唤起、润滑、满意度和性高潮均受到损害。体毛对身体的影响、外貌的社会影响和性吸引力这些方面对其影响很大。性生活满意度受损，而性生活的重要性与非 PCOS 女性相似。PCOS 的身体症状，如多毛症、肥胖、月经不规律和不孕，可能导致女性缺乏吸引力，从而影响性行为。

如有需要，应根据症状表现有针对性地进行治疗，可能涉及药物治疗或心理疗法，以促进精神健康。随着研究的深入，我们对 PCOS 症状的认识越来越细致，因此需要根据患者的不同需求，定期更新现有的 PCOS 患者管理指南。

PCOS 会通过多种方式影响人们的生活质量：BMI 过高、负面的文化信仰、低劣的医疗服务质量、对 PCOS 相关问题的认识不足，以及需要长时间地与医务人员进行咨询。

PCOS 患者有很高的进食障碍风险，因此应该考虑对这些患者进行进食障碍的筛查，以免漏诊或误诊。

建议在 PCOS 患者中筛查阻塞性睡眠呼吸暂停（OSA），因为过度肥胖会使这些患者患 OSA 及其并发症的风险增加。尽管不建议对所有 PCOS 患者进行子宫内膜癌的常规筛查，但是对于那些子宫内膜增厚、雌激素暴露过度、体重增加、阴道异常出血的患者推荐进行筛查是有必要的。可通过不同的影像学方法进行筛查。

参考文献

1. Miazgowski T, Martopullo I, Widecka J, Miazgowski B, Brodowska A. National and regional trends in the prevalence of polycystic ovary syndrome since 1990 within Europe: the modeled estimates from the Global Burden of Disease Study 2016. Arch Med Sci. 2019;17(2):343-351.
2. Dashti S, Latiff LA, Hamid HA, et al. Sexual dysfunction in patients with polycystic ovary syndrome in Malaysia. Asian Pac J Cancer Prev. 2016;17(8):3747-3751.
3. Eftekhar T, Sohrabvand F, Zabandan N, et al. Sexual dysfunction in patients with polycystic ovary syndrome and its affected domains. Iran J Reprod Med. 2014;12(8):539-546.
4. Ercan CM, Coksuer H, Aydogan U, et al. Sexual dysfunction assessment and hormonal correlations in patients with polycystic ovary syndrome. Int J Impot Res. 2013;25(4):127-132.
5. Veras AB, Bruno RV, de Avila MA, Nardi AE. Sexual dysfunction in patients with polycystic ovary syndrome: clinical and hormonal correlations. Compr Psychiatry. 2011;52(5):486-489.
6. Hahn S, Janssen OE, Tan S, et al. Clinical and psychological correlates of quality-of-life in polycystic ovary syndrome. Eur J Endocrinol. 2005;153(6):853-860.
7. Elsenbruch S, Hahn S, Kowalsky D, et al. Quality of life, psychosocial well-being, and sexual satisfaction in women with polycystic ovary syndrome. J Clin Endocrinol Metab. 2003;88(12):5801-5807.
8. Janssen O, Hahn S, Tan S, et al. Mood and sexual function in polycystic ovary syndrome. Semin Reprod Med. 2008;26(1):45-52.

第二十九章 非洲多囊卵巢综合征的全球应对方式

一、引言

多囊卵巢综合征（PCOS）是一种复杂的慢性遗传性多系统疾病，常合并生殖、代谢和社会心理问题。患者易出现一系列并发症，如不孕症、心血管疾病（CVD），以及子宫内膜癌/卵巢恶性肿瘤。这些对健康产生的重要且深远的影响使 PCOS 具有研究价值。有研究表明，遗传和环境因素（久坐不动的生活方式和西方化的饮食习惯）通过雄激素合成失调和胰岛素抵抗（IR）促进 PCOS 病理生理学过程。遗传和环境因素的复杂相互作用进一步导致了 PCOS 的各种表型，以及种族、地域差异，因此有必要探索其基因 – 环境相关性。由于人类在世界各地生活的环境各不相同，因此需要仔细研究这些差异，以制定适当的管理原则和指南。

非洲是世界第二大洲，其人口超过 13 亿，也是人口第二多的大洲。然而，它仍然是世界上最贫穷和最不发达的大洲。这在撒哈拉以南地区最为明显，那里约有 50% 的人口生活在贫困线以下。全球 PCOS 的患病率呈上升趋势，非洲也不例外。

PCOS 的表型识别、诊断和管理在全球范围内存在差异。差异取决于认知、成本、医疗机构可及性、利益相关者参与、临床指南的可用性，以及求医行为（HSB）等因素。随着这些因素在非洲许多地区的变化，非传染性疾病（NCD）的患病率正在迅速赶上大部分疾病（传染性疾病和营养不良相关疾病），这可能是因为人们的生活方式转变为西方饮食，以及养成了久坐的习惯。

随着对 PCOS 作为影响女性健康重要因素的认知不断提高，对非洲 PCOS 的研究逐渐增加，但仍难以满足需求。文化和传统是非洲人生活的重要组成部分，超过 85% 的非洲人寻求传统药物治疗疾病，这进一步使治疗复杂化。因此，关于非洲大多数领域的 PCOS 数据仍然缺乏。

本章旨在重点介绍非洲 PCOS 的各个方面，探讨 PCOS 在非洲的患病率、独特的临床特征、诊断和治疗方案、HSB 及面临的挑战。

二、患病率

作为一种综合征，PCOS 是由一系列症状诊断的。在排除具有相似症状和体征的疾病后即可做出诊断。这使得 PCOS 的患病率难以统计，因为临床工作者面对的是多种

PCOS 表型。值得注意的是，临床转诊的 PCOS 患者比非转诊者的症状更严重。与非转诊患者相比，临床转诊的患者常（存在偏倚）表现出更完整的 PCOS 表型（表型 A），其多毛症和肥胖更严重、血清雄激素水平更高。一项系统回顾和荟萃分析证实了转诊偏倚的存在并得出结论，转诊的 PCOS 患者总体上肥胖程度更高，症状更重。转诊偏倚会影响患病率研究。有显著症状或更易寻求医疗干预的女性比其他 PCOS 女性的数据更易获得。女性因下巴或胸部长出毛发而就诊的可能性小于跌倒后骨折。这导致 PCOS 等临床疾病的患病率研究变得复杂。

绝大多数（并非全部）关于 PCOS 患病率的研究来自北美、欧洲、中东、南亚和澳大利亚。南美洲、俄罗斯、大洋洲岛屿国家（美拉尼西亚、密克罗尼西亚和波利尼西亚）或非洲的重要数据缺失。非洲是黑种人女性的家园，关于非洲 PCOS 患病率的研究存在空白，现有研究仅显示其他大洲黑种人女性的患病率。不过，一项荟萃分析显示黑种人女性患 PCOS 的风险更高，患 PCOS 的黑种人女性患代谢综合征（MetS）的风险更高。

总体而言，现有数据表明，需要在世界范围内对非选择（无偏倚）人群进行严谨的流行病学研究，以确定所研究区域中该疾病的真实患病率和表型。通过此类研究，种族/民族、环境、社会经济和营养差异对 PCOS 的发展、并发症、表型和患病率的影响将更加清晰。此类研究对于确定基因型与表型之间的关系至关重要，并促进人们更好地理解这种疾病的分子机制。开展良好的流行病学研究也可能为该疾病的进化史提供线索，从而发现潜在的 PCOS 核心因素。了解某个地区 PCOS 对公共卫生和经济的影响可能有助于制定有效的公共卫生和预防政策。

三、临床表现

PCOS 的症状和体征通常与雄激素过多及排卵功能障碍有关，下丘脑 – 垂体 – 卵巢（HPO）轴受到影响。典型的临床特征包括月经不规律、长期无排卵、多毛症、不孕症/低生育力和（或）多囊卵巢形态。根据临床表现和特征，2012 年美国国立卫生研究院主办的 PCOS 循证研讨会（表 29.1）提出了 PCOS 的不同表型。此外，PCOS 还与代谢异常有关，包括糖耐量减低（IGT）/空腹血糖受损、2 型糖尿病（T2DM）、MetS、超重/肥胖、动脉粥样硬化性血脂异常、全身炎症、非酒精性脂肪性肝病（NAFLD）、高血压和凝血功能障碍。PCOS 还具有重要的心理影响，将在后文详细讨论。

表 29.1 多囊卵巢综合征的表型

表型	特征
A	高雄激素血症、排卵功能障碍、多囊卵巢形态
B	高雄激素血症与排卵功能障碍
C	高雄激素血症与多囊卵巢形态
D	排卵功能障碍与多囊卵巢形态

PCOS 的各种表型存在种族差异。与美国白种人相比，患有 PCOS 的非裔美国人有更高的 MetS 患病率。然而，通过比较美国西班牙裔女性与非西班牙裔的黑种人和白种人女性，Engmann 等发现，在高雄激素血症（HA）和代谢方面，西班牙裔女性的 PCOS 表型最严重。他们的研究发现，非西班牙裔黑种人女性的表型比西班牙裔女性轻，另外在某些方面，比非西班牙裔白种人女性更轻。在非洲的研究中，一项对尼日利亚不孕女性的研究发现，16.7% 的女性患有 PCOS，与卵巢正常的不孕女性相比，这些患者的多毛症、无排卵伴月经稀发、血清睾酮水平升高的发生率更高。在对坦桑尼亚妇科门诊的不孕女性进行的类似研究中发现，PCOS 的患病率较高（32%），超过 3/4（78%）的女性存在多囊卵巢，75% 的女性患有稀发排卵/无排卵，超过一半（56%）的女性患有多毛症。然而，即使在非 PCOS 的患者中，也有 10.3% 的人存在多囊卵巢。在肯尼亚一家三级转诊医院的妇科门诊就诊的 131 名月经稀发或闭经的患者中，约 1/3（37.4%）的患者根据鹿特丹标准被诊断为 PCOS。与未患 PCOS 的患者相比，PCOS 患者的卵巢平均体积更大，总睾酮水平更高。

因此，尽管 PCOS 的许多特征跨越国界、种族和文化，但 PCOS 的临床表现和临床影响存在种族差异，与遗传和环境因素相关。

（一）社会心理和文化

PCOS 是一种影响女性生活的慢性疾病，与各种形式的重大心理合并症有关（方框 29.1）。女性性别、肥胖和不孕症是焦虑症与抑郁症的独立危险因素。同时具有这些表现的女性 PCOS 患者发生心理障碍的风险更高。由于多毛症与消极体象，对体形的不满在 PCOS 患者中更为常见。值得注意的是，PCOS 患者的心理疾病可能未被发现，这将会影响他们的生活质量。因此对于医务工作者来说，有必要了解 PCOS 管理的社会心理方面的知识。

方框 29.1　多囊卵巢综合征的心理合并症

- 焦虑症：29%～50%，非 PCOS 的女性为 18%
- 抑郁症：57%，非 PCOS 的女性为 7%
- 无助感
- 社交恐惧症风险增加，社交和日常生活困难
- 痛苦的慢性情绪压力
- 焦虑情绪增加
- 自杀意念
- 双相情感障碍
- 注意缺陷障碍/多动障碍

值得注意的是，非洲的大多数人群都高度重视外表，异常的外貌变化会对生活在其中的个人与家庭产生重大影响。在美国进行的一项研究比较了 PCOS 患者和非 PCOS 的青春期女性，发现与非 PCOS 女性相比，PCOS 女性焦虑症、抑郁症和注意缺陷障

碍 / 多动障碍的患病率明显更高。此外，研究发现 PCOS 对黑种人女性的心理影响比白种人女性小，可能是由于心理障碍的诊断标准差异或在不同种族 / 民族的人群中获取精神卫生医疗的困难程度不同。患有 PCOS 的非洲女性因痤疮、多毛症、月经不规律、肥胖和不孕症等生理表现而有病耻感，这影响了她们在社会生活中的文化融合和生存。

在传统的非洲社会中，生育力受到高度尊重，被视为一种义务。在非洲的许多地区，它是正常与财富的标志，低生育力被视为禁忌语。尼日利亚的一项研究发现，患有不孕症的女性比没有不孕症的女性精神疾病发病率更高。这与歧视、缺乏家庭支持和人工流产史密切相关。在加纳的 100 名不孕症女性中，近 2/3（62%）的人患有抑郁症，这与较低的社会经济地位显著相关。此外，对卢旺达不孕夫妇进行的一项调查发现，不孕夫妇出现婚姻破裂、性功能障碍和家庭暴力的比例明显高于有生育力的夫妇。这些研究表明，PCOS 患者可能因生育问题被边缘化，从而导致心理疾病。

尽管关于非洲 PCOS 种族 / 民族差异的研究有限，但通过从全球其他地区和对具有与 PCOS 相似表现的女性进行的研究可以得出结论，PCOS 对非洲女性及其家庭具有显著的临床、社会心理和文化影响。因此，治疗过程中不仅要关注躯体症状，还要对心理社会和文化方面进行评估。

（二）求医行为

不寻求医疗帮助的原因有很多。阻碍人们就医的因素包括语言、经济能力、可行性和可接受性。贫穷、病耻感、缺乏知识和误导性信息可能是影响非洲患者就医的重要文化和社会经济因素（图 29.1）。

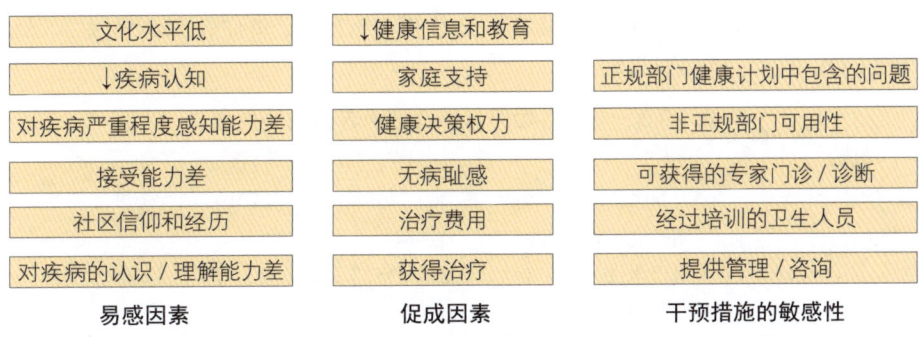

图 29.1 影响社区人群求医行为的因素：非洲多囊卵巢综合征管理面临的挑战

诊断 PCOS 及其相关临床表现的困难，进一步增加了 HSB 的复杂性。超过半数的 PCOS 患者在确诊前看了 3 个或 3 个以上的医师，不到 1/4 的患者对诊断时提供的有关生活方式管理和药物治疗 PCOS 的相关信息感到满意，超过 50% 的患者没有接受任何有关 PCOS 长期并发症的相关信息或情绪支持与咨询。大多数 PCOS 患者不太可能继续接受昂贵的治疗，因为还有其他更重要的事情。在非洲更是如此，这是一个饱受贫困和传统习俗困扰的大洲，甚至有采用宗教祈祷 / 宗教习俗的传统方式来治疗肺结核病等"精神传播疾病"的做法。家庭内部的文化因素与已婚/同居夫妇之间的权力斗争有关，也可能决定HSB，通常是男性决定女性是否应该寻求治疗。85%的非洲人每天的生活费不足5.5美元，这就不难解释为何一个月经不规律、下巴长出毛发的患者不愿意支付医疗费用。

由于贫困、病耻感，以及对PCOS的临床表现了解不足等因素，非洲PCOS女性可能无法获得理想的HSB。

随着网络信息获取越来越便利，越来越多的都市年轻女性开始意识到PCOS引发的体貌异常，并通过对比网络虚拟形象（近乎完美的肤质和体态特征），主动寻求医疗帮助以改善外貌。面对这类因不同诉求而就医的群体，就非洲女性是否会为可能影响日常生活的症状求医而简单下定结论显然有失偏颇（图29.1）。

四、治疗方式

由于非洲PCOS患者所面临的固有挑战，很难决定用哪种治疗方式能减轻她们的痛苦。如前所述，结核病等疾病被认为是精神类疾病且可以通过神灵仪式或宗教祈祷治愈。非洲医学专家的相对缺乏进一步加剧了PCOS患者就医的局限性。非洲缺乏临床内分泌学家、临床遗传学家、生理学家、细胞治疗从业者、生殖内分泌学家或对内分泌感兴趣的妇科医师等从业人员。一些地区执业的普通妇科医师很少与内分泌学家共同管理PCOS患者，他们更喜欢单独管理患者。这些因素限制了非洲治疗PCOS的可用方式。

（一）面临的挑战

在了解到PCOS是一种具有重要的临床和社会心理影响的多系统疾病后，更重要的是要认识到全球不同地区对其认知、接受程度和治疗方面存在较大差异。表29.3概述了非洲PCOS患者面临的具体挑战。

表29.3 非洲多囊卵巢综合征患者面临的挑战

挑战	讨论
对传染病关注度较高	对包括多囊卵巢综合征在内的非传染性疾病（NCD）的关注较少
缺乏PCOS相关数据	由于缺乏资金和意识，研究有限
求医行为	出现急性/严重症状才会就诊，而不是寻求预防性的长期治疗。因此，PCOS患者就诊较晚，并伴有并发症/合并症
病耻感与信仰	PCOS的表现与病耻感和错误的信念/神话有关
缺乏知识	政府、医疗机构人员及公众对PCOS的了解不足
缺乏专家	缺乏经验丰富的专科医师与亚专科医师
医疗机构分布集中	大多数专业设施与亚专科医师位于主要城镇
治疗费用问题	健康保险有限，大部分治疗需自费，激素检测和PCOS的管理是昂贵的
缺乏指南	大多数非洲国家没有PCOS诊断和管理指南
实验室基础设施和人员有限	激素检测准确性差，提供专业服务的实验室较少，而且距离区域中心较远
国际基金	大部分基金用于传染病和有限的非传染性疾病；PCOS没有优先级
专科医师与亚专科医师分布	乡村的专科医师/亚专科医师很少，多数在大城市或由资助项目招募

在传染病肆虐的非洲，对 NCD 的关注有限。随着 NCD 负担的增加，以及全球对这一问题的认识提高，非洲的研究越来越多，但速度比所需慢得多。因此，缺乏关于 PCOS 流行病学、诊断和管理的数据，特别是来自资源匮乏的撒哈拉以南非洲国家的数据。

尽管有限的研究正在评估非洲 PCOS 的 HSB，但在非洲大部分地区，慢性 NCD 的 HSB 是治疗性的而不是预防性的，这意味着患者诊断较晚，随访较差。Idriss 等在塞拉利昂的一项研究中发现，尽管城市和农村地区的社区成员和领导人掌握了足够的常见 NCD 基本知识，但只有在出现严重症状时才会加强应对。他们还发现，寻求治疗受到以往经验、个人和社会对方法适当性的信仰、医疗机构的可及性与成本，以及疾病特定因素（如急性症状）的影响。

与 PCOS 表现（如低生育力）相关的病耻感，尤其是在社会经济水平较低的环境中，可能会进一步影响非洲的 HSB。尼日利亚的一项对公务员的研究发现，适当 HSB 的概率很高。然而，在社会经济地位较低的人群中，缺乏医疗保险和受教育水平低与较少就诊相关。

PCOS 在非洲面临的另一个挑战是缺乏利益相关方提供的科普、专业知识和支持。在大多数非洲国家，特别是在撒哈拉以南地区，内分泌学 / 生殖内分泌学是一个小众的专业，因此绝大多数 PCOS 患者主要由妇产科医师而不是由多学科团队管理，且管理的重点倾向于 PCOS 的生殖方面，对代谢和社会心理因素的关注有限。此外，公共卫生部门对 PCOS 的研究，以及提供的资金和关注很少，而这是大多数非洲国家医疗需求的主要部分。

（二）诊断方面的挑战

在非洲国家，低生育力被视为主要健康问题，但缺乏 PCOS 的临床指南。因此，它不是最低医疗服务的一部分。缺乏指南意味着诊断困难。因此，许多患者被延迟诊断或无法被诊断。这就增加了 PCOS 并发症的风险，包括低生育力、功能失调性子宫出血、子宫内膜癌，以及代谢、心血管疾病和社会心理合并症。

在任何资源贫乏的环境中，由于实验室基础设施不足和专业人员缺乏，达到 PCOS 的治疗标准具有挑战性。2003 年鹿特丹标准是诊断 PCOS 最常用的标准，在排除其他疾病（高催乳素血症、甲状腺疾病、迟发性先天性肾上腺皮质增生症或分泌雄激素的肿瘤）后，至少符合 3 个标准中的 2 个［临床和（或）生化 HA、慢性稀发排卵 / 无排卵、多囊卵巢形态］。对于疑似 PCOS 的患者，至少需要评估睾酮水平、硫酸脱氢表雄酮（DHEAS）、促甲状腺激素（TSH）、催乳素、17-羟孕酮（17-OHP）、经阴道超声（评估多囊卵巢形态和子宫内膜形态），必要时进行子宫内膜活检。

代谢评估也是诊断 PCOS 的一部分，其中包括糖耐量评估（建议使用 75 g 口服葡萄糖耐量试验）、胰岛素水平和脂质谱。这些评估需要良好的实验室支持 PCOS 的检测、监测、控制和管理。在中低收入国家难以获得有质量保证的实验室结果，导致诊断延迟或误诊，治疗无效，影响患者的安全。大多数实验室集中在主要城市/城镇，由私人运营或属于中央转诊机构，从而限制了绝大多数公立、综合和地区转诊医院进行激素检测。此外，与这些医疗机构的距离和贫困造成了非洲PCOS治疗的不平等。中低收入国家（LMIC）接受了大量资金支持（如来自联合国机构和非营利组织），但其中不包括对PCOS的识别、诊断和管理的资金支持。这进一步减少了非洲人获得公平治疗的机会。

许多LMIC严重缺乏专业的医务人员，导致由非专业人员，如临床技术员和非专业医师治疗PCOS等复杂疾病。由于PCOS的症状差异较大且医务人员专业知识不足，出现了误诊和漏诊。此外，少数受过培训的专科医师和亚专科医师集中在大城市或被非政府组织项目招募，导致区域性医师短缺。

（三）管理方面的挑战

除了接触专家的机会有限之外，非洲PCOS患者在病情管理方面还面临其他挑战。整个社会和医学界都缺乏认识（主要是因为缺乏有组织的教育和专家），阻碍了对治疗的有效探索。贫穷本身是求医的主要障碍，而且相对于非紧急的慢性疾病，其他更严重的医疗状况可能会被优先医治。另一个障碍是缺乏适当的医疗设施。以芬兰为例，其2014—2017年孕产妇死亡率稳定在每10万活产中有3例死亡，而肯尼亚同期死亡率却高达每10万活产中有300例以上死亡，且每年仅下降1%。这就引出了一个问题：芬兰在孕产妇护理方面是否要比这些国家好一百倍？通过时间变化来观察和理解这一点很有趣，因为它把我们带到了1900—1904年，芬兰的产妇死亡率为每10万例活产中有240例死亡，仍低于以下国家2017年的孕产妇死亡率：安哥拉、吉布提、卢旺达、缅甸、加蓬、科摩罗、莫桑比克、苏丹、赤道几内亚、加纳、塞内加尔、布基纳法索、马达加斯加、肯尼亚、马拉维、乌干达、刚果、多哥、贝宁、埃塞俄比亚、斯瓦蒂尼、津巴布韦、刚果民主共和国、厄立特里亚、海地、尼日尔、坦桑尼亚、喀麦隆、莱索托、布隆迪、马里、几内亚、冈比亚、科特迪瓦、阿富汗、利比里亚、几内亚比绍、毛里塔尼亚、中非共和国、索马里、尼日利亚、塞拉利昂、乍得和南苏丹。其中只有2个国家不在非洲。2001—2003年，在东非肯尼亚沿海省的某个农村地区，只有5.4%的婴儿出生在医疗机构内。当如此重要的对抗疗法（孕产妇护理）变成关键问题时，关注非洲的PCOS管理似乎要求过高了。

五、建议和结论

PCOS有多种临床和生化表现，作为一种公认的疾病，大多数医务人员都意识到它的存在。鹿特丹标准是诊断该疾病最常用的标准。随着诊断的标准化和之后的疾病定义，亚临床疾病更易被识别，医务人员更容易诊断这种疾病。

截至本章撰写时，非洲尚无负责PCOS教育的全洲性机构（针对医护人员或患者）。

此类"教育"可包括为专业人士制定诊断与管理指南等。此类机构的建立有助于非洲本土专业文献的发表，促进在利益相关群体中传播 PCOS 相关知识，并为政府政策制定提供依据。在互联网普及的推动下，"地域限制"已难以成为信息传播不足的借口。健康教育还应面向患者群体，为其提供疾病知识、最佳就医途径及自我管理策略。建立患者互助组织是重要举措，此类组织可通过提供循证信息、同伴支持、提升公众认知及倡导以女性为中心的医疗服务为 PCOS 患者赋能。全球许多互助组织已与医疗机构及研究者建立合作，在疾病倡导与认知提升方面贡献显著。此类合作为跨领域协作创造契机，使循证信息得以惠及更多专业群体及其支持对象。强有力的全洲性政策组织还可推动 PCOS 教育纳入地方医学课程。随着更多医护人员对 PCOS 的认知提升，PCOS 的早期识别率将随之提高，从而加速提升患者生活质量。医学界对 PCOS 的重视必将催生更多专科人才，促进多学科团队的形成以支持患者群体。政策制定者与互助组织可借势优化转诊体系，使大量 PCOS 患者获得多学科协作的专业诊疗服务。

提高认知的另一优势在于推动鉴别诊断。随着临床医师对 PCOS 诊断能力的增强，实验室检测需求将激增，进而促进检测中心网络化布局，形成区域性病理采集网络。PCOS 诊疗率的提升可能吸引商业医疗保险关注，为非洲大陆医疗公平性建设创造新机遇。

由于非洲缺乏关于 PCOS 的数据，因此在实现 PCOS 患者的早期诊断和适当管理方面仍有较大改善空间。严谨的研究可以帮助填补现有的知识空白，进一步指导和改善 PCOS 女性的诊断和管理。

参考文献

1. El Hayek S, Bitar L, Hamdar LH, Mirza FG, Daoud G. Polycystic ovarian syndrome: an updated overview. Front Physiol. 2016;7:124. doi:10.3389/FPHYS.2016.00124.
2. Charifson MA, Trumble BC. Evolutionary origins of polycystic ovary syndrome: an environmental mismatch disorder. Evol Med Public Health. 2019;2019:50-63. doi:10.1093/emph/eoz011.
3. Unluturk U, Harmanci A, Kocaefe C, Yildiz BO. The genetic basis of the polycystic ovary syndrome: a literature review including discussion of PPAR-γ. PPAR Res. 2007;2007:49109. doi:10.1155/2007/49109.
4. Genotype Environment Interaction - An Overview. ScienceDirect Topics; 2021. Available at: https://www.sciencedirect.com/topics/medicine-and-dentistry/genotype-environment-interaction.
5. United Nations Department of Economics and Social Affairs The World Population Prospects: 2015 Revision. United Nations; 2015. https://www.un.org/en/development/desa/publications/world-population-prospects-2015-revision.html#:~:text=The%20current%20world%20population%20of,2015%20Revision%E2%80%9D%2C%20launched%20today.
6. United Nations. Economic Commission for Africa (2004). Unlocking Africa's trade potential in the global economy : policy paper. [Addis Ababa] :. © UN.ECA,. https://hdl.handle.net/10855/5506"
7. World Health Organization, 2016. Report on the Status of Major Health Risk Factors for Noncommunicable Diseases: WHO African Region, 2015 [Online]. Available at: https://www.afro.who.int/publications/report-status-major-health-risk-factors-noncommunicable-diseases-who-african-region-0.
8. Ntumy M, Maya E, Lizneva D, Adanu R, Azziz R. The pressing need for standardization in epidemiologic

studies of PCOS across the globe. Gynecol Endocrinol. 2019;35(1):1-3. doi:10.1080/09513590.2018.1488958.
9. Kofi-Tsekpo M. Institutionalization of African traditional medicine in health care systems in Africa. Afr J Health Sc. 2004;11(1-2):i-ii. doi:10.4314/AJHS.V11I1.30772.
10. Ezeh U, Yildiz BO, Azziz R. Referral bias in defining the phenotype and prevalence of obesity in polycystic ovary syndrome. J Clin Endocrinol Metab. 2013;98(6):E1088-E1096. doi:10.1210/JC.2013-1295.
11. Lizneva D, Kirubakaran R, Mykhalchenko K, et al. Phenotypes and body mass in women with polycystic ovary syndrome identified in referral versus unselected populations: systematic review and meta-analysis. Fertil Steril. 2016;106(6):1510-1520.e2. doi:10.1016/J.FERTNSTERT.2016.07.1121.
12. Ding T, Hardiman PJ, Petersen I, et al. The prevalence of polycystic ovary syndrome in reproductive-aged women of different ethnicity: a systematic review and meta-analysis. Oncotarget. 2017;8(56):96351-96358. doi:10.18632/ONCOTARGET.19180.
13. Maya ET, Guure CB, Adanu RMK, et al. Why we need epidemiologic studies of polycystic ovary syndrome in Africa. Int J Gynecol Obstet. 2018;143(2):251-254. doi:10.1002/IJGO.12642.
14. Alur-Gupta S, Lee I, Chemerinski A, et al. Racial differences in anxiety, depression, and quality of life in women with polycystic ovary syndrome. F S Rep. 2021;2(2):230-237. doi:10.1016/J.XFRE.2021.03.003.
15. Azziz R, Woods KS, Reyna R, Key TJ, Knochenhauer ES, Yildiz BO. The prevalence and features of the polycystic ovary syndrome in an unselected population. J Clin Endocrinol Metab. 2004;89(6):2745-2749. doi:10.1210/JC.2003-032046.
16. Knochenhauer ES, Key TJ, Kahsar-Miller M, Waggoner W, Boots LR, Azziz R. Prevalence of the polycystic ovary syndrome in unselected black and white women of the southeastern United States: a prospective study. J Clin Endocrinol Metab. 1998;83(9):3078-3082. doi:10.1210/JCEM.83.9.5090.
17. Hillman JK, Johnson LNC, Limaye M, Feldman RA, Sammel M, Dokras A. Black women with polycystic ovary syndrome (PCOS) have increased risk for metabolic syndrome and cardiovascular disease compared with white women with PCOS. Fertil Steril. 2014;101(2):530-535. doi:10.1016/J.FERTNSTERT.2013.10.055.
18. Witchel SF, Oberfield SE, Peña AS. Polycystic ovary syndrome: pathophysiology, presentation, and treatment with emphasis on adolescent girls. J Endocr Soc. 2019;3(8):1545-1573. doi:10.1210/JS.2019-00078.
19. Johnson TRB, Kaplan LK, Ouyang P, Rizza RA, National Institutes of Health Evidence-based methodology workshop on polycystic ovary syndrome. Bethesda, Maryland: National Institutes of Health; 2012. https://prevention.nih.gov/sites/default/files/2018-06/FinalReport.pdf.
20. Anagnostis P, Tarlatzis BC, Kauffman RP. Polycystic ovarian syndrome (PCOS): long-term metabolic consequences. Metabolism. 2018;86:33-43. doi:10.1016/J.METABOL.2017.09.016.
21. Hadjiconstantinou M, Mani H, Patel N, et al. Understanding and supporting women with polycystic ovary syndrome: a qualitative study in an ethnically diverse UK sample. Endocr Connect. 2017;6(5):323. doi:10.1530/EC-17-0053.
22. Moulana M. Persistent risk: psychological comorbidity in polycystic ovary syndrome. Endocrinol Metab Int J. 2020;8(6):139-141. doi:10.15406/EMIJ.2020.08.00297.
23. Moulana M, Lim CS, Sukumaran AP. High risk of psychological disorders: anxiety and depression in adolescent girls with polycystic ovary syndrome. Endocrinol Metab Int J. 2020;8(3):73-77. doi:10.15406/emij.2020.08.00282.
24. Engmann L, Jin S, Sun F, et al. Racial and ethnic differences in the polycystic ovary syndrome (PCOS) metabolic phenotype. Am J Obstet Gynecol. 2017;216(5):493.e1. doi:10.1016/J.AJOG.2017.01.003.
25. Oriji VK. Prevalence of polycystic ovary syndrome (PCOS) among infertile women attending fertility clinic at a university teaching hospital in Nigeria. J Gynecol Womens Health. 2019;15(5):555922. doi:10.19080/JGWH.2019.15.555922.
26. Pembe AB, Abeid AM. Polycystic ovaries and associated clinical and biochemical features among women with infertility in a tertiary hospital in Tanzania. Tanzan J Health Res. 2009;11(4):175-180.

27. The Rotterdam ESHRE/ASRM-Sponsored PCOS Consensus Workshop Group. Revised 2003 consensus on diagnostic criteria and long-term health risks related to polycystic ovary syndrome. Hum Reprod. 2004;19:41-47. Available at: https://doi.org/10.1093/humrep/deh098.
28. Odera FO. (2019). Prevalence of Polycystic Ovary Syndrome Among Women Presenting with Amenorrhea and Oligomenorrhea at the Kenyatta National Hospital [Online]. Available at: http://erepository.uonbi.ac.ke/bitstream/handle/11295/108179/Odera_Prevalence%20of%20polycystic%20ovary%20syndrome%20among%20women%20presenting%20with%20amenorrhea%20and%20oligomenorrhea%20at%20the%20kenyatta%20national%20hospital.pdf?sequence=1&isAllowed=y.
29. Wijeyaratne CN, Dilini Udayangani SA, Balen AH. Ethnic-specific PCOS. Expert Rev Endocrinol Metab. 2013;8(1):71-79.
30. Kocełak P, Chudek J, Naworska B, et al. Psychological disturbances and quality of life in obese and infertile women and men. Int J Endocrinol. 2012;2012:236217. doi:10.1155/2012/236217.
31. Elsenbruch S, Benson S, Hahn S, et al. Determinants of emotional distress in women with polycystic ovary syndrome. Hum Reprod. 2006;21(4):1092-1099. doi:10.1093/HUMREP/DEI409.
32. Deeks AA, Gibson-Helm ME, Teede HJ. Anxiety and depression in polycystic ovary syndrome: a comprehensive investigation. Fertil Steril. 2010;93(7):2421-2423. doi:10.1016/J.FERTNSTERT.2009.09.018.
33. Benson S, Hahn S, Tan S, et al. Prevalence and implications of anxiety in polycystic ovary syndrome: results of an internet-based survey in Germany. Hum Reprod. 2009;24(6):1446-1451. doi:10.1093/HUMREP/DEP031.
34. Scaruffi E, Gambineri A, Cattaneo S, Turra J, Vettor R, Mioni R. Personality and psychiatric disorders in women affected by polycystic ovary syndrome. Front Endocrinol. 2014;5:185. doi:10.3389/FENDO.2014.00185.
35. Klipstein KG, Goldberg JF. Screening for bipolar disorder in women with polycystic ovary syndrome: a pilot study. J Affect Disord. 2006;91(2-3):205-209. doi:10.1016/J.JAD.2006.01.011.
36. Hergüner S, Harmancı H, Toy H. Attention deficit-hyperactivity disorder symptoms in women with polycystic ovary syndrome. Int J Psychiatry Med. 2015;50(3):317-325. doi:10.1177/0091217415610311.
37. Makanjuola AB, Elegbede AO, Abiodun OA. Predictive factors for psychiatric morbidity among women with infertility attending a gynaecology clinic in Nigeria. Afr J Psychiatry (South Africa). 2010;13(1):36-42.
38. Alhassan A, Ziblim AR, Muntaka S. A survey on depression among infertile women in Ghana. BMC Womens Health. 2014;14(1):42. doi:10.1186/1472-6874-14-42.
39. Dhont N, van de Wijgert J, Coene G, Gasarabwe A, Temmerman M. 'Mama and papa nothing': living with infertility among an urban population in Kigali, Rwanda. Hum Reprod. 2011;26(3):623-629. doi:10.1093/HUMREP/DEQ373.
40. Al Shamsi H, Almutairi AG, Al Mashrafi S, Al Kalbani T. Implications of language barriers for healthcare: a systematic review. Oman Med J. 2020;35(2):e122. doi:10.5001/OMJ.2020.40.
41. Goudge J, Gilson L, Russell S, Gumede T, Mills A. Affordability, availability and acceptability barriers to health care for the chronically ill: longitudinal case studies from South Africa. BMC Health Serv Res. 2009;9:75. Available at: https://doi.org/10.1186/1472-6963-9-75.
42. Msoka EF, Orina F, Sanga ES, et al. Qualitative assessment of the impact of socioeconomic and cultural barriers on uptake and utilisation of tuberculosis diagnostic and treatment tools in East Africa: a cross-sectional study. BMJ Open. 2021;11(7):e050911. doi:10.1136/BMJOPEN-2021-050911.
43. Gibson-Helm M, Teede H, Dunaif A, Dokras A. Delayed diagnosis and a lack of information associated with dissatisfaction in women with polycystic ovary syndrome. J Clin Endocrinol Metab. 2017;102(2):604-612. doi:10.1210/JC.2016-2963.
44. World Bank Blogs. 85% of Africans Live on Less than $5.50 Per Day. 2019. Available at: https://blogs.worldbank.org/opendata/85-africans-live-less-550-day.
45. Idriss A, Diaconu K, Zou G, Senesi RG, Wurie H, Witter S. Rural–urban health-seeking behaviours for non-communicable diseases in Sierra Leone. BMJ Global Health. 2020;5(2):e002024. doi:10.1136/

BMJGH-2019-002024.

46. Pebolo FP, Grace AA, Gasthony A. Polycystic ovarian syndrome: diagnostic challenges in resource-poor settings, Ugandan perspectives. PAMJ Clin Med. 2021;5:41. Available at: https://doi.org/10.11604/PAMJ-CM.2021.5.41.26386.
47. Azziz R, Marin C, Hoq L, Badamgarav E, Song P. Health care-related economic burden of the polycystic ovary syndrome during the reproductive life span. J Clin Endocrinol Metab. 2005;90(8):4650-4658. doi:10.1210/JC.2005-0628.
48. Nkengasong JN, Yao K, Onyebujoh P. Laboratory medicine in low-income and middle-income countries: progress and challenges. Lancet (London, England). 2018;391(10133):1873-1875. doi:10.1016/S0140-6736(18)30308-8.
49. Benediktsson H, Whitelaw J, Roy I. Pathology services in developing countries a challenge. Arch Pathol Lab Med. 2007;131:1636-1639.
50. Finland Maternal Mortality Rate 2000-2021. MacroTrends; 2021. Available at: https://www.macrotrends.net/countries/FIN/finland/maternal-mortality-rate.
51. Kenya Maternal Mortality Rate 2000-2021. MacroTrends; 2021. Available at: https://www.macrotrends.net/countries/KEN/kenya/maternal-mortality-rate.
52. Högberg U. The decline in maternal mortality in Sweden: the role of community midwifery. Am J Public Health. 2004;94(8):1312-1320. doi:10.2105/AJPH.94.8.1312.
53. Maternal Mortality Rates and Statistics. Unicef Data; 2017. Available at: https://data.unicef.org/topic/maternal-health/maternal-mortality/.
54. Cotter K, Hawken M, Temmerman M. Low use of skilled attendants' delivery services in rural Kenya. J Health Popul Nutr. 2006;24(4):467. Available at: https://www.ncbi.nlm.nih.gov/pmc/articles/PMC3001150/.
55. Avery J, Ottey S, Morman R, Cree-Green M, Gibson-Helm M. Polycystic ovary syndrome support groups and their role in awareness, advocacy and peer support: a systematic search and narrative review. Curr Opin Endocr Metab Res. 2020;12:98-104. doi:10.1016/J.COEMR.2020.04.008.

第三十章 北美洲多囊卵巢综合征的现状分析

一、引言

北美洲面积约为 24 230 000 km²,是第三大洲,人口数量约占世界人口总数的 10%,其已发展成为世界上经济非常发达的地区之一。该大洲不仅人均收入全球最高,而且食物摄入量也是最高,这也导致了北美洲超重和肥胖人群较多。

多囊卵巢综合征(PCOS)通常表现为一系列代谢紊乱、皮损、妇科异常症状和体征等共同构成的综合征,症状可轻可重。美国生殖医学协会(ASRM)限定 PCOS 应具备以下 3 个表现中的 2 个:高雄激素血症(临床表现或者生化指标提示为 HA)、稀发排卵/无排卵、多囊卵巢。在美国,接近 7% 的育龄女性患有 PCOS,这也导致了每年用于治疗 PCOS 及其并发症的医疗费用达到了 40 亿美金,大大加剧了医疗的经济负担。

二、美国女性的多囊卵巢综合征相关疾病

(一)皮肤性损害

1. 多毛症和痤疮

在美国,约有 70% 的多毛症女性同时患有 PCOS,因此多毛为其常见症状。多毛症定义为上唇、下颌、乳晕、胸部、背部,以及下腹部等部位终毛呈男性型分布。阿拉巴马大学一项研究报道显示,在美国,有 74% 的多毛症女性同时患有 PCOS。HA 还表现为痤疮,其分布与多毛症相同,主要分布于颈部、胸部、下颌部、上腹部。对于那些常规治疗效果不佳,或者过了青春期依然不改善的痤疮,应予以警惕,并需要进一步评估。

2. 脱发

在美国,受脱发困扰的人群中,PCOS 是最常见的病因之一。西奈山医学院的一项研究报道显示,38.5% 的脱发女性同时存在 HA 的问题。

(二)排卵功能障碍/月经不规律

排卵功能障碍通常临床表现为月经周期少于 26 天或者大于 35 天,或者 1 年不足 9 个月经周期。一项针对亚拉巴马州育龄女性的入职体检的前瞻性研究表明,22.8% 的女性

患有月经失调。黑种人女性月经失调发生率为 25.1%，而在白种人女性中，这一比例为 20.5%。Haitz 等对 20～39 岁的美国女性进行了一项研究，观察到腰臀比越大，罹患月经不规律的风险越高。该研究还表明，月经周期正常的 PCOS 患者的代谢紊乱程度较低。

（三）代谢综合征

根据美国国家胆固醇教育计划成人治疗指引（NCEP ATP3），出现以下 5 条异常情况中的 3 条，即可诊断代谢综合征（MetS）：女性腰围大于 88 cm，空腹血糖（FBG）达到 110 mg/dL，空腹血清甘油三酯达到 150 mg/dL，血清高密度脂蛋白（HDL）低于 50 mg/dL，血压不低于 130/85 mmHg。据报道，美国患有 PCOS 的女性中，MetS 的发病率约为 43%，这一数字远高于该地区非 PCOS 女性 24% 的 MetS 发病率。而在世界其他地区，这种发病率甚至更低，如意大利，仅有 8.2% 的患有 PCOS 的女性同时患有 MetS。这些数据可能与美国人的饮食习惯及肥胖的高发有关，进而也印证了生活方式对 MetS 及 PCOS 的深远影响。据观察，同时患有 MetS 及 PCOS 的美国女性比单独患有 PCOS 者更容易出现严重 HA 相关症状。在美国，患有 PCOS 的患者中，最常见的是 HDL 降低的情况，这种现象高达 68%，其次是体重指数（BMI）升高（67%）、高血压（45%）、高甘油三酯血症（35%）及 FBG 异常（4%）。MetS 患者罹患 2 型糖尿病（T2DM）及心血管并发症的风险增加。

（四）胰岛素抵抗及高胰岛素血症

高胰岛素血症是一个重要的外在因素，因其加重了 PCOS 患者的 HA 症状。众所周知，即使没有肥胖的问题，因导致胰岛素抵抗（IR）的疾病存在 [如糖尿病（DM）]，患者通常也会存在 PCOS。Legro 等报道称，在患有 PCOS 的美国女性中，糖耐量减低的发生率为 31.1%，而在年龄及 BMI 均匹配的对照组中，其发生率仅为 7.8%。另一项研究表明，患有 PCOS 的西班牙裔女性，其 IR 程度高于同样患有 PCOS 的非西班牙裔女性。

（五）血脂异常

在美国，以高甘油三酯及低 HDL 为特征的血脂异常，在 PCOS 患者中常见。一项比较了美国人及意大利人饮食习惯的研究报道显示，尽管总摄入量相似，美国女性的饱和脂肪摄入量是意大利女性的 2 倍。由于存在饮食及生活习惯上的差异，70%～90% 的美国 PCOS 患者存在血脂异常的现象。美国匹兹堡大学对美国 PCOS 的女性进行了大规模队列研究，其结果表明，在美国，血脂异常患者较早发病，甚至很多 45 岁以前就出现了血脂异常。

（六）糖尿病

在美国，患有 PCOS 的女性中，DM 发生率可以高达 7.5%，而健康年轻人群仅为 0.7%。一项针对美国年轻女性的大型队列研究显示，20 多岁患有 PCOS 的女性，到了 50 岁以后，更容易罹患 DM 及血脂异常，而且这种增加的风险与她们的 BMI 无关。

（七）癌症

1. 乳腺癌

众所周知，较高的循环性类固醇激素水平可以增加罹患乳腺癌的风险。一项针对威斯康星州、马萨诸塞州、新罕布什尔州 50～75 岁乳腺癌患者的大型病例对照研究显示，高雄激素相关疾病，如 PCOS，会增加罹患乳腺癌的风险。

2. 卵巢癌

在美国，卵巢癌是女性癌症死亡的第四大原因。卵巢癌还与 PCOS 患者中雄激素的暴露增加有关。此外，PCOS 患者中经常出现的肥胖问题也与卵巢癌的发生呈正相关。

3. 子宫内膜癌

长期无排卵导致高水平雌激素缺乏孕酮拮抗作用。因此，子宫内膜长期暴露在较高雌激素水平下，会导致子宫内膜增生，甚至增加患子宫内膜癌的风险。PCOS 患者的肥胖、高胰岛素血症、高雄激素血症和胰岛素样生长因子 -1 分泌增加都是子宫内膜癌的已知风险因素。一项针对患有子宫内膜癌的美国女性的大型队列研究表明，其中 39% 的患者有月经不规律史，33% 的患者有 DM 病史，56% 的患者合并肥胖，而这些症状经常与 PCOS 相关。

（八）多囊卵巢综合征患者的生育力问题

PCOS 患者无排卵通常导致不孕症的发生，这也是美国女性低生育力最常见的原因。据 ASRM 报道，PCOS 患者的不孕率高达 70%～80%。因此 ASRM 建议，PCOS 的患者在试孕 6 个月失败后，即可开始进行不孕的相关检查。

（九）多囊卵巢综合征患者的妊娠丢失问题

显然，雌激素、雄激素及胰岛素均可以影响子宫内膜，进而导致 PCOS 患者的妊娠丢失。据报道，在美国 PCOS 患者的妊娠丢失率高达 30%～40%，远高于无 PCOS 女性的 10%～15%。除了我们观察到的激素和代谢异常之外，妊娠状态的女性和 PCOS 患者的血液还处于高凝状态；这些因素累积在一起都会导致妊娠丢失。

（十）静脉血栓栓塞性疾病

深静脉血栓（deep vein thrombosis，DVT）和肺栓塞（pulmonary embolism，PE）均属于静脉血栓栓塞（venous thromboembolism，VTE）。PCOS 患者体内的高胰岛素水平会导致纤溶酶原激活物抑制物 -1 水平升高，而后者在抑制纤溶方面起着重要作用。一项针对 PCOS 女性的病例对照研究显示，PCOS 患者的 VTE 患病率远高于非 PCOS 患者。此外，研究显示 PCOS 患者使用口服避孕药（OC）有一定保护作用。

（十一）心血管疾病

PCOS 患者体内的高胰岛素水平会促进胆固醇向动脉平滑肌细胞的转运，并增加这些细胞中的胆固醇合成。这使多囊患者罹患心血管疾病（CVD）及脑血管疾病的风险增加。PCOS 患者的 HA 也会增加心血管疾病的患病风险。匹兹堡大学的一项针对 125 名 PCOS 患者及 142 名对照组美国女性的病例对照研究，使用了颈动脉超声对内膜中层厚度（intima-media thickness，IMT）进行评估，评估结果显示，患有 PCOS 的女性其颈动脉 IMT 明显高于未患病女性。

美国心脏协会（AHA）将患有 PCOS 的女性分为"PCOS 相关 CVD 危险组""PCOS 相关 CVD 高危组"。

- 危险组女性包括：腹型肥胖、高血压、血脂异常、糖耐量异常、有 CVD 家族史、亚临床血管病变和吸烟的女性。
- 高危组女性包括：患 T2DM、MetS、肾脏及血管疾病的女性。

PCOS 会增加患者罹患 CVD 及脑血管疾病的风险，因此需要积极控制症状，同时加强疾病筛查和监测。

（十二）胃肠及肝脏问题

胰岛素抵抗及高胰岛素血症会增加脂肪组织中的脂肪分解及肝脏脂肪组织的重新合成，这两者都会导致流向肝脏的游离脂肪酸（FFA）增加，从而造成肝脏脂肪堆积，进而导致许多 PCOS 患者出现非酒精性脂肪性肝病（NAFLD）。在加利福尼亚州进行的一项研究发现，30% 的 PCOS 女性患者体内的转氨酶（NAFLD 标志物）水平升高。另一项在北卡罗来纳州进行的研究报道显示，15% 的 PCOS 患者转氨酶异常，肝脏活检显示患有非酒精性脂肪性肝炎（NASH）。一项针对美国 PCOS 女性的回顾性研究显示，55% 患有 PCOS 的女性同时患有脂肪肝；值得注意的是，在这 55% 的女性中，有近 40% 的人体形偏瘦。NAFLD 使患者面临肝病加重的风险。Carmina 等指出，需要对 PCOS 患者进行肝脏评估，也应评估 NAFLD 女性患者是否同时患有 PCOS。

（十三）睡眠障碍

无论是否存在肥胖问题，IR 与阻塞性睡眠呼吸暂停（OSA）及白天过度嗜睡（excessive daytime sleepiness，EDS）均密切相关。与健康对照组相比较，PCOS 患者（无论肥胖与否）OSA 患病率明显升高。Vgontzas 等指出，PCOS 患者罹患 OSA 的概率是健康对照组的 30 倍；同时 80% 的 PCOS 患者（无论肥胖与否）患有 EDS，而对照组这一比例仅为 25%。PCOS 患者还经常被报道存在入睡困难问题。这可能是应激系统激活所致。合并 OSA 的 PCOS 患者的代谢紊乱也比无 OSA 的 PCOS 患者更加严重。芝加哥大学对 PCOS 女性进行了一项研究，结果显示患病组 OSA 的发生率为 56%，而对照组仅为 19%。

（十四）心境障碍

雄激素分泌过多及性激素结合球蛋白（SHBG）降低共同导致了 PCOS 患者体内游离睾酮水平升高。Weiner 等在对美国女性的研究中发现，睾酮水平异常的女性更容易发生情绪低落。这也支持了一个观点，即 PCOS 患者的精神状况不佳并不只是由身体症状造成的。PCOS 女性的心理健康失调，尤其是心境障碍非常普遍。众所周知，PCOS 会降低患者的健康状况，因为其各种症状会加重患者对月经、容颜、生育力问题，以及对未来出现并发症的担忧。所有这些都会导致精神、躯体及性满意度的下降。

（十五）抑郁症

患有 PCOS 的女性抑郁症的患病风险显著升高。美国一项纵向前瞻性研究报道显示，患有 PCOS 的女性发生抑郁症的比例为 35%，而健康对照组为 10%。即使不考虑肥胖及生育力问题，美国女性罹患抑郁症的风险也更高。这些数据表明，有必要对 PCOS 患者进行积极的抑郁症筛查。

（十六）焦虑症

据报道，在美国患有 PCOS 的女性有 15% 存在焦虑症。在美国的研究人群中，担心体重增加及减肥困难比担心多毛症更容易引起焦虑，这可能与高收入国家更容易获得激光脱毛等先进的皮肤美容服务有关。

（十七）进食障碍

与健康对照组相比，患有 PCOS 的女性同时患有进食障碍的风险更高。美国一项研究表明，PCOS 女性合并进食障碍比例可达 14%。肥胖会加重 PCOS 的临床表现，PCOS 的患者经常就减肥进行咨询。患有进食障碍的女性减重会非常困难，进而影响她们的身心健康。

三、诊断

ASRM 推荐结合病史、体格检查、血液检测、超声检查来诊断 PCOS。医疗保健人员应尽可能地寻找 HA 的临床表现或实验室指标，如 PCOS 女性的多毛症。在询问 PCOS 患者病史时经常被提及的就是月经不规律，可以表现为闭经，定义为月经周期超过 199 天，或者月经稀发周期延长为 35～199 天。超声检查多用于评估多囊卵巢；高达 61% 的 PCOS 患者可以通过超声或者腹腔镜发现多囊卵巢。肥胖是指体重指数达到 30～40 kg/m^2，而重度肥胖是指体重指数超过 40 kg/m^2。在 PCOS 患者中肥胖也很常见，尤其在美国，据一项大型研究报道显示，肥胖患病率为 45%，而重度肥胖为 31%。根据美国妇产科学会的建议，除了糖耐量筛查排除 T2DM，以及监测血脂外，每次就诊应评估患者的血压情况。

美国的一项研究显示，北美洲的医疗保健人员在 PCOS 的诊断上存在很大差异。在初次接诊时开具的检查中，87% 的医师进行了促甲状腺激素（TSH）的检测，78% 进行了血清催乳素检测。在评估代谢状况时，61% 的医师检测了血脂，60% 检测了血糖，41% 检测了空腹胰岛素，25% 检测了糖化血红蛋白。

四、治疗（根据美国生殖医学协会的建议）

对于 PCOS 患者的管理应从整体上把控，同时解决患者的身体和精神症状。

（一）生活方式干预

在采取药物干预措施的同时，还应提供有关减重、运动、戒酒、戒烟的咨询。

（二）代谢

二甲双胍常用于治疗 PCOS，其不但能改善胰岛素敏感性，也有助于改善月经不规律。

（三）皮肤问题

1. 激素控制

抑制性激素的分泌通常是治疗 PCOS 相关皮肤损害的重点，因为这些皮肤损害大多源于循环中高雄激素水平。通常使用复方口服避孕药（COC）来达到这一目的。

2. 外周雄激素阻断剂

通过应用螺内酯、非那雄胺、氟他胺等雄激素阻断剂来抑制外周雄激素。

3. 美容治疗

激光疗法是治疗多毛症的一种物理性疗法。

（四）月经不规律

OC 常用于改善 PCOS 患者的月经不规律及激素状况。

（五）多囊卵巢综合征与生育力

对于有不孕症治疗需求的、肥胖的 PCOS 女性，一线治疗就是减肥。首选枸橼酸氯米芬诱导排卵；对枸橼酸氯米芬无效的患者通常需要注射促性腺激素。对于这些枸橼酸氯米芬治疗无效的患者，也可以用腹腔镜卵巢打孔术替代促性腺激素治疗，如果依然无效，一般推荐体外受精。

（六）基于社区的研究

美国的一项随机试验证实，为患者提供基于社区的临床试验及生活习惯改善，相对于单纯生活方式干预，更能提高患者生活质量，减少抑郁症状，更有效地减重。

五、并发症及族群构成

鉴于北美洲族群构成多元，在诊疗 PCOS 时，充分考虑不同族群患者并发症易感性的差异至关重要。中东或地中海血统的女性，多毛症更易发；与南欧或东欧女性相比，南亚和西班牙裔女性更易出现糖耐量异常；黑种人和西班牙裔女性更易出现肥胖和代谢问题；CVD 更常见于黑种人女性；在西班牙裔女性中，T2DM 及代谢疾病发生率更高，这可能与遗传倾向或饮食和生活方式的改变相关。

六、美国青少年多囊卵巢综合征

我们经常针对成人的 PCOS 进行研究及治疗，然而青少年女性也会发生 PCOS。儿童期出现的肥胖可能会增加 PCOS 的患病风险，雄激素分泌过高，以及 SHBG 被抑制相关的 HA，其与肥胖导致的胰岛素抵抗相关。在美国，PCOS 是导致青少年女性出现内分泌肥胖综合征的主要原因。据报道，PCOS 青少年女性肥胖率为 60%，而健康对照组肥胖率仅为 18%。

由于正常青春期发育与 PCOS 的某些症状是重叠的，因此在这一人群中甄别 PCOS 的患者是极具挑战性的。月经不规律、无排卵周期、卵巢多发滤泡、雄激素水平浓度高于正常等现象经常出现，这使得早期疾病识别对于大多数医师来说都是一个挑战。此外，由于第二性征发育的 Tanner 分级存在个体差异，通过体格检查来评估 HA 也很困难。

虽然痤疮在这个年龄阶段很常见，但是否会持续到成年，以及是否会对治疗产生抵抗性还需要进一步评估。

青春期的月经不规律定义为初潮第 1 年月经周期超过 90 天，第 2～3 年月经周期小于 21 天或超过 45 天，之后的 3 年月经周期小于 21 天或超过 35 天。然而，只有 40% 的月经不规律的女性真正患有 PCOS。

半数以上的 HA 青春期女性可能会患有多毛症，然而这种现象在青春期刚刚启动时可能并不明显。Baumann 等建议，对于肥胖、多毛症、痤疮、脱发，以及月经不规律等症状的青春期少女，应警惕 PCOS 的发生，因为其可能是该疾病发生的唯一特征性表现。而且，出现这些症状意味着患 CVD、血脂异常、T2DM 的风险增加。Lewy 等对美国青少年女性进行了一项研究，结果表明 HA 女性的外周血胰岛素敏感性降低了 50%，这使她们罹患 T2DM 的风险大大增加。

（一）美国青少年多囊卵巢综合征的诊断

约翰斯·霍普金斯大学的一项研究调查了美国医师对青少年 PCOS 的诊治情况。研究发现，大多数医师会对初潮后 1～2 年月经不规律的少女进行检查。通常会给患者进行血清检查，包括黄体生成素（LH）、卵泡刺激素（FSH）、睾酮、催乳素、孕酮、脱氢表雄酮（DHEA）、血糖等。

（二）美国青少年多囊卵巢综合征的治疗

青少年 PCOS 患者的推荐治疗方案与成人相似，包括改变生活方式、应用胰岛素增敏剂及 COC。在美国，大多数医疗保健人员都会使用二甲双胍和孕酮。另一项研究评估了北美洲青少年 PCOS 患者的治疗方法，研究表明 98% 的医师会使用口服避孕药，90% 的医师建议患者进行生活方式干预，如改变饮食习惯和运动。一项针对美国患有 PCOS 的青少年女性的小型研究表明，接受认知行为治疗的患者体重减轻的幅度及心境障碍的缓解更明显。

七、北美洲多囊卵巢综合征与肥胖

肥胖影响着美国 1/3 以上的成人及 20% 的育龄女性。研究表明，当增加食物分量时，人们可能不自觉摄入更多，这种增多的摄入甚至可以达到 30%。Nestly 和 Young 的研究表明，美国的食物分量较前增加了 2～5 倍。在美国，快餐的分量比欧洲要大。

1970年以来,为了应付不断增加的人口体重,食物的分量也在成比例增加,这也导致了超重和肥胖人口不断增加。

(一)患有多囊卵巢综合征的肥胖女性的病理生理学

在出现无排卵和HA症状之前,往往会出现体重增加的病史,这表明肥胖与PCOS之间存在着联系。肥胖会对女性生殖系统产生各种影响,而其发生率越来越高,这对为这些患者提供生育力保健的医师来说是一个挑战。脂肪组织会分泌一些脂肪细胞因子(如瘦素、胃促生长素、脂连蛋白、抵抗素)来影响性腺功能。作为被研究最多的脂肪细胞因子,瘦素通过抑制卵泡发育、刺激下丘脑-垂体性腺轴、调节早期胚胎发育来影响性腺功能。众所周知,瘦素通过作用于卵泡细胞受体,减少卵泡膜及颗粒细胞中胰岛素诱导的类固醇生成。此外,其还通过抑制LH水平来减少颗粒细胞中雌激素的生成。所有这些都导致了肥胖女性生殖潜能的下降和生殖功能的改变。在肥胖的女性中,脂连蛋白水平下降,并与胰岛素水平呈负相关,这可能是肥胖女性中出现IR及HA的重要原因。

总之,HA及高胰岛素血症是肥胖的主要后果。HA通过诱导颗粒细胞凋亡导致排卵障碍。据报道,肥胖的青春期女性HA的患病率较高,这使她们面临罹患PCOS的风险。

(二)肥胖对女性的影响

一项针对超过7000名美国女性的大型队列研究显示,超重和肥胖女性即使月经周期正常,其生育力也会比体重指数正常的女性低。在一些肥胖的人群中PCOS的发生率可以高达30%,尽管原因依然有待评估。肥胖女性的PCOS症状会加重,代谢紊乱,以及对生育的影响也会更加严重(图30.1)。

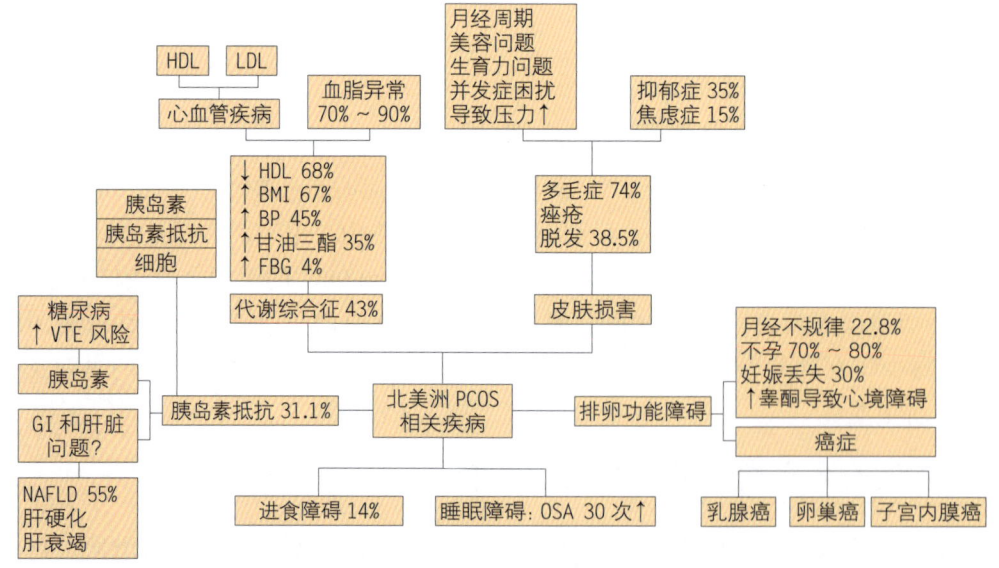

BMI,体重指数;BP,血压;FBG,空腹血糖;GI,胃肠道;HDL,高密度脂蛋白;LDL,低密度脂蛋白;NAFLD,非酒精性脂肪性肝病;OSA,阻塞性睡眠呼吸暂停;VTE,静脉血栓栓塞。

图30.1 北美多囊卵巢综合征及其相关疾病

参考文献

1. Schaetzl RJ, Zelinsky W, Hoff man PF, Watson JW. North America. Encyclopedia Britannica. 2022. https://www.britannica.com/place/North-America
2. James PT, Leach R, Kalamara E, Shayeghi M. The worldwide obesity epidemic. Obes Res. 2001;9(suppl 11):228S-233S.
3. Williams T, Mortada R, Porter S. Diagnosis and treatment of polycystic ovary syndrome. Am Fam Physician. 2016;94(2):106-113.
4. Cırık DA, Dilbaz B. What do we know about metabolic syndrome in adolescents with PCOS? J Turk Ger Gynecol Assoc. 2014;15(1):49.
5. Azziz R, Marin C, Hoq L, Badamgarav E, Song P. Health care-related economic burden of the polycystic ovary syndrome during the reproductive life span. J Clin Endocrinol Metab. 2005;90(8):4650-4658.
6. Archer JS, Chang RJ. Hirsutism and acne in polycystic ovary syndrome. Best Pract Res Clin Obstet Gynaecol. 2004;18(5):737-754.
7. Azziz R. The evaluation and management of hirsutism. Obstet Gynecol. 2003;101(5):995-1007.
8. Housman E, Reynolds RV. Polycystic ovary syndrome: a review for dermatologists: part I. Diagnosis and manifestations. J Am Acad Dermatol. 2014;71(5):847.e1-847.e10.
9. Baumann EE, Rosenfield RL. Polycystic ovary syndrome in adolescence. Endocrinologist. 2002;12(4):333-348.
10. Futterweit W, Dunaif A, Yeh HC, Kingsley P. The prevalence of hyperandrogenism in 109 consecutive female patients with diffuse alopecia. J Am Acad Dermatol. 1988;19(5):831-836.
11. Strowitzki T, Capp E, von Eye Corleta H. The degree of cycle irregularity correlates with the grade of endocrine and metabolic disorders in PCOS patients. Eur J Obstet Gynecol Reprod Biol. 2010;149(2):178-181.
12. Azziz R, Woods KS, Reyna R, Key TJ, Knochenhauer ES, Yildiz BO. The prevalence and features of the polycystic ovary syndrome in an unselected population. J Clin Endocrinol Metab. 2004;89(6):2745-2749.
13. Hartz AJ, Rupley DC, Rimm AA. The association of girth measurements with disease in 32,856 women. Am J Epidemiol. 1984;119(1):71-80.
14. Apridonidze T, Essah PA, Iuorno MJ, Nestler JE. Prevalence and characteristics of the metabolic syndrome in women with polycystic ovary syndrome. J Clin Endocrinol Metab. 2005;90(4):1929-1935.
15. Ford ES, Giles WH, Dietz WH. Prevalence of the metabolic syndrome among US adults: findings from the third National Health and Nutrition Examination Survey. JAMA. 2002;287(3):356-359.
16. Carmina E, Napoli N, Longo RA, Rini GB, Lobo RA. Metabolic syndrome in polycystic ovary syndrome (PCOS): lower prevalence in southern Italy than in the USA and the influence of criteria for the diagnosis of PCOS. Eur J Endocrinol. 2006;154(1):141-145.
17. Wang ET, Calderon-Margalit R, Cedars MI, et al. Polycystic ovary syndrome and risk for long-term diabetes and dyslipidemia. Obstet Gynecol. 2011;117(1):6.
18. Legro RS, Kunselman AR, Dodson WC, Dunaif A. Prevalence and predictors of risk for type 2 diabetes mellitus and impaired glucose tolerance in polycystic ovary syndrome: a prospective, controlled study in 254 affected women. J Clin Endocrinol Metab. 1999;84(1):165-169.
19. Kauffman RP, Baker VM, DiMarino P, Gimpel T, Castracane VD. Polycystic ovarian syndrome and insulin resistance in white and Mexican American women: a comparison of two distinct populations. Am J Obstet Gynecol. 2002;187(5):1362-1369.
20. Carmina E, Legro RS, Stamets K, Lowell J, Lobo RA. Difference in body weight between American and Italian women with polycystic ovary syndrome: influence of the diet. Hum Reprod. 2003;18(11):2289-2293.
21. Berneis K, Rizzo M, Lazzaroni V, Fruzzetti F, Carmina E. Atherogenic lipoprotein phenotype and low-density lipoproteins size and subclasses in women with polycystic ovary syndrome. J Clin Endocrinol Metab. 2007;92(1):186-189.

22. Talbott EO, Guzick DS, Sutton-Tyrrell K, et al. Evidence for association between polycystic ovary syndrome and premature carotid atherosclerosis in middle-aged women. Arterioscler Thromb Vasc Biol. 2000;20(11):2414-2421.
23. Ehrmann DA, Barnes RB, Rosenfield RL, Cavaghan MK, Imperial J. Prevalence of impaired glucose tolerance and diabetes in women with polycystic ovary syndrome. Diabetes Care. 1999;22(1):141-146.
24. Hankinson SE, Eliassen AH. Endogenous estrogen, testosterone and progesterone levels in relation to breast cancer risk. J Steroid Biochem Mol Biol. 2007;106(1-5):24-30.
25. Baron JA, Weiderpass E, Newcomb PA, et al. Metabolic disorders and breast cancer risk (United States). Cancer Causes Control. 2001;12(10):875-880.
26. Risch HA. Hormonal etiology of epithelial ovarian cancer, with a hypothesis concerning the role of androgens and progesterone. J Natl Cancer Inst. 1998;90(23):1774-1786.
27. Kuper H, Cramer DW, Titus-Ernstoff L. Risk of ovarian cancer in the United States in relation to anthropometric measures: does the association depend on menopausal status? Cancer Causes Control. 2002;13(5):455-463.
28. Soliman PT, Oh JC, Schmeler KM, et al. Risk factors for young premenopausal women with endometrial cancer. Obstet Gynecol. 2005;105(3):575-580.
29. Giudice LC. Endometrium in PCOS: implantation and predisposition to endocrine CA. Best Pract Res Clin Endocrinol Metab. 2006;20(2):235-244.
30. Laven JS, Imani B, Eijkemans MJ, Fauser BC. New approach to polycystic ovary syndrome and other forms of anovulatory infertility. Obstet Gynecol Surv. 2002;57(11):755-767.
31. Practice Committee of the American Society for Reproductive Medicine. Definitions of infertility and recurrent pregnancy loss: a committee opinion. Fertil Steril. 2013;99(1):63.
32. Lentscher JA, Slocum B, Torrealday S. Polycystic ovarian syndrome and fertility. Clin Obstet Gynecol. 2021;64(1):65-75.
33. Jakubowicz DJ, Iuorno MJ, Jakubowicz S, Roberts KA, Nestler JE. Effects of metformin on early pregnancy loss in the polycystic ovary syndrome. J Clin Endocrinol Metab. 2002;87(2):524-529.
34. Okoroh EM, Hooper WC, Atrash HK, Yusuf HR, Boulet SL. Is polycystic ovary syndrome another risk factor for venous thromboembolism? United States, 2003-2008. Am J Obstet Gynecol. 2012;207(5):377.e1-377.e8.
35. Defronzo RA, Ferrannini E. Insulin resistance, a multifaceted syndrome responsible for NIDDM, obesity, hypertension, dyslipidemia, and atherosclerotic cardiovascular disease. Diabetes Care. 1991;14:173-194.
36. Cobin RH. Cardiovascular and metabolic risks associated with PCOS. Intern Emerg Med. 2013;8(1):61-64.
37. Talbott EO, Guzick DS, Sutton-Tyrrell K, et al. Evidence for association between polycystic ovary syndrome and premature carotid atherosclerosis in middle-aged women. Arterioscler Thromb Vasc Biolo. 2000;20(11):2414-2421.
38. Mosca L. Guidelines for prevention of cardiovascular disease in women: a summary of recommendations. Prev Cardiol. 2007;10:19-25.
39. Wild S, Pierpoint T, McKeigue P, Jacobs H. Cardiovascular disease in women with PCOS at long-term follow-up: a retrospective cohort study. Clin Endocrinol. 2000;522:595-600.
40. Utzschneider KM, Kahn SE. The role of insulin resistance in nonalcoholic fatty liver disease. J Clin Endocrinol Metab. 2006;91(12):4753-4761.
41. Schwimmer JB, Khorram O, Chiu V, Schwimmer WB. Abnormal aminotransferase activity in women with polycystic ovary syndrome. Fertil Steril. 2005;83(2):494-497.
42. Setji TL, Holland ND, Sanders LL, Pereira KC, Diehl AM, Brown AJ. Nonalcoholic steatohepatitis and nonalcoholic fatty liver disease in young women with polycystic ovary syndrome. J Clin Endocrinol Metab. 2006;91(5):1741-1747.
43. Gambarin-Gelwan M, Kinkhabwala SV, Schiano TD, Bodian C, Yeh HC, Futterweit W. Prevalence of nonalcoholic fatty liver disease in women with polycystic ovary syndrome. Clin Gastroenterol Hepatol. 2007;5(4):496-501.

44. Carmina E. Need for liver evaluation in polycystic ovary syndrome. J Hepatol. 2007;47(3):313-315.
45. Vgontzas AN, Legro RS, Bixler EO, Grayev A, Kales A, Chrousos GP. Polycystic ovary syndrome is associated with obstructive sleep apnea and daytime sleepiness: role of insulin resistance. J Clin Endocrinol Metab. 2001;86(2):517-520.
46. Chrousos GP. The role of stress and the hypothalamic–pituitary–adrenal axis in the pathogenesis of the metabolic syndrome: neuro-endocrine and target tissue-related causes. Int J Obes. 2000;24(2):S50-S55.
47. Sam S, Ehrmann DA. Pathogenesis and consequences of disordered sleep in PCOS. Clin Med Insights Reprod Health. 2019;13:1179558119871269.
48. Tasali E, Van Cauter E, Hoff man L, Ehrmann DA. Impact of obstructive sleep apnea on insulin resistance and glucose tolerance in women with polycystic ovary syndrome. J Clin Endocrinol Metab. 2008;93(10):3878-3884.
49. Weiner CL, Primeau M, Ehrmann DA. Androgens and mood dysfunction in women: comparison of women with polycystic ovarian syndrome to healthy controls. Psychosom Med. 2004;66:356-362.
50. Himelein MJ, Thatcher SS. Polycystic ovary syndrome and mental health: a review. Obstet Gynecol Surv. 2006;61:723-732.
51. Hahn S, Janssen OE, Tan S, et al. Clinical and psychological correlates of quality-of-life in polycystic ovary syndrome. Eur J Endocrinol. 2005;153:853-860.
52. Kerchner A, Lester W, Stuart SP, Dokras A. Risk of depression and other mental health disorders in women with polycystic ovary syndrome: a longitudinal study. Fertil Steril. 2009;91(1):207-212.
53. Hollinrake E, Abreu A, Maifeld M, Van Voorhis BJ, Dokras A. Increased risk of depressive disorders in women with polycystic ovary syndrome. Fertil Steril. 2007;87(6):1369-1376.
54. Fauser BC, Tarlatzis BC, Rebar RW, et al. Consensus on women's health aspects of polycystic ovary syndrome (PCOS): the Amsterdam ESHRE/ASRM-Sponsored 3rd PCOS Consensus Workshop Group. Fertil Steril. 2012;97(1):28-38.
55. Glueck CJ, Dharashivkar S, Wang P, et al. Obesity and extreme obesity, manifest by ages 20–24 years, continuing through 32–41 years in women, should alert physicians to the diagnostic likelihood of polycystic ovary syndrome as a reversible underlying endocrinopathy. Eur J Obstet Gynecol Reprod Biol. 2005;122(2):206-212.
56. Bonny AE, Appelbaum H, Connor EL, et al. Clinical variability in approaches to polycystic ovary syndrome. J Pediatr Adolesc Gynecol. 2012;25(4):259-261.
57. Romualdi D, De Cicco S, Tagliaferri V, Proto C, Lanzone A, Guido M. The metabolic status modulates the effect of metformin on the antimullerian hormone-androgens-insulin interplay in obese women with polycystic ovary syndrome. J Clin Endocrinol Metab. 2011;96(5):E821-E824.
58. Moghetti P, Castello R, Negri C, et al. Metformin eff ects on clinical features, endocrine and metabolic profiles, and insulin sensitivity in polycystic ovary syndrome: a randomized, double-blind, placebo-controlled 6-month trial, followed by open, long-term clinical evaluation. J Clin Endocrinol Metab. 2000;85(1):139-146.
59. Archer JS, Chang RJ. Hirsutism and acne in polycystic ovary syndrome. Best Pract Res Clin Obstet Gynaecol. 2004;18(5):737-754.
60. Thessaloniki ESHRE/ASRM-Sponsored PCOS Consensus Workshop Group. Consensus on infertility treatment related to polycystic ovary syndrome. Hum Reprod. 2008;23(3):462-477.
61. Rofey DL, Szigethy EM, Noll RB, Dahl RE, Lobst E, Arslanian SA. Cognitive–behavioral therapy for physical and emotional disturbances in adolescents with polycystic ovary syndrome: a pilot study. J Pediatr Psychol. 2009;34(2):156-163.
62. Anderson AD, Solorzano CMB, McCartney CR. Childhood obesity and its impact on the development of adolescent PCOS. Semin Reprod Med. 2014;32(3):202-213.
63. Roe AH, Prochaska E, Smith M, Sammel M, Dokras A. Using the Androgen Excess–PCOS Society criteria to diagnose polycystic ovary syndrome and the risk of metabolic syndrome in adolescents. J Pediatr. 2013;162(5):937-941.

64. Warren-Ulanch J, Arslanian S. Treatment of PCOS in adolescence. Best Pract Res Clin Endocrinol Metab. 2006;20(2):311-330.
65. Peña AS, Witchel SF, Hoeger KM, et al. Adolescent polycystic ovary syndrome according to the international evidence-based guideline. BMC Med. 2020;18(1):1-16.
66. Lewy VD, Danadian K, Witchel SF, Arslanian S. Early metabolic abnormalities in adolescent girls with polycystic ovarian syndrome. J Pediatr. 2001;138(1):38-44.
67. Guttmann-Bauman I. Approach to adolescent polycystic ovary syndrome (PCOS) in the pediatric endocrine community in the USA. J Pediatr Endocrinol Metab. 2005;18(5):499-506.
68. Rofey DL, Szigethy EM, Noll RB, Dahl RE, Lobst E, Arslanian SA. Cognitive–behavioral therapy for physical and emotional disturbances in adolescents with polycystic ovary syndrome: a pilot study. J Pediatr Psychol. 2009;34(2):156-163.
69. US Department of Health and Human Services. Overweight and Obesity Statistics. National Institute of Diabetes and Digestive and Kidney Diseases; 2015.
70. Broughton DE, Moley KH. Obesity and female infertility: potential mediators of obesity's impact. Fertil Steril. 2017;107(4):840-847.
71. Steenhuis IH, Leeuwis FH, Vermeer WM. Small, medium, large or supersize: trends in food portion sizes in The Netherlands. Public Health Nutr. 2010;13(6):852-857.
72. Young LR, Nestle M. The contribution of expanding portion sizes to the US obesity epidemic. Am J Public Health. 2002;92(2):246-249.
73. Young LR, Nestle M. Portion sizes and obesity: responses of fastfood companies. J Public Health Policy. 2007;28(2):238-248.
74. Littlejohn EE, Weiss RE, Deplewski D, Edidin DV, Rosenfield R. Intractable early childhood obesity as the initial sign of insulin resistant hyperinsulinism and precursor of polycystic ovary syndrome. J Pediatr Endocrinol Metab. 2007;20(1):41-52.
75. Metwally M, Li TC, Ledger WL. The impact of obesity on female reproductive function. Obes Rev. 2007;8(6):515-523.
76. Moschos S, Chan JL, Mantzoros CS. Leptin and reproduction: a review. Fertil Steril. 2002;77:433-444.
77. Brannian JD, Hansen KA. Leptin and ovarian folliculogenesis: implications for ovulation induction and ART outcomes. Semin Reprod Med. 2002;20:103-112.
78. Spicer LJ. Leptin: a possible metabolic signal affecting reproduction. Domest Anim Endocrinol. 2001;21:251-270.
79. Gil-Campos M, Canete RR, Gil A. Adiponectin, the missing link in insulin resistance and obesity. Clin Nutr. 2004;23:963-974.
80. Billig H, Chun SY, Eisenhauer K, Hsueh AJ. Gonadal cell apoptosis: hormone-regulated cell demise. Hum Reprod Update. 1996;2:103-117.
81. Gesink Law DC, Maclehose RF, Longnecker MP. Obesity and time to pregnancy. Hum Reprod. 2007;22(2):414-420.
82. Alvarez-Blasco F, Botella-Carretero JI, San Millán JL, EscobarMorreale HF. Prevalence and characteristics of the polycystic ovary syndrome in overweight and obese women. Arch Intern Med. 2006;166(19):2081-2086.
83. Broughton DE, Moley KH. Obesity and female infertility: potential mediators of obesity's impact. Fertil Steril. 2017;107(4):840-847.